Jefferson Hospital
Laboratory Department
P.O. Box 18119
Pittsburgh, PA 15236

kjeldsberg's
Body Fluid Analysis

edited by

Jerry W Hussong, MD
Associate Professor of Pathology
Chief Medical Officer
ARUP Laboratories Inc
Department of Pathology
University of Utah Health Sciences

Carl R Kjeldsberg, MD
Professor of Pathology & Medicine
ARUP Laboratories Inc
Department of Pathology
University of Utah Health Sciences

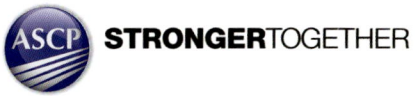

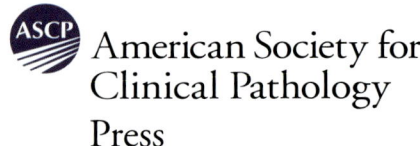

Publishing Team
Aimee Algas Alker (editorial)
Erik Tanck (design/production)
Joshua Weikersheimer (publishing direction)

Special illustration acknowledgments

- Katherine Henning (synovial fluid, p137; salivary glands, p207; sweat glands, p214)
- Kate Lamy (amniotic fluid, p31; CSF circulation, p45)
- Madeline Myung Sun Lee, MS (male genital tract, p161; urinary tract, p179; anatomy of the eye, p209)

Print ISBN 978-089189-5824
E-book ISBN 978-089189-6241

Notice
Trade names for equipment and supplies described herein are included as suggestions only. In no way does their inclusion constitute an endorsement or preference by the American Society for Clinical Pathology. The ASCP did not test the equipment, supplies, or procedures and therefore urges all readers to read and follow all manufacturers' instructions and package insert warnings concerning the proper and safe use of products.

Copyright © 2015 by the American Society for Clinical Pathology

All rights reserved. No part of this publication may be reproduced, stored in a retrieval system, or transmitted in any form or by any means, electronic, mechanical, photocopying, recording, database, online or otherwise, without the prior written permission of the publisher.

19 18 17 16 15   5 4 3 2 1

Printed in Singapore

Contributors

- Douglas T Carrell, PhD, HCLD, Director of IVF & Andrology Laboratories, Professor of Surgery (Urology), Obstetrics & Gynecology, and Human Genetics, University of Utah — Chapter 8

- Michael B Cohen, MD, Professor of Pathology, Vice Chair for Faculty Development, Ombudsman for Health Sciences, University of Utah — Chapters 2, 5, 6 & 9

- Marc R Couturier, PhD, Assistant Professor of Pathology, Medical Director of Parasitology/Fecal Testing, Infectious Disease Rapid Testing, and Microbial Immunology, ARUP Laboratories, University of Utah — Chapters 2, 3, 4, 5, 6, 7, 9 & 10

- Benjamin R Emery, M Phil, TS, University of Utah — Chapter 8

- Jordan D Farley, BS, University of Utah — Chapter 8

- David G Grenache, PhD, D(ABCC), Associate Professor of Pathology, Medical Director, Chemistry Division, Special Chemistry & Endocrinology/Manual Electrophoresis, ARUP Laboratories, University of Utah — Chapters 2, 3, 4 & 5

- Jerry W Hussong, MD, Associate Professor of Pathology, Chief Medical Officer/Director of Laboratories, ARUP Laboratories, University of Utah — Chapters 1, 2 & 10

- Carl R Kjeldsberg, MD, Professor of Pathology & Medicine, ARUP Laboratories, University of Utah — Chapters 3, 4, 5, 6, 7 & 9

- Allen N Lamb, PhD, FACMG, Medical Director, Cytogenetics, ARUP Laboratories, University of Utah — Chapters 2 & 3

- Sherrie L Perkins, MD, PhD, Professor of Pathology, Division Chief, Clinical Pathology, Director of Hematopathology, ARUP Laboratories, University of Utah — Chapters 2 & 4

- Monis B Shamsi, PhD, IVF & Andrology Laboratories, University of Utah — Chapter 8

- Ella Sorensen, BA, MT(ASCP), Medical Technologist Specialist, ARUP Laboratories, University of Utah — Chapter 2

- Joely A Straseski, PhD, D(ABCC), Assistant Professor of Pathology, Medical Director, ARUP Laboratories, University of Utah — Chapters 2, 6, 7, 9 & 10

Acknowledgments

We gratefully acknowledge the many fine contributions by Joseph Knight, MD, who was the coauthor of the *Body Fluids* book for the first 3 editions.

We gratefully appreciate Meryl Haber, MD, Scottsdale, Arizona, for generously sharing his outstanding collection of urinary sediments—cells, casts & crystals—of which many are included in the chapter on urine.

Janet Oertli, MT(ASCP) and Ted Pysher, MD in the Pathology Department at the Primary Children's Hospital, IHC, Salt Lake City, Utah, kindly made available their collection of CSF slides.

Michael Berry, Senior Cytotechnologist, ARUP Laboratories, Salt Lake City, Utah, made available his teaching collection of cytology specimens.

Sally Hill, MT, QCYM(ASCP) assisted with generation of flow cytometry histograms.

Joe Marty, MS, MT(ASCP) took several of the synovial fluid crystal microphotographs.

Dr Archana Agarwal, Department of Pathology & ARUP Laboratories, Salt Lake City, Utah, reviewed and made suggestions for the molecular section of Chapter 2.

Dr Elaine Lyon, Department of Pathology and ARUP Laboratories, Salt Lake City, Utah contributed images, reviewed, and made suggestions for the cystic fibrosis testing section in Chapter 10.

Susan Driggs, Melissa Anderson, Blythe Boston, Shaun Bowers, Rob Blaylock, MD, Kumar Pokharel, Jennifer Salmon, Milly Weaver, Val Evans, JoD Fontenot, Chris Lehman, MD, and Lori Wilson provided assistance with various laboratory procedures.

We greatly acknowledge Joshua Weikersheimer, Director of ASCP Press, for excellent assistance in all aspects of this publication.

Most of all, we are grateful for the support and love from our families: Gillean, Tanya, Kristina, Brian and Jane.

Preface

It has been over a decade since the last edition of *Body Fluids* was published. During that time there have been many requests and inquiries about updating this text. Since then, many new testing modalities have been developed; many others have been improved.

The new *Kjeldsberg's Body Fluid Analysis* has been reworked and expanded. Chapters on urine and specialized body fluids have been included. In addition, a complete chapter is devoted to testing methodologies. In order to provide the most current information about the laboratory analyses, many new authors, representing most subspecialties, have been added; they also bring new specialized analysis, especially molecular pathology expertise, to bear.

This printed text will be complicated by an appbook version, which, among other embellishments, will give the reader access to many more illustrations of morphologic variation than could ever be included in the printed text itself.

Kjeldsberg's Body Fluid Analysis was written for a diverse audience including students, residents, fellows, pathologists, medical technologists, microbiologists, and chemists. It may also be very useful to internal medicine specialists, surgeons, rheumatologists, obstetricians/gynecologists, and hematologists/oncologists. We have tried to present the concepts with a simple, straightforward approach, providing sufficient information for practical application without creating an unreadable encyclopedia of data.

Jerry W Hussong, MD
Carl R Kjeldsberg, MD

Contents

Preface iv

1: Overview 1

2: Laboratory Methods 3

General principles 3

Specimen collection, requirements & stability 4
  Amniotic fluid 4
  Cerebrospinal fluid 4
  Serous fluids 5
  Synovial fluid 5
  Urine 5

Gross (macroscopic) examination 6
  Amniotic fluid 6
  Cerebrospinal fluid 6
  Serous fluids 6
  Synovial fluid 6
  Urine 7

Microscopic examination 7
  Manual cell count 7
    Equipment and reagents 7
    Procedure (using improved Neubauer hemocytometer) 7
  Automated cell counts 9
  Cell concentration & cytospin preparation 9
    Equipment and reagents 9
    Procedure 9
  Slide staining 10

Differential cell counts & cytomorphology 10
  Cell block preparations 11
Synovial fluid crystal identification 11
  Procedure 12
  Types of crystals 14

Chemistry 17

Microbiology 18
  Microbiologic methods 18
  Bacteriological techniques 18
    Gram stain 19
    Bacterial culture 19
    Acid-fast bacilli & fungal culture 19

Immunophenotyping 20
  Immunohistochemistry 20
  Flow cytometry 23

Molecular testing 26

Cytogenetics 26
  Body fluid specimen types & transportation of samples .. 26
  Specimen processing 27
  Harvesting of metaphase cells, slide preparation, and chromosome & FISH analysis 27
  Reporting of results 28

Artifacts & pitfalls 28

Key points 28

References 29

3: Amniotic Fluid — 31

Anatomy & pathophysiology 31

Clinical indications for amniotic fluid testing 32

Specimen collection, requirements & stability 32
- Gross examination 33
- Microscopic examination 33

Premature rupture of membranes . . .33

Chemical analysis 34
- α fetoprotein (AFP) 34
- Cholinesterase 35
- Bilirubin 35
- Pulmonary surfactants 36
  - Lecithin to sphingomyelin ratio 37
  - Lamellar body count 37
  - Phosphatidylglycerol 38
- Chemical markers of ruptured membranes 38
  - Placental α microglobulin-1 38

Prenatal diagnosis of chromosomal abnormalities 39

Microbiologic examination 41
- Vertically transmitted infections 41

Artifacts & pitfalls 42

Key points 42

References 43

4: Cerebrospinal Fluid — 45

Anatomy & pathophysiology 45

Clinical indications & recommended laboratory studies 46

Specimen collection, requirements & stability 47

Gross examination 49

Microscopic examination 50
- Cell counts 51
- Differential count 53

CSF normal cytology 54

Abnormal cytology 59

CSF analysis for malignancy 63
- Acute leukemia 63
- Chronic leukemias 65
- Malignant lymphomas 65
- Primary CNS tumors 66
- Metastatic malignancies 67

Chemical analysis 69
- Total protein & albumin 69
- Glucose 69
- Lactate 70
- C reactive protein 70
- Immunoglobulins 70
- Myelin basic protein 71
- Transferrin 71
- Bilirubin 71
- Adenosine deaminase 72
- Tumor markers 72
- Brain injury markers 73
- Electrolytes and acid-base balance 73
- Neurodegenerative disease markers 74

Microbiologic examination 74
- Bacterial meningitis 75
- Viral meningitis 77
- Fungal meningitis 78
- Tuberculous meningitis 80
- Free living amoebic infections 80
- Parasitic meningitis/meningoencephalitis 81
- Neuroborreliosis 81
- Neurosyphilis 82

Artifacts & pitfalls 83

Key points 83

References 84

5: Pleural & Pericardial Fluid — 89

- Anatomy & pathophysiology 89
- Specimen collection 90
- Pleural biopsy 91
- Transudates & exudates 91
- Recommended tests 92
- Gross examination 92
- Cell count 93
- Microscopic examination 93
- Clinical considerations 108
- Malignant disorders 109
- Chemical analysis 111
  - Total protein & lactate dehydrogenase 111
  - Glucose 112
  - pH 112
  - Lipids 112
  - Adenosine deaminase 112
  - Amylase 113
  - Tumor markers 113
  - Complement, rheumatoid factor & antinuclear antibody 113
- Microbiologic examination 114
- Artifacts & pitfalls 116
- Key points 116
- References 117

6: Peritoneal Fluid — 119

- Anatomy & pathophysiology 119
- Specimen collection & clinical indications 119
- Recommended tests 120
- Gross examination 120
- Cell counts 121
- Microscopic examination & clinical considerations 121
  - Malignancies 124
- Chemical analysis 129
  - Protein & albumin 129
  - Bilirubin, urea nitrogen & creatinine 129
  - Amylase & lipase 130
  - Cholesterol & triglycerides 130
  - Lactate dehydrogenase (LDH) 130
  - pH 131
  - Lactate 131
  - Glucose 131
  - Alkaline phosphatase 131
  - Electrolytes 131
  - Markers of malignancy 131
- Microbiologic examination 132
- Special studies 133
- Artifacts & pitfalls 134
- Key points 134
- References 134

7: Synovial Fluid — 137

- **Anatomy & pathophysiology** — 137
- **Specimen collection, requirements & stability** — 138
- **Laboratory studies** — 139
- **Gross examination** — 139
- **Cell counts** — 141
- **Microscopic examination & clinical considerations** — 141
- **Crystal examination, identification & clinical considerations** — 146
- **Chemical & immunologic analysis** — 151
  - Glucose — 151
  - Protein — 151
  - Uric acid — 152
  - Enzymes — 152
  - Lactate — 152
  - Lipids — 153
  - pH — 153
  - Immunologic analysis — 153
  - Newer biomarkers — 154
- **Microbiologic examination** — 154
  - Lyme arthritis — 156
- **Artifacts & pitfalls** — 157
- **Key points** — 157
- **References** — 158

8: Seminal Fluid — 161

- **Normal human reproductive physiology** — 161
- **Semen analysis** — 162
  - Preanalytic considerations — 163
- **Gross examination of semen** — 164
- **Microscopic examination of semen** — 164
  - Sperm count — 164
  - Sperm motility — 165
  - Sperm morphology — 166
  - Sperm viability — 167
  - Leukocytes & immature germ cells — 168
- **Antisperm antibody testing** — 168
  - Immunobead assay — 169
  - Mixed agglutination assay — 169
  - ELISA assay for antisperm antibodies — 169
- **Assays of sperm functional ability** — 169
  - Sperm penetration assay — 169
  - Acrosome reaction assays — 170
  - Hemizona assay — 170
- **Assessment of reactive oxygen species (ROS)** — 171
- **Sperm DNA damage assays** — 172
  - Acridine orange test — 172
  - Sperm chromatin structure assay — 172
  - Terminal deoxynucleotidyl transferase mediated dUTP nick end labeling (TUNEL) assay — 172
  - Sperm chromatin dispersion (SCD) — 172
  - The comet assay — 173
  - Sperm aneuploidy testing by fluorescent in situ hybridization (FISH) — 174
- **Artifacts & pitfalls** — 175
- **Key points** — 175
- **References** — 176

9: Urine — 179

Anatomy & pathophysiology — 179
Clinical indications & considerations & recommended laboratory studies — 180
Specimen collection, requirements & stability — 180
Gross examination — 181
- Appearance — 181
- Color — 181
- Clarity — 181
- Odor — 181
- Volume — 181
- Specific gravity & osmolality — 181

Cell counts — 182
Microscopic examination — 182
- Epithelial cells — 182
- Nonepithelial cells — 185
- Microorganisms — 187
- Crystals — 189
- Casts — 194
- Other — 197

Chemical analysis — 198
- pH — 198
- Protein — 198
- Albumin — 199
- Glucose — 199
- Ketones — 199
- Nitrite — 200
- Leukocyte esterase — 200
- Blood — 200
- Bilirubin & urobilinogen — 200

Microbiologic examination — 201
- Bacterial urinary tract infections — 201
- Urinalysis markers as a screen for UTI — 201
- Culture — 201
- Viral detection — 202
- Parasitic evaluation — 203
- Urinary antigen testing — 203
- Molecular detection of sexually transmitted infections — 203

Special studies — 204
- Calculi — 204
- Bladder tumor antigens — 204
- FISH — 205
- Other — 205

Artifacts & pitfalls — 205
Key points — 205
References — 205

10: Specialized Body Fluids — 207

Saliva — 207
- Specimen collection, requirements & stability — 207
- Chemical analysis — 208
- Cortisol — 208
- Sex steroids — 208
- Toxicology — 208
- Microbiologic testing — 209
- HIV — 209
- CMV — 209
- HCV — 209

Fluids of the eye — 209
- Vitreous fluid — 209
- Aqueous fluid — 210
- Specimen collection, requirements & stability — 210
- Chemical analysis — 210
- Glucose & glucose metabolism — 211
- Insulin & c-peptide — 211
- Electrolytes — 211
- Creatinine & urea nitrogen — 212
- Alcohols — 212
- Special studies — 212

Postmortem interval   212
- Microbiologic examination of vitreous fluid & endophthalmitis — 212
  - Bacterial endophthalmitis — 213
  - Mycobacterial endophthalmitis — 213
  - Fungal endophthalmitis — 213
  - Viral infections — 213
  - Parasitic infections — 214

Sweat — 214
- Specimen collection, requirements & stability — 215
- Chemical analysis — 215

Sweat chloride   215
- Molecular testing — 217

Artifacts & pitfalls — 217
Key points — 217
References — 217

kjeldsberg's
Body Fluid Analysis

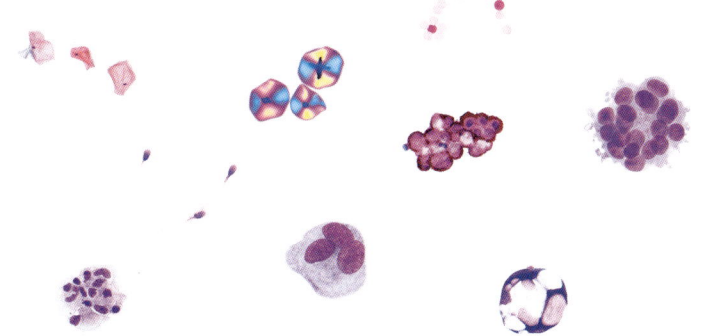

Hussong JW

Overview
Chapter 1

The examination of body fluids provides essential information for the care and treatment of patients. This evaluation encompasses many disciplines, involves multiple steps, and requires the integration of numerous data elements into the analysis f1.1. The evaluation of body fluids typically includes gross examination, microscopic examination, cell and differential counts, chemical analysis and microbiology studies. In addition, numerous ancillary studies including flow cytometry, molecular analysis and cytogenetics have now become more readily available and are used more frequently in the evaluation of many body fluids.

Although many new testing modalities are currently available for the evaluation of body fluids, morphologic evaluation still remains the cornerstone in the workup and diagnoses of these specimen types. It is imperative that laboratory professionals develop and maintain morphologic expertise as it is the morphologic examination of body fluids that often directs and guides additional testing and serves as the foundation for accurate interpretation and diagnosis. Still today, morphologic evaluation in conjunction with chemical analysis and microbiology studies are the most important components of body fluid evaluation.

Important indications for the evaluation of body fluids are
1. to determine the etiology of the fluid accumulation
2. to distinguish between benign and malignant processes

Appropriate laboratory testing and specimen utilization is therefore essential for differentiating between the numerous potential disease processes and etiologies. The following chapters provide both an overview of common testing for each body fluid type but also highlight the unique features that must be considered. The individual body fluid chapters provide review of the morphologic features, chemical analysis and microbiologic evaluation for each fluid type. Additionally, more complex testing techniques are also presented as is appropriate to the specific fluid type. Many of the body fluid types discussed are difficult to replace and would put the patient at increased risk of complications with recollection; therefore, appropriate care must be taken to properly handle and test all body fluid specimens. As often numerous tests are requested for an individual body fluid sample, it is important not to waste any of the submitted specimen to be sure that ample specimen is available to complete all of the requested testing. There will be occasions, however, in which the submitted sample will not be of sufficient volume to allow for all of the testing that has been requested. In such instances, there must be communication between the testing laboratory and the submitting clinician to prioritize testing. The treating clinician will be the most familiar with the patient and the diagnostic considerations and will be best able to make decisions regarding test prioritization.

Chapter 2 is dedicated to laboratory methodology. It provides an overview of testing considerations and reviews the basic principles in the processing and evaluation of body fluids. In contrast to the previous edition, this text presents the principles and description of body fluid laboratory testing methodologies together within a single chapter. It includes a brief review of synovial fluid crystal analysis. The remaining chapters cover specific body fluid types and their unique features. New chapters have been added, including a chapter on urine and specialized body fluids. The chemical analysis and microbiology sections of the chapters have been expanded to provide the reader with current testing options and strategies. The urine chapter

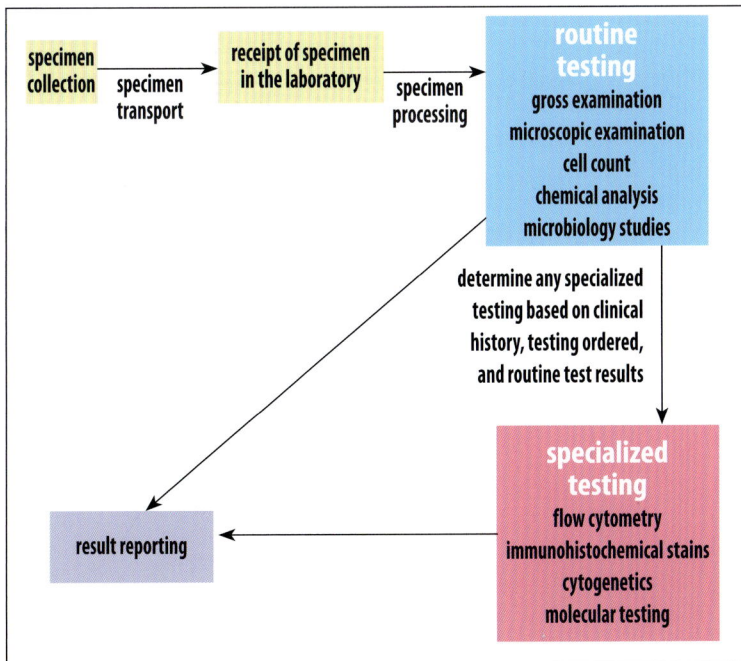

f1.1 Algorithm for body fluid processing

emphasizes morphologic evaluation and reviews many of the common findings that will be encountered during urinalysis. The chapter on specialized body fluids introduces and discusses basic concepts for the evaluation of saliva, vitreous and sweat, including a brief discussion on the workup of cystic fibrosis. The seminal fluid chapter has been expanded and includes testing recommendations and current testing strategies.

During the last several years, numerous tests for the evaluation of body fluids, which were previously manual and labor intensive, have now become automated. Part of this automation has come about due to the increased need of laboratories to become more efficient with cost containment. Such utilization measures are among the most current topics discussed by laboratory directors and administrators and will continue to be an important aspect of laboratory medicine and health care delivery. Similar to the testing of other specimen types, the use of automated analyzers in the testing of body fluids must strictly follow manufacturers' guidelines and be employed only for those body fluid types cleared and specified in the "intended use" statement for the device. If the laboratory modifies the approved testing device or a testing kit, performance specifications, including accuracy, precision, sensitivity, specificity, reference intervals and reportable range of test results, must be established before specimen testing and reporting of patient results. Quality control measurements must also be in place to assure the proper functioning of the testing instrumentation.

The testing of body fluid specimens is subject to the same quality measures and patient safety risks as testing done in the clinical laboratory on all other specimen types. Numerous preanalytic, analytic and postanalytic variables influence sample testing and results. Examples of preanalytic variables include test ordering, patient and specimen identification, and specimen collection and transport. Analytic variables include specimen viability, instrument function and Q/C. Result reporting, result communication, error correction and specimen storage are postanalytic variables. Other factors that can affect laboratory testing and result reporting include administrative oversight and leadership, properly trained personnel, laboratory information systems, instrumentation, physical facilities and process control.

Furthermore, the evaluation and testing of body fluids requires the laboratory to follow the same laboratory standards and regulations, including test validation, quality assurance/quality control and proficiency testing (PT). Laboratory testing activities are under federal regulation through CLIA '88. All laboratories must comply with all of the provisions of CLIA. Laboratories must be licensed and accredited according to both federal and state requirements. In addition, laboratories must adhere to the standards of the Health Insurance Portability and Accountability Act (HIPAA), which was enacted in 1996 and protects the confidentiality of health information while allowing its exchange in appropriate circumstances. Additionally, all clinical laboratories within the United States must have a designated laboratory director who is professionally responsible and legally accountable for the testing results. The laboratory director oversees all of the activities of the laboratory.

Numerous proficiency testing options are now available for body fluids from accreditation agencies such as the College of American Pathologists (CAP). Some of these require laboratory testing of specific analytes and others are pictures or images that require morphologic identification of the cellular elements. Similar to other proficiency testing, the submitted results are scored and a summary report is sent back to the testing laboratory. When proficiency testing is not available for specific analytes, interlaboratory exchange programs can be utilized for result comparison. In addition, as a given specimen may be evaluated in multiple areas of the laboratory, such as morphologic examination in both the hematology and cytology areas, it is important to have a system in place to regularly compare results within the same laboratory.

Throughout the last several years numerous important ancillary techniques have been developed and are more commonly utilized to evaluate body fluids. Many of these ancillary tests are now more universally available. These include flow cytometry, FISH analysis, karyotyping, and molecular testing. Furthermore, microbiology testing has also changed significantly and not infrequently utilizes molecular testing modalities. However, in spite of the numerous advancements in testing techniques and strategies now available, many time honored procedures, eg, the Gram stain and cytologic/morphologic examination, remain immensely important and should not be overlooked.

A thorough understanding of body fluid evaluation and testing by laboratory personnel is essential. Such knowledge provides the members of the laboratory team the ability to produce high quality testing results and assist their clinical colleagues with test selection, testing sequence and prioritization. It is through high quality laboratory testing that we contribute to the care of patients and serve as vital members of the health care delivery team. Morphologic examination along with appropriate laboratory testing serves as the cornerstone of patient care and directs the diagnosis and downstream therapies of patients.

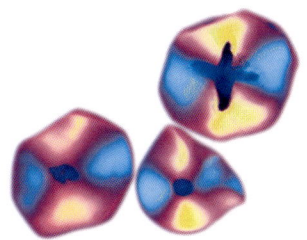

Hussong JW, Sorensen E, Perkins SL, Couturier MR, Grenache DG, Lamb AN, Straseski JA, Cohen MB

Laboratory Methods
Chapter 2

Analysis of body fluids often includes many routine techniques including gross examination, cell count, differential count, chemical analysis, microbiologic testing and cytologic examination. Although some of the principles of body fluid evaluation have remained constant over the years, in the past decade or so, many newer technologies have emerged that require more specialized testing methodologies and instrumentation. This chapter reviews specimen requirements and routine laboratory techniques used in the evaluation of body fluids. Also discussed are preanalytic, analytic and postanalytic variables that need to be considered in the evaluation of body fluids and how they can affect specimen testing and result reporting.

This chapter has been designed to describe a uniform process for body fluid handling, triaging and evaluation and includes many basic principles. It will outline common and necessary testing techniques from receipt of the body fluid at the testing facility to reporting of the results to the health care provider. In addition to general testing modalities, more specialized ancillary studies may need to be performed on some specimens. These may include but are not limited to flow cytometry, immunohistochemistry, cytogenetics and molecular studies. Although many testing methodologies apply to several body fluid types regardless of source, where appropriate, specific testing considerations will be described as it relates to unique features of the individual body fluid type. A section on synovial fluid crystal analysis is also included to aid the reader in the identification of common crystals and associated disorders. The techniques for the preparation and evaluation of seminal fluid will be discussed separately in Chapter 8. Similarly, the requirements and evaluation of unique body fluids such as vitreous and saliva will be discussed in Chapter 10.

General principles

The methods for obtaining most extravascular body fluids are considerably more complex than those for collecting a peripheral blood specimen. The process is often uncomfortable and potentially places the patient at risk [PMID 23396954, PMID 23543985, PMID 23716522]. Every attempt should be made to understand the clinical history and associated pertinent laboratory tests ordered for the submitted specimen.

The laboratory has little control over what information is submitted on the requisition form or how much specimen is submitted. However, in some instances, laboratory personnel may need to answer questions from clinicians and ancillary support staff regarding specimen submission and test selection to optimize fluid collection and minimize the potential for inadequate specimen collection. Furthermore, laboratory personnel must make every attempt to anticipate the most efficient utilization of the submitted specimen so that as much accurate and useful information can be obtained as in many situations repeat collection cannot be accomplished.

In general, body fluid specimens should be transported at ambient temperature (room temperature) to the laboratory as soon as possible as degradation of the cellular component of the specimen begins almost immediately upon collection. Transport time and temperature are preanalytic variables that can affect the integrity of the specimen t2.1 [PMID 10705825]. Transporting of specimens through pneumatic tubes may result in too much shaking or agitation of the specimen resulting in specimen degradation [PMID 22467320, PMID 15117440]. Individual institutional guidelines regarding specimen transport and the use of pneumatic tubes should be developed as appropriate and documented in the standard operating procedure (SOP).

t2.1	Preanalytic, analytic & postanalytic variables affecting body fluid analysis & result reporting		
Preanalytic		**Analytic**	**Postanalytic**
Collection method		Specimen viability/integrity	Result reporting
Specimen handling		Insufficient specimen	Report delivery
Specimen labeling		Instrument failure	Specimen storage
Collection vessel		QC	
Anticoagulant used			
Transport time & temperature			

Body fluid specimens should be received properly labeled with the patient name, birthdate, identifying number, date and time of collection, location (unit), fluid source and tests ordered (which may be indicated on an accompanying requisition form or ordered electronically). Occasionally, specimens will be received unlabeled or insufficiently labeled for proper identification. In this situation the submitting unit should be notified and a new specimen should be requested.

Occasionally specimens cannot be recollected and individual institutions should establish a policy regarding identification, labeling and testing of such specimens. Testing should never be performed and results released without complete confidence of the specimen identity.

Specimen collection, requirements & stability

The type of vessel used for specimen collection is also important. Fluids must be collected in vessels manufactured from materials that do not affect testing results. Collection of body fluids in glass tubes, for example, can result in cellular adherence and inaccurate cell or differential counts. Various transport container types may be needed depending on the testing performed and specimen source. Fluid specimens of large volume, such as pleural or peritoneal fluids, may need to be aliquoted into smaller containers for transport to the laboratory.

Body fluid analysis should be performed as soon as possible upon receipt of the specimen in the laboratory. Most body fluids are stable for 2-4 hours at ambient temperature or up to 24 hours refrigerated [PMID 10973869, PMID 21998343, PMID 23537933, PMID 8990255]. Crystals may remain stable for up to 48-72 hours or more in refrigerated specimens [PMID 11959769, PMID 23872540]. Ideally, body fluid samples for microbiologic studies should be inoculated into blood culture bottles at collection or transported at ambient temperature to the laboratory immediately for processing. If this is not possible, refrigeration of the specimen is recommended. Some organisms, however, are fastidious and temperature sensitive and may not remain viable with refrigeration.

All body fluid types need to be collected with a volume sufficient to perform all of the tests ordered. Clotting invalidates an accurate cell count and frozen samples are unacceptable for cell count because freezing lyses the cells. If the volume of the sample received is insufficient to perform all requested tests, the ordering provider should be contacted to prioritize the tests desired.

After completion of initial testing, the remaining specimen should be stored refrigerated in the event further or repeat testing is necessary. Each laboratory must decide and document in its SOP, how long each sample type is to be retained and stored.

Amniotic fluid

Analysis of amniotic fluid provides useful information for fetal evaluation. Numerous laboratory tests including fetal lung maturity analysis, and fetal chromosome evaluation can guide the clinician on the progress of the pregnancy and alert the provider and parents of potential problems or abnormalities. Amniotic fluid is typically obtained by transabdominal amniocentesis and the indication and subsequent laboratory testing depends on the gestational age. t2.2 outlines the specimen requirements for amniotic fluid collection.

t2.2 Specimen requirements for amniotic fluid

Test	Recommended anticoagulant	Suggested volume*	Additional comments
Fetal lung maturity	None	6-7 mL	Specimen should be refrigerated to prevent degradation of phospholipids
Chemical analysis	None	3-5 mL	Specimen should be protected from light for bilirubin testing
Cytogenetics/ karyotyping	None	6-7 mL	Specimens should be kept at ambient temperature
Microbiology studies and Gram stain	None	3-5 mL	Use of an anticoagulant with a bactericidal or bacteriostatic effect is unacceptable; transfer of the fluid directly into blood culture bottles after collection is recommended

*No more than 30 mL in total of amniotic fluid should be removed as it may precipitate premature labor or spontaneous rupture of membranes. Smaller volumes may be adequate depending on the testing ordered. The first 1-2 mL removed should be discarded because it may be contaminated with blood and maternal cells.

Cerebrospinal fluid

Careful examination of the cerebrospinal fluid (CSF) is extremely important and may provide essential diagnostic information. The specimen must be properly collected and processed in order to obtain accurate testing results. Cerebrospinal fluid specimens should be divided into 3-4 samples collected in sequentially labeled sterile plastic tubes t2.3. The tendency of mononuclear phagocytes and polymorphonuclear leukocytes to adhere to uncoated glass can result in the lowering of the total cell count as well as distortion of the differential count. Although tube order may vary somewhat, ideally, tube 1 should be used for chemical analysis and immunologic studies, tube 2 for microbiologic studies and Gram stain, tube 3 for cell count and differential count, and tube 4 for cytologic examination and other studies. Tube 1, however, should never be used for microbiologic studies because it may be contaminated with skin flora. The suggested collection sequence also reduces the possibility of contamination from peripheral blood, which can invalidate the cell count as well as the immunologic and chemical findings. If a traumatic tap has occurred, serial tubes will show a progressive decrease in the number of red blood cells (RBCs). In true pathologic/hemorrhagic conditions, the tubes will be uniform in color throughout. Some have advocated spectrophotometry in the evaluation and diagnosis of subarachnoid hemorrhage [PMID 23729569]. If significant hemorrhage has occurred due to a traumatic tap, correction for peripheral blood contamination may need to be employed.

t2.3 Specimen requirements & suggested tube collection sequence for cerebrospinal fluid

Test	Recommended anticoagulant	Suggested volume†	Collection sequence
Chemical analysis and immunologic studies	None	1-3 mL	Tube 1
Microbiology studies and Gram stain	None	3-5 mL‡	Tube 2
Cell count and differential count*	None	1-3 mL	Tube 3§
Cytologic examination and other studies	None	5-10 mL	Tube 4

*If a traumatic tap is suspected, cell counts can also be performed on tube 1 and the results compared to tube 3
†Suggested volumes for adult patients; smaller volumes may be adequate depending on the testing performed
‡Greater volume may be needed for acid fast bacilli (AFB) cultures
§Some suggest that the cell and differential count be performed on the last tube in the collection sequence

Serous fluids

There are numerous indications for the laboratory evaluation of serous fluids. They include differentiating between transudates and exudates, distinguishing between malignant and nonmalignant effusions and providing a specific etiology for the patient's effusion. Serous fluids including pleural, pericardial and peritoneal fluids have similar specimen requirements t2.4. These specimens are often collected in large volumes that require aliquoting into smaller containers preferably prior to transport to the laboratory. If aliquoting is required, the specimen must be adequately mixed by gentle agitation prior to aliquoting and before cell and differential counts are performed.

t2.4 Specimen requirements for serous fluids (pleural, pericardial & peritoneal)

Test	Recommended anticoagulant	Suggested volume*	Additional comments
Cell count and differential count	EDTA	3-5 mL	
Chemical analysis such as total protein, LDH, amylase	Sodium heparin or none	5-8 mL	
Microbiology studies and Gram stain	None	8-10 mL†	Use of an anticoagulant with a bactericidal or bacteriostatic effect is unacceptable; transfer of the fluid directly into blood culture bottles after collection is recommended
Cytologic examination (including smears, cytospin preparations, cell blocks), other studies‡	None	15-100 mL	Specimens anticoagulated with heparin and EDTA are acceptable

*Suggested volumes for adult patients; smaller volumes may be adequate depending on the testing performed and source of specimen
†Larger volumes may be necessary for AFB cultures
‡Larger volumes may be required for cytologic examination of some samples; flow cytometry requires either no anticoagulation of the serous fluid or, if the specimen is contaminated with blood, anticoagulation with EDTA, sodium heparin or ACD

Synovial fluid

Thorough evaluation of synovial fluid specimens may be limited due to the volume of the joint fluid or effusion that can be obtained by the submitting clinician. Ideally, 3-5 mL samples will allow adequate testing of cell and differential counts and crystal evaluation as well as chemical analysis respectively t2.5. Specimens for chemical and complement analysis should be centrifuged as soon as possible after receipt in the laboratory to remove all of the cells as cells in the synovial fluid can alter the chemical composition. At least 5 mL of synovial fluid is preferable for microbiologic analysis. Importantly, it must be recognized that useful information can also be obtained from smaller volumes of synovial fluid and every attempt must be made to provide as much useful information as possible to the treating physician even on limited samples. For example, small volumes of synovial fluid may allow for adequate microbiologic examination and determination of the presence and identification of crystals. Microbiologic specimens must be submitted sterile without the use of anticoagulants. Anticoagulants with bactericidal or bacteriostatic properties, in particular, should not be used. Anaerobic transfer tubes or blood culture bottles are recommended. Submission of additional specimen in a clean sterile tube may be used for fungal and acid-fast bacterial cultures, as clinically indicated. Microbiologic samples should not be refrigerated if they are going to be processed within 4 hours of collection as this may compromise organism growth and identification. Crystals may remain stable for up to 48-72 hours in refrigerated specimens, if more immediate analysis is not possible [PMID 11959769, PMID 23872540].

t2.5 Specimen requirements for synovial fluid

Test	Recommended anticoagulant	Suggested volume*	Additional comments
Cell count and differential count, crystal identification, wet mounts	Liquid EDTA, sodium heparin	3-5 mL	Oxalate, powdered EDTA and powdered lithium heparin are unacceptable anticoagulants as they may form crystals
Chemical analysis such as total protein, glucose, CH50	None	3-5 mL	
Microbiology studies and Gram stain	None	>5 mL	Use of an anticoagulant with a bactericidal or bacteriostatic effect is unacceptable; transfer of the fluid directly into blood culture bottles after collection is recommended

*Suggested volumes for adult patients; smaller volumes may be adequate depending on the testing performed

Urine

Urinalysis can provide significant information regarding the health of the urinary tract system as well as allow detection of systemic disease processes. In most cases, obtaining a urine specimen is noninvasive and creates minimal distress to the patient. In some patients, however, urine collection must be obtained through more invasive procedures such as catheterization or suprapubic aspiration. Appropriate collection and evaluation is important to provide the greatest amount of information to the treating clinician. Specimen requirements for urine specimens are outlined in t2.6. Ideally, submission of urine samples to the laboratory for testing should occur within 2 hours. The volume of the urine sample received must be recorded.

t2.6 Specimen requirements for urine			
Test	Recommended anticoagulant	Suggested volume*	Additional comments
Chemical analysis	None	3-5 mL	
Sediment examination	None	3-5 mL	Boric acid may be used as a preservative if specimen transport will be delayed
Microbiology studies and Gram stain	None	3-5 mL	Use of an anticoagulant with a bactericidal or bacteriostatic effect is unacceptable

* Suggested volumes for adult patients. For some laboratory tests, a 24 hour urine sample will be necessary.

Gross (macroscopic) examination

Gross (macroscopic) examination of all body fluids employs similar strategies but varies somewhat in utility and process. Specific features routinely recorded for each body fluid type are outlined below. For all body fluids, the volume of the specimen received should be recorded. Please refer to the individual chapters for a more complete description of the typical gross and microscopic findings for each body fluid type and their significance.

Amniotic fluid

Gross examination of amniotic fluid should be performed before and after centrifugation. The color as well as the presence or absence of meconium should be noted. Most midtrimester amniotic fluids are colorless. Discoloration of amniotic fluid is more commonly secondary to the presence of blood than meconium. If blood is present, it may be helpful or necessary to determine the source of the blood (fetal vs maternal). This information may guide the appropriate therapy. The presence and extent of fetal red blood cells in maternal peripheral blood have historically been determined by a Kleihauer-Betke stain and more recently by flow cytometry assays [PMID 17053464, PMID 17878734, PMID 22231030]. The Kleihauer-Betke stain can also be used to evaluate amniotic fluid for the presence of fetal red blood cells. If meconium is present, the extent can be classified as thin (light), moderate or thick (heavy). Thick meconium has been associated with increased risk of meconium aspiration syndrome [PMID 17896254, PMID 24551662].

Cerebrospinal fluid

Gross examination of CSF includes inspecting the sample for color, clarity, and the presence of clots. Recording of the color of the specimen before centrifugation and the color of the supernatant after centrifugation is recommended. Normal CSF does not clot, appears clear and colorless and has a viscosity similar to water. If disease is present, the color may be altered and the fluid may appear cloudy, turbid, viscous, or clotted. Some have suggested that the recording of turbidity or cloudiness is unnecessary as cell counts are routinely reported [ISBN 1-56238-614X]. Pigmentation (also referred to as xanthochromia) usually refers to a pale pink to yellow color in the supernatant of centrifuged CSF specimens. It is typically due to lysis and breakdown of hemoglobin. Other causes, however, include hyperbilirubinemia and metastatic melanoma. There is ongoing debate as to the usefulness of reporting color or pigmentation in CSF specimens. Traditionally the presence of CSF pigmentation has been utilized to suggest subarachnoid or intracerebral hemorrhage or infarction. Pigmentation, however, can been seen as an artifact of specimen collection or due to contamination of the collecting tube or needle with detergent. Artifactual CSF pigmentation is more commonly observed in traumatic taps, particularly if centrifugation and analysis are delayed. In addition, some studies suggest that visual evaluation for pigmentation is inferior to spectrophotometry for the diagnosis of subarachnoid hemorrhage [PMID 23800427, PMID 24448178]. Each individual laboratory will have to decide for themselves on the utility of reporting color/pigmentation as part of the gross examination of CSF specimens. Commonly reported colors for CSF include yellow, orange, pink, red, brown and green. Refer to Chapter 4 for the description of the significance of the various colors. Clarity is often reported as clear, hazy, cloudy, turbid or bloody. Turbidity or cloudiness begins to appear with a white blood cell count >200 cells/μL or a red cell count of 400/μL. It should be noted that these terms are somewhat arbitrary and some guidelines have advocated not reporting turbidity in CSF specimens as it commonly reflects cell counts [ISBN 1-56238-614X].

Serous fluids

Serous fluids are typically colorless to pale yellow in color. The color, however, is influenced by the presence of blood or hemorrhage, protein, and cellular content. The significance of the presence of blood or hemorrhage varies between the source of the serous fluid being examined and whether the effusion was associated with a traumatic tap. In addition to color, the clarity of the specimen should also be recorded. Depending upon whether the serous fluid represents a transudate or exudate, the degree of turbidity of the specimen can vary significantly. Milky appearing serous fluids may suggest a chylous effusion that typically results from blockage or disruption of lymphatic flow. Causes for chylous effusions include trauma, infections, lymphoma and carcinoma. Turbid but not chylous effusions may also be associated with infection or malignancy.

Synovial fluid

The gross examination of synovial fluid includes reporting of color and clarity. Normal synovial fluid is colorless but often appears pale yellow in color due to the presence of degraded hemoglobin from degenerating RBCs. Septic joint fluid may appear yellow, brown or even green depending on the inflammatory response and organisms present. The clarity of normal synovial fluid is clear or transparent. Increased inflammatory cells can change the clarity of the specimen. The presence of crystals, synovial lining elements and metals or plastics from patients with prosthetic joints, can also result in changes in clarity and may result in opacity. Highly viscous synovial fluids are often difficult to work with. In this situation, addition of hyaluronidase may reduce the viscosity and make the fluid easier to analyze [PMID 16025090, PMID 22955210, PMID 5654509].

Urine

Routine urinalysis includes the reporting of gross (macroscopic) findings including color and clarity. Normal urine can be a wide range of colors depending upon its concentration and the medical condition of the patient. Typical reporting of colors includes yellow, red, orange and brown, although other colors may be seen. Normal urine is clear but may become cloudy due to precipitation of phosphates in alkaline urine and urates in acidic urine. Clarity is often recorded as clear, hazy, cloudy, turbid or flocculent. The specific gravity or osmolarity of the urine specimen is commonly determined.

Microscopic examination

Microscopic evaluation of body fluids can include manual or automated cell counts, differential counts, and evaluation of fluids for crystals, organisms, casts or neoplastic cells. An abbreviated discussion on manual and automatic cell counts and a description of crystal identification is provided below. Entire textbooks have been devoted to the microscopic evaluation of many of the body fluids and the reader is encouraged to refer to them for a more complete description.

Manual cell count

The examination of body fluids for red blood cells (RBCs) and total nucleated cells (TNCs) is routinely performed. Light microscopy with stains that enhance cell recognition or phase microscopy can be utilized. Below is a description of a manual cell counting procedure. Individual laboratories or institutions may have varying procedures for performing manual cell counts.

Equipment and reagents

- Certified pipettes or commercial diluting systems
- Test tubes for dilutions
- Capillary (microhematocrit) tubes, plain or Pasteur pipettes
- Hemocytometer and thick coverslip
- Petri dish
- Moist paper
- Wood applicator sticks
- Microscope
- Hyaluronidase with toluidine blue (0.05%)
- Isotonic saline

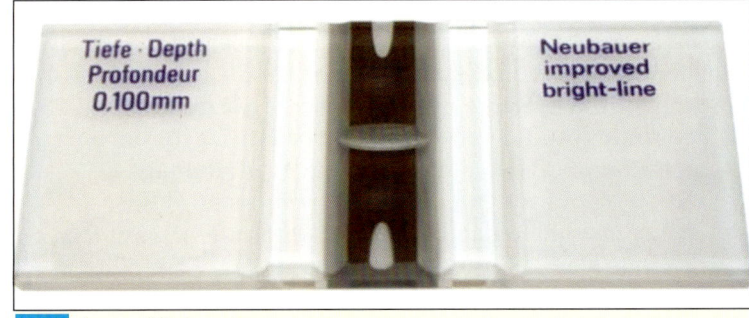

f2.1 Improved Neubauer hemocytometer

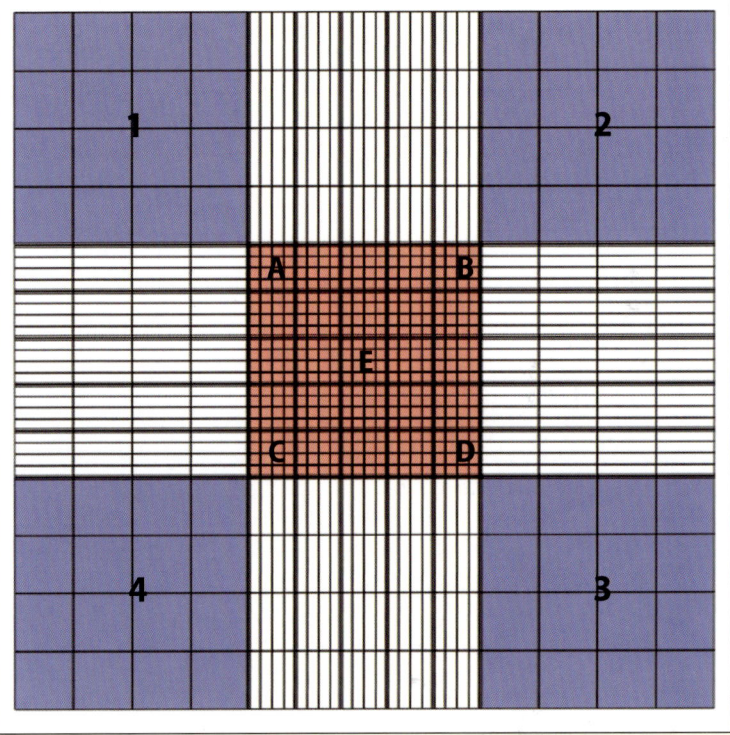

f2.1 Grid of improved Neubauer hemocytometer. 0.1 mm deep (from coverglass down to chamber)
1, 2, 3, 4 = total nucleated cell (TNC) large counting squares; each measures 1 mm × 1 mm & has a volume of 0.1 µL.
A, B, C, D, E = RBC small counting squares; each measures 0.2 mm × 0.2 mm & has a volume of 0.004 µL
(for calculations see p 8)

Procedure (using improved Neubauer hemocytometer)

Manual cell counts are performed on body fluids using a counting chamber consisting of a microscopic slide with a grid etched onto the surface. While the improved Neubauer hemocytometer i2.1 is the most widely used, other chambers are still used in some laboratories. The grid of a Neubauer chamber is divided into 9 large squares, each with an area of 1 mm² and a depth of 0.1 mm f2.1. The center large square is further subdivided into 25 smaller squares. A thick coverslip specifically designed for the hemocytometer must be used to attain accurate counts.

- The sample should be thoroughly mixed to assure an even distribution of cells. Gentle inversion at least 10× by hand is sufficient for most fluids but viscous and turbid specimens require increased mixing for accurate results. Rocking on a mechanical rocker should not exceed 5 minutes to prevent damage to cells except for extremely viscous synovial fluids, which may be rocked for up to 10 minutes. Extremely viscous synovial fluids may need to be treated with hyaluronidase prior to cell count analysis.

- If the sample is clear, no dilution is necessary. If the sample is cloudy or turbid, a dilution is made using isotonic saline, isotonic diluent or hyaluronidase with toluidine blue. Both RBCs and TNCs remain intact with these diluting fluids. For enumerating nucleated cells (NCs), some laboratories prefer dilution with Turk solution (gentian violet dye with acetic acid) that lyses RBCs and stains the nuclei of the NCs for easier visualization. The diluent should be checked for contamination.

- The College of American Pathologists (CAP) requires that dilutions be made using certified pipettes or commercial dilution systems. **t2.7** gives suggested dilutions depending on the appearance of the fluid.

t2.7 Suggested body fluid dilutions for cell counts based on appearance

Fluid appearance	Suggested dilution
Clear	No dilution
Slightly to moderately turbid	1:3, 1:5, 1:10, 1:20
Very turbid or grossly bloody	Start with 1:20
Serially dilute up to 1:100 for TNCs and up to 1:200 for RBCs	

RBC = red blood cell; TNC = total nucleated cell

- Both sides of a clean, dry hemocytometer are charged with the well mixed specimen using a hematocrit tube or Pasteur pipette. The chamber is allowed to fill by capillary action until the volume of fluid just covers the mirrored surface. The hemocytometer is placed in a moist paper lined petri dish with the hemocytometer resting on 2 applicator sticks to prevent contact with the paper until the cells have settled (~5-10 minutes). Both RBCs and TNCs can be counted on the same chamber.

- The entire chamber is scanned on 10 times for the presence of cell clumps. If present, note "The count may be affected by the presence of clumps." Scan at least 10 fields on 10× and 40× to evaluate for debris. If debris is present, there should be a note, such as "The count may be affected by the presence of debris."

- Based on the number of TNCs and RBCs present, determine an appropriate area of the hemocytometer to count. Ideally, a total of 50-200 cells should be counted on each side of the hemocytometer. All counts should be done in duplicate using 40× power.

t2.8 gives guidelines for the area to be counted based on the number of cells present on each side of the hemocytometer.

t2.8 Suggested guidelines for counting of TNCs & RBCs based on the number of cells present

Cells per chamber side	Squares counted	Area counted
<200 in 9 large squares (entire chamber)	All 9 squares	9 mm^2
>200 in 9 large squares	4 corner squares	4 mm^2
>200 cells in 1 large square	5 small squares within center large square	0.2 mm^2
Cells crowded and overlapping	Consider a higher dilution	

Volume = area × depth (0.1 mm)
1 mm^3 = 1 μL

The total cells counted per μL are calculated using the following formula:

$$\text{Total cells/μL} = \frac{\text{\# cells counted} \times \text{dilution factor}}{\text{\# squares counted} \times \text{volume of each square}}$$

- When few TNCs are present in a specimen with much higher RBC numbers or vice versa, it may be necessary to make different dilutions for RBCs and TNCs. The higher dilution will introduce error especially when there are <50 cells (RBCs or TNCs) in 9 squares.

- Count cells in a regular pattern across the area to be counted. Count squares on both the left and right side of the chamber to minimize variability due to differences in cell distribution.

- Cells that touch the left and upper double boundary lines but not those cells that touch the right and bottom double boundary lines should be counted.

- When the boundary line is a triple line, all of the cells within the square and those touching the middle line inward are counted.

- Count the same number of squares on both sides of the chamber and average the raw cell counts.

- Repeat the procedure if duplicate counts >50 cells do not agree within 10%, or if counts <50 cells differ by >5 cells.

- Include in the RBC count:
  - RBCs with distinct outlines with halos & clear centers
  - Crenated RBCs (cells with many fine pointed projections)
  - Ghost RBCs with intact circular membranes; they can appear to have granular hemoglobin at their margins

- Include in the total nucleated cell (TNC) count:
  - Lymphocytes, monocytes/macrophages, mesothelial cells, synovial lining cells, PMNs, blasts, lymphoma cells, nucleated RBCs

- Do not include in the count
  - Broken cells, sheets or clumps of tumor cells
  - Tissue cells
  - Distinguishable tumor cells (nonhematopoietic)

Automated cell counts

For decades, the manual hemocytometer method has been the standard for enumerating total nucleated cells and red blood cells in body fluids.

Laboratories are under increasing pressure to provide accurate testing in a more cost effective manner. This has lead to the development of many automated methods that have more rapid, less labor intensive testing methods. Automating body fluid cell counts is desirable but caution is required to validate these methods and assure their clinical accuracy.

Various instruments have been validated for performing automated body fluid cell counts. Examples include the Beckman-Coulter LH750, Advia 2120, Iris iQ200, Sysmex-5000, and Abbot Cell-Dyn. The methodology utilized by these instruments is diverse and includes technologies such as impedance, digital imaging, flow cytometry, and light scatter. Each instrument manufacturer gives guidelines as to which body fluid types have been approved by regulatory agencies to perform on their instrument. Laboratories should always follow the manufacturer's guidelines for testing, including which fluids have clearance and an "intended use" statement for analysis. CLSI gives a detailed protocol for validation of methods that have not been approved. Recently a plethora of studies evaluating these automated methods has been published [PMID 14649464, PMID 19095566, PMID 19228639, PMID 20236183, PMID 21836038, PMID 23647736]. They include comparison of cell counts on cerebrospinal, serous, and synovial fluids obtained by automated methods and by manual counts on the hemocytometer. Most studies suggest sufficient correlation but disagreement continues on the accuracy and appropriateness of using automated methods for low cell count specimens. While some studies suggest linear ranges to 0, others show unacceptable rates of error in low ranges and suggest a lower limit of detection for specific instruments. Automated CSF nucleated counts have been especially problematic because normal CSF nucleated counts are extremely low (0-5/µL for adults and 0-30/µL for neonates). The separation between normal and disease conditions is narrow and depends on the ability of the method to provide accurate and reproducible results in low ranges. If the test system is modified beyond the specifications of the manufacturer, performance specifications including accuracy, precision, sensitivity, specificity, reportable range of testing results and reference intervals must be established before reporting of patient results.

Cell concentration & cytospin preparation

Numerous methods have been described for concentrating body fluid cells. These include centrifugation with smears made from the resuspended sediment. Cytocentrifugation has become the preferred method for most laboratories. Wedge or push smears should not be used as these methodologies often impact the integrity of the cellular component. Cytocentrifuge preparations are air dried and therefore suitable for Wright-Giemsa staining as well as various cytochemical and immunohistochemical staining procedures.

A cytocentrifuge is a low speed, low acceleration centrifuge suitable for making concentrated thin layer cell preparations from body fluids. It is especially well suited for low cellularity body fluid specimens. The cytocentrifuge consists of a rotating carrier and multiple assemblies mounted on the carrier for rotation. Individual assemblies consist of a sample chamber, and a slide overlaid with a filter card that provides an absorbent seal all held together with a clip.

As the rotor of the centrocentrifuge starts spinning, centrifugal force moves the sample toward the slide. Cells are randomly deposited directly on the slide and the filter card absorbs the accompanying liquid. Cells are typically concentrated 20 fold by cytocentrifugation [ISBN 1-56238-614X]. Below is an example procedure for preparing cytospin slides of body fluids.

Equipment and reagents

- Microscope slides with premarked circle(s): single or double 8 mm circle
- Cytospin chambers (disposable)
- Filter cards (blotter), prepunched (filter card may be attached to chamber)
- Cytospin clips
- Transfer pipettes
- Cytocentrifuge
- 22% bovine serum albumin
- buffered hyaluronidase

Procedure

- Label slides with patient's name, identification number, date, and fluid source. Assemble the sample chamber, filter card, and slide with the slide clip and place in cytospin. Depending on the appearance of the fluid, varied drops may be used.
  - Clear fluid, 5-10 drops
  - Cloudy fluid, 1-3 drops
  - Bloody fluid, 5-10 drops of a 1:5 saline dilution

  Using a different number of drops on the 2 sections of a double chamber or on each of 2 slides is often helpful in obtaining optimal cell distribution. A pullapart smear may be prepared for highly viscous fluids such as some synovial fluids.

- Except for synovial fluids, add 1 or 2 drops of 22% bovine serum albumin to the bottom of the sample chamber. This will reduce the cell distortion and increase yield.

- Add 1-10 drops of fluid (or properly diluted fluid) into the sample chamber with a Pasteur or plastic transfer pipette. Cap sample chambers to minimize possible aerosol.

- Spin at 1,500 rpm for ~5 minutes (other speeds and time may be acceptable if validated).

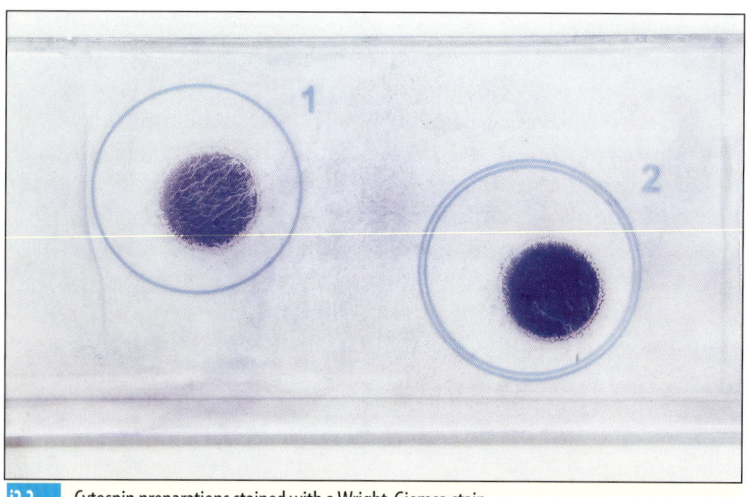

i2.2 Cytospin preparations stained with a Wright-Giemsa stain

- Carefully remove the slides, filter cards, and sample chambers together. If not using a premarked slide, mark a circle around the concentrate on the back of the slide with a crayon or marker.
- Air dry the slides before staining.
- Stain the slides for morphologic evaluation (see below and i2.2).
- Coverslip the stained slide using mounting media as a sealant.

It should be noted that extensive cellular distortions may be seen as a result of the cytocentrifugation process. These artifacts can be minimized by establishing the optimal speed and time of centrifugation, using an optimal cellular concentration and with the addition of albumin to the specimen. In addition, some changes and artifacts occur while the specimen is in the collection vessel.

Slide staining

There are only a few commonly used stains in the morphologic examination of body fluids. The most common is a Romanowsky stain. There are several variants of this stain, which are based on the preparation of air dried smears/cytospin slides. In most hematology labs, this is the Wright or Wright-Giemsa stain. A quicker version of the Wright stain is the Diff-Quik stain. A very good Romanowsky stain is the May-Grunwald-Giemsa (MGG) stain but obtaining high quality reagents for this stain in the United States has been a challenge. The second most common stain is the Papanicolaou stain that was originally developed for the examination of vaginal and cervical-vaginal specimens. It is an alcohol based stain and requires "wet smears," and includes 3 principal reagents, hematoxylin (nuclear), and 2 cytoplasmic counter stains: eosin and orange G. The cytology literature discusses 2 variants, a regressive and a progressive process that differ in nuclear staining technique. Based largely on the work with fine needle aspiration biopsies (FNABs), advantages of both stains have been recognized and in many settings offer complimentary morphologic information t2.9. The Romanowsky stain provides information about the cytoplasm and the background, eg, stroma, and the Papanicolaou stain provides excellent nuclear detail used in assessing malignancy. Romanowsky stains are preferred for evaluation of hematologic malignancies. Other stains such as the Gram stain and AFB stains may be performed to evaluate for microorganisms (see below). Staining quality is extremely important for accurate diagnosis. Fluctuations in staining buffer pH, for example, can affect the staining quality.

t2.9 Usefulness of Romanowksy & Papanicolaou stains

Morphologic observation	Romanowsky (includes Wright-Giemsa)	Papanicolaou
Nuclear detail	+	+++
Keratin	+	+++
Cytoplasmic mucin	++	+/-
Cytoplasmic granules	++	+/-
Extracellular mucin/matrix	+++	+
Other extracellular features	+++	+/-

Differential cell counts & cytomorphology

A differential cell count should be performed on stained smears made from concentrated cells and not from cells in a hemocytometer. A "chamber differential" (performed in a counting chamber) is unsatisfactory, as cell types are difficult to correctly identify in the wet preparations. Concentration of the fluid sample onto a smear/slide, by cytocentrifugation, will provide a larger number of cells for examination and proper staining will allow for more accurate cellular identification.

Morphologically, a smear made from concentrated cells is also superior to push smears. Push smears are not recommended for body fluid cellular examination because with this technique, cells often do not remain intact. The use of these direct (push) smears is being formally discouraged by the College of American Pathologists (CAP), with cytocentrifugation being its recommended method.

The Wright-Giemsa stain is excellent for studying cellular morphologic characteristics, especially those of hematopoietic cells. It is a polychromatic stain composed of basic and acidic dyes. Some cellular structures take up acidic dyes and stain red, some take up basic dyes and stain blue, and others take up both acidic and basic dyes.

A Wright-Giemsa stained slide used for a differential cell count is first scanned using both low power (10×) and then a higher power (40×) objective. The distribution of the various cell types, presence of cell clumping, organisms, debris, and/or crystals should be noted. The cells on the preparation should be distributed with sufficient spacing between cells for adequate visualization. If the cells are overcrowded and morphology distorted, making them difficult to identify, the cytocentrifuge procedure should be repeated using fewer drops of fluid or a higher dilution. The procedure should also be repeated whenever the cell recovery on the cytospin preparation does not correlate with the number of cells obtained by the cell count.

An oil immersion objective of even higher power (50× or 100×) is used to verify any abnormal findings noted on scanning and to perform a differential cell count. A differential count includes counting and subclassifying 100 nucleated cells and reporting each subclass as a percentage of the total cells. If <100 cells are present, the number counted should be recorded. Absolute numbers can be reported and/or converted to a percentage.

Each laboratory should define the subclasses of nucleated cells to be routinely reported. One example might include reporting:

- PMNs (including immature & pyknotic forms)
- Lymphocytes
- Mononuclear cells (including monocytes, macrophages, mesothelial cells, synovial lining cells & excluding lymphocytes)
- Other possible categories (blasts, lymphoma cells, plasma cells, variant lymphocytes & unidentifiable cells)

A comment section should be included for reporting the presence of hemosiderin, hematoidin crystals, hemophagocytosis, lining cells, malignant cells or other significant findings.

Organisms such as bacteria, yeast, fungi, and parasites, when present, should be documented, including whether they are intra or extracellular. A Gram stain should be used to confirm the presence of organisms.

Nucleated red blood cells (nRBCs) are not included in the differential but counted separately. If nRBCs have been included in the TNC enumeration, and if >10 nRBCs/100 TNC are counted, a corrected TNC should be performed. Broken cells, sheets or clumps of tumor cells, tissue cells including squamous epithelial, endothelial, cartilage, neural tissue/neurons, and germinal matrix cells are not counted in the differential count but should be noted as a comment.

All slides with unusual findings, or atypical, unidentified, or suspected neoplastic cells, should be reviewed by a pathologist. Each laboratory will have to determine the specific morphologic or clinical parameters for physician slide review of body fluids. It is common that aliquots of the same sample are being analyzed morphologically in the hematology and cytopathology laboratories concurrently. As much as is feasible, the morphologic interpretation of each individual specimen from the various laboratory sections (hematology and cytopathology) should be compared for quality assurance and sampling error.

Each body fluid type will have typical cellular constituents that must be recognized in addition to the presence of unusual or neoplastic cellular elements. The reader should refer to the individual chapters for the common and important cytomorphologic findings of each body fluid type.

Cell block preparations

For further morphologic examination and if specimen volume permits, cell blocks should be prepared and used as an adjunct to smear/cytospin evaluation [PMID 16604559, PMID 364975]. This process involves concentrating the cellular component or sediment from the submitted sample, processing the specimen including fixation, and embedding it in a paraffin block. Histologic sections are then prepared in a manner similar to tissue sections. Sections from the prepared cell block can also be utilized for immunohistochemical staining.

Synovial fluid crystal identification

Identification of crystals in synovial fluid is one of the most useful laboratory studies in the evaluation of arthritides. It is essential that all synovial fluids be carefully examined for crystals using appropriate techniques and that the examiner has experience in crystal identification. Improper identification of crystals can result in incorrect patient therapies or procedures. Although there is a myriad of crystal types that can be seen in synovial fluid, the most commonly seen are monosodium urate (MSU), calcium pyrophosphate dihydrate (CPPD), cholesterol, steroid, apatite, phosphate, and oxalate t2.10. It is important to realize that numerous substances or artifacts can resemble crystals and lead to misinterpretation t2.11.

t2.10 Common synovial fluid crystals		
Crystal	**Clinical disorder**	**Laboratory findings**
Monosodium urate (MSU)	Urate gout	Negatively birefringent, needlelike (intra- or extracellular)
Calcium pyrophosphate dihydrate (CPPD)	CPPD deposition disease; pseudogout, pyrophosphate gout, chondrocalcinosis	Positively birefringent, rhombohedral but may have other shapes (intra- or extracellular), often seen without polarized microscopy
Basic calcium phosphates Hydroxyapatite Octacalcium Tricalcium (whitlockite) Hydroxyl phosphate dihydrate (brushite)	Apatite gout	Usually not identified with conventional polarized microscopy Alizarin red S stain (nonspecific but causes crystals containing calcium to stain orange in bright field microscopy and bright red with polarized light microscopy)
Calcium oxalate Monohydrate (whewellite) Calcium oxalate (weddelite)	Primary oxalosis, chronic renal failure (renal dialysis patients)	Small, variably birefringent, bipyramidal (may be seen in urine)
Cholesterol	Cholesterol gout (chronic effusions, rheumatoid arthritis, osteoarthritis)	Large, rectangular notched plates or occasionally needles
Lipid crystals	Rheumatoid arthritis, trauma, atraumatic acute arthritis	Maltese cross, needles, positive birefrigent
Charcot-Leyden crystals	Hypereosinophillic syndromes with synovitis	Bipyramidal hexagons
Hematoidin	Hemarthrosis, sickle cell arthropathy	Golden rhomboids in bright field light

t2.11	Artifacts that may be seen during examination of synovial fluids for crystals

Glass fragments
Dust particles
Fibers
Lipid from degenerated cells
Talc/starch from gloves
Drying artifact
Lint
Collagen fibrils
Cartilage fragments
Metal fragments from prosthesis
Scratches in glass slide
Anticoagulants including lithium heparin and powdered EDTA
Medications including corticosteroids

A variety of techniques are available for crystal identification; however, microscopic examination with a standard laboratory microscope equipped with a polarizer, analyzer, and red compensator is all that is necessary for routine analysis t2.12. The necessary attachments can be purchased as kits from microscope manufacturers such as Leica, Nikon and Olympus. To facilitate accurate identification of crystals, it is important that a high quality microscope with polarizing lenses and a red compensator be used f2.2.

t2.12	Crystal identification techniques
Techniques	**Use**
Bright field microscopy	Evaluates stained specimens and wet preparations for apatite and colored crystals
Polarized microscopy	Identifies MSU and CPPD crystals
Polarized light with compensator	Differentiates MSU and CPPD crystals
Alizarin red S staining	Crystals containing calcium will stain orange with bright field microscopy and bright red with polarized light microscopy
Infrared spectroscopy	Determines chemical composition
X ray diffraction	Elucidates chemical structure (requires a large amount of crystals)

Procedure

Synovial fluid crystal examination must include a wet mount and both an unstained and stained cytocentrifuge preparation.

Wet prep

Synovial fluid is gently mixed and a small drop of the fluid placed on a clean microscope slide with a glass coverslip placed on top of the drop of fluid.

Cytocentrifuge preparation

A cytocentrifuge slide is prepared using the techniques described previously. After drying, the unstained slide is examined for crystals. Additionally, the slide is examined for crystals after staining with Wright-Giemsa stain. The stained slide can also be used to perform a differential count. Alternatively, 2 cytospin slides can be made with both stained and unstained slides examined for crystals.

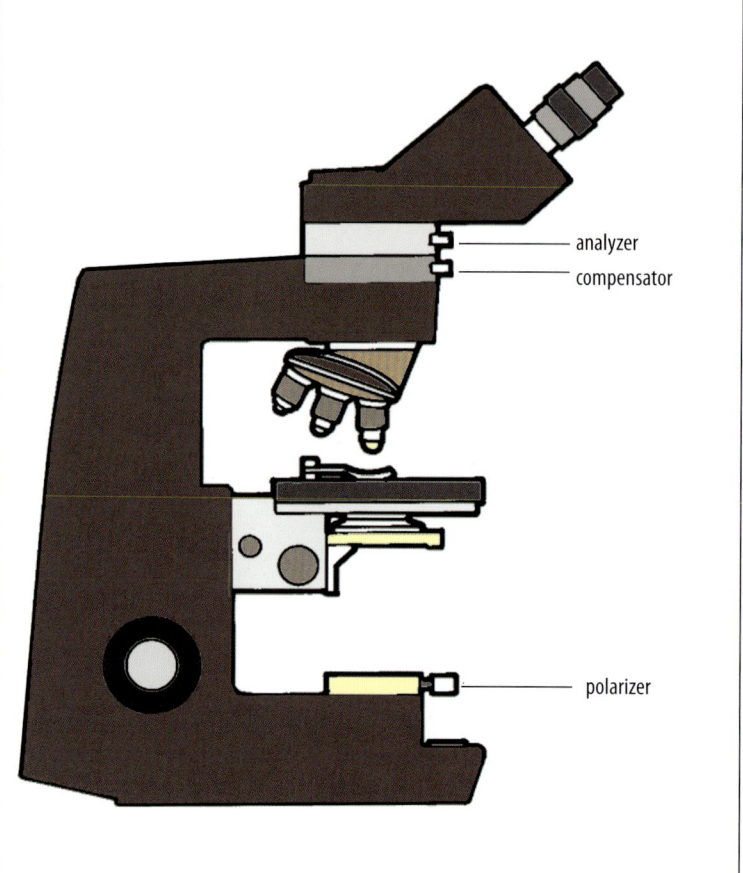

f2.2 Schematic diagram of a microscope illustrating the position of the polarizer, analyzer & compensator

- The specimen is first examined using bright field light microscopy to detect the presence or absence of globules or chunks of material that may represent hydroxyapatite crystals. Cells, fibrils, lipids, hematin, CPPD, and other crystals may also be seen. Initial review of synovial fluids by bright field light microscopy may help in correlating findings with compensated polarized light microscopy. For example, hematin crystals can be mistaken for CPPD crystals by compensated polarized light microscopy, but this is less likely to occur if the golden hematin crystals are initially recognized with bright field light microscopy. Lowering the microscope condenser or using phase microscopy will aid in finding crystals with bright field light microscopy.

- If unknown crystals are present, the synovial fluid may be stained with alizarin red S. After adding 1 drop of filtered alizarin red S stain solution to 1 drop of synovial fluid on a glass slide, the specimen is coverslipped and examined. With bright field light microscopy, crystals containing calcium stain orange. With polarized light microscopy, the crystals appear bright red. Alizarin red S staining may be useful for identifying phosphate crystals that contain calcium. Shiny, refractile, coinlike clumps that stain positive with alizarin red S staining are most likely to be hydroxyapatite crystals. CPPD crystals do not stain as strongly as do hydroxyapatite crystals. The presence of CPPD crystals must be confirmed by compensated polarized light microscopy. Alizarin red S does not, however, distinguish the different types of calcium crystals. If the specimen stains positive with alizarin red S, then any 1 of the several calcium crystals, including calcium oxalate, may be present t2.10. The other calcium phosphate crystals are more difficult to identify and require specialized equipment that is available only in highly specialized laboratories. There is not agreement on the clinical importance of detecting and identifying calcium phosphate crystals other than CPPD crystals.

- Polarized microscopy is primarily used to detect MSU or CPPD crystals. Calcium oxalate, lipid crystals, cholesterol, steroids, starch, and artifacts may also be detected by polarized microscopy.

- A standard laboratory bright light microscope with 2 additional filters (a polarizer and an analyzer) is used for synovial fluid crystal identification. The polarizer is placed between the light source and the microscope stage. The analyzer must be placed above the specimen. Its placement, however, depends on the microscope design.

- Light from the source exits in multiple directions. Polarizing lenses act as filters. Only light traveling in 1 plane exits a polarizing lens. The second polarizing lens used is called the analyzer f2.2. When the analyzer is placed so that it is perpendicular to the first polarizing lens, the light path is essentially blocked. This is called maximum extinction.

- When a birefringent crystal is placed in the polarized light path, the light is refracted. The light refracted by the crystal can now exit through the second polarizing lens or analyzer. When looking through the microscope, this birefringent crystal will appear as a bright area against the background. With rotation of the polarizing lens, the background will become dark i2.3. With polarized light microscopy, MSU and CPPD crystals appear white i2.4, i2.5. To further identify MSU or CPPD crystals, the red compensator is added.

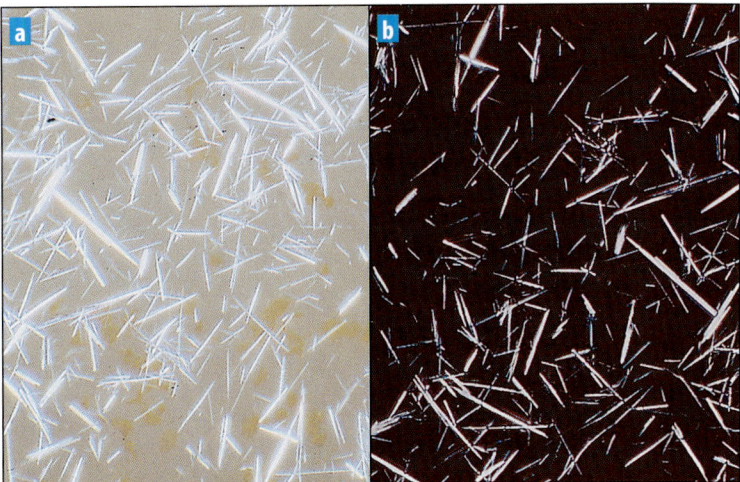

i2.3 **a** & **b** show the background & MSU crystals under polarizing lenses with **b** representing the polarizing lenses rotated to obtain maximum extinction

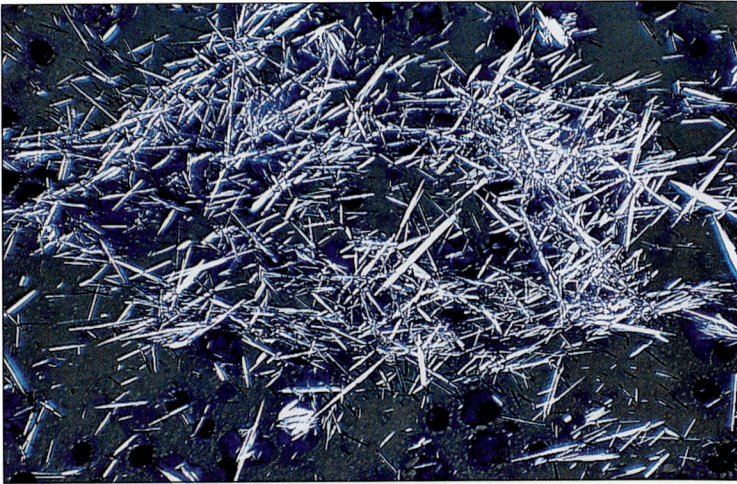

i2.4 Intracellular & extracellular MSU crystals, which appear needlelike (Wright-Giemsa stain, polarized light)

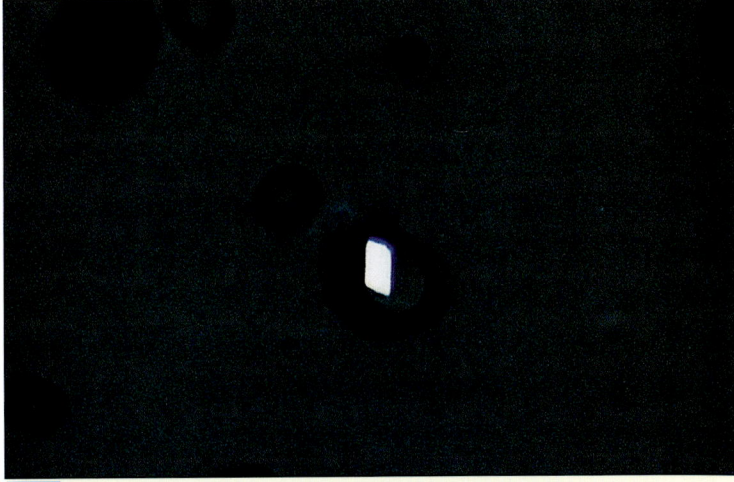

i2.5 Typical intracellular CPPD crystal (Wright-Giemsa stain, polarized light)

2: Laboratory Methods

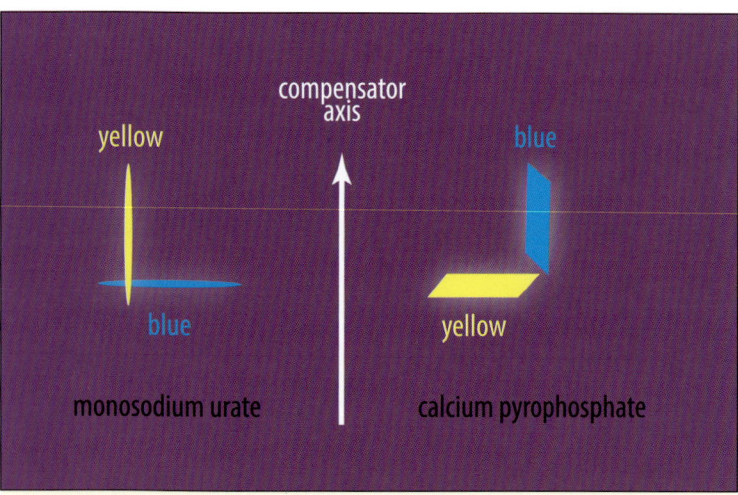

f2.3 2-dimensional schematic representation of MSU & CPPD crystals when viewed under a compensated polarized light microscope. MSU crystals appear yellow when parallel to the compensator, while CPPD crystals appear blue when parallel to the compensator.

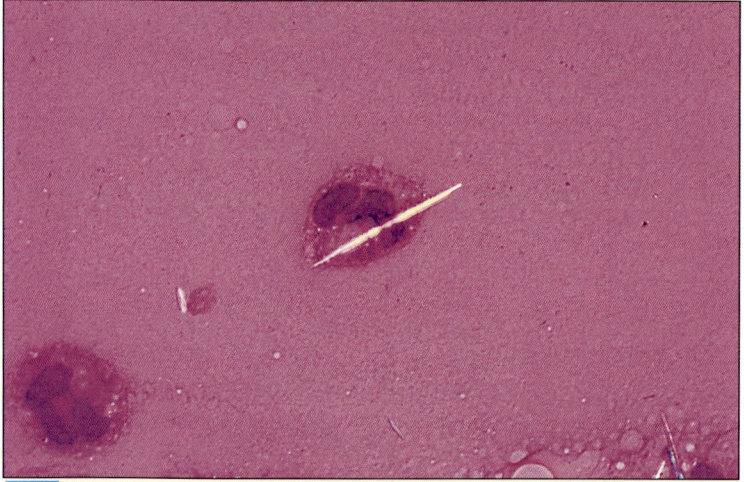

i2.6 Intracellular MSU crystal. The crystal is yellow when parallel to the red compensator (Wright-Giemsa stain, compensated polarized light).

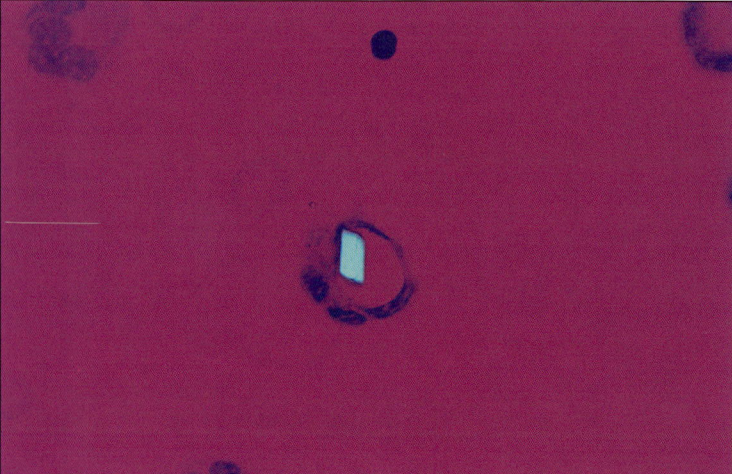

i2.7 CPPD crystal appears blue when parallel to the axis of the red compensator (Wright-Giemsa stain, compensated polarized light)

- Polarized light microscopy with a compensator is used to identify and confirm the presence or absence of MSU and CPPD crystals. The red compensator retards light so that birefringent crystals produce visibly different colors. The colors produced by MSU and CPPD are opposite. When the microscope and crystals are properly oriented, MSU crystals will appear yellow when parallel to the compensator and blue when perpendicular to the compensator. CPPD crystals will be opposite. They will appear blue when parallel to the compensator and yellow when perpendicular to the axis of the compensator f2.3 i2.6-i2.7.

- The patient's sample is first examined under low power (10× objective). If the light intensity is too strong, weakly birefringent crystals such as CPPD may not be seen. After crystals have been found under low power, they should be examined under high power (40× or 100×). By using compensated polarized microscopy, any MSU or CPPD crystals that are present can be identified. The presence of other crystals may also be reported. The number of crystals present is estimated as few, moderate, or many, and the crystals are described as intracellular, extracellular, or both. Sometimes it takes a careful search to identify CPPD crystals because of their weak birefringence or small size. An experienced observer will often be able to distinguish the needlelike MSU crystals from rhombohedral shaped CPPD crystals. It is important to confirm the initial impression, however, with compensated polarized light microscopy. Occasionally, a rhombohedral CPPD crystal may be viewed on its side and resemble an MSU crystal. MSU and CPPD crystals may occur together.

Types of crystals

- MSU crystals are easily recognized with polarized light microscopy when present in adequate numbers. They appear as elongated needlelike crystals i2.8. The ends of the crystals are tapered to a sharp point. The central part of the crystals is thicker. They are ~2-20 µm long and 0.2-1.0 µm thick. Their presence is confirmed with the use of a red compensator. Their needlelike appearance and the negative birefringence seen with a red compensator is all that is routinely necessary for their identification. MSU crystals appear yellow when parallel to the red compensator and blue when perpendicular to the compensator. They may appear intracellular, extracellular, or both. Sometimes MSU crystals are small and are few in number. At least 15 minutes should be spent examining synovial fluid for crystals before a negative result is given to the clinician.

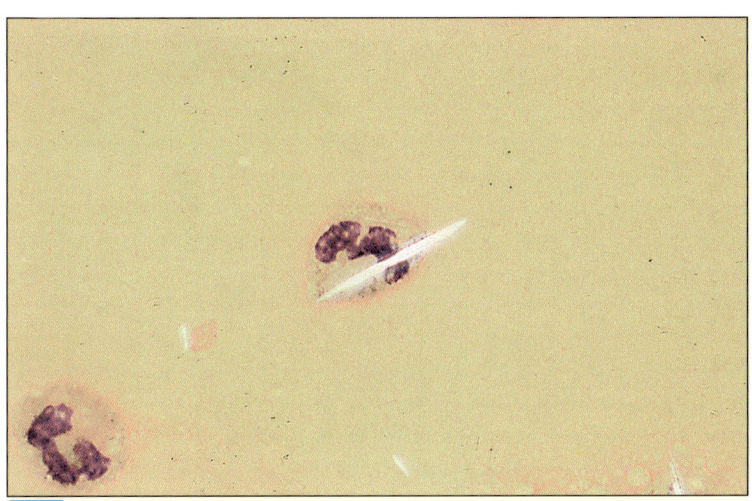

i2.8 Intracellular needle shaped MSU crystal (Wright-Giemsa stain, polarized light)

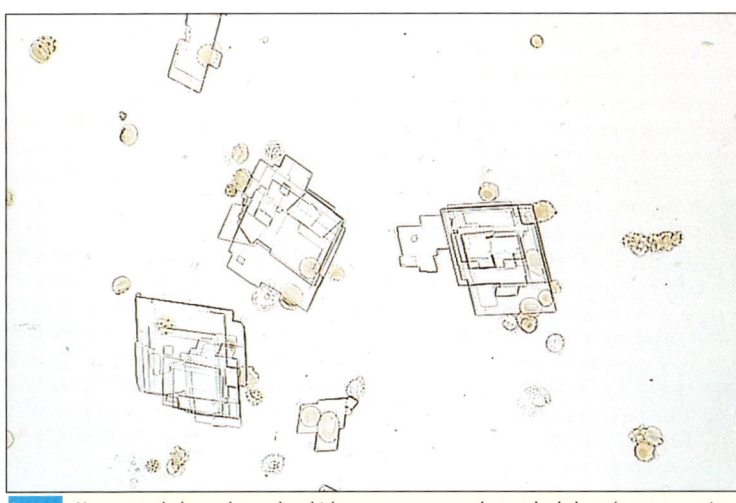

i2.10 Numerous cholesterol crystals, which appear as rectangular notched plates (wet preparation, bright field light)

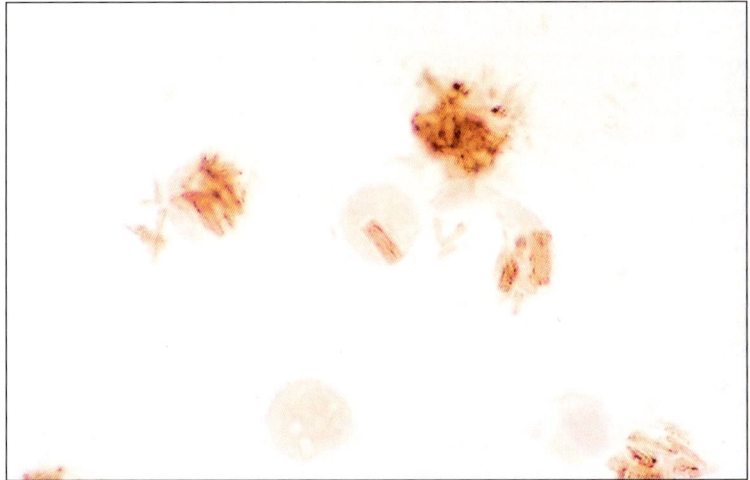

i2.9 CPPD crystals stained with alizarin red S stain

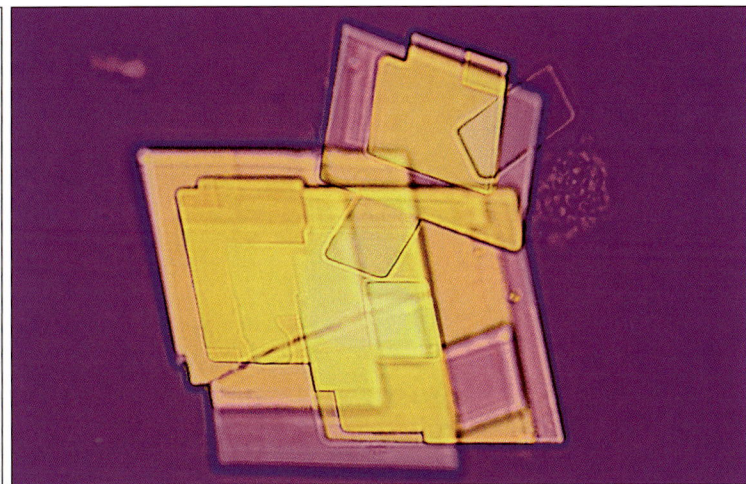

i2.11 The same specimen as i2.10 viewed with polarized compensated light (wet preparation)

- CPPD crystals appear rhombohedral with polarized light microscopy. CPPD crystals are ~2-20 μm long and 1-4 μm wide. Occasionally a CPPD crystal may be observed on its side and be mistaken for an MSU crystal by polarized light microscopy. CPPD birefringence with a red compensator, however, is opposite that seen with MSU crystals. CPPD crystals that are parallel to the red compensator appear blue while CPPD crystals that are perpendicular to the compensator appear yellow. CPPD crystals may be intracellular, extracellular, or both. They are not as strongly birefringent as MSU crystals. If the microscope light source is too bright, CPPD crystals may be missed.

- Hydroxyapatite crystals occur in patients with osteoarthritis and rheumatoid arthritis. They are not pathognomonic for any specific disease entity. With bright field light microscopy, they vary in shape but may appear as globules, 2-10 μm wide that are usually not birefringent with polarized light microscopy. The crystals may be intracellular or extracellular. They stain positive with alizarin red S stain. Other calcium containing phosphate crystals, including CPPD crystals, will also stain with alizarin red S stain i2.9. Other phosphate crystals can be seen in synovial effusions. With the exception of CPPD, none of the phosphate crystals are considered pathognomonic of a specific disease process.

- Cholesterol crystals are seen infrequently. They usually appear as rectangular notched plates or rings i2.10, i2.11. Cholesterol rich effusions are rare. If present, they usually occur in a patient with longstanding rheumatoid arthritis. Cholesterol rich synovial fluid may grossly appear purulent. When viewed under a bright light, cholesterol rich fluids will have a scintillating appearance and a milky yellow to brown color.

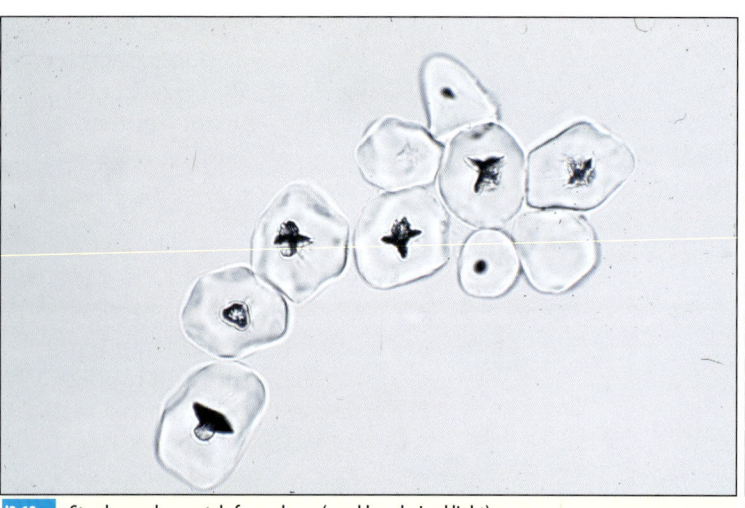

i2.12 Starch powder crystals from gloves (weakly polarized light)

i2.14 Oxalate crystal (wet preparation, bright field light microscopy)

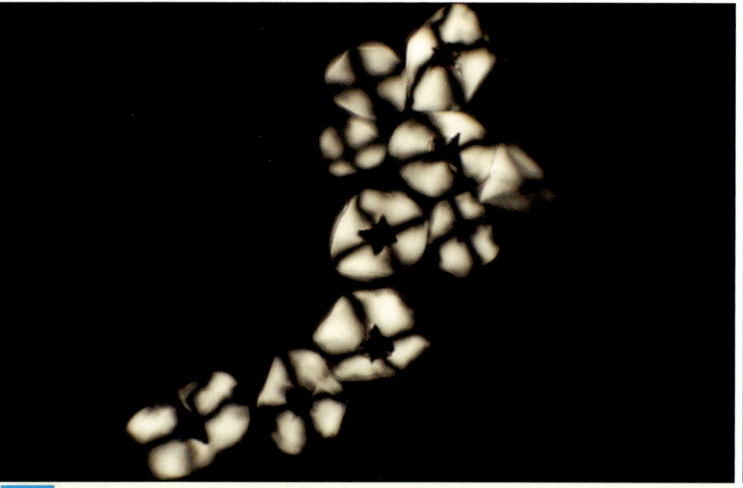

i2.13 Starch powder crystals from gloves (polarized light)

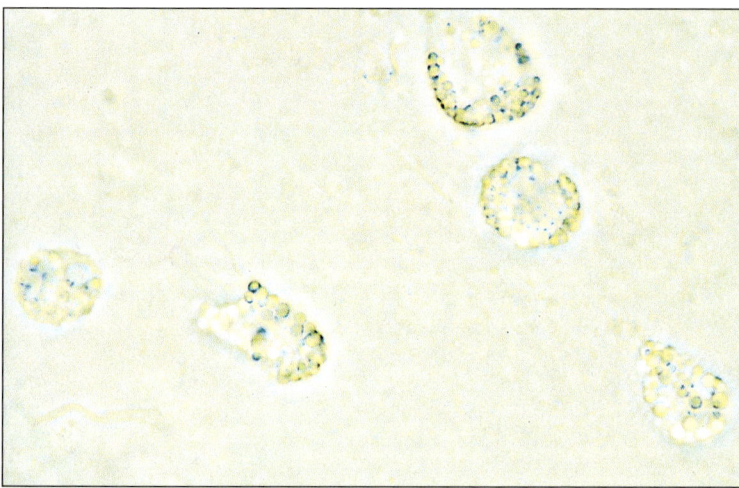

i2.15 Lipid liquid crystals, which appear as small intracellular inclusions of neutral fat (bright field light microscopy)

- Starch crystals from surgical gloves may be seen in synovial effusions i2.12, i2.13. With polarized light microscopy, these crystals appear as bright Maltese crosses. Starch crystals should not be mistaken for the more significant spheroid aggregates of MSU crystals.

- Calcium oxalate crystals may be seen in the synovial fluid from renal dialysis patients and in patients with primary oxalosis. These crystals are usually small and bipyramidal or small and pleomorphic i2.14. They may have strong birefringence or no birefringence. They are positive with alizarin red S stain as are other crystals containing calcium.

- Lipids may be crystalline or noncrystalline and are seen in chronic effusions and in chylous effusions i2.15. With polarized light microscopy, crystalline lipids are strongly birefringent and appear as Maltese crosses.

- Corticosteroid crystals represent one of the more common artifacts in synovial fluid that may be mistaken for MSU crystals. Such crystals may be seen for several weeks or months after the injection of corticosteroids into joint cavities or the surrounding connective tissue. Knowing whether a patient has a history of corticosteroid injections is therefore important in the evaluation of joint fluids i2.16.

- Hematin crystals may be seen in synovial effusions with hemarthrosis. Hematin is a degradation product of hemoglobin. Red blood cells in synovial effusions are phagocytosed by macrophages and the enzymatic degradation of hemoglobin may result in the production of hematin crystals. These crystals are commonly rhombohedral, 2-8 μm in length, and appear golden with bright field light microscopy i2.17. They may also be irregularly shaped. Their presence suggests that significant joint hemorrhage has occurred. Hematin crystals can be mistaken for CPPD crystals because of their rhombohedral shape but can be differentiated by their lack positive birefringence and detection on bright field light microscopy.

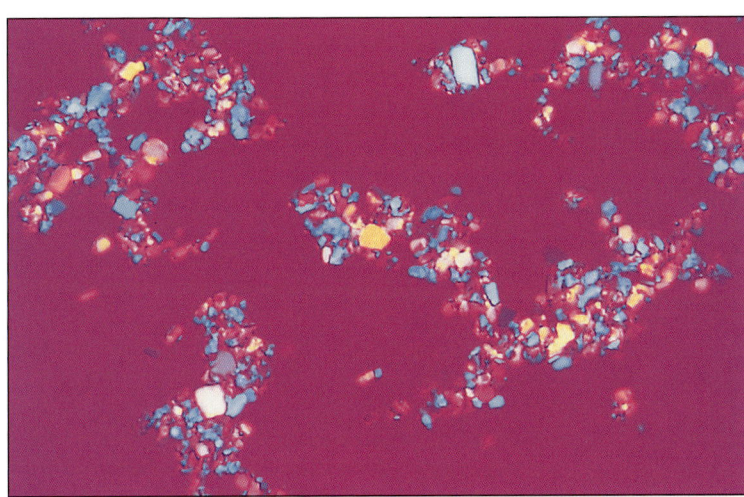

i2.16 Corticosteroid crystals seen after corticosteroid injections. They can be confused with MSU & CPPD crystals (wet preparation, polarized compensated light).

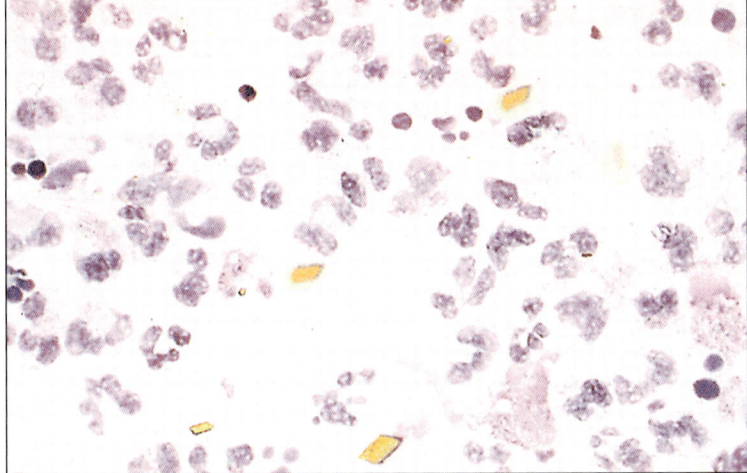

i2.17 Hematin crystals found in hemorrhagic synovial fluid (Wright-Giemsa stain).

A variety of artifacts may be seen in synovial effusions with polarized light microscopy t2.11. By using clean microscope slides and coverslips, many common artifacts may be eliminated. Clinically significant crystals should not have irregular outlines or broken and jagged edges. In cases where it is difficult to determine the type or nature of the crystalline material present, consultation from a more experienced observer may be helpful.

Numerous casts, crystals and calculi can also be identified within the urine and are briefly discussed within Chapter 9. The reader should also refer to more specialized texts for complete review of the types, composition and clinical significance.

Chemistry

Clinical laboratories may receive requests to analyze body fluids for a variety of chemical constituents. Before performing the analysis there are several caveats that must first be considered. Foremost, requests for testing analytes in "nonstandard" body fluids should be critically evaluated for clinical utility prior to performing testing. Analyte/body fluid combinations are context dependent therefore, analyte concentration or detection may offer useful clinical information in 1 type of body fluid but not another. For example, the clinical usefulness of measuring glucose in cerebrospinal fluid is well established while the utility of determining its concentration in amniotic fluid is questionable. This is particularly important because clinical decisions may be based on the test result.

If the method used for detecting or quantifying the analyte is commercially available and approved/cleared by a regulatory agency (eg, the Food and Drug Administration [FDA]), then the manufacturer will provide information regarding the intended use of the test, including the types of body fluids for which the method can be used. The use of a body fluid not specifically indicated in the product insert can be considered a "nonstandard" body fluid. Such testing of a nonstandard body fluid is considered by some regulatory agencies to be a method modification, and thus renders the assay unapproved/cleared. Such modifications will influence decisions regarding the analytical validation experiments that should be performed prior to clinical testing (as indicated below).

Another consideration is the matrix of the body fluid sample [CLSI EP14-A2]. The sample matrix refers to all the components of a sample except the analyte, including things like the amount of protein and lipid present, the relative abundance of water, sample viscosity, etc. The matrix of the body fluid sample being analyzed is important because of its influence on the measurement of the analyte and the result obtained. This "matrix effect" is caused by any variation in the composition of the biological sample being tested that differs from the matrix for which the method was designed. Many (but not all) commercially available methods are designed specifically for measuring analytes in serum or plasma. The use of such methods with body fluids that have a different matrix from serum or plasma may not produce equivalent measurements.

As is the case with any clinical test, an analytical validation of a method's performance with matrix appropriate samples is necessary prior to using that method to test patient specimens. The information presented here is not intended to be a comprehensive description of the components of an analytical validation as this information is readily available from other sources. Presented is a brief description of the experiments that should be considered when validating a method for use with a nonstandard body fluid.

Validation experiments to consider include those to determine precision, accuracy, analytical measuring range, analytical sensitivity, analytical specificity, and the determination of a reference interval. Which experiments to perform will be influenced by whether or not the method is approved/cleared by a regulatory body such as the FDA.

Precision experiments are required to determine the reproducibility of the method. Guidance is available for designing and performing precision experiments and for interpreting the data [CLSI EP05-A2]. Because the between-individual sample matrix of body fluids can be extremely variable, it is important to consider if the experiments will be performed on a single representative fluid or if several representative fluids will be utilized. While the former provides a simpler pathway to evaluating precision the latter will likely provide a more robust estimate of imprecision.

Accuracy experiments determine the ability of the method to produce a result that reflects the true quantity of the analyte. Matrix effects can have a substantial influence on method accuracy. One approach to determine accuracy is to perform recovery experiments. A known quantity of the analyte is added to the body fluid sample and percent recovery is calculated from the concentration of the measured analyte. It is important to keep the volume of the added analyte low relative to the volume of the body fluid sample (eg, <10%) in order to minimize altering the matrix of the body fluid. The percent recovery must be evaluated against acceptance criteria that meets the medical requirements of the test and can vary between analytes and type of body fluid.

The linearity of the method for a specific body fluid type should be determined in order to demonstrate the concentration range over which the analyte can be accurately measured. Linearity experiments can be performed by combining body fluid samples with both low and high concentrations of the specific analyte in different ratios in order to obtain several samples that bracket the intended analytical measuring range [CLSI EP06-A].

The analytical sensitivity of the method is often used to describe the lowest analyte concentration that can be measured. Evaluating the analytical sensitivity of a method is commonly done by repeated measurements on a sample containing a low quantity of the analyte [CLSI EP17-A2]. The coefficient of variation is calculated from the results and evaluated for acceptability. Note that for several analytes, determining analytical sensitivity may not be necessary if clinically relevant results are associated only with increased body fluid concentrations.

Analytical specificity experiments can help to identify possible interferences and their influence on measurement accuracy. Common sources of interference are bloody samples (hemolysis) and those with increased concentrations of bilirubin (icterus) or lipid (lipemia). Depending on their source, some body fluid samples may contain high concentrations of hyaluronic acid that can increase sample viscosity. The addition of hyaluronidase may be used to decrease viscosity and therefore potential interference from hyaluronidase should be investigated in those cases. Analytical specificity can be evaluated by measuring the analyte before and after addition of known quantities of a specific interfering substance to a body fluid sample that does not already contain the interferent [CLSI C56-A].

Establishing appropriate reference intervals is often challenging and nowhere is this more evident than with body fluid analysis, particularly for analytes measured in nonstandard body fluids. Body fluids are not normally obtained from healthy individuals so it is nearly impossible to identify a reference interval from this population. One alternative is to use a sufficient number of body fluid samples submitted for clinical testing and correlate the result with the clinical outcome. The goal of this effort is to establish a reference interval (or cutoff) from individuals who do not have the condition for which the body fluid analysis is indicated. In most cases, this is as close to a "healthy" population that one can come for body fluid analysis. Another option is to evaluate the scientific and medical literature for information that can provide insight into appropriate intervals or cutoffs. However, a major limitation of this approach is the lack of assay standardization or harmonization; therefore intervals or cutoffs identified in the literature are likely to be method specific and not easily transferred. In situations for which no reference interval can be established, it may be useful to recommend comparing the concentration of the analyte in a body fluid to its concentration in a serum or plasma sample obtained at the same time as the body fluid.

Proficiency testing (PT) is an important component of a quality management system and helps to ensure that test results are valid. While there are commercially available programs that offer body fluid PT for numerous analytes, formal PT programs are not available for all, particularly those used for analytes measured in nonstandard body fluids. In this situation, an alternative method of PT must be implemented. One way to perform alternate assessment is to send aliquots of body fluid samples to another laboratory. This approach provides useful information only when both laboratories utilize the same method for analysis. Alternatively, the split samples can be retested within the laboratory but a major limitation of this approach is its inability to evaluate accuracy.

Refer to each individual chapter for a discussion of commonly evaluated analytes specific to that body fluid type.

Microbiology

Microbiologic methods

Microbiologic testing of sterile body fluids is a crucial step in the interrogation of suspected infectious diseases. Historically, body fluids were primarily tested microbiologically using cultures and stains. The ongoing evolution of microbiology has led to not only improved culture and staining approaches, but also indirect detection modalities such as antigen detection (most commonly used in CSF and urine) and real time polymerase chain reaction (PCR) (useful in most, if not all body fluids).

Bacteriologic techniques

First considering the traditional culture and stain based approach to infectious disease, specimen collection and transport is paramount to achieve sensitive testing results. Microorganism viability is a major limiting factor of culture, and many of the infectious agents found in sterile body fluids are often fastidious by nature. Specimens should be collected in a sterile collection tube for immediate transport to the clinical microbiology laboratory or directly inoculated into blood culture bottles [ISBN 978-1555816780]. Alternatively, if available, the specimen should be collected in an anaerobic transport tube to maximize the recovery of aerobes, microaerophiles, and anaerobes [ISBN 978-1555816780]. Care should be taken when receiving other collection tubes in the laboratory for culture, as growth of many organisms can be inhibited by the use other media types (eg, *Neisseria gonorrhoeae* by sodium polyanethol sulfonate [SPS]) [ISBN 978-1555816780]. In many cases, recollection of the specimen is required for appropriate culture conditions to be achieved, or referral to a nonculture based method (eg, PCR) may be appropriate if an additional specimen cannot be collected. These specimens may still be of utility for primary staining purposes; however the results should carry a strongly worded interpretation that explains the potential limitations of the media type on the testing.

Gram stain

Primary Gram stains of body fluids can be performed from the raw specimen itself, or in the case of nonpurulent specimens and especially CSF, using a cytocentrifugation slide chamber [ISBN 978-1555816780]. The use of cytocentrifugation allows for improved sensitivity of the Gram stain, particularly when a low organism burden is suspected (eg, *Listeria monocytogenes* or *Streptococcus pneumoniae* in CSF specimens) [ISBN 978-1555816780, Perry 1995]. Another advantage to cytocentrifugation is that the sample volume required to prepare the stain is low, allowing for additional adjunct testing to be performed on volume limited specimens. Since interpretation of the Gram stain often is the most crucial first step in guiding empiric therapy in infectious processes, a sensitive method allows the lab to detect more true infections and visualize more organisms in which to accurately assign morphological identification.

Bacterial culture

The solid media used to recover bacteria in body fluid specimens has been largely unchanged over several decades, though the specimen preparation methods have evolved. In all circumstances, nonselective media are the most appropriate choice for primary, direct to plate culture of body fluids and for specimens that have been enriched from blood culture bottles (discussed below). The use of a nonselective media allows for the widest breadth of culture recovery of insulting organisms. Generally speaking, a sheep blood agar plate and/or a chocolate agar plate are inoculated and incubated to recover aerobic organisms [ISBN 978-1555816780]. For anaerobic culture, a blood based agar (such as Columbia blood and/or Brucella blood) is adequate to recover many cultureable anaerobic organisms [ISBN 978-1555816780]. Mixed aerobic/anaerobic polymicrobial infections are often encountered in body fluids, especially peritoneal fluid (associated with bowel perforations), and therefore both aerobic and anaerobic cultures should be set up to achieve the most accurate and informative culture results [Troidle 2006]. Importantly, the use of nonselective media in routine culture will also allow for the recovery of yeast such as *Candida* species.

Though traditionally body fluids were directly inoculated onto solid media, this has been largely supplanted in favor of specimen concentration before solid media inoculation or liquid enrichment in blood culture bottles. The College of American Pathologists (CAP) requires centrifugation of body fluids for cultures in all CAP accredited laboratories. This technique has dramatically increased the sensitivity over traditional direct from specimen inoculation to solid media [ISBN 978-1555816780]. Studies have also established increased sensitivity of culture by inoculating an aliquot of the primary specimen in a blood culture bottle and holding the specimen in an automated blood bottle incubator [PMID 10385010, PMID 21459855, PMID 3049220]. Continuous monitoring blood culture machines allow for these specimens to be incubated for extended periods of time (10-14 days or more) in order to recover slow growing fastidious organisms such as *Propionibacterium acnes*. These extended incubations would generally not be possible with solid media culture, as the agar will often dry out in the incubator. Many commercial blood culture bottles contain SPS, and therefore the manufacturer recommended minimum volume of blood should be substituted with sterile body fluid as this ensures that the SPS is diluted to noninhibitory concentrations [ISBN 978-1555815271]. If very small volumes of body fluids are received, inoculation of blood bottles is not appropriate and solid agar culture should be performed from the concentrate instead.

An attractive aspect of blood culture bottle enrichment is that these broths can often support the growth of many fastidious organisms and provides an enrichment of the organism for subsequent subculture to solid medium. If organisms that do not readily grow in liquid culture are suspected (eg, *Neisseria gonorrheae*), a chocolate agar plate should be inoculated from the original specimen concentrate, or if only blood culture bottles were received in the laboratory, a sample from the blood culture broth can be immediately inoculated onto chocolate agar when the specimen arrives in the laboratory [ISBN 978-1555815271]. If a blood culture bottle has visible growth by Gram stain or the automated blood culture incubator signals growth in the bottle, but the organism does not grow upon subculture to solid media, then direct sequencing of the bacterial 16S rRNA gene from the growth within the blood bottle media may be performed [PMID 11574575]. This procedure should only be performed in a laboratory that has thoroughly validated this methodology.

A significant limitation of the blood bottle inoculation is that the quantitative nature of a solid media culture is lost, and the clinician will need to interpret the culture results in the clinical context more judiciously. For example, an organism that could represent a skin flora contaminant (eg, coagulase negative *Staphylococcus*, *Propionibacterium acnes*) may result in only a single colony on solid media culture, whereas the liquid culture will quickly be overgrown with the organism, making its significance more challenging to interpret. Generally speaking however, if a sterile body fluid is properly collected and processed, the presence of any growth would be deemed significant.

Acid-fast bacilli & fungal culture

In addition to routine bacterial organisms in sterile body fluids, occasionally acid-fast bacilli (AFB; ie, *Mycobacterium* species) and fungi are primary pathogens of concern, and this is frequently site specific (eg, *Cryptococcus* species in CSF) and patient specific (eg, patients with a specific underlying immunodeficiencies are at higher risk of invasive fungal disease). Sterile body fluids submitted for AFB culture and stain should be collected in sterile, leakproof, laboratory approved containers without any fixatives or preservatives [ISBN 978-1555816780]. Specimens should be transported at 4°C in <24 hours, unless immediate inoculation (<1 hour) is possible, in which case specimens should be maintained at room temperature [ISBN 978-1555816780]. AFB specimens from nonsterile sites often require additional preparation vs routine bacteriology cultures in that specimens should be decontaminated to prevent bacterial overgrown on/in the AFB media. Sterile body fluids should not undergo decontamination before culturing to avoid an unnecessary loss in sensitivity [ISBN 978-1555815271, ISBN 978-1555816780]. The sensitivity of AFB culture and stain is increased when the primary specimen is concentrated, and stains and culture are prepared from the specimen concentrates rather than the raw fluid. CSF specimens containing very small numbers of mycobacteria and large volumes of fluid should be concentrated prior to inoculation [ISBN 978-1555815271, ISBN 978-1555816780].

There are multiple stains available for AFB, including the Kinyoun and Ziehl-Neelson stain, and auramine O stain. The former 2 stain mycolic acid and allow for bright field visualization of AFB, while the auramine O stain targets mycolic acid, but is detected by fluorescent microscopy. In terms of culture, there are many commercially available liquid and solid media for AFB. The media used is typically left to the individual laboratory; however the general consensus is that setup of AFB cultures to at least both solid and liquid media yields the best overall results since some organisms grow better in liquid, while others cannot grow in liquid media at all [ISBN 978-1555816780]. As the spectrum of clinically significant AFB continues to widen, additional culture conditions may need to be considered in specific clinical scenarios (eg, blood containing medium for *Mycobacterium haemophilum*).

Fungal infections are relatively uncommon in sterile body fluids. They can, however, occur, particularly in immunocompromised hosts such as transplant patients, HIV patients, and most recently in healthy patients receiving contaminated steroid injections that were directly injected into large joints and the CSF [PMID 23083312]. Direct staining of sterile fluids for fungal elements can be performed using KOH/calcofluor white (fluorescence readout). While this stain does not allow for immediate identification of the offending mold, the fluorescence output allows for easier detection than a color based stain. In certain cases, the morphology may allow a mold to be broadly classified as a zygomycete, yeast, or simply "other mold." Staining has limited sensitivity in most sterile fluids and should always be combined with culture based detection methods. If the specimen has limited volume, the stain should be omitted in favor of culture. Importantly, culture allows for ultimate identification of the mold based on morphology (classical growth morphology and microscopic stain), biochemical profile, 18S rRNA sequencing, and most recently matrix assisted laser desorption/ionization time of flight (MALDI-TOF) mass spectrometry [PMID 23573782]. Culture for fungi should include a rich, selective media for optimal recovery of pathogenic mold in order to reduce bacterial contamination (more important for nonsterile specimens) as well as a nonselective media to allow optimal, unimpeded growth of fungi [PMID 23083312]. The major limitation of fungal cultures is the common slow growth rate of molds and the need for sporulation to occur for accurate morphological identification. In some cases, the turnaround time can exceed the appropriate clinical window for proper antifungal therapy. The preliminary detection of a mold is therefore paramount in patient care, with specific identification allowing for tailored antifungal therapy and prognostic implications.

Additionally, antigen detection, DNA hybridization probes, or PCR may be included (particularly for dimorphic fungi such as *Coccidioides immitis*, *Histoplasma capsulatum*, and *Blastomyces dermatitidis*). These methods are further discussed in the context of the specific body fluid in each applicable chapter. Direct nucleic acid sequencing of sterile body fluids for mold is not currently recommended.

Immunophenotyping

Numerous techniques are available for immunophenotyping the cellular components of body fluids. The most commonly utilized are immunohistochemistry and flow cytometry (for hematopoietic cells). As often the evaluation of the cellular components in body fluids requires further investigation beyond cytologic examination, immunophenotyping can provide additional information about cellular origin and differentiation as well as the cellular constituents within the body fluid specimen.

Immunohistochemistry

Immunohistochemistry (IHC) is a method for identifying and localizing specific protein antigens in tissues or cells based on recognition of specific antigenic epitopes by antibodies. Detection of the antigen-antibody binding reaction can be used to characterize and visualize the protein in cells or tissues. Both polyclonal and monoclonal antibodies may be used, although monoclonal antibodies are considered more specific. Use of immunohistochemistry has several applications including tumor diagnosis (based on the identification of tumor specific proteins), providing prognostic information about a tumor, or identification of possible therapeutic targets. For body fluids, IHC can be carried out on either cytospin preparations of unfixed cells prepared directly from the body fluid (see above) or on fixed specimens (such as cell block preparations).

Initially immunohistochemical detection of the antigen-antibody binding was done using immunofluorescent probes requiring detection by a fluorescent microscope, but currently most IHC staining is colormetric allowing interpretation and detection by conventional microscopy. Procedural modifications have increased the detection sensitivity of antibody binding by use of multiple step detection techniques based on sequential enzymatic reactions, heat or enzymatic unmasking of antigenic epitopes or amplification methods to allow detection of low density antigens. These techniques have greatly improved the sensitivity of IHC in detecting specific proteins.

Most clinical IHC staining uses an indirect or sandwich procedure that utilizes sequential binding of antibodies to allow for amplification of the detection signal. In the indirect method, an unlabeled primary antibody that reacts directly with the cellular antigen of interest is first applied. Then a secondary antibody of high binding affinity and specificity that is directed against the species specific immunoglobulin of the primary antibody is reacted to the primary antibody. The detection conjugation moiety is attached to the secondary antibody, thereby enhancing binding specificity of the primary antibody by having the capacity for several of the detection molecules binding to the antigen of interest, and effectively amplifying the detection signal.

Antibody detection is usually by a peroxidase/antiperoxidase (PAP) detection method whereby an antibody directed against horseradish peroxidase will bind to the antigen and produce a small and very stable brown, blue or black colored complex that can be easily detected by light microscopy. In addition to the horseradish peroxidase PAP detection method, several other approaches have been used for detection of the antigen antibody complex that create a different colorimetric product or are useful in specific tissues or clinical settings. The biotin-avidin conjugation (ABC) method utilizes biotin that is chemically linked to the primary antibody to produce a biotinylated conjugate for antigen binding that will localize and concentrate biotin at the antibody target site. Avidin can then be conjugated to the horseradish peroxidase moiety, and avidin will bind to the biotinylated antibody. This will localize the peroxidase at the site of antigen binding and takes advantage of the high affinity of avidin and biotin binding to amplify the signal and reaction sensitivity. One drawback of the ABC approach occurs when the tissue/cellular elements contain significant amounts of endogenous biotin (such as in liver cells) that may increase nonspecific or false positive staining. Another approach to staining utilizes the alkaline phosphatase-antialkaline phosphatase detection (APAAP) method. This technique substitutes the PAP complex with an APAAP complex and is useful for staining of tissues or cells with high levels of endogenous peroxidase. The APAAP method gives rise to a bright red or blue color for detection and is particularly useful when there are high numbers of myeloid cells that have a high degree of endogenous peroxidase which may be difficult to completely block when using horseradish peroxidase approaches. In addition, this method can be used as a secondary staining procedure to allow double labeled immunohistochemical staining with tissue/cells already stained with another antibody using PAP complex. This allows identification of 2 separate targets in a single slide.

In order for the immunohistochemical methods outlined above to be successful, the antibody binding epitope of the antigen of interest must be available for binding. Initial studies with IHC were done on fresh tissues, but were limited by the poor preservation of histologic details allowing for localization of the antigen-antibody complex binding. Attempts to use IHC on fixed tissues/sections have found some variability in the avidity of antibody-antigen binding, probably reflecting that the protein conformation of the antigen of interest has been altered by fixation of the tissue or tissue processing. It is thought that formalin or formaldehyde fixation (as is commonly used for cell block preparations of body fluids) causes alterations in the tertiary and quaternary structures of a protein, although the primary and secondary structures remain intact. The longer that a tissue remains in a fixative, the more the protein structure is affected and the greater the impact on IHC staining due to impaired antigen-antibody affinity and binding. These changes in protein structure may lead to the inability of the antibody to detect and bind to the antigen. Therefore, many fixed tissues will require some sort of antigen retrieval (AR) process in an attempt to restore the tertiary structures of the antigenetic epitope to make it more accessible to antibody binding and IHC staining.

A variety of antigen retrieval techniques have been developed using either heat or enzymatic approaches. Heat methods involve using a pressure cooker, water bath or microwave to heat the buffer or water covering the slides containing the tissue sections. Usually the sections are heated between 90°C and 120°C in either distilled water or a buffered solution. Unmasking or restoration of the structure of the antigenic epitopes is influenced by such parameters as the heating temperature, heating time, as well as the pH of the antigen retrieval solution. Thus different approaches may need to be used for each individual antigenic epitope of interest and thus determined by the individual testing laboratory. Treatment of tissue sections with a variety of enzymes such as trypsin or neuraminidase will also enhance the staining of specific antigen epitopes. However, enzymes also tend to degrade normal cellular proteins and often adversely impact normal histologic or cytologic features. The heat induced AR techniques are now, by far, the most widely used as they are easily performed and have less tendency to distort morphologic features.

Immunohistochemistry has a variety of uses including identification of tumor or cellular origin as well as identification of prognostic markers, therapeutic targets and infectious agents. One of the major uses of IHC is determination of tumor histogenetic origin by identification of specific staining characteristics that help to characterize the cell of origin for a neoplasm. This is particularly helpful in poorly differentiated tumors where the type of tumor may not be identifiable by specific morphologic features and in fluids where morphologic features may be lost. Often a combination of morphologic and immunophenotypic findings is required to allow for a definitive diagnosis to be rendered. It is important that a battery of antibodies be used in making a diagnosis with IHC staining. Characterization of malignancies requires the ability to differentiate carcinomas from hematopoietic neoplasms or sarcomas. Usually this requires a panel of immunohistochemical stains that help to define the tissue of origin by identifying tumor specific antigens. The choice of specific antibodies will be dependent on the pathologist's initial morphologic impression and the differential diagnosis based on the clinical history and morphological features of the tumor. The pathologist will utilize a panel of antibodies specifically chosen to identify or exclude specific tumor types. For example, initially a screening panel may be used, such as a pancytokeratin to identify a carcinoma and CD45 to identify lymphoma

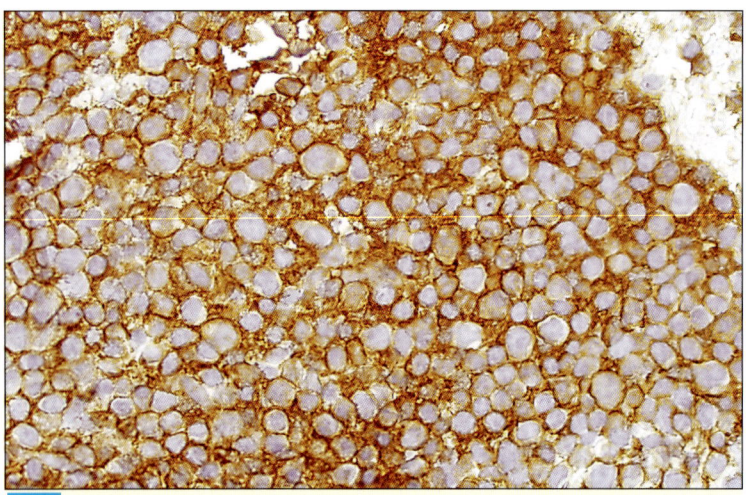

i2.18 CD20 immunohistochemical stain highlighting (brown color) the majority of the cells in this cell block section, containing a B cell lymphoma

or other hematopoietic neoplasms. Additional stains may then be added to further refine and narrow the diagnosis. Although it is beyond the scope of this chapter to discuss the workup of a wide variety of neoplasms, some of the currently available specific antibodies useful in identification of specific classes of tumors are presented in t2.13, t2.14, t2.15.

The use of immunohistochemical methods for determination of prognosis and choice of therapy is best established in breast carcinoma. IHC staining to demonstrate the presence of estrogen receptors (ER), progesterone receptors (PR) as well as overexpression of the human epidermal receptor protein 2 (HER2) impacts therapy, prognosis and helps our understanding of the biology of the disease.

Use of IHC to identify specific therapeutic targets is very useful for the treatment of non-Hodgkin lymphoma (NHL) and targeted therapies are also becoming more common in solid tumors. One of the first widely used targeted therapies was immunotherapy using monoclonal anti CD20 (rituximab) for treatment of many subtypes of CD20 positive mature B cell lymphomas i2.18. Other lymphoid targets, such as CD22 (epratuzimab), CD30 (SGN-30), CD40 (SGN-40), CD80 (galiximab) and CD52 (alemtuzumab) have also been exploited.

The identification of specific immune targets may provide alternative approaches to therapy that may be instituted clinically. For example, acute myeloid leukemias that express the CD33 antigen may be amenable to treatment with an anti CD33 targeted therapy as a second line approach or in patients that are unable to tolerate intensive chemotherapeutic approaches.

Another application of IHC is identification of infectious agents. Several antibodies have been developed that may be used to identify infectious agents including herpes viruses, cytomegalovirus, Epstein-Barr virus, some bacterial agents (such as *Helicobacter pylori*) and some fungi. This may provide a useful adjunct to cultures and other microbiologic techniques for identification of infectious agents in body fluids.

t2.13 Antibodies useful in hematolymphoid disorders

Antibodies	Reactivity
General hematolymphoid antibodies	
CD45 (LCA)	Hematolymphoid cells, but negative in Reed-Sternberg/Hodgkin cells
Hodgkin lymphoma	
CD30 (Ki1)	Reed-Sternberg/Hodgkin cells
CD15 (LeuM1)	Reed-Sternberg cells
CD20	Some Reed-Sternberg cells
Non-Hodgkin lymphoma B cell	
CD20	Mature B cell antigen
CD79a	Pan B cell antigen (including blasts and plasma cells)
CD19	B cell antigen positive in B lymphoblasts & mature B cells
PAX-5	Nuclear B cell antigen in most B cells
κ/λ light chains	Mature B cells and plasma cells
Non-Hodgkin lymphoma T cell	
CD2	Pan T cell marker
CD3	Pan T cell marker
CD4	T helper cell marker
CD5	Pan T cell marker
CD7	Pan T cell marker
CD8	T suppressor cell marker
CD45RO	Pan T cell marker
CD43	Pan T cell marker, relatively nonspecific as also seen in several other hematopoietic malignancies
Other antibodies useful in non-Hodgkin lymphoma	
ALK	Fusion protein seen in some anaplastic large cell lymphomas
Cyclin D1	Fusion protein seen in mantle cell lymphomas, some plasma cell neoplasms
Bcl2	Overexpression seen in follicular lymphoma
CD1a	T lymphoblasts & Langerhans cells
CD10 (CALLA)	Germinal center lymphocytes & lymphoblasts
CD30	Activation marker seen in some lymphomas, characteristic in anaplastic large cell lymphoma & Hodgkin lymphoma
CD56/CD57	NK cells
TIA1	NK cells and cytotoxic T lymphocytes
Perforin/granzyme B	Cytotoxic T cells
Terminal deoxynucleotidyl transferase (TdT)	DNA polymerase seen in blasts, in particular lymphoid blasts
Epstein-Barr virus latent membrane protein (EBV-LMP)	Viral protein marking EBV infection useful in diagnosis of T/NK neoplasms and immunosuppression related lymphomas
Myeloid/monocytic neoplasms	
CD34	Blast marker useful in acute myeloid & lymphoid leukemias
CD117 (c-kit)	Myeloid marker seen in myeloid malignancies & other immature myeloid cells
CD15	Myelomonocytic cells
CD33	Myelomonocytic cells
CD68	Monocytic cells, histiocytes
Lysozyme	Myeloid cells
Plasma cells	
CD138	Plasma cells
CD79a	Pan B cell marker including B lymphoblasts & plasma cells
κ/λ light chains	Identifies clonality in plasma cells
Erythroid	
Glycophorin	Erythroid cells
Hemoglobin A	Erythroid cells

t2.14 Antibodies useful in the workup of nonhematolymphoid neoplasms

Antibodies	Reactivity
Breast tumors	
Calponin	Reactive in myoepithelial cells, used to evaluate stromal invasion
P63	Specific nuclear staining for myoepithelial cells used to evaluate stromal invasion in breast carcinoma
E-cadherin	Transmembrane protein essential for cell to cell adhesion, may be useful to differentiate ductal from lobular carcinomas of the breast
Gross cystic disease fluid protein 15 (GCDFP15)	Found in breast, salivary gland, apocrine glands and Paget disease of skin, vulva & prostate
Estrogen receptor (ER) Progesterone receptor (PR)	Positive in normal breast tissue and infers response to hormonal therapy if expressed by breast carcinomas
Gastrointestinal tumors	
CD117	Positive in gastrointestinal stromal tumors, mast cells, hematopoietic blasts
HepPar1	Positive in hepatocytes and hepatocellular carcinoma
Synaptophysin	Positive in a variety of neuroendocrine tumors
Chromogranin A	Positive in a variety of neuroendocrine tumors
Helicobacter pylori	Identifies *H pylori* organisms, strongly associated with lymphoid hyperplasia, gastric lymphoma and gastric adenocarcinoma
Skin tumors	
S100	Positive in melanoma, neural tumors, Langerhans cells and some histiocytic proliferations
HMB45 Melan A	Positive in melanocytes, nevi and melanomas
Other tumors	
p16	Positive in neoplasms associated with human papillomavirus such as invasive squamous carcinoma of the cervix, squamous intraepithelial lesions and cervical adenocarcinoma
Ki67	Indicates proliferation index, correlates with tumor grade and could be used as predictor of recurrence in urothelial carcinoma
CD10	Positive in endometrial stromal tumors
CA125	Positive in normal endometrium, primary nonmucinous epithelial ovarian cancers
CD99	Positive in round blue cell tumors including peripheral sheath tumors, Ewing sarcoma, and sex cord tumors
Wilms tumor 1 (WT1)	Tumor suppressor function, positive in Wilms tumor, desmoplastic small round cell tumor, mesothelioma, ovarian surface epithelium, serous carcinoma of the ovary
Human chorionic gonadotropin (hCG)	Positive in choriocarcinoma and some dysgerminomas
Human placental lactogen (hPL)	Positive in choriocarcinoma and variants of trophoblastic tumor
Vimentin	Not considered to be cell type specific but can be useful as control marker
Desmin	Positive in striated muscle and rhabdomyosarcoma
CD34	Positive in hematopoietic progenitor cells, vascular tumors including angiosarcoma and hemangioendothelioma, dermatofibrosarcoma protuberans, spindle cell lipoma and solitary fibrous tumor
CD31	Positive in vascular endothelial lining cells and tumors including angiosarcoma, and hemangioma
CD68	Positive in fibrohistiocytic lesions
GFAP	Positive in gliosis, gliomas; CNS parenchyma

t2.14 Antibodies useful in the workup of nonhematolymphoid neoplasms (continued)

Metastatic carcinoma of unknown primary	
CK7, CK20	Cytokeratins commonly used in the differential diagnosis of carcinomas
Thyroglobulin	Positive in thyroid carcinomas
Placental alkaline phosphatase (PLAP)	A marker of malignant germ cell tumors, especially dysgerminoma and embryonal carcinoma
α fetoprotein (AFP)	Positive in yolk sac tumor and hepatocellular carcinoma
Thyroid transcription factor 1 (TTF1)	Positive in thyroid, thyroid tumors and lung carcinomas
Villin	Positive in the brush border of the intestine and the proximal renal tubular epithelium
CDX2	Highly sensitive and specific for intestinal differentiation, can be seen in some ovarian, urinary bladder and endometrioid carcinomas
Prostate specific antigen (PSA)	Positive in prostatic adenocarcinoma
Renal cell carcinoma antigen	Positive in primary renal carcinomas
Calretinin	Positive in mesothelioma
HHV8	Associated with Kaposi sarcoma, primary effusion lymphoma, and multicentric Castleman disease

t2.15 Keratin stains that may help identify tissue of origin in tumor cells

Keratin antigen	Antibody clone	Molecular weight (kD)	Tissue expression
CK7	OV-TL 12/30	54	Lung carcinoma (small and non-small cell types) Breast Transitional cell carcinoma Endometrial carcinoma Mesothelioma
CK20	K20	46	Most gastrointestinal carcinomas Ovarian mucinous carcinoma Biliary carcinoma Transitional cell carcinoma Merkel cell carcinoma
Cocktails of keratin peptides			
Pancytokeratin	AE1/AE3		Carcinomas of simple and complex epithelium
CK8	CAM 5.2		All carcinomas of simple (nonstratified) epithelium, ductal and pseudostratified epithelium

Flow cytometry

Immunophenotyping by flow cytometry is typically utilized to evaluate cells of hematopoietic origin. This technique requires evaluation of single cells suspended in fluid media and is therefore optimal for the analysis of hematopoietic cells. A stream of single file cells is produced from cellular suspensions by hydrodynamic differential pressures creating a laminar flow configuration f2.4. During analysis, individual cells pass through a light source (laser beam with a specific wavelength) and various cellular parameters are measured simultaneously. These include cell size (forward light scatter), nuclear and cytoplasmic complexity (side light scatter) and most importantly the presence of surface and/or cytoplasmic antigens (through fluorochrome conjugated antibody light emission) f2.5. Fluorochrome conjugated antibodies bind with specific

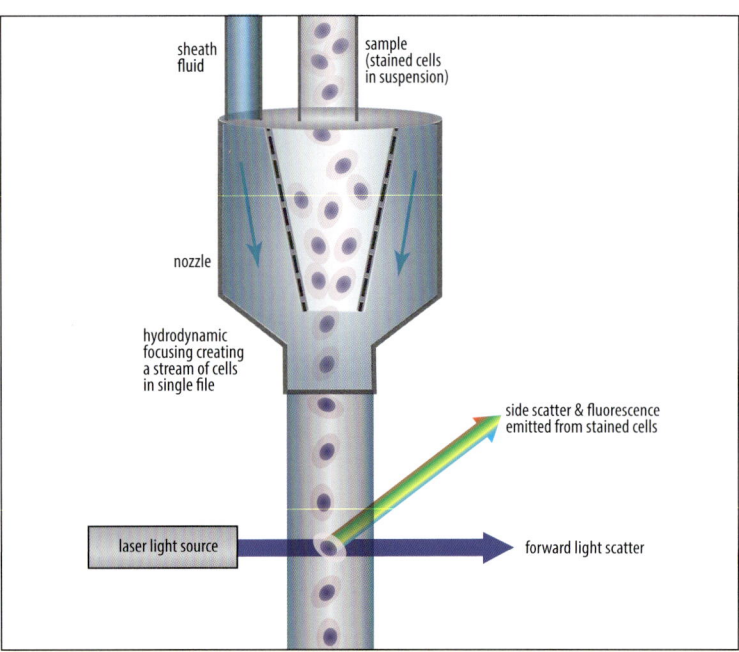

f2.4 Schematic of cellular flow through the flow cytometer

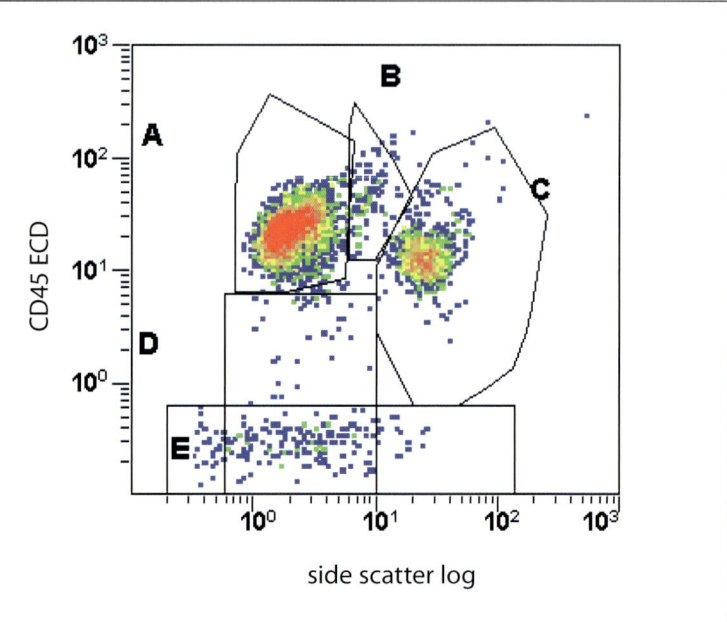

f2.6 CD45 vs side scatter flow cytometry histogram; common gating strategy to separate and identify cellular populations (**a** lymphocytes, **b** monocytes, **c** granulocytes, **d** blasts, **e** cellular debris).

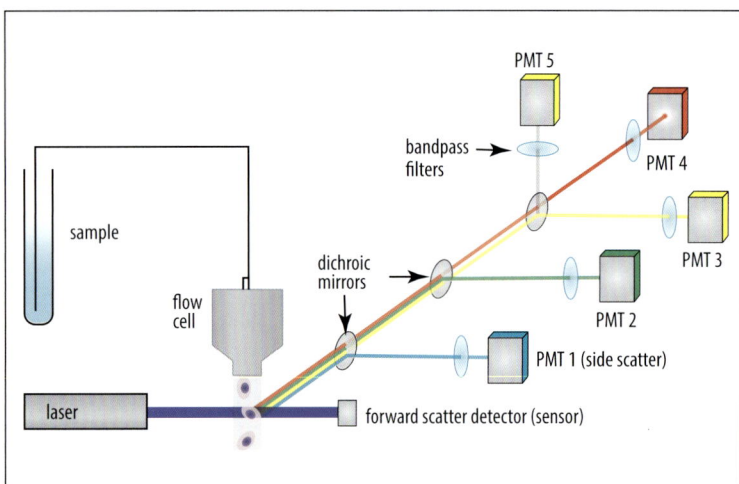

f2.5 Schematic diagram of a flow cytometer; as fluorochrome labeled cells pass through the light source (laser beam), emitted light is directed to photomultiplier tubes (PMTs) by mirrors and filters for detection and processing

cellular antigens upon incubation with the cells of interests. Unbound antibody is rinsed away and the individual cells are evaluated as they pass single file through a beam of light (laser). Cells that have bound fluorochrome conjugated antibodies emit wavelengths of light as they pass through and absorb incident light from the laser. The emitted light from the fluorochrome is detected by both photomultiplier tubes and photodiodes, after it passes through a series of lens, filters and mirrors. The detected light signals are converted into digital signals, processed by computer software, and displayed in dotplots or histograms for analysis **f2.6**. Individual fluorochromes and fluorochrome conjugates have unique light emission spectra (and color), which allows detection of unique patterns of antigen expression based upon which fluorochrome conjugated antibodies bind to the cell and are excited as the cell passes through the laser beam **t2.16**. While it is common to evaluate 5-6 antigens (fluorochrome conjugated antibody-antigen complexes) simultaneously on each cell, some commercially available flow cytometers have multiple lasers with different emitting wavelengths that can evaluate up to 10-12 fluorochrome conjugated antibodies simultaneously. Based upon the excited fluorochrome conjugated antibodies that attach to the individual cells (leukocytes), the characteristics of the leukocytes in the body fluid can be determined by evaluating a series of histograms generated by the analysis. In addition, normal and abnormal antigen expression patterns, including the presence of mature or immature hematopoietic cell populations, can be identified. One of the most useful aspects of flow cytometry is evaluation of B cell populations for aberrant expression (such as CD5 or CD10) as well as identification of monotypic or monoclonal B cell populations. Clonal B cell populations typically express a predominance of either κ or λ light chains or do not express surface light chains at all. This is in contrast to normal B cell populations, which typically have κ:λ ratios ranging from 0.8:1 to 4.0:1. **t2.17** lists common antigens that can be evaluated by flow cytometry. In addition, **f2.7** shows a series of histograms in which a monotypic CD5+ B cell population was identified.

Flow cytometry is an ancillary technique ideal for evaluating hematopoietic cells in body fluids. As it requires a single cell suspension for analysis, body fluids must be anticoagulated with EDTA, sodium heparin or ACD if they are contaminated with blood that may cause clotting. In addition, the volume of specimen that is required for the analysis can vary greatly. In cellular body fluid specimens, 1-3 mL of fluid is adequate in most cases. In paucicellular specimens, as is common in cerebrospinal fluid, larger sample volumes may be required or evaluation of only a limited/targeted panel of antigens may be necessary.

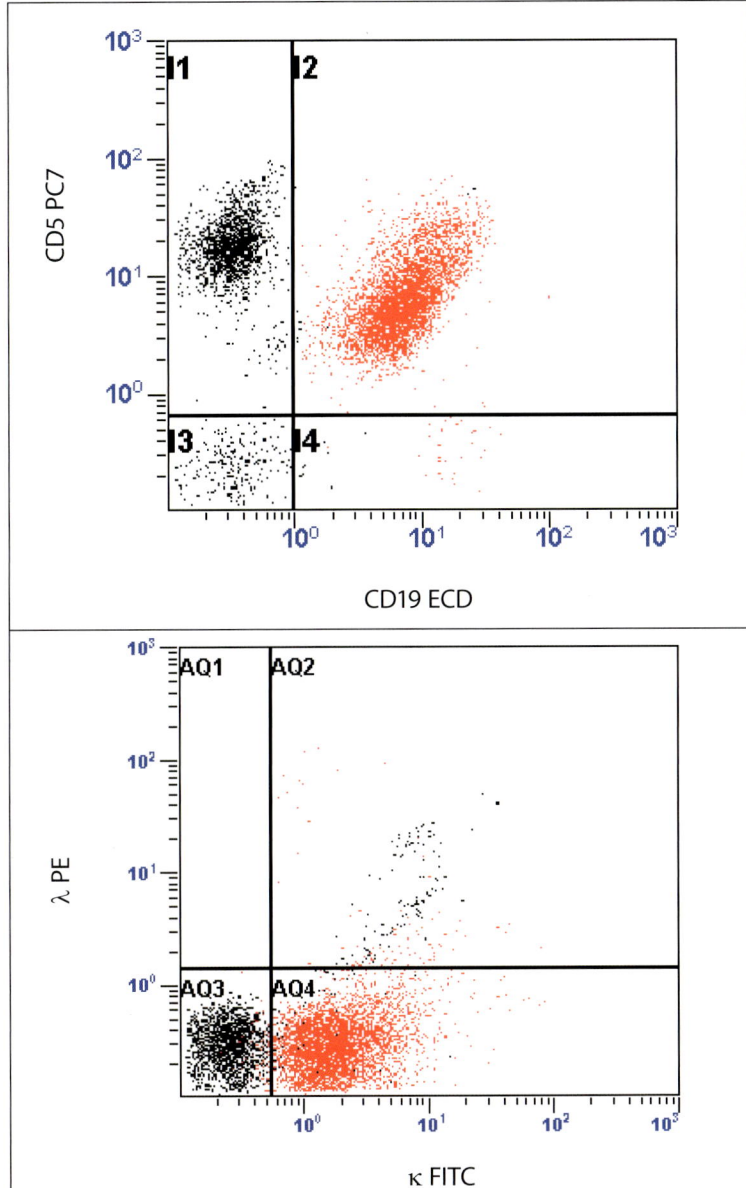

f2.7 **a** CD19 vs CD5 flow cytometry histogram. The CD19 positive B cell population (highlighted in orange) coexpresses CD5. The CD5+ CD19– events (highlighted in black) represent T cells. **b** κ vs λ flow cytometry histogram. The CD19/CD5 coexpressing population from **a** shows κ monotypia (highlighted in orange)

t2.16 Approximate excitation & emission wavelengths & color of fluorochromes

Fluorochrome	Excitation wavelength (nm)	Emission wavelength (nm)	Color
Fluorescein isothiocynate (FITC)	488	520	Green
Phycoerythrin (PE)	488	575	Orange
PE-Texas red (ECD)	488	613	Red-orange
PE-cyanin 5.1 (PC5)	488	667	Red
PE-cyanin 7 (PC7)	488	780	Far red
Texas red	600	615	Red
Allophycocyanin	600	655	Red
Cyanin 5	633	670	Red

t2.17 Common antigens evaluated by flow cytometry

Antibodies	Reactivity
CD45 (LCA)	Expressed by hematopoietic cells, often used in combination with side scatter as a gating strategy to separate populations of hematopoietic cells of different lineages
Lymphoid markers	
CD2	Pan T cell, NK cell marker
CD3	Pan T cell marker
CD4	T helper cell marker, also expressed by monocytes
CD5	Pan T cell marker
CD7	Pan T cell, NK cell marker
CD8	T suppressor cell marker
CD10 (CALLA)	Germinal center lymphocytes, follicular lymphoma, Burkitt lymphoma, some large B cell lymphomas, B lymphoblasts, hematogones
CD19	Pan B cell marker including B lymphoblasts
CD20	Mature B cell marker
CD22	Pan B cell marker
CD30	Seen in some lymphomas, including anaplastic large cell lymphoma
CD38	Prognostic marker in chronic lymphocytic leukemia, also expressed by plasma cells
CD56/CD57	NK cells, CD56 also expressed by some neoplastic plasma cells
CD103	Hairy cell leukemia
αβ/γδ	T cell receptors, expressed by subsets of T cells
κ/λ	Expressed by mature B cells and plasma cells, useful to assess clonality
Terminal deoxynucleotidyl transferase (TdT)	Lymphoid blasts, occasionally myeloid blasts
Myelomonocytic markers	
CD13	Myeloid and monocytic marker
CD15	Myeloid and monocytic marker
CD33	Myeloid and monocytic marker
CD34	Blast marker, including both myeloid and lymphoid blasts
CD117	Immature myeloid marker, mast cells
Myeloperoxidase	Marker of myeloid origin
Plasma cell markers	
CD38	Plasma cells
CD138	Plasma cells
κ/λ light chains	Expressed by mature B cells and plasma cells, useful to assess clonality
Erythroid markers	
Glycophorin	Erythroid cells
Megakaryocytic markers	
CD42	Megakaryocytic differentiation
CD61	Megakaryocytic differentiation

Molecular testing

Molecular testing has become an important ancillary methodology to evaluate a wide variety of medical conditions, and, in some instances, has become the preferred method of testing.

Infectious disease testing, in particular, has benefited tremendously by this advancement, particularly for difficult to culture or nonculturable pathogens (eg, Epstein-Barr virus, JC virus). Molecular testing has also facilitated the diagnosis and characterization of numerous hematopoietic disorders.

In general, molecular testing can be broken down into 3 general applications: hybridization/probe based signal amplification, direct nucleic acid amplification, and nucleic acid sequencing.

Direct detection of target nucleic acids by nucleic acid probe based hybridization is a relatively simple method that can be performed with rapid turnaround time. A common example is in situ hybridization, in which a complementary nucleic acid probe is hybridized to a specific target sequence present in the tissue sample on a glass slide. Signal detection can be obtained by radioisotopic or colorimetic methods. Such testing can also be performed on cytospin preparations that allows for the use of this technique for body fluid evaluation. These assays are relatively free from laboratory contamination issues and can often be performed on specimens that may otherwise be inhibitory to target amplification methods. In addition, it allows direct visualization (localization) of the target sequence in tissue sections. Examples of in situ hybridization studies include detection of Epstein-Barr virus or human papillomavirus.

Molecular amplification of nucleic acids can be achieved by multiple technologies including traditional polymerase chain reaction (PCR) of variable sized nucleic acid sequences and real time PCR by fluorescent DNA binding dyes or molecular probe based amplification. Alternatively, for RNA targets, reverse transcription (RT) can be incorporated into the reaction to allow for transcription of target RNA into cDNA, which can then be amplified and detected in subsequent reactions. Traditional PCR requires 2 DNA oligonucleotides that are complementary to a target nucleic acid sequence. These oligonucleotides are used to amplify a specific sequence of target DNA and the resultant end products are qualitatively analyzed by electrophoresis through an agarose gel. Real time PCR uses fluorescence detection (either fluorescent intercalating dyes or probes) to detect the amplified target in "real time" as the reactions are occurring. Real time PCR targets are typically much shorter DNA sequences than conventional PCR assays, with probe based assays offering generally the shortest target sequences. Short sequences can be amplified using probes since the sequences of the 2 primers plus the probe provide increased overall target specificity. The short size of the targets allows for more rapid cycling time and in many cases, easier quantitation of the target nucleic acid. In the case of infections of sterile body fluids, the presence of a target nucleic acid sequence indicates an infection by the offending organism of interest. The specificity and sensitivity of molecular methods is entirely dependent on the design of the nucleic acid primers and in the case of some real time PCR methods, the probe sequence. For this reason, most PCR testing has been achieved by laboratory developed tests; however FDA cleared tests have been developed on several commercially available thermocyclers, and several companies are now selling FDA cleared systems that require little to no end user proficiency in molecular biology. Examples of PCR based tests used in the clinical setting, would also include the detection of B cell or T cell gene rearrangements in the evaluation of lymphomas. More recently, numerous PCR testing platforms have become available for use and specific platforms aimed at CSF testing are in development.

Direct target sequencing allows for specific DNA sequences to be amplified and analyzed 1 nucleic acid at a time (eg, Sanger sequencing). This can be performed directly from a clinical specimen to look for specific mutations associated with a given condition. In hematologic malignancies, an example would be evaluation for *JAK2* exon 12 mutation. In the case of infectious disease testing, a cultured organism's DNA can be sequenced to obtain accurate identification. Such sequencing of specific genes has expanded the list of pathogens identified in culture for routine bacteria, AFB, and fungi as well. In fact, many isolates/identifications previously described by traditional culture and biochemical analysis have proven to be inaccurate when compared to sequence analysis.

Among the newest iterations of sequencing, is so called "next generation sequencing," or NGS. NGS is high throughput sequencing that allows the sequencing of RNA or DNA more quickly than previous methods such as Sanger sequencing. Numerous commercially available NGS technologies are currently available. These instruments have revolutionized the field of nuclei acid sequencing with the ease and speed of determining DNA sequences. The challenge, however, remains how to analyze, evaluate and interpret such large volumes of information that now are becoming readily produced. An additional barrier to implementation in fields such as infectious disease testing is the very long turnaround time to clinically actionable results that is reflected by the immense bioinformatics component of this analysis.

Cytogenetics

Although cytogenetics has a limited role in the evaluation of most body fluids, the basic concepts and utility are presented below. The processing of samples is similar regardless of specimen type. Cytogenetic analysis requires living cells that are either (1) induced to divide in culture, allowing metaphase cells to be collected for chromosome analysis, or (2) used for fluorescence in situ hybridization (FISH) analysis on uncultured interphase cells.

Body fluid specimen types & transportation of samples

Body fluid sample types processed by the cytogenetics laboratory for constitutional studies may include amniotic fluid cells (amniocytes) and cells from cystic hygroma fluid, fetal pleural effusion fluid, and fetal urine. Cells from pleural effusions, and more rarely CSF samples, may be used for lymphoma/leukemia studies.

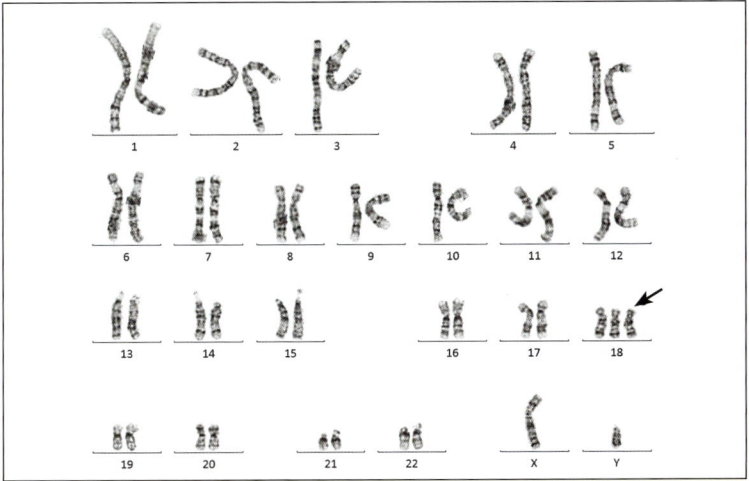

i2.19 Karyogram with trisomy 18 from amniocytes

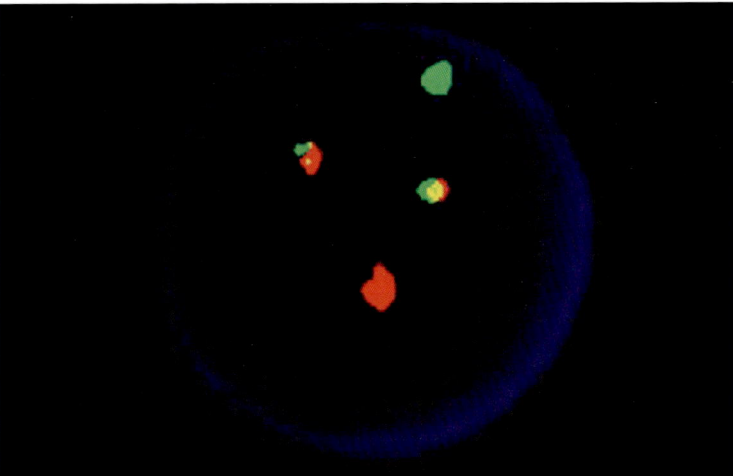

i2.20 FISH analysis: MYC break apart probe at 8q24 (Abbott Molecular). The red is proximal (centromeric) & the green is distal (telomeric) to the *MYC* gene. The separation of the colors occurs due to a translocation of *MYC* with an unidentified partner.

Amniotic fluid (AF) should be transported to the testing laboratory in sterile tubes (15 mL screw top) with minimal delay at room (ambient) temperature, avoiding extremes in temperature, especially increased temperatures (see additional comments in Chapter 3). Cystic hygroma fluid, fetal urine, fetal pleural effusion fluid, and cerebrospinal fluid should also be handled and transported in a similar manner.

Specimen processing

Body fluid specimens are centrifuged to collect all cells. For cystic hygroma and fetal pleural effusion fluids, both phytohemagglutinin (PHA) stimulated suspension cultures for any white cells present and attachment cultures for any fibroblasts or other cell types are established for constitutional studies. For amniotic fluid and fetal urine samples, cells are only set up as attachment cultures. Uncultured cells from any of these fluids may be used for interphase FISH analysis. As total cell numbers may be low, a combination of conventional cytogenetics and FISH provides the greatest diagnostic yield on cystic hygroma and fetal urine fluids. [PMID 11641692, PMID 12509716].

Cell culture of amniotic fluid cells requires specialized supplemented tissue culture medium to support optimal growth of amniocytes. Cells are placed on a coverslip in a small culture dish and allowed to attach and grow. Cells from cystic hygromas, fetal pleural effusions, and fetal urine are generally cultured in the same supplemented medium used for amniocytes.

For lymphoma/leukemia studies, cells from pleural effusion and cerebrospinal fluid samples may be used. For cancer studies, different types of culture media with different growth factors are used in an attempt to favor the growth of abnormal clones based on the disease type—lymphoid or myeloid—and based on the specific disease. The cytogenetics laboratory usually performs a cell count and inoculates cultures with a specific number of cells. Growth in culture is usually for different lengths of time, such as 24, 48, and/or 72 hours. Due to the lower cellularity of CSF samples, performing only FISH on uncultured cells instead of attempting to grow more cells in culture may yield results in a higher percentage of samples.

Harvesting of metaphase cells, slide preparation, and chromosome & FISH analysis

Collecting cells in metaphase involves adding colcemid to the culture medium to disrupt the mitotic spindle and prevents the cells from progressing beyond metaphase. Metaphase cells are then treated with a hypotonic salt solution (KCl) to cause the cell to swell, moving the chromosomes apart. The cells are then fixed with Carnoy fixative (3:1 methanol:acetic acid).

The fixed cell pellet can then be placed on slides, and with the appropriate humidity and drying rate, well spread metaphase chromosome preparations are obtained. After additional drying in an oven, the chromosome slides are treated with trypsin and stained (Wright stain; Giemsa stain), allowing the banded chromosomes to be visualized (usually referred to as G banded preparations).

Chromosomes in metaphase spreads are then counted and analyzed either through the microscope or on computer screens of captured images. Automated systems can scan and capture images at high resolution, eliminating the task of manual scanning, counting, and analysis through the microscope. Karyograms are prepared electronically by cutting or separating the individual chromosomes and arranging these in pairs (1-22 and the sex chromosomes, X and Y, i2.19. Analysis involves a band by band assessment of each chromosome pair as compared to an idealized representation of each chromosome (ideogram) at the 400, 450, or 550 or greater band levels [ISBN 978-3318022537].

The banding level for chromosomes derived from leukemia/lymphoma samples tends to be in the 350-400 band range. Due to the lower banding level and, in general, poorer quality of the chromosome preparations, many rearrangements may be difficult to detect, requiring FISH for diagnosis. Chromosomes from amniocytes and other fluids may be in the 400-450 range (this is contrasted with most constitutional studies on PHA stimulated blood chromosomes that are usually at the 550 band level).

FISH is also useful for the detection of clonal abnormalities present in the interphase cells from cancer samples that may be difficult to stimulate to divide in culture and be available for metaphase chromosome analysis i2.20. FISH probes are limited to providing information about very specific regions or translocations (1 or a few loci if several FISH probes are used), so a combination of metaphase chromosome and interphase FISH analysis are often used to detect and monitor clonal abnormalities.

For constitutional samples, FISH is often performed on metaphase cells when a specific syndrome is suspected, for example, DiGeorge syndrome/velo-cardio-facial syndrome associated with a 22q11.21 deletion. This may be performed on any of the sample types listed above. FISH for rapid aneuploidy screening for chromosomes 21, 18, 13, X and Y may be performed on interphase cells from amniotic fluid, cystic hygroma, fetal pleural effusion, and fetal urine samples.

Specific details regarding the requirements for the number of cells counted and analyzed for each sample type for chromosome and FISH analysis are specified by the College of American Pathologists (CAP) Cytogenetics checklist and by American College of Medical Genetics and Genomics (ACMG) Standards and Guidelines for Clinical Genetics Laboratories—Clinical Cytogenetics.

Chromosomal microarray analysis (CMA) is used to both complement and, more recently, replace conventional chromosome analysis for some sample types. CMA is performed on the same specimens as discussed above and uses DNA isolated from uncultured and/or cultured cells. Specimen requirements and transport are the same as for chromosome testing.

Reporting of results

Many laboratories attempt to have 2-3 different cytogenetic technologists review the chromosomes before the final review by a certified doctoral level cytogeneticist. Following completion of the analysis by cytogenetic technologists, a review is performed by a more experienced senior level technologist who also analyzes the karyotype and prepares the report. The case is then submitted to a doctoral level cytogeneticist for final analysis, review, and result reporting.

Artifacts & pitfalls

- Thick and poorly stained cytospin preparations can lead to misinterpretation and difficulty in distinguishing between benign & malignant cellular components
- Inappropriate use of collection vessels and anticoagulants may lead to false negative microbiology studies
- Dust particles, talc, fibers and other artifacts can be misinterpreted as crystals in synovial fluids

Key points

- Evaluation of body fluid samples often includes gross examination, cell count, differential count, chemical analysis, microbiologic testing and microscopic examination
- Collection method, specimen handling, collection vessel, and transport time & temperature are preanalytic variables that influence sample testing and accurate testing results
- Synovial fluid crystal analysis often requires bright field microscopy as well as polarized & compensated light microscopy
- Cell block preparations of body fluids can be used for histologic sections & immunohistochemical studies
- Flow cytometry is a useful ancillary testing technique for immunophenotyping hematopoietic cells

References

PMID 10385010 Ferrer A, Osset J, Alegre J, et al [1999] Prospective clinical and microbiologic study of pleural effusions. *Eur J Clin Microbiol Infect Dis* 18(4):237-41

PMID 10705825 Narayanan S. The preanalytic phase. An important component of laboratory medicine. *Am J Clin Pathol*. 2000 Mar;113(3):429-52

PMID 10973869 Froom P, Bieganiec B, Ehrenrich Z et al [2000] Stability of common analytes in urine refrigerated for 24 h before automated analysis by test strips. *Clin Chem* 46(9):1384-6

PMID 11574575 Qian Q, Tang YW, Kolbert CP et al [2001] Direct identification of bacteria from positive blood cultures by amplification and sequencing of the 16S rRNA gene: evaluation of BACTEC 9240 instrument true-positive and false-positive results *J Clin Microbiol* 39(10):3578-82

PMID 11641692 Donnenfeld AE, Lockwood D, Lamb AN [2001] Prenatal diagnosis from cystic hygroma fluid: the value of fluorescence in situ hybridization. *Am J Obstet Gynecol* 185(4):1004-8

PMID 11959769 Galvez J, Saiz E, Linares LF et al [2002] Delayed examination of synovial fluid by ordinary and polarized light microscopy to detect and identify crystals. *Ann Rheum Dis* 61(5):444-7

PMID 12509716 Donnenfeld AE, Lockwood D, Custer T et al [2002] Prenatal diagnosis from fetal urine in bladder outlet obstruction: success rates for traditional cytogenetic evaluation and interphase fluorescence in situ hybridization. *Genet Med* 4(6):444-7

PMID 14649464 Aulesa C, Mainar I, Prieto M et al [2003] Use of the Advia 120 hematology analyzer in the differential cytologic analysis of biological fluids (cerebrospinal, peritoneal, pleural, pericardial, synovial, and others). *Lab Hematol* 9(4):214-4

PMID 15117440 Sodi R, Darn SM, Stott A [2004] Pneumatic tube system induced haemolysis: assessing sample type susceptibility to haemolysis. *Ann Clin Biochem* 41(Pt3):237-40

PMID 16025090 Sugiuchi H, Ando Y, Manabe M et al [2005] Measurement of total and differential white blood cell counts in synovial fluid by means of an automated hematology analyzer. *J Lab Clin Med* 146(1):36-42

PMID 16604559 Das K [2006] Serous effusions in malignant lymphomas: a review. *Diag Cytopathol* 34(5):335-47

PMID 17053464 Dziegiel M, Nielsen L, Berkowicz A [2006] Detecting fetomaternal hemorrhage by flow cytometry. *Curr Opin Hematol* 13(6):490-5

PMID 17878734 Savithrisowmya S, Singh M, Kriplani A et al [2008] Assessment of fetomaternal hemorrhage by flow cytometry and Kleihauer-Betke test in Rh-negative pregnancies. *Gynecol Obstet Invest* 65(2):84-8

PMID 17896254 Khazardoost S, Hantoushzadeh S, Khooshideh M et al [2007] Risk factors for meconium aspiration in meconium stained amniotic fluid. *J Obstet Gynaecol* 27(6):577-9

PMID 19095566 Glasser L, Murphy CA, Machan JT [2009] The clinical reliability of automated cerebrospinal fluid cell counts on the Beckman-Coulter LH750 and Iris iQ200. *Am J Clin Pathol* 131:58-63

PMID 19228639 Walker RJ, Nelson LD, Dunphy BW et al [2009] Comparative evaluation of the Iris iQ200 body fluid module with manual hemacytometer count. *Am J Clin Pathol* 131(3):333-8

PMID 20236183 Paris A, Nhan T, Cornet E et al [2010] Performance evaluation of the body fluid mode on the platform Sysmex XE-5000 series automated hematology analyzer. *Int J Lab Hematol* 32(5):539-47

PMID 21459855 Menzies SM, Rahman NM, Wrightson JM, et al [2011] Blood culture bottle culture of pleural fluid in pleural infection. *Thorax* 66(8):658-62

PMID 21836038 Goubard A, Marzouk M, Canoui-Poitrine F et al [2011] Performance of the Iris iQ200 Elite analyser in the cell counting of serous effusion fluids and cerebrospinal drainage fluids. *J Clin Pathol* 64:1123-27

PMID 21998343 Rosenling T, Stoop MP, Smolinska A et al [2011] The impact of delayed storage on the measured proteome and metabolome of human cerebrospinal fluid. *Clin Chem* 57(12):1703-11

PMID 22231030 Kim Y, Makar R [2012] Detection of fetomaternal hemorrhage. *Am J Hematol* 87(4):417-23

PMID 22467320 Evliyaoglu O, Toprak G, Tekin A et al [2012] Effect of pneumatic tube delivery system rate and distance on hemolysis of blood specimens. *J Clin Lab Anal* 26(2):66-9

PMID 22955210 Jayadev C, Rout R, Price A et al [2012] Hyaluronidase treatment of synovial fluid to improve assay precision for biomarker research using multiplex immunoassay platforms. *J Immunol Methods* 386(1-2):22-30

PMID 23083312 Kauffman CA, Pappas PG, Patterson TF [2013] Fungal infections associated with contaminated methylprednisolone injections. *N Engl J Med* 368(26):2495-500

PMID 23396954 Almolla J, Balconi G [2011] Interventional ultrasonography of the chest: Techniques and indications. *J Ultrasound* 14(1):28-36

PMID 23537933 Simonsen AH, Bahl JM, Danborg PB et al [2013] Pre-analytical factors influencing the stability of cerebrospinal fluid proteins. *J Neurosci Methods* 215(2):234-40

PMID 23543985 Katz MJ, Peters MN, Wysocki JD et al [2013] Diagnosis and management of delayed hemoperitoneum following therapeutic paracentesis. *Proc (Bayl Univ Med Cent)* 26(2):185-6

PMID 23573782 Posteraro B, De Carolis E, Vella A et al [2013] MALDI-TOF mass spectrometry in the clinical mycology laboratory: identification of fungi and beyond. *Expert Rev Proteomics* 10(2):151-64

PMID 23647736 Danise P, Maconi M, Rovetti A et al [2013] Cell counting of body fluids: comparison between 3 automated haematology analysers and the manual microscope method. *Int J Lab Hematol* 35(6):608-13

PMID 23716522 Shostak E, Brylka D, Krepp J et al [2013] Bedside sonography for detection of postprocedure pneumothorax. *J Ultrasound Med* 32(6):1003-9

PMID 23729569 Nagy K, Skagervik I, Tumani H et al [2013] Cerebrospinal fluid analyses for the diagnosis of subarachnoid haemorrhage and experience from a Swedish study. What method is preferable when diagnosing a subarachnoid haemorrhage? *Clin Chem Lab Med* 51(11):2073-86

PMID 23800427 Smith A, Wu AH, Lynch KL et al [2013] Multi-wavelength spectrophotometric analysis for detection of xanthochromia in cerebrospinal fluid and accuracy for the diagnosis of subarachnoid hemorrhage. *Clin Chim Acta* 424:231-6

PMID 23872540 Tausche A, Gehrisch S, Panzner I et al [2013] A 3-day delay in synovial fluid crystal identification did not hinder the reliable detection of monosodium urate and calcium pyrophosphate crystals. *J Clin Rheumatol* 19(5):241-5

PMID 24448178 Marshman LA, Duell R, Rudd D et al [2014] Intra- and inter-observer agreement in visual inspection for "xanthochromia": implications for subarachnoid haemorrhage diagnosis, CT validations studies, and for "Walton's rule." *Neurosurgery* epub

PMID 24551662 Mundhra R, Agarwal M [2013] Fetal outcome in meconium stained deliveries *J Clin Diagn Res* 7(12):2874-6

PMID 3049220 Runyon BA, Canawati HN, Akriviadis EA [1998] Optimization of ascitic fluid culture technique. *Gastroenterology* 95:1351-1355

PMID 364975 Dekker A, Bupp P [1978] Cytology of serous effusions. An investigation into the usefulness of cell blocks versus smears. *Am J Clin Pathol* 70(6):855-60

PMID 5654509 Palmer D [1968] Total leukocyte enumeration in pathologic synovial fluids. *Am J Clin Pathol* 49(6):812-4

PMID 8990255 Ashwood ER [1997] Standards of laboratory practice: evaluation of fetal lung maturity. National Academy of Clinical Biochemistry. *Clin Chem* 43(1):211-4

ISBN 1-56238-614X CLSI [2006] *Body Fluid Analysis for Cellular Composition; Approved Guideline*. CLSI document H56-A. Clinical and Laboratory Standards Institute

ISBN 978-1555815271 York MK, Thomson RB Jr [2007] Body fluid cultures (excluding blood, cerebrospinal fluid, and urine). In: *Clinical Microbiology Procedures Handbook*, 3e. ASM Press, p3.5.1-3.5.8

ISBN 978-1555816780 Baron EJ, Thomson RB Jr [2011] Specimen collection, transport, and processing: bacteriology. In: *Manual of Clinical Microbiology*, 10e. ASM Press, p228-271

ISBN 978-3318022537 Shaffer LG, McGowan-Jordan J, Schmid M ed [2012] *ISCN 2013: An International System for Human Cytogenetic Nomenclature*. S Karger

CLSI C56-A CLSI [2012] *Hemolysis, Icterus, and Lipemia/Turbidity Indices as Indicators of Interference in Clinical Laboratory Analysis; Approved Guideline.* CLSI document C56-A. Clinical and Laboratory Standards Institute

CLSI EP05-A2 CLSI [2004] *Evaluation of Precision Performance of Quantitative Measurement Methods; Approved Guideline*, 2e. CLSI document EP05-A2. Clinical and Laboratory Standards Institute

CLSI EP06-A CLSI [2003] *Evaluation of Linearity of Quantitative Measurement Procedures: A Statistical Approach; Approved Guideline.* CLSI document EP06-A. Clinical and Laboratory Standards Institute

CLSI EP14-A2 CLSI [2005] *Evaluation of Matrix Effects; Approved Guideline*, 2e. CLSI document EP14-A2. Clinical and Laboratory Standards Institute

CLSI EP17-A2 CLSI [2012] *Evaluation of Detection Capability for Clinical Laboratory Measurement Procedures; Approved Guideline.* CLSI document EP17-A2. Clinical and Laboratory Standards Institute

American College of Medical Genetics (ACMG) [2010] Standards and guidelines for clinical genetics laboratories, section E. www.acmg.net/StaticContent/SGs/Section_E_2011.pdf

CAP [2013] Cytogenetics Checklist. www.cap.org/apps/docs/laboratory_accreditation/checklists/new/cytogenetics checklist

Perry JL [1995] Utility of cytocentrifugation for direct examination of clinical specimens. *Clin Microbiol Newsl* 17:29-32

Troidle L, Finkelstein F [2006] Treatment outcome of CPD-associated peritonitis. 2006: *Ann Clin Microbiol Antimicrob* 5(6), http://www.ann-clinmicrob.com/content/5/1/6

Grenache DG, Lamb AN, Couturier MR, Kjeldsberg CR

Amniotic fluid
Chapter 3

Anatomy & pathophysiology

Amniotic fluid is the fluid that surrounds the fetus shortly after conception and throughout the remainder of pregnancy **f3.1**. The source of amniotic fluid is dynamic and changes during gestation. In early pregnancy, it is an ultrafiltrate of maternal plasma. By midgestation, amniotic fluid is composed largely of fetal urine as well as fluids that diffuse through the fetal skin (prior to kertinization) and from the fetal lungs.

As the source of the amniotic fluid changes, so too does its composition. The concentration of sodium, chloride, and uric acid are higher and the concentration of urea and creatinine are lower in the 1st trimester when the fluid is derived largely from maternal plasma. As the pregnancy progresses, the concentration of these analytes change in opposite directions. The amount of particulate matter in the amniotic fluid increases over time. Very little is present in the 1st trimester, but large numbers of cells can be observed by 16 weeks' gestation, having been shed from tissue surfaces of the amnion **i3.1** and fetus. Later in gestation, surfactant rich lamellar bodies from the fetal lungs and lanugo (the very fine, soft, and usually unpigmented hair that appears on the body of the fetus) contribute to the haziness of the fluid. At term, large particles of vernix caseosa (sebum and desquamated epithelial cells) may be present. Although the fetus does not normally defecate in utero, a severely stressed fetus may pass its first stool, called meconium, that consists of materials ingested by the fetus (primarily intestinal epithelial cells, lanugo, and mucus) and bile from the fetal liver.

Amniotic fluid has several functions that are required for normal fetal growth and development. These include

1. protecting the fetus from trauma and infection and maintaining a constant temperature
2. preventing umbilical cord compression between the fetus and uterus
3. serving as a source of fluid and nutrients for the fetus
4. providing adequate space for fetal movements that permits development of the lungs and the musculoskeletal system

The volume of amniotic fluid increases with increasing gestational age reaching peak volumes at 33 weeks' gestation. Actual volumes vary considerably across pregnancies. The 5th, 50th, and 95th, percentiles at 33 weeks' gestation are approximately 300 mL, 800 mL, and 1,900 mL, respectively [PMID 4637037]. Amniotic fluid volumes are a function of fluid production and

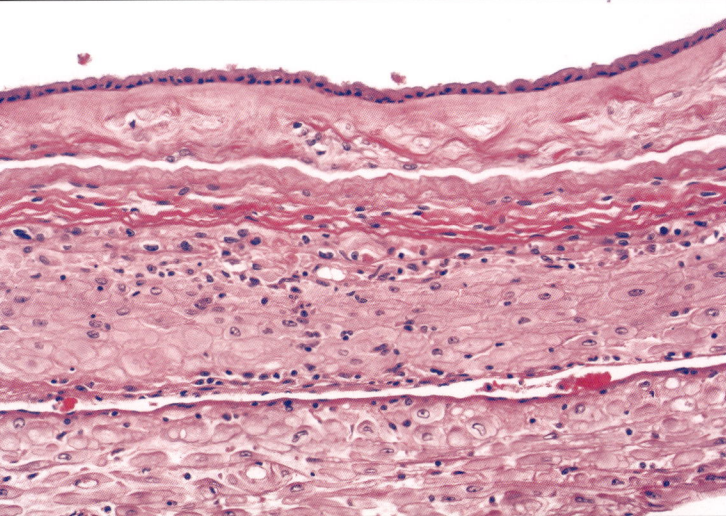

f3.1 The anatomic relationships of the fetus and the amniotic fluid

i3.1 The amnion, the innermost layer of the amniotic cavity, is lined by a single layer of epithelial cells (top layer) that resides on a basement membrane

clearance. Near term, fluid production is largely from fetal urine and fetal lung liquids and clearance is via fetal swallowing and intramembranous fluxes. Intramembranous fluxes are the exchange of water and solutes between amniotic fluid and fetal blood and take place primarily on the fetal surface of the placenta. In the 3rd trimester, fluid flows are very dynamic (approximately 1,000 mL/day) such that the amniotic fluid is replaced twice each 24 hours.

The volume of amniotic fluid is an indicator of the fetal condition because variations in fetal homeostasis such as urine production, swallowing, and lung liquid secretion influence the fluid volume. Abnormal amniotic fluid volumes are associated with several pregnancy related pathologies. Hydramnios or polyhydramnios refers to an increased volume of amniotic fluid (>2 liters) and is associated with fetal malformations, particularly of the central nervous system (spina bifida and anencephaly) or the gastrointestinal tract (esophageal atresia). Oligohydramnios refers to a decreased volume of amniotic fluid and has several etiologies. It is rare in the 1st trimester and the cause is not known, but when it does occur the prognosis for a successful pregnancy is poor. In the 2nd trimester the cause is often due to disorders of the fetal urinary system. Oligohydramnios in the 3rd trimester is often associated with preterm premature rupture of membranes or with uteroplacental insufficiency.

Clinical indications for amniotic fluid testing

Clinical tests performed on amniotic fluid include
1. prenatal genetic testing
2. determining fetal lung maturity
3. identifying infection
4. determining the degree of fetal hemolytic anemia
5. testing for open neural tube defects
6. evaluating the integrity of fetal membranes t3.1

t3.1 Clinical tests, their clinical indications & approximate weeks' gestation for amniotic fluid tests

Test(s)	Indication	Weeks' gestation
Bilirubin (ΔOD_{450})	Hemolytic disease of the newborn	14-40
α fetoprotein Acetylcholinesterase	Open neural tube defects	15-25
Karyotype Fluorescence in situ hybridization Chromosomal microarray analysis	Prenatal genetic testing	16-22
Lecithin to sphingomyelin ratio Lamellar body count Phosphatidylglycerol	Fetal lung maturity	32-38
Placental α macroglobulin-1 Insulinlike growth factor binding protein-1	Premature rupture of membranes	Varies
Culture Gram stain Molecular testing	Infectious disease	Varies

Specimen collection, requirements & stability

Amniocentesis is the technique used for withdrawing amniotic fluid from the uterine cavity using a needle inserted into the uterus through the abdomen. It is most commonly performed at 15-20 weeks' gestation. Major complications of amniocentesis are infection, premature rupture of membranes, direct or indirect injury to the fetus, and fetal loss. The true rate of pregnancy loss associated with amniocentesis is uncertain. When the procedure is performed under ultrasound guidance, reported rates of fetal loss range from about 1/100-1/1,000 procedures. A practice bulletin from the American College of Obstetricians and Gynecologists state a procedure related loss rate of 1/300-1/500 [PMID 18055749]. Amniocentesis can be performed earlier or later in gestation. Higher fetal loss and complication rates are seen when performed prior to 15 weeks' gestation. Maternal complications are rare.

After the maternal abdomen is cleaned with an antiseptic solution, a 20-22 gauge needle of 8.9 cm in length is inserted into the uterine cavity. Amniocentesis is usually performed with sonographic guidance to prevent the needle from being inserted into the maternal bladder, placenta, umbilical cord, or the fetus. The first few mL of fluid may contain maternal cells and so this is often discarded to prevent ambiguous cytogenetic studies. The total volume of amniotic fluid collected should be based on the gestational age of the fetus. In the 2nd trimester, this volume is usually 2-30 mL that is aspirated into sterile syringes. Women with Rh(D)– blood types should receive anti D immune globulin after the procedure to prevent alloimmunization.

The type of testing to be performed on amniotic fluid will determine how the sample should be processed. Samples for cytogenetic studies should be kept at room temperature and submitted to the laboratory within 24 hours as the ability to successfully culture amniocytes in vitro decreases with time. If the sample is inadvertently frozen, DNA may be recovered for microarray, quantitative PCR, or single gene testing. Tests for the assessment of open neural tube defects (α fetoprotein and acetylcholinesterase) can utilize samples kept at room temperature (required if cytogenetic studies are also needed), refrigerated, or frozen. Samples for amniotic fluid bilirubin testing must be protected from light as bilirubin is degraded by exposure to light. Fetal lung maturity tests require samples to be refrigerated to prevent the degradation of phospholipids. Frozen samples are considered to be unacceptable for lamellar body count testing [PMID 20716798].

It is sometimes necessary to determine if an amniotic fluid sample submitted to the laboratory is, in fact, urine. The concentration of creatinine in the amniotic fluid is close to that of plasma so high concentrations suggest that the sample is urine. Similarly, the concentrations of total protein and glucose in the amniotic fluid are considerably higher than in normal urine so their measurement can also be informative. A rapid method of distinguishing between the 2 fluid types is with the protein and glucose tests on a urine dipstick. Amniotic fluid will yield detectable amounts of both of these analytes while normal urine would not.

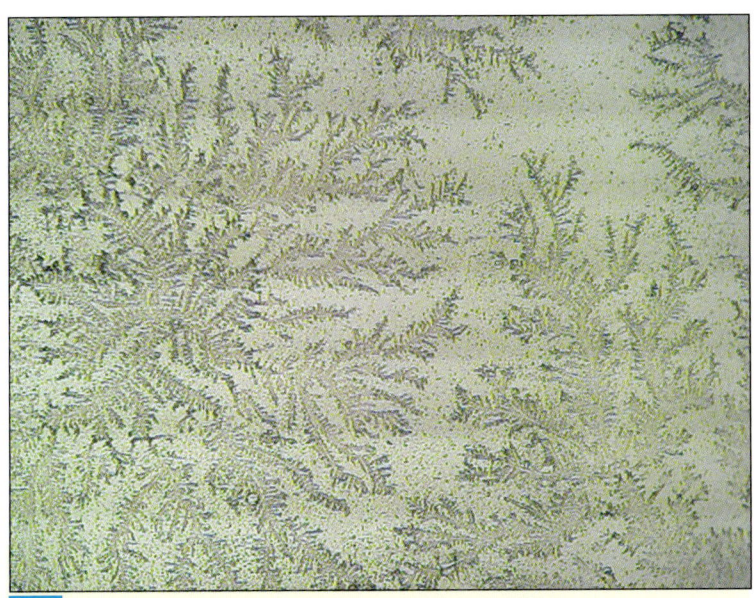

i3.2 Fernlike crystals indicate that the specimen contains amniotic fluid

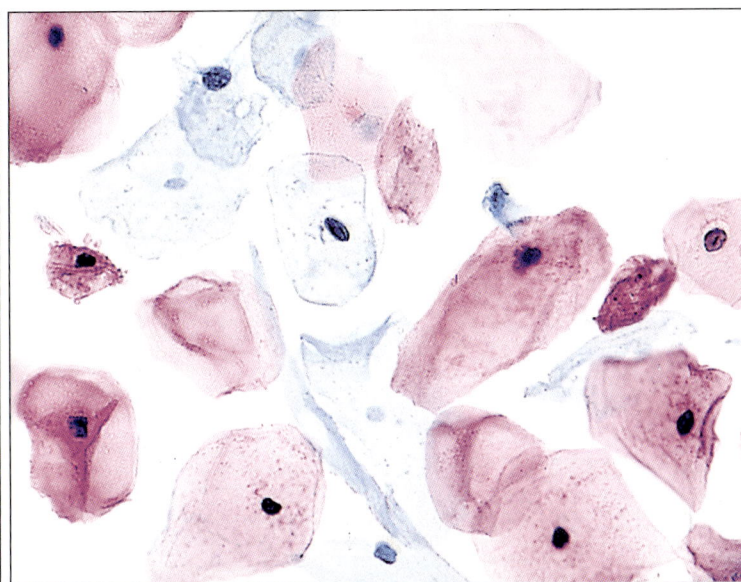

i3.3 Superficial & intermediate squamous epithelial cells in amniotic fluid (Papanicolaou stain)

Gross examination

The appearance of the amniotic fluid should be noted. If blood is present it is usually due to maternal origin. Amniotic fluid that appears green or brown in the 2nd trimester suggests an intraamniotic hemorrhage that occurred prior to the amniocentesis and is associated with a higher rate of miscarriage or fetal death [PMID 3717234, PMID 2130841].

Microscopic examination

The cytologic examination of amniotic fluid is of limited clinical value compared to other procedures to be described. Microscopic examination of a specimen, however, may provide additional information in the diagnoses of ruptured membranes and chorioamnionitis (see below). Fetal sex can be determined by performing fluorescence in situ hybridization (FISH) on uncultured cells [PMID 1609805] or by extracting DNA and performing quantitative PCR [PMID 22467160].

Premature rupture of membranes

The premature rupture of membranes (PROM) is a common obstetrical problem complicating 5-10% of all pregnancies and is defined as the rupture of amniotic membranes prior to the start of labor or regular uterine contractions [PMID 17400872]. Approximately 5% of PROM cases occur before 37 completed weeks' gestation and is designated as preterm premature rupture of the membranes (PPROM). PROM is associated with an increased incidence of chorioamnionitis and prematurity as well as increased perinatal and maternal morbidity and mortality.

In the majority of women, the diagnosis of PROM can be based on history and with a speculum examination. In approximately 10% of all cases, the diagnosis of ruptured membrane is difficult to establish. The gold standard test for diagnosing PROM is amniocentesis with infusion of a dilute indigo carmine dye into the amniotic cavity. PROM is diagnosed by the detection of the dye in the vagina within 30 minutes of infusion. While the test is very accurate it is invasive, expensive, and may itself cause PROM or other complications like infection. Less invasive, "classic" methods for diagnosing PROM include visual observation of pooling amniotic fluid during speculum examination, oligohydramnios determined by ultrasound, pH testing of pooled fluid (the nitrazine test), and the fern test. However, these methods are limited by rather poor sensitivity and specificity when applied to women for whom a diagnosis of PROM is not certain [Palmer 2007]. Chemical markers of PROM are described later in this chapter.

The fern test is named for the pattern of crystallization that occurs when amniotic fluid is placed on a glass slide and allowed to air dry. A sample of vaginal secretions from the posterior vaginal pool is placed on a clean glass slide and the sample evenly spread to create a thin smear. The specimen is allowed to dry and then examined under a low power (10×) magnification. The presence of fernlike crystals indicates that the specimen contains amniotic fluid i3.2. The presence of blood, urine, cervical mucus, vaginal noninfectious leukorrhea, sperm, and even fingerprints may produce a false positive result. False negative results may result during prolonged rupture of membranes (longer than 24 hours) or if only a small quantity of amniotic fluid has leaked. Although it is rapid and simple to perform, the National Academy of Clinical Biochemistry concluded that there was limited evidence regarding its sensitivity and specificity when utilized in women for whom membrane status was definitively known [Palmer 2007]. Further, its performance deteriorates when used to evaluate women whose membrane integrity was uncertain.

Other tests that have been used to identify amniotic fluid found in the vagina include examining the fluid for amniotic fluid cells using a Papanicolaou stain or a Nile blue dye. With a Papanicolaou stain the fetal cells show a variable staining pattern with colors ranging from emerald green to orange or pink i3.3. In contrast, the vaginal cells are uniformly green or blue green. With the Nile blue dye (a metachromatic fat stain, oxane sulfate) the fetal stains are

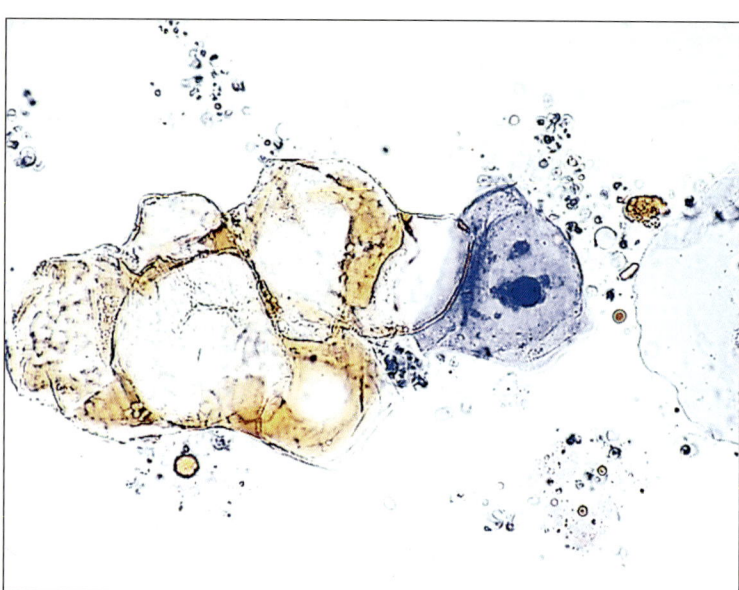

i3.4 Orange yellow staining cells are fetal epidermal cells (Nile blue dye)

orange yellow, due to the presence of lipid on the surface of the cell (vernix), and the vaginal cells are blue i3.4.

The Gram stain is described in the section "Microbiologic examination" later in this chapter.

Chemical analysis

As with other body fluids, the chemical makeup of amniotic fluid is complex. Furthermore, its composition varies considerably as gestation proceeds. In the very early stages of pregnancy, its composition mimics that of maternal serum. As pregnancy progresses, the concentration of some analytes decreases (eg, total protein, sodium, glucose, chloride, bilirubin), while that of others progressively increases (eg, potassium, creatinine, urea, uric acid, amylase, pulmonary surfactants) [ISBN 978-158829-2704]. A reliable interpretation of these values depends not only on accurate analyte measurements and gestational age estimation, but also on whether the patient has a normal volume of amniotic fluid. These variables make interpreting many biochemical tests results difficult. While the amniotic fluid concentrations of many different analytes (eg, electrolytes, metabolites, enzymes, hormones) have been investigated over the years, relatively few have demonstrated clinical utility.

α fetoprotein (AFP)

AFP is a 69,000 Da glycoprotein synthesized first by the fetal yolk sac and then by the fetal liver. Although its physiologic function is not known, it may function as a carrier protein similar to that of albumin. AFP concentrations in fetal serum increase up to 3 mg/mL (3,000 μg/mL) by 9 weeks' gestation and then slowly decrease to about 200 μg/mL by 32 weeks' gestation. AFP synthesis ceases at about the time of delivery, and serum concentrations fall rapidly thereafter.

From the fetus, AFP gains access to the amniotic fluid primarily via the urine following renal filtration. The changes in amniotic fluid AFP concentrations parallel those in serum but are approximately 2-3 orders of magnitude lower (~2 μg/mL by 32 weeks' gestation). However, in various congenital anomalies, amniotic fluid AFP concentrations are considerably increased. The most common of these anomalies is an open neural tube defect (NTD) in which there is an anatomic lesion that is in direct contact with the amniotic fluid. Other causes of increased amniotic fluid AFP concentrations include multiple gestation, fetal demise, congenital nephrosis, or other fetal structural defects (eg, omphalocele, gastroschisis).

NTDs occur when the lateral edges of the neural plate fail to properly fuse by the 27th day after conception. Failure of the tube to completely fuse is invariably followed by a malformation of the surrounding mesodermal structures. Anencephaly is the most severe NTD and involves the absence of brain, skull, and scalp and affected infants die in utero or shortly after delivery. Spina bifida falls into 1 of 3 categories: spina bifida occulta, spina bifida cystica with meningocele, and spina bifida cystica with meningomyelocele. The severity of complications (paralysis, orthopedic abnormalities, bowel and bladder incontinence, etc) is a function of where on the spine the defect is located and whether or not the defect is open or closed. Open defects, which account for approximately 80% of all NTDs, are not covered by skin and are the only NTDs that can be detected by AFP testing.

Testing for amniotic fluid AFP is typically preceded by AFP testing in maternal serum as a screening test for an open NTD. Screening for NTDs is optimally performed between 16 and 18 weeks' gestation but can be done from 15 to 25 weeks' gestation. Because the concentration of AFP in maternal serum is dynamic during the screening window, it is expressed as the multiple of the median (MoM) by dividing an individual's AFP result by the median AFP concentration for the relevant gestational age (by day). Median values must be established by each laboratory using the AFP method used for screening and the reference population that is screened. Use of the MoM also allows comparison of results across laboratories and avoids analytical variation due to method differences. The maternal serum AFP MoM is interpreted against a cutoff MoM that maximizes diagnostic sensitivity and specificity. For most open NTD screening programs this cutoff is 2.0 or 2.5 MoM. A cutoff of 2.0 will detect 75-90% of open spina bifida cases with a false positive rate of 2-5% while these rates are 65-80% and 1-3%, respectively, with a 2.5 cutoff [PMID 15915088]. Both cutoffs will detect nearly all cases of anencephaly.

Women with maternal serum AFP results above the cutoff should be offered diagnostic testing, usually high resolution ultrasound to observe the fetus for defects and, if none are observed, amniocentesis for amniotic fluid AFP and acetylcholinesterase testing.

Due to its considerably higher concentration in amniotic fluid compared to maternal serum, amniotic fluid AFP is a much better predictor of an open NTD. Provided that the laboratory has established amniotic fluid AFP medians, amniotic fluid AFP testing can be performed and interpreted up to 25 weeks' gestation. An abnormal result is defined as an amniotic fluid AFP MoM that is >2.0 [PMID 15915088]. This cutoff produces a detection rate for open spina bifida of 96-99% and a false positive rate of 2-5% [PMID 2483269].

Maternal serum and amniotic fluid AFP is measured using commercially available automated immunoassays.

Cholinesterase

Cholinesterases are enzymes that catalyze the hydrolysis of choline esters. Acetylcholinesterase (AChE) is distributed in the gray matter of the central nervous system, where it terminates synaptic transmission by specifically hydrolyzing the neurotransmitter acetylcholine. AChE is also present in red blood cells but its function there is unknown. Pseudocholinesterase (PChE) is distributed in the white matter of the central nervous system and in the blood. Although it has no known physiological function PChE is of pharmacologic importance because, unlike AChE, PChE is capable of hydrolyzing exogenous carboxylic or phosphoric acid esters such as those found in succinylcholine, aspirin, ester type local anesthetics, amitriptyline, cocaine, heroin, and several anticonvulsant drugs.

Amniotic fluid normally contains PChE but not AChE. Due to the high abundance of AChE in cerebrospinal fluid, a fetus with an open NTD will leak AChE into the amniotic fluid. As indicated above, increased amniotic fluid AFP is not specific for open NTD so the measurement of AChE in amniotic fluid is used as a confirmatory test for open NTD in cases where the amniotic fluid AFP concentration is increased. The diagnostic sensitivity of an amniotic fluid AFP MoM >2.0 in conjunction with the detection of amniotic fluid AChE for open NTD is 99% [PMID 9316128]. Amniotic fluid AChE is also present in ~80% of fetuses with abdominal wall defects.

Contamination of amniotic fluid with fetal blood, but not maternal blood, can result in elevated AFP and detectable AChE [PMID 7126503]. As such, all AChE+ samples should also be tested for the presence of hemoglobin F, commonly performed, qualitatively, by radial immunodiffusion.

Polyacrylamide gel electrophoresis is used for the detection of amniotic fluid AChE. Amniotic fluid from unaffected pregnancies contains only PChE. When present, AChE migrates anodally to PChE. Both enzyme bands are revealed by incubating the gel with copper ions and acetylcholine, a substrate for AChE and PChE. The presence of AChE must be confirmed by demonstrating its inhibition using the selective inhibitor 1,5-bis(4-allyldimethylammoniumphenyl) pentan-3-one dibromide (BW284c51).

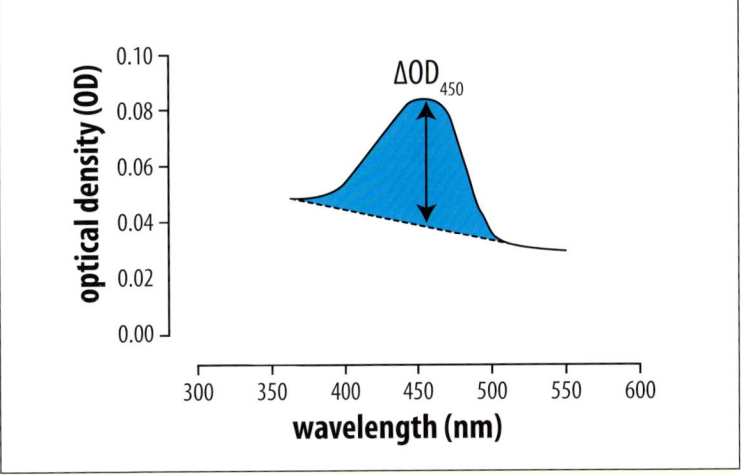

f3.2 Absorption spectrophotometry scan of amniotic fluid for determining the ΔOD_{450}. The dashed line represents the baseline drawn between 350 and 550 nm. The difference between the optical density of the curve and the dashed line at 450 nm is the ΔOD_{450} value.

Bilirubin

During normal pregnancy, amniotic fluid bilirubin peaks between 19 and 22 weeks' gestation at a concentration of 1.6-1.8 mg/L with lower concentrations observed before and after this peak. These low concentrations do not permit bilirubin to be measured using standard chemical techniques. Bilirubin can be measured, directly, using absorption spectrophotometry between wavelengths of 350 and 550 nm. Bilirubin absorbs light maximally at 450 nm so the extent to which the absorbance curve deviates from a baseline (drawn between the optical density readings at 350 and 550 nm) at this wavelength is proportional to the bilirubin concentration. This change in absorbance is frequently referred to as the ΔOD_{450} f3.2.

Clinically the measurement of the ΔOD_{450} is used to assess the severity of fetal anemia in pregnancies affected by hemolytic disease of the newborn (HDN). HDN occurs when maternal IgG molecules with specificity to paternally inherited fetal red blood cell antigens cross the placenta and cause the destruction of fetal red blood cells. Maternal sensitization occurs upon exposure of the maternal immune system to fetal red blood cells either from antepartum or intrapartum fetomaternal hemorrhage. Maternal sensitization often occurs during the first pregnancy with a fetus that expresses the red blood cell antigens. Although this first fetus is at low risk of developing HDN, future antigen positive fetuses are at high risk.

Although several red blood cell antigens can cause HDN, most alloimmunizations are directed against the rhesus (Rh) and Kell blood group systems. The introduction of effective prophylaxis with anti D immune globulin in 1968 dramatically decreased the incidence of HDN in developed countries, yet failure to receive anti D prophylaxis can still occur. In developing countries without prophylaxis, 14% of affected pregnancies result in stillbirth and 50% of surviving infants will die shortly after birth or develop serious morbidities [PMID 21037283].

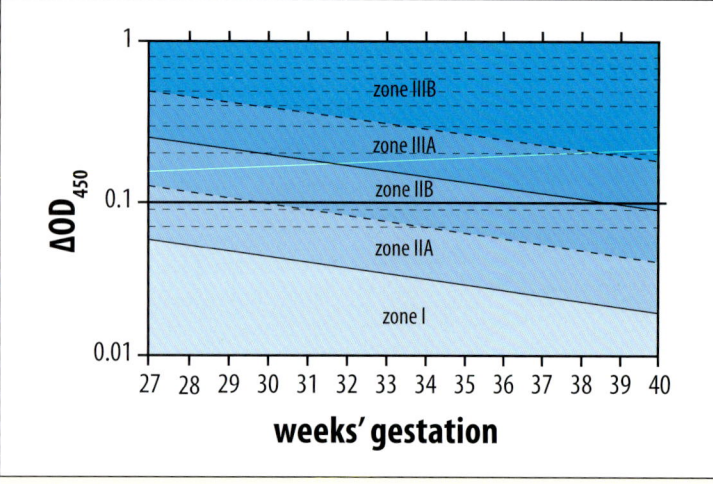
f3.3 The Liley chart for interpreting the ΔOD_{450}

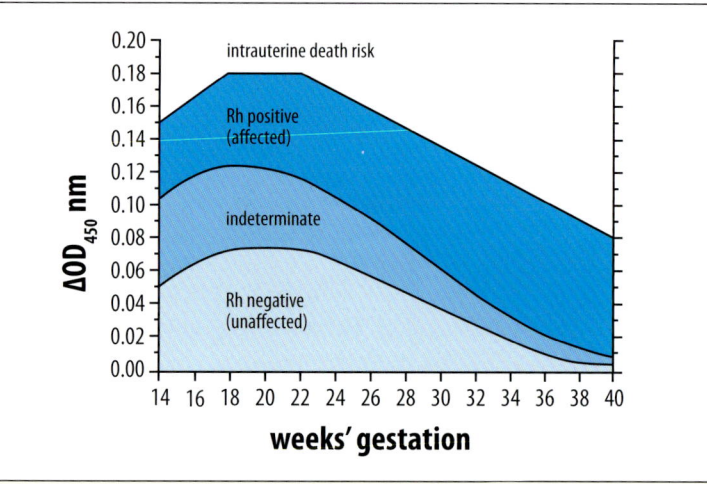
f3.4 The Queenan chart for interpreting the ΔOD_{450}

Bilirubin concentration determined by the ΔOD_{450} is not in mass concentration and so the ΔOD_{450} result is interpreted with either the Liley f3.3 or the Queenan chart f3.4, both of which require knowledge of the gestational age at which the sample was obtained. The Liley chart, developed in 1961 from sensitized pregnancies beginning at 27 weeks' gestation, was divided into 3 zones (I, II, and III) with zones II and III divided into 2 equal subzones (A and B). Results falling with zone I are associated with fetuses without anemia or who are mildly affected. Results in zone II suggest fetuses with moderate anemia although anemia may range from mild to severe. Results in zone III represent fetuses with severe anemia.

The Liley chart was not developed from pregnancies prior to 27 weeks' gestation and charts with linearly extrapolated zones before 27 weeks should not be used, as these will underestimate the severity of fetal anemia [PMID 12220785]. The Queenan chart, developed in 1993 from amniotic fluid specimens collected between 14 and 40 weeks' gestation, is a better estimator of fetal anemia [PMID 12220785]. The Queenan chart is divided into 4 zones, the lowest and highest of which represent fetuses with no to mild anemia and those with severe HDN, respectively. Between these 2 extremes is a zone that represents fetus with all possible outcomes although higher results suggest a greater risk of severity.

Regardless of which chart is used for result interpretation, serial testing to identify ΔOD_{450} trends are more informative than single determinations. Decreasing results are associated with mild disease and stable or increasing results suggested severe anemia.

The use of Doppler ultrasonography as a noninvasive method of determining fetal anemia was first described in 2000. This technique measures the peak velocity of systolic blood flow in the fetal middle cerebral artery [PMID 16837679]. A faster rate of blood flow indicates a more severely anemic fetus. In light of the availability of this noninvasive assessment, the use of amniocentesis to determine the ΔOD_{450} result is nearly obsolete.

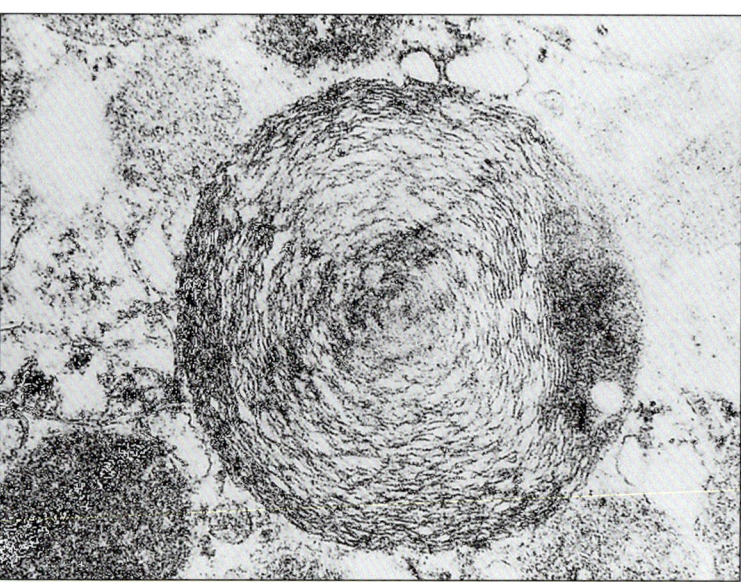
i3.5 Lamellar body. Electron micrograph shows the symmetric layers of protein & phospholipid.

Pulmonary surfactants

Surface tension in the hydrated lung works to oppose lung inflation and promote the collapse of alveoli. Pulmonary surfactant prevents atelectasis in the newborn infant by decreasing alveolar surface tension through the creation of a lipid rich monolayer phase that separates alveolar gas from the liquid surfaces of epithelial cells. This stabilizes alveoli and allows lung volumes to be maintained at expiration.

Pulmonary surfactant is synthesized by type II pneumocytes and packaged into storage granules called lamellar bodies beginning around 25 weeks' gestation i3.5 [PMID 16303123]. As secreted from lamellar bodies, pulmonary surfactant is a heterogeneous mixture of approximately 90% phospholipids and 10% protein. The most abundant phospholipids are dipalmitoylphosphatidylcholine (PC or lecithin) and phosphatidylglycerol (PG). Other pulmonary surfactants such as phosphatidylinositol, phosphatidylethanolamine, and sphingomyelin are much less abundant.

Lecithin in the amniotic fluid becomes detectable around 25 weeks' gestation and then steadily increases to its peak at week 36. In contrast, the synthesis of PG occurs much later, near week 35, and increases to term [PMID 16303123].

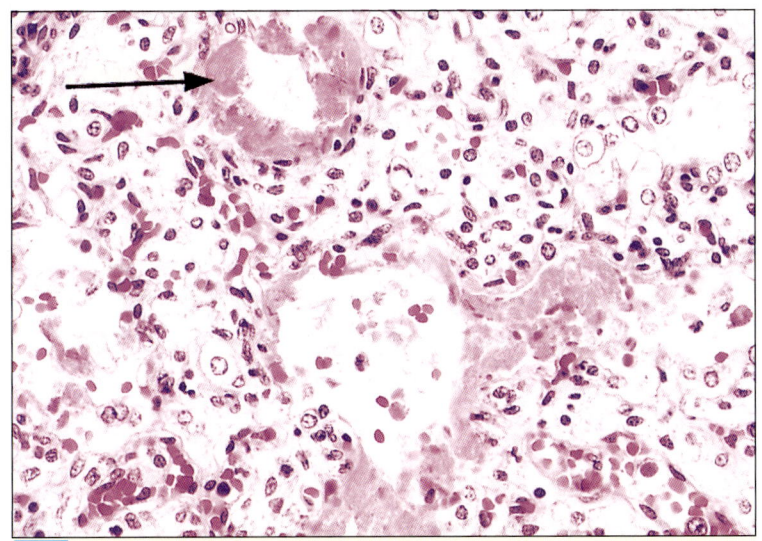

i3.6 Hyaline membrane disease. Histologic section of lung showing air spaces lined by pink hyaline membranes (arrow) with adjacent atelectasis (H&E stain).

Because fetal lung liquids contribute to amniotic fluid, the measurement of pulmonary surfactants and/or the enumeration of lamellar bodies in amniotic fluid have been used for the assessment of fetal lung maturity and the prediction of respiratory distress syndrome (RDS) of the newborn.

RDS results from a deficiency of pulmonary surfactant that leads to higher surface tension within the alveoli, causing alveolar collapse and impaired gas exchange. The result is neonatal hypoxia, with further worsening of pulmonary status manifested by acidosis and increased shunting within the lungs. Signs of RDS include neonatal tachypnea, grunting, inspiratory thoracic retractions, and cyanosis, often occurring within several hours of birth. The characteristic histology seen in infants who die from RDS was the source of the historical name for RDS: hyaline membrane disease. Waxy appearing layers of hyaline membrane i3.6 line the collapsed alveoli and the lungs show evidence of hemorrhage, overdistension of the airways, and necrotic pneumocytes.

Overall, the diagnostic sensitivity of all FLM tests is approximately 95-98% but the overall specificity is poor and ranges from 50-80%. Due to the low prevalence of RDS, the negative predictive value of any FLM test is very high (>95%). As such, a negative test result can be relied upon as a very good predictor of lung maturity [PMID 16303123].

While several tests of fetal lung maturity have been developed over the last few decades, only 3 continue to be in routine use today.

Lecithin to sphingomyelin ratio

The lecithin to sphingomyelin (L:S) ratio was the first biochemical test for assessing the maturity of the fetal lungs. It describes the relative change in the concentration of lecithin to that of sphingomyelin in amniotic fluid as determined by thin layer chromatography (TLC). Although low, the concentration of amniotic fluid sphingomyelin remains relatively constant throughout the last trimester of pregnancy and therefore serves as an internal standard against which the concentration of lecithin can be compared. The L:S ratio increases with increasing gestational age and, therefore, with the maturity of the fetal lung.

Although numerous variations to the original TLC procedure have been described, the essential elements remain the same. The test requires a minimum of 3-4 mL of amniotic fluid that is centrifuged briefly at low speed to remove debris while preserving phospholipid content. The specimen is mixed with methanol followed by lipid extraction into chloroform and applied to a TLC plate along with controls and markers that will show the locations of the various phospholipid components. The plate is developed in a solvent system containing chloroform, methanol, 2-propanol, triethylamine, and water. The phospholipids are visualized by using cupric acetate and phosphoric acid followed by charring. The lecithin and sphingomyelin bands are quantified densitometrically and the relative intensity of each band is expressed as a ratio. Common to all the methodological variations is that TLC is technique dependent. A ratio cutoff of 2.0 is frequently used as the decision point to indicate fetal lung maturity t3.2. However, the absence of a single, standardized procedure combined with the numerous analytical variations of the original procedure requires that all laboratories that perform the L:S ratio validate their method and their cutoff with a clinical outcome study.

t3.2 Fetal lung maturity test cutoffs commonly used to indicate pulmonary maturity

Test	Cutoff	Interpretation
Lecithin to sphingomyelin ratio	<2.0	Not mature
	≥2.0-2.5	Mature
Lamellar body count	<50,000/µL*	Not mature
	≥50,000/µL	Mature
Phosphatidylglycerol	Absent	Not mature
	Present	Mature

*Maturity cutoff varies according to method used to enumerate lamellar bodies

A commercially available method for performing the L:S ratio is available but the test is time consuming, requires considerable expertise to perform, and is imprecise (CVs of ~20%), even in laboratories that process a large number of samples.

Because blood has an L:S ratio between 1.5 and 2.0, amniotic fluid specimens contaminated with blood will cause the amniotic fluid LS to reflect that range. Similarly, meconium contaminated specimens are unacceptable because meconium produces an LS ratio of 1.1-3.6.

Lamellar body count

Lamellar bodies range in size from 1.7 to 7.3 fL, which is comparable to the 5-7 fL size range of blood platelets. This similarity permits the use of a standard automated hematologic cell counter to quantify the number of lamellar bodies in amniotic fluid as the lamellar body count (LBC). Some of the common methods used for platelet counting, which are also applied to the LBC, include optical and classical impedance methods. Additionally, some automated cell counters employ both impedance and optical methods for counting platelets. It is important to note that an LBC determined by these techniques may be comparable, although not always identical.

In the impedance method, the amniotic fluid sample is diluted in a current conducting solution. The lamellar bodies within the sample are drawn through a small aperture positioned between 2 sensing electrodes connected across a direct current potential. As each lamellar body passes through the aperture, it produces a momentary increase in impedance resulting in an electrical pulse. The number of pulses indicates the LBC, while the amplitude of the pulse is proportional to the lamellar body volume. The upper and lower pulse height thresholds are selected to ensure that only particles within a specific volume range are counted.

In optical counting, lamellar bodies in the diluted sample are hydrodynamically focused in a flow cell and illuminated by a narrow beam of laser light. The light scattered by each lamellar body is captured by a photodetector and converted to an electrical pulse, the total number of which is proportional to the LBC. Pulse amplitude is proportional to lamellar body volume. The number of pulses within a predetermined size range yields the corresponding LBC.

Amniotic fluid specimens for LBC should be mixed gently before testing but not centrifuged as this will lower the LBC. A consensus maturity cutoff of >50,000/μL was published in 2001 [PMID 11165603] when the Beckman Coulter brand of automated cell counters predominated in clinical laboratories. It is now well known that the different manufacturers' brands of automated cell counters do not produce similar LBC results. As such, instrument specific maturity cutoffs are required for LBC result interpretation t3.2 [CLSI 2011].

Contamination of the amniotic fluid specimen with whole blood can, paradoxically, cause a decrease in the LBC. This is likely due to the formation of a fibrin matrix that can trap lamellar bodies and prevent them from being enumerated [PMID 20716798]. Conversely, the presence of meconium causes a false increase in the LBC due to the presence of particles in meconium that are counted as platelets.

Phosphatidylglycerol

Despite its low relative contribution to total pulmonary surfactant, PG has also been used as an indicator of fetal lung maturity. PG is considered to be a late marker of lung maturity because it appears in the amniotic fluid several weeks after that of lecithin. The incorporation of the detection of PG by TLC as part of the L:S ratio was pursued due to the rather poor diagnostic specificity of the L:S ratio. The modified test utilized 2 dimensional TLC to determine the L:S ratio as well as the relative amounts of disaturated lecithin, phosphatidylinositol and phosphatidylglycerol in amniotic fluid. This "lung profile" offered advantages over the L:S ratio by enhancing the accuracy of a ratio >2.0 and decreasing the rate of false immature results.

An immunochemical approach to the detection of PG is also available. This slide agglutination test utilizes polyclonal anti PG antibodies to agglutinate PG following its incorporation into reagent liposomes. The test is simple to perform and the presence of absence of agglutination is determined by visible inspection. Visible agglutinates indicate the presence of PG and the result is interpreted as being indicative of fetal lung maturity t3.2.

A major advantage of PG as a marker of lung maturity is that it is not present in blood or meconium. Thus, the detection of PG can still be determined in amniotic fluid specimens contaminated with blood or meconium.

Chemical markers of ruptured membranes

The premature rupture of membranes (PROM) is described earlier in this chapter. Biomarkers that are present in high concentration in the amniotic fluid but are low to absent in other body fluids are ideal candidates for detecting PROM. While several biomarkers have been explored, few have proved themselves to be clinically useful.

Placental α microglobulin-1

Placental α microglobulin-1 (PAMG-1) is a placental glycoprotein secreted into the amniotic fluid, where it is present at a high concentration (2,000-25,000 ng/mL) relative to that of maternal blood (5-25 ng/mL) or cervicovaginal fluid with intact membranes (0.05-2 ng/mL). A commercial test for PAMG-1 that exploits these large differences in concentration has been developed for clinical use as an aid for the detection of premature rupture of membranes (PROM).

The test is an immunochromatographic test that utilizes 2 monoclonal antibodies for the rapid detection of PAMG-1 in cervicovaginal fluid. The specimen is collected using a polyester swab that is placed into the vagina and the collected fluid is eluted off the swab by rinsing it in a vial containing a buffer solution. The test strip is placed into the buffer for 10 minutes, and the test result is determined by visual inspection of a test and a control line (both are observed in the presence of PROM) on the lateral flow device. The analytical limit of detection of the test is 5 ng/mL.

Compared to classic methods of detecting PROM, the detection of PAMG-1 is sensitive (~95%) and specific (~99%) [PMID 23000696].

Insulinlike growth factor binding protein-1

Insulinlike growth factor binding protein-1 (IGFBP-1) is a 25,000 dalton glycoprotein expressed and secreted by several tissues including the decidualized endometrium. It is the predominant binding protein of insulinlike growth factor in fetal and maternal blood and amniotic fluid. It is 100-1,000× more concentrated in the amniotic fluid compared to maternal serum.

It is also an immunochromatographic test that utilizes 2 monoclonal antibodies with specificity to human IGFBP-1. The sample is collected as described above and the test strip placed into the buffer for 5 minutes. Test results are determined by visual inspection of a test and a control line (both are observed in the presence of PROM) on the lateral flow device. The analytical limit of detection of the test is 25 ng/mL.

Similar to PAMG-1, the sensitivity of IGFBP-1 is ~88% and its specificity is ~96%. A metaanalysis of PAMG-1 and IGFBP-1 concluded that PAMG-1 is the more accurate of the 2 markers for identifying PROM [PMID 23314505].

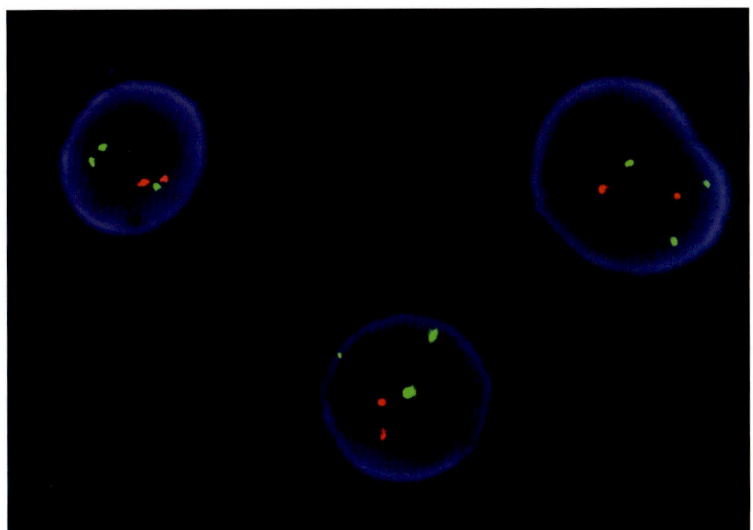

i3.7 Trisomy 13 by FISH of uncultured amniocytes (interphase cells) with FISH probes for chromosomes 13 (green) & 21 (red), showing 3 copies of the chromosome 13 specific probe (probes from the AneuVysion kit, Abbott Molecular, Inc)

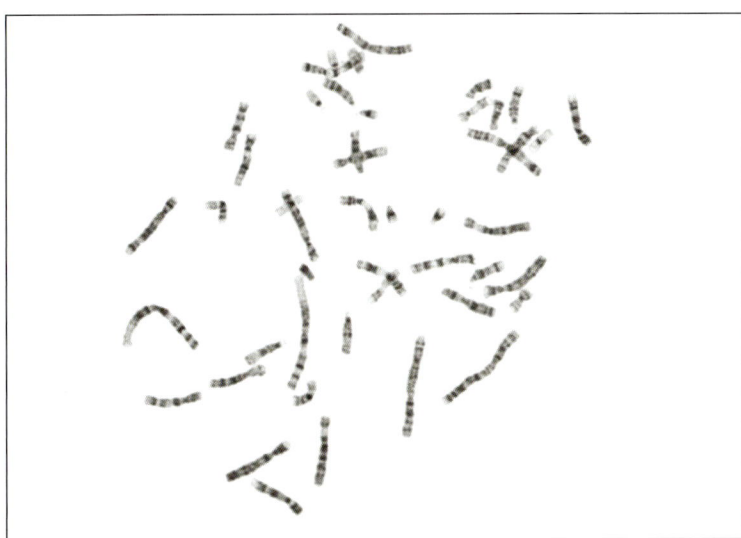

i3.8 Metaphase spread of the G banded chromosomes as they appear through a microscope (trisomy 21)

Prenatal diagnosis of chromosomal abnormalities

Prenatal diagnosis for genetic diseases can be performed on uncultured or cultured amniotic fluid cells (amniocytes). Amniocentesis for genetic analysis is generally performed between 16-22 weeks' gestation. The cells in the fluid, amniocytes, are a mixture of cell types that appear to be derived from epithelial surfaces such as the fetal skin, urogenital, respiratory, and gastrointestinal tracks and amniotic membranes, umbilical cord, and potentially trophoblasts [Van Dyke 2010]. Therefore, the cells may be from the fetus or the extraembryonic tissues (membranes, cord, and trophoblasts). Amniotic fluid samples from pregnancies past 30 weeks' gestation, collected due to abnormal ultrasound findings discovered later in the pregnancy, can be difficult to grow in culture due to the presence of accumulated cell debris and other materials. Also, the quality of the DNA obtained from these cells may be less than optimal, creating challenges in producing valid test results.

The amniotic fluid is centrifuged to concentrate the cells, which also allows for the assessment of blood in the sample, usually of maternal origin. The amniocytes may be processed directly (uncultured) or set up in culture for chromosome, biochemical, or DNA for single gene analysis. Testing performed on uncultured cells can be useful for rapid aneuploidy testing by fluorescence in situ hybridization (FISH) i3.7 [PMID 1609805], by extracted DNA [PMID 22467160], or by microarray analysis [PMID 23215555]. Backup cultures should be established if repeat or additional testing is needed. The presence of maternal blood in the sample makes the analysis on uncultured cells for rapid FISH or molecular techniques difficult and requires cultured cells to avoid the potential of contaminating maternal blood.

Cell culture of amniocytes involves specialized supplemented tissue culture medium to support optimal amniocyte growth [Van Dyke 2010] and is necessary to obtain dividing cells for conventional cytogenetic analysis. For culture, cells are placed on a coverslip in a small culture dish and allowed to attach and grow. Only a small proportion of the

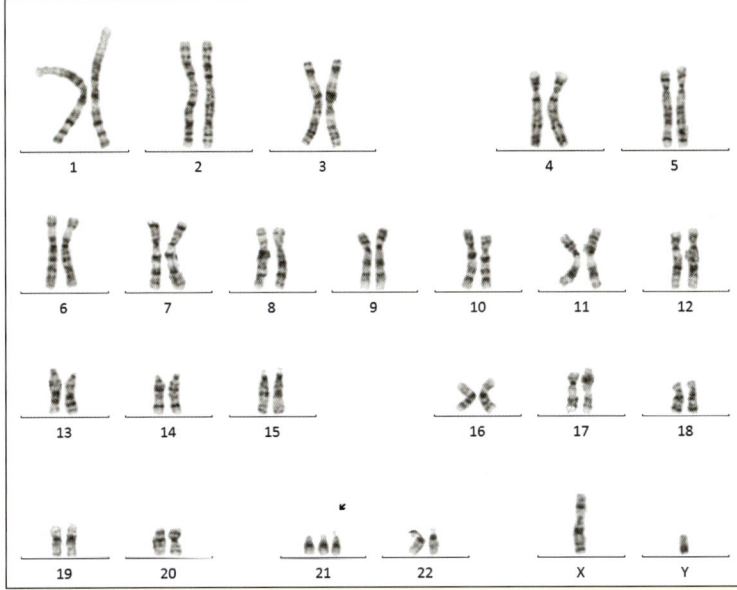

i3.9 A karyogram of G banded chromosomes from a patient with Down syndrome (trisomy 21)

amniocytes are capable of attaching, and these grow as individual colonies in the primary culture. Cells that fail to attach and grow in culture may be collected when culture media is changed for the first time, providing an additional source of cells for interphase FISH testing or DNA extraction. The cultures are monitored over time and the cells are harvested in situ by collecting dividing cells with colcemid treatment. This is followed by hypotonic treatment and fixation with Carnoy fixative (3:1 methanol:acetic acid) and the spreading of chromosomes on the coverslip. Following appropriate drying of the preparation, the coverslip/slides are treated by banding with trypsin and staining. Chromosomes are then counted and analyzed through the microscope or on a computer screen using digital images i3.8. Karyograms are prepared by separating and arranging the chromosomes in pairs i3.9.

Maternal cell contamination testing should be a routine part of any molecular testing, including microarray analysis, both for uncultured and cultured samples. Uncultured

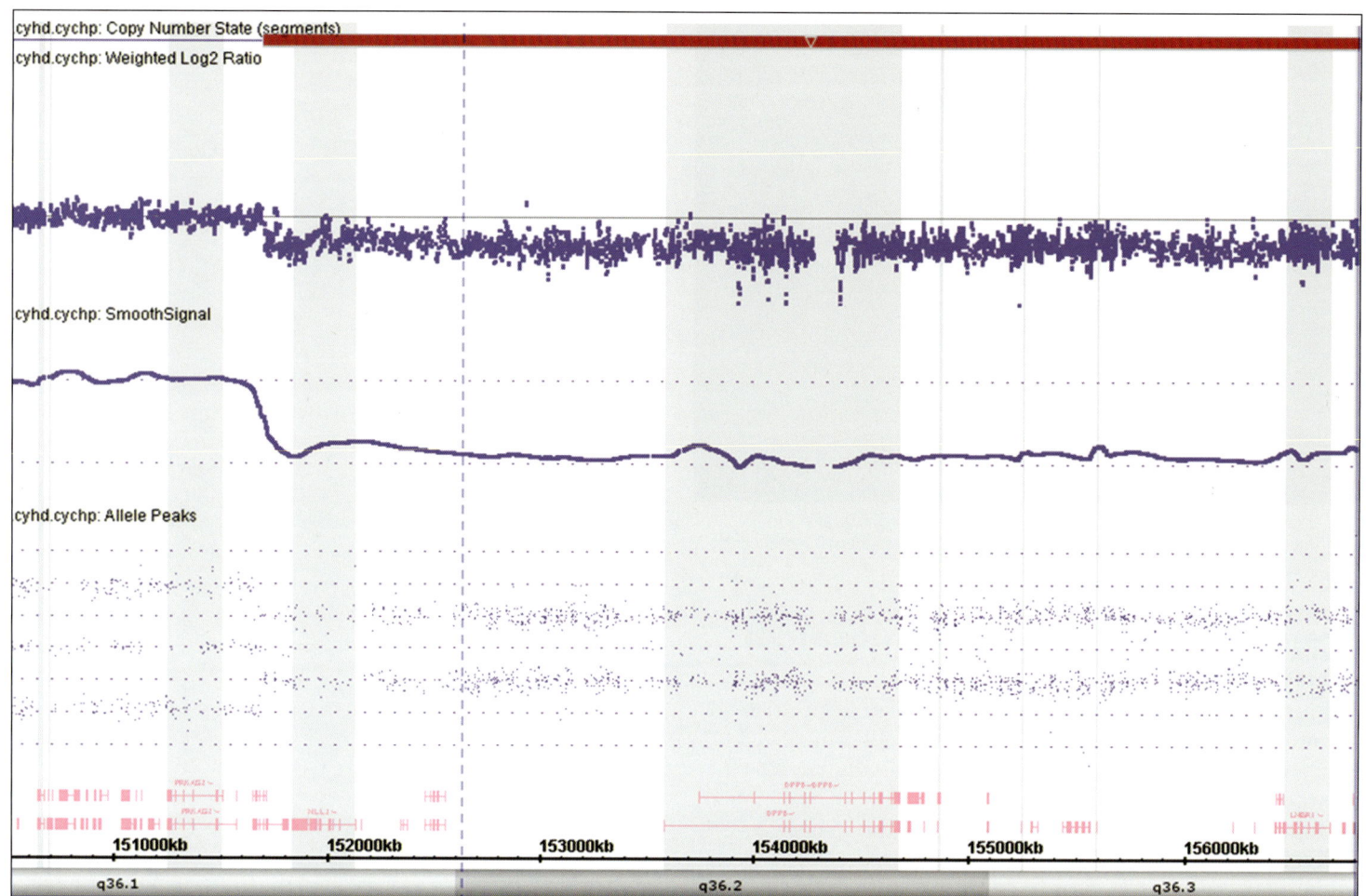

f3.5 Genomic microarray analysis of DNA extracted from cultured amniocytes detects a 7.4 Mb deletion of the terminal region of chromosome 7 (7q36.1 to 7q36.3; chr7: 151697825-159119707) that includes the gene SHH associated with holoprosencephaly. The clinical indication for this study was an abnormal ultrasound with findings of holoprosencephaly and absent corpus callosum. The deletion (red bar) is indicated by a shift in the weighted log2 ratio and a drop of the smooth signal (copy number) from 2 copies to 1 copy of the distal chromosome 7 long arm. The allele (SNP) peaks track for most of the chromosome shows 3 tracks for the presence of heterozygosity (AA, AB, BB). In the region of the deletion (hemizygous) there is only one allele (A or B), so only 2 tracks are indicated. The last track (in pink) shows the genes in the region. Affymetrix CytoScan HD array and CHAS software.

cells may have maternal white blood cells present that can negatively interfere with DNA based tests. Maternal cell contamination due to maternal white blood cells is not generally of concern for cells grown in culture as these do not attach to the culture dish surface and are generally eliminated when the culture media is changed. As additional testing usually requires more cells, or follows routine chromosome analysis, subculturing may be necessary to expand the number of cells. A potential risk of subculturing is the expansion of any maternal fibroblasts that may be present.

Indications for invasive prenatal testing include
1. advanced maternal age (35 years or greater)
2. abnormal noninvasive prenatal testing results (biochemical or cell free DNA testing)
3. abnormal ultrasound findings
4. a parent (or parents) that carry a balanced chromosome abnormality
5. a previous child with a chromosome abnormality
6. an increased risk for a single gene and/or metabolic disorder

There are now a large number of single gene conditions that may be detected prenatally. Testing for metabolic disorders may still need to be performed antenatally based on quantitation of metabolites if the gene, or the mutation specific to the family, has not been identified.

Most indications for prenatal chromosome diagnosis have been based on the risk for a whole chromosome abnormality (aneuploidy) and other large structural chromosome rearrangements. The development and widespread implementation of chromosomal microarray analysis (CMA) in postnatal patients with indications of multiple congenital anomalies, intellectual disability, developmental delays, or autism has revealed a whole new level of submicroscopic anomalies **f3.5** [PMID 21841781]. This significantly increases the diagnostic yield from 2-3% due to whole chromosome aneuploidies and large rearrangements to a 10-15% abnormal detection rate of clinically significant copy number changes, and has led to CMA replacing routine G banded chromosome analysis as a first tier test for most postnatal studies [PMID 20466091]. A large prenatal study demonstrated that CMA also improves the detection rate of clinically significant abnormalities above the common aneuploidies in the prenatal population [PMID 23215555]. The detection rates were increased by 1.5% in women of

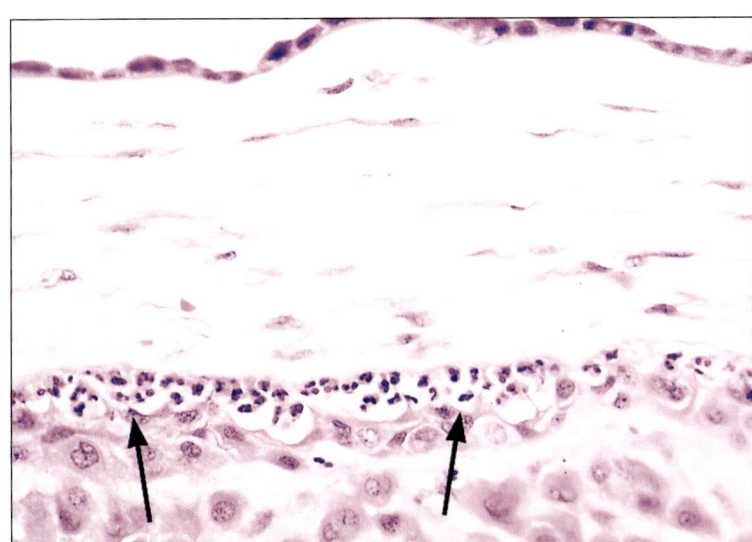

i3.10 Chorioamnionitis. The histologic diagnosis is made by finding polymorphonuclear leukocytes between the amnion & chorion of the membranes (arrows; H&E stain).

advanced maternal age and in those with abnormal noninvasive prenatal testing by biochemical screening and by 6% in those with abnormal ultrasound [PMID 23215555]. Thus, noninvasive screening programs that detect large chromosome anomalies (eg, aneuploidies) and routine prenatal chromosome analysis do not address these additional submicroscopic pathogenic copy number variants detected by CMA [PMID 23168792]. The American College of Obstetricians and Gynecologists recommends that 1) women undergoing an invasive prenatal procedure with a fetus that has structural anomalies detected by ultrasound have CMA and 2) women with a structurally normal fetus undergoing an invasive prenatal procedure have either karyotyping or CMA [PMID 24264715].

Microbiologic examination

Infections of the amniotic space are relatively common, complicating 1-2% of pregnancies [PMID 9067792].

Premature rupture of membranes and prolonged labor are the risk factors considered most significant for developing chorioamnionitis i3.10 due to ascending bacterial invasion of the amniotic fluid [PMID 21672080]. Cesarean sections are often performed on a prophylactic basis in cases of premature rupture of membranes and labor that fails to progress to avoid such complications, though it is not clear that this reduces neonatal infection rates [PMID 16437525].

Amniotic fluid may be collected passively during labor or via amniocentesis for infectious disease testing. Specimens should be collected in anaerobic transport tubes and maintained at room temperature. If chorioamnionitis is suspected, then Gram stain and culture are the standard diagnostic tools used to identify the infection. The cytocentrifuged Gram stain should be used to improve sensitivity (see Chapter 2), as the bacterial burden (like other sterile body fluids) may be low in amniotic fluid. In the case of a patient in active labor, the Gram stain may provide the only timely clinical information that can be used to refine empiric therapy. Typically, antimicrobial therapy is broad and covers aerobic Gram negative and Gram positive organisms, as well as anaerobes, since the laboratory results are typically not available for either the stain or culture before empiric therapy is started [PMID 21672080].

The spectrum of bacteria found in amniotic fluid is quite wide, including Gram positive and Gram negative aerobes and anaerobes, as well as cell wall deficient bacteria (eg, *Mycoplasma* and *Ureaplasma*) [PMID 22137615]. The latter are problematic for primary Gram stain, as they do not retain crystal violet or safranin, and will not be readily detected. Cultures should be set up for routine aerobic bacteria as well as anaerobic bacteria using nonselective media such as a routine blood based agar as well as chocolate agar (to enhance recovery of fastidious organisms). Culture of *Mycoplasma* and *Ureaplasma* requires specific media for growth (eg, A7, A8) and collection (viral/universal transport media or a *Mycoplasma/Ureaplasma* specific medium) and culture is insensitive, despite being the gold standard [PMID 23587772]. The time to growth may also take up to a week or more, limiting the clinical utility of this culture in guiding patient management. Due to the difficulties with culture, *Mycoplasma* and *Ureaplasma* are often not considered in culture orders, but should always be considered in the differential diagnosis and treated empirically [PMID 23587772]. Molecular detection of genital *Mycoplasma* species and *Ureaplasma* may alleviate the turnaround time limitations, but it is only performed in limited reference laboratories [PMID 23587772].

Molecular studies have shown that many anaerobes that have been identified as pathogens of the amniotic space cannot easily be recovered even under routine anaerobic culture conditions using anaerobic transport media. The true breadth and magnitude of these infections is not currently well defined. Molecular studies have shown that fastidious organisms such as *Sneathia sanguinigenes* and *Leptotrichia* species can be present in amniotic fluid, but are unable to be cultured using standard media and anaerobic atmosphere [PMID 22137615, PMID 7548574, PMID 18971361]. The 2 closely related genera have been associated with preterm labor and fetal demise, making their detection all the more important [PMID 18971361, PMID 17522272]. Currently there is no commercially available assay available that provides molecular detection of these or other fastidious anaerobes. For this reason, empiric therapy typically includes metronidazole to cover the majority of anaerobes, irrespective of whether they are expected to be identified in culture or not.

Vertically transmitted infections

There are several vertically transmitted infections that can cause significant developmental defects, fetal distress, spontaneous abortion, and fetal demise t3.3. These pathogens include (but are not limited to) human cytomegalovirus (CMV), *Toxoplasma gondii*, human herpes simplex viruses (HSV) 1 & 2, rubella virus, parvovirus B19, certain enteroviruses, human immunodeficiency virus, syphilis, certain hepatitis viruses, and bacteria (such as group B streptococci [GBS], enteric Gram negative rods, and *Listeria*). Many of these infections are initially tested by serological markers via specific detection of IgM antibodies in serum collected during the acute phase of symptoms, or by demonstrating seroconversion of IgG in paired sera appropriately collected at least 2 weeks apart. In the case of CMV, IgG avidity testing is also useful to more accurately detect seroconversion and estimate a more discrete time of acquisition [PMID 9086155]. Because CMV is very prevalent, and many individuals are IgG seropositive, determining the time in which seroconversion occurred is paramount to gauging the relevance of these antibodies to pregnancy. If the serological pattern is suspicious for acute or recent acquisition, then testing of the amniotic fluid by a highly specific molecular assay may be indicated in some cases [PMID 22275111].

t3.3 Vertically transmitted infections of clinical concern during pregnancy

Bacteria	Viruses	Parasites
Brucella abortus	Enteroviruses	Toxoplasma gondii
Chlamydia trachomatis	Hepatitis B, C, and E	
Enteric Gram negative rods (eg, E coli, Citrobacter, Enterobacter)	Human cytomegalovirus	
Group B streptococci	Human herpes simplex virus 1 & 2	
Listeria monocytogenes	Human immunodeficiency virus	
Neisseria gonorrheae	Human papillomavirus	
Mycoplasma species	Parvovirus B19	
Treponema pallidum	Rubella virus	

In the event that an amniocentesis is performed as standard of care, the specimen can be used to interrogate for the pathogens specifically indicated by serological assays. CMV and *Toxoplasma* have been studied extensively for detection of the pathogens in amniotic fluid, while other organisms described are not readily tested for by PCR, but may be under specific consultation by an infectious disease specialist [PMID 22275111]. These assays are typically research use only assays, and should be appropriately validated for use on amniotic fluid. Consultation with the laboratory is imperative to determine what collection media/tube/temperature combination is validated for the assay. In the case of GBS PCR, one study demonstrated superior detection of GBS in amniotic fluid from women with premature rupture of membranes vs culture [PMID 23390279]. The GBS PCR, unlike culture, can be performed and resulted in only a few hours; however it is unclear whether this test would provide sufficient evidence to warrant not treating for GBS despite a negative test result since the therapy is relatively benign and provides significant protection against GBS mediated neonatal sepsis.

Artifacts & pitfalls

- The presence of blood, urine, cervical mucus & noninfectious leukorrhea can give a false positive fern test
- Contamination of amniotic fluid with fetal blood can result in elevated AFP and detectable ACheE
- In light of Doppler ultrasonography as a noninvasive method, the use of amniocentesis to determine the ΔOD450 result is nearly obsolete
- Contamination of the amniotic fluid specimen with whole blood can cause, paradoxically, a decrease in LBC
- Presence of meconium causes false increase in LBC

Key points

- Clinical tests are performed on amniotic fluid for
  - prenatal genetic testing
  - determining fetal lung maturity
  - identifying infection
  - determining the degree of fetal hemolytic anemia
  - testing for open neural tube defects
  - evaluating the integrity of fetal membranes.
- Amniotic fluid cells may be used for the rapid detection of aneuploidy detection by fluorescence in situ hybridization or by quantitative PCR following DNA extraction
- Microbiologic test results are crucial for directing pathogen specific therapy; however, empiric therapy is required in cases of PROM

References

PMID 11165603 Neerhof MG, Dohnal JC, Ashwood ER et al [2001] Lamellar body counts: a consensus on protocol. *Obstet Gynecol* 97(2):318-320

PMID 12220785 Moise KJ [2002] Management of rhesus alloimmunization in pregnancy. *Obstet Gynecol* 100(3):600-611

PMID 15915088 Bradley LA, Palomaki GE, McDowell GA, ONTD Working Group, ACMG Laboratory Quality Assurance Committee [2005] Technical standards and guidelines: prenatal screening for open neural tube defects. *Genet Med* 7(5):355-369

PMID 1609805 Klinger K, Landes G, Shook D et al [1992] Rapid detection of chromosome aneuploidies in uncultured amniocytes by using fluorescence in situ hybridization (FISH). *Am J Hum Genet* 51(1):55-65

PMID 1609805 Klinger K, Landes G, Shook D et al [1992] Rapid detection of chromosome aneuploidies in uncultured amniocytes by using fluorescence in situ hybridization (FISH). *Am J Hum Genet* 51(1):55-65

PMID 16303123 Grenache DG, Gronowski AM [2006] Fetal lung maturity. *Clin Biochem* 39(1):1-10

PMID 16437525 Dare MR, Middleton P, Crowther CA et al [2006] Planned early birth versus expectant management (waiting) for prelabour rupture of membranes at term (37 weeks or more). *Cochrane Database Syst Rev* (1):CD005302

PMID 16837679 Oepkes D, Seaward PG, Vandenbussche FPHA et al [2006] Doppler ultrasonography versus amniocentesis to predict fetal anemia. *New Engl J Med* 355(2):156-164

PMID 17400872 ACOG Committee on Practice Bulletins-Obstetrics [2007] ACOG Practice Bulletin No. 80: premature rupture of membranes. Clinical management guidelines for obstetrician-gynecologists. *Obstet Gynecol* 109(4), 1007–1019

PMID 17522272 *J Clin Microbiol* Thilesen CM, Nicolaidis M, Lökebö JE et al [2007] *Leptotrichia amnionii*, an emerging pathogen of the female urogenital tract. *J Clin Microbiol* 45(7):2344-7

PMID 18055749 American College of Obstetricians and Gynecologists [2007] ACOG Practice Bulletin No. 88, Invasive prenatal testing for aneuploidy. *Obstet Gynecol* 110(6):1459-1467

PMID 18971361 Han YW, Shen T, Chung P et al [2009] Uncultivated bacteria as etiologic agents of intra-amniotic inflammation leading to preterm birth. *J Clin Microbiol* 47(1):38-47

PMID 20466091 Miller DT [2010] Consensus statement: chromosomal microarray is a first-tier clinical diagnostic test for individuals with developmental disabilities or congenital anomalies. *Am J Hum Genet* 86(5):749-764

PMID 20716798 Lockwood CM, Crompton JC, Riley JK et al [2010] Validation of lamellar body counts using 3 hematology analyzers. *Am J Clin Pathol* 134(3):420-428

PMID 21037283 Zipursky A, Paul VK [2011] The global burden of Rh disease. *Arch Dis Child Fetal Neonatal Ed* 96(2):F84-5

PMID 2130841 Isada NB, Koppitch FC 3rd, Johnson MP et al [1990] Does the color of amniotic fluid still matter? *Fetal Diagn Ther* 5(3-4):165-167

PMID 21672080 Czikk MJ, McCarthy FP, Murphy KE [2011] Chorioamnionitis: from pathogenesis to treatment. *Clin Microbiol Infect* 17(9):1304-11

PMID 21841781 Cooper GM et al [2011] A copy number variation morbidity map of developmental delay. *Nat Genet* 43(9):838-846

PMID 22137615 DiGiulio DB [2012] Diversity of microbes in amniotic fluid. *Semin Fetal Neonatal Med* 17(1):2-11

PMID 22275111 Adams LL, Gungor S, Turan S et al [2012] When are amniotic fluid viral PCR studies indicated in prenatal diagnosis? *Prenat Diagn* 32(1):88-93

PMID 22467160 Mann K, Ogilvie CM [2012] QF-PCR: application, overview and review of the literature. *Prenat Diagn* 32(4):309-314

PMID 23000696 van der Ham DP, van Teeffelen ASP, Mol BWJ [2012] Prelabour rupture of membranes: overview of diagnostic methods. *Curr Opin Obstet Gynecol* 24(6):408-412

PMID 23168792 ACOG [2012] Committee opinion no 545: noninvasive prenatal testing for fetal aneuploidy, *Obstet Gynecol* 120(6):1532-1534

PMID 23215555 Wapner RJ [2012] Chromosomal microarray versus karyotyping for prenatal diagnosis, *N Engl J Med* 367(23):2175-2184

PMID 23314505 Ramsauer B, Vidaeff AC, Hösli I et al [2013] The diagnosis of rupture of fetal membranes (ROM): a meta-analysis. *J Perinat Med* 41(3):233-240

PMID 23390279 Bourgeois-Nicolaos N, Cordier AG, Guillet-Caruba C et al [2013] Evaluation of the Cepheid Xpert GBS assay for rapid detection of group B Streptococci in amniotic fluids from pregnant women with premature rupture of membranes. *J Clin Microbiol* 51(4):1305-6

PMID 23587772 Capoccia R, Greub G, Baud D [2013] *Ureaplasma urealyticum, Mycoplasma hominis* and adverse pregnancy outcomes. *Curr Opin Infect Dis* 26(3):231-40

PMID 24264715 American College of Obstetricians and Gynecologists [2013] Committee opinion no. 581: the use of chromosomal microarray analysis in prenatal diagnosis. *Obstet Gynecol* 122(6):1374-1377

PMID 2483269 Wald N, Cuckle H, Nanchahal K [1989] Amniotic fluid acetylcholinesterase measurement in the prenatal diagnosis of open neural tube defects. Second report of the Collaborative Acetylcholinesterase Study. *Prenat Diagn* 9(12):813-29

PMID 3717234 Zorn EM, Hanson FW, Greve LC et al [1986] Analysis of the significance of discolored amniotic fluid detected at midtrimester amniocentesis. *Am J Obstet Gynecol* 154(6):1234-1240

PMID 4637037 Queenan JT, Thompson W, Whitfield CR et al [1972] Amniotic fluid volumes in normal pregnancies. *Am J Obstet Gynecol* 114(1):34-38

PMID 7126503 Barlow RD, Cuckle HS, Wald NJ et al [1982] False positive gel-acetylcholinesterase results in blood-stained amniotic fluids. *BJOG* 89(10):821-826

PMID 7548574 Hillier SL, Krohn MA, Cassen E et al [1995] The role of bacterial vaginosis and vaginal bacteria in amniotic fluid infection in women in preterm labor with intact fetal membranes. *Clin Infect Dis* 20Suppl2:S276-8

PMID 9067792 Casey BM, Cox SM [1997] Chorioamnionitis and endometritis. *Infect Dis Clin North Am* 11(1):203-22

PMID 9086155 Grangeot-Keros L, Mayaux MJ, Lebon P et al [1997] Value of cytomegalovirus (CMV) IgG avidity index for the diagnosis of primary CMV infection in pregnant women. *J Infect Dis* 175(4):944-6

PMID 9316128 Crandall BF, Chua C [1997] Risks for fetal abnormalities after very and moderately elevated AF-AFPs. *Prenat Diagn* 17(9):837-841

ISBN 978-158829-2704 Gronowski AM [2004] *Handbook of Clinical Laboratory Testing During Pregnancy*. Humana Press; Appendix, t3

CLSI [2011] *Assessment of Fetal Lung Maturity by the Lamellar Body Count; Approved Guideline*. CLSI document C58-A. Clinical and Laboratory Standards Institute

Palmer OM, Grenache DG, Gronowski AM [2007] The NACB Laboratory Medicine Practice Guidelines for Point of Care Reproductive Testing. *Point of Care: The Journal of Near-Patient Testing & Technology* 6(4):265-272

Van Dyke DL [2010] Chapter 4. Amniotic fluid cell culture. In: Milunsky A, Milunsky JM, ed. *Genetic Disorders and the Fetus*, 6e. Wiley-Blackwell, p138-159

3: Amniotic Fluid

Perkins SL, Couturier MR, Grenache DG, Kjeldsberg CR

Cerebrospinal Fluid
Chapter 4

Anatomy & pathophysiology

The brain and spinal cord are protected by 3 meningeal membranes: the dura mater (outermost), arachnoid mater, and pia mater (innermost). Cerebrospinal fluid (CSF) is present in the space between the arachnoid membrane and the pia mater and circulates through this space over the central hemispheres and the spinal cord **f4.1**. The cerebral ventricles are the major CSF containing reservoir. CSF is primarily produced by the choroid plexus found within the lateral, 3rd and 4th brain ventricles by ultrafiltration of plasma and secretion by specialized choroid epithelial cells that have microvilli on the surface into the ventricular spaces. CSF may also be formed outside the choroid plexus in the cerebral subarachnoid spaces, ependymal lining of the ventricles, as well as by the brain parenchyma itself, although these secondary sites are thought to produce much less of the CSF volume than does the choroid plexus [PMID 22100360]. CSF circulates in a consistent manner through the ventricular system through the lateral ventricles to the 3rd ventricle and into the 4th ventricle. Most of the CSF will then flow into the subarachnoid spaces surrounding the brainstem with only a small amount entering into the spinal canal. Impediments to normal CSF circulation, such as cysts or tumors, may lead to hydrocephalus (often termed obstructive hydrocephalus) [PMID 19410151, PMID 22100360, PMID 23832074]. CSF is reabsorbed through the arachnoid villi and arachnoid granulations into the venous sinuses and ultimately into the bloodstream, although some data suggest CSF may also be reabsorbed through capillary walls [PMID 20435061]. Thus, the arachnoid villi form an interface between the CSF and the blood. Blockage of resorption by cellular debris from hemorrhage or infection collecting in the arachnoid villi will also lead to hydrocephalus (often termed communicating hydrocephalus), although the causes of hydrocephalus are often multifactorial and not always easily divided into simple communicating or obstructive subtypes, particularly in children [PMID 23215851, PMID 19410151, PMID 21928018].

Total CSF volumes range from 90-155 mL in an adult, 60-100 mL in children and 10-60 mL in infants. In adults, ~500-650 mL/day or 20-27 mL/hour of CSF is produced and circulated, with largest volumes being produced in the early morning hours. This represents complete replacement of the CSF every 5-6 hours [ISBN 978-141602-9083]. CSF acts as a protective cushion for the central nervous system tissue and protects it from abrupt changes in pressure. It also, by cellular exchange mechanisms, provides a means to collect waste, circulate nutrients and provide a homeostatic environment for nervous tissue. In addition, CSF will act as a buffer between the blood and central nervous system (blood-brain barrier). The blood-brain barrier consists of choroid plexus epithelium as that is in direct contact with the endothelium of capillaries and will regulate the passage of various substances into the brain. Some substances, such as glucose, will diffuse readily into the brain whereas others, including many medications and larger proteins, will be excluded. Average values for the measured normal components of the

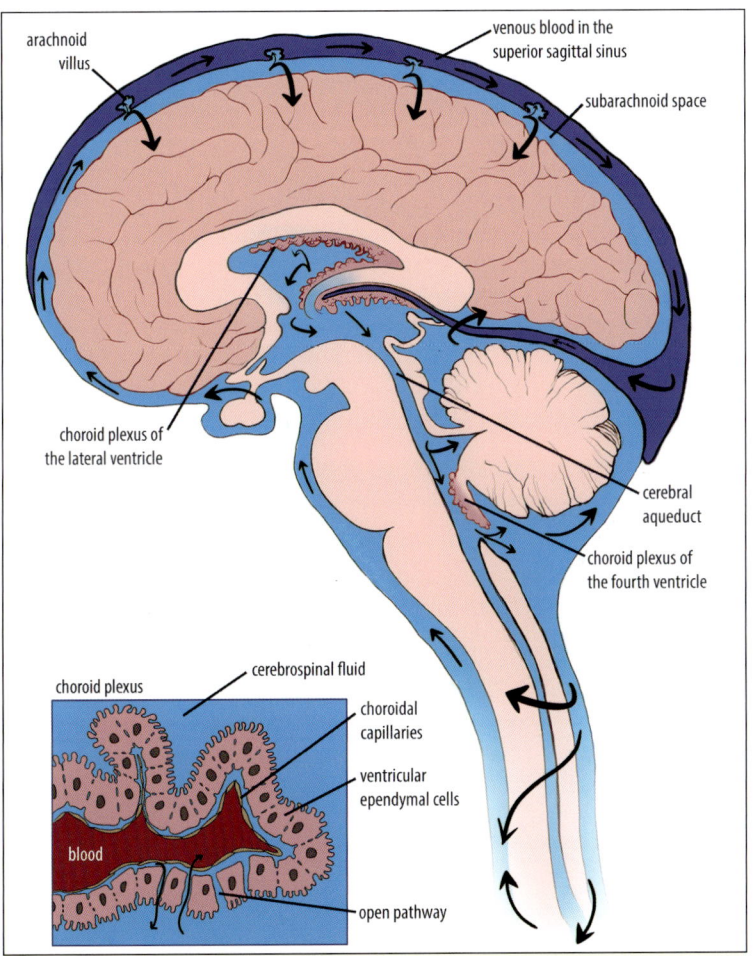

f4.1 Schematic diagram to illustrate the circulation patterns for CSF in the brain and spinal cord; cyan=CSF, red=arterial blood, dark blue=venous blood

CSF compared to plasma are presented in **t4.1**. Breakdown of the blood-brain barrier occurs in a number of pathologic conditions, including inflammation or meningitis, brain tumors and infarction. In these conditions constituents in the blood or brain may leak into the CSF and changes to expected reference values for solutes and other CSF components **t4.2** may be observed [PMID 19664713, PMID 18040800].

t4.1	**Average solute concentrations in CSF & plasma**	
Solute	**Plasma**	**CSF**
Na^+ (mEq/kg)	150.00	147.00
K^+ (mEq/kg)	4.63	2.86
Mg^{2+} (mEq/kg)	1.61	2.23
Ca^{2+} (mEq/kg)	4.70	2.28
Cl^- (mEq/kg)	99.00	113.00
HCO_3^- (mEq/kg)	26.80	23.30
pCO_2 (mm Hg)	35-45	45-50
Total protein (mg/dL)	6987.20	39.20
Glucose (mg/dL)	96.20	59.70
Osmolality (mOsm/kg)	289.00	289.00
pH	7.41	7.31

Adapted from IBSN 978-1-4160-2908-3

t4.2	**Reference values for cerebrospinal fluid**	
Component*	**Conventional units**	**SI units**
Albumin	10-30 mg/dL	100-300 mg/L
Calcium	2.1-2.7 mEq/L	1.05-1.35 mmol/L
Chloride	115-130 mEq/L	115-130 mmol/L
Glucose	50-80 mg/dL	2.75-4.40 mmol/L
Lactate	9-26 mg/dL	1.13-3.23 mmol/L
Lactate dehydrogenase	0-25 U/L at 37°C	NA
Leukocyte count: adults[†]	0-5 mononuclear cells/µL	$0-0.005 \times 10^9$/L
Leukocyte count: neonates	0-30 mononuclear cells/µL	$0-0.0030 \times 10^9$/L

Data partially adapted with permission from Krieg AF, Kjeldsberg CR ; except where noted, reference values apply to adults; NA = not applicable
*Reliable values for most enzymes have not yet been established.
[†]Children have intermediate leukocyte values >20/µL the 1st year of life & >10/µL until adolescence

Clinical indications & recommended laboratory studies

The indications for performing a lumbar puncture and examination of the CSF can be divided into 4 major categories: suspected meningeal infection, subarachnoid hemorrhage, malignancy and demyelinating diseases **t4.3**. CSF examination, including morphologic, chemical and/or microbiologic studies, is often used to identify and diagnose specific conditions. In addition, lumbar puncture may provide an avenue for introducing treatment.

The identification of infectious causes of meningitis/meningoencephalitis, particularly bacterial meningitis, is one of the most important indications for CSF examination and requires collection of materials for cultures or molecular testing to make a definitive diagnosis. The specificity and sensitivity of CSF examination for other conditions, such as identification of malignancy or hemorrhage is less, and the use of imaging techniques may obviate the need for CSF examination to make a diagnosis in many cases. Chemical analysis of CSF, including testing for markers of demyelinating diseases, will often provide supportive evidence of a clinical diagnosis or help to exclude other differential diagnostic considerations [PMID 3520526, PMID 22278331, PMID 16545048].

t4.3	**Indications for lumbar puncture**
Suspected conditions	
Infections: bacterial, viral, fungal, parasitic Meningitis, encephalitis, syphilis	
Tumors Acute leukemia or lymphoma Primary CNS tumors Metastatic disease	
Demyelinating disorders Multiple sclerosis, Guillame-Barré syndrome	
Subarachnoid hemorrhage	
Therapy	
Intrathecal chemotherapy for malignancies	
Intrathecal antibiotics for infections	
Introduction of anesthesia	
Introduction of contrast materials for radiology	
Removal of fluid to relieve pressure or blood from hemorrhage	

Based on differential diagnostic considerations and clinical scenario, the recommended tests for cerebrospinal fluid will differ. **t4.4** identifies those laboratory tests that should be routinely performed in all CSF examinations. Other testing should be utilized, as appropriate or clinically indicated, to address specific differential diagnostic considerations **t4.4**. It should be noted that CSF examination and specific testing has varying sensitivities and specificities with regards to establishing a diagnosis **t4.5**. For example, when infection is suspected, appropriate staining for organisms and cytologic examination, cultures and tests for bacterial and fungal antigens or DNA testing becomes essential to diagnosis. In viral infections, the morphologic examination of CSF may allow exclusion of bacterial or fungal infection and new technologies, such as PCR for viral species, may allow for definitive diagnosis (as discussed later).

t4.4	**Laboratory tests on cerebrospinal fluid**
Routine	
Opening CSF pressure	
Cell count (total & differential)	
Glucose (CSF:plasma ratio)	
Protein	
When indicated	
Cultures (bacteria, fungi, viruses, *Mycobacterium tuberculosis*)	
Stains (Gram stain, acid-fast stain on cytospin)	
Fungal, bacterial, viral & parasitic serologies	
Molecular testing (polymerase chain reaction) for bacteria, fungi & viruses	
Cytology	
Protein electrophoresis	
Myelin basic protein	
Fibrin derivative D-dimer	

t4.5	Diseases detected by routine laboratory examination of CSF
High sensitivity, high specificity	
Bacterial, tuberculous, & fungal meningitis, some causes of viral meningitis	
High sensitivity, moderate specificity	
Some causes of viral meningitis	
Subarachnoid hemorrhage	
Multiple sclerosis	
Central nervous system syphilis	
Infectious polyneuritis	
Paraspinal abscess	
Moderate sensitivity, high specificity	
Meningeal malignancy (either primary or metastatic)	
Moderate sensitivity, moderate specificity	
Intracranial hemorrhage	
Viral encephalitis	
Subdural hematoma	

Sensitivity = the ability of a test to detect disease when it is present
Specificity = the ability of a test to exclude disease when it is not present

Specimen collection, requirements & stability

Obtaining CSF for purposes of diagnostic examination requires proper collection and processing in order to obtain the optimal samples to provide required diagnostic information. It is essential that a sufficient amount of CSF is collected to allow for performance of desired laboratory testing, and appropriate clinical information should also be submitted to the laboratory [PMID 16545048, PMID 22278331]. In addition, the differential diagnostic considerations and specific features associated with the collection procedure (eg, traumatic tap) may alter the sample collection strategy or volumes of samples collected. Therefore, it is essential that a clear sample collection strategy, as well as mechanisms for expeditiously handling and testing the specimen, be determined before specimen collection is initiated [PMID 3520526, PMID 22278331, ISBN 978-141602-9083].

Cerebrospinal fluid may be collected by a variety of procedures. Most commonly, CSF is collected by lumbar puncture. In addition, use of cisternal, lateral cervical puncture, external ventricular drainage and collection of CSF from shunts or ventricular cannulas may also be utilized [ISBN 978-141602-9083]. Collection of CSF requires understanding of the underlying anatomy and patient positioning as has been well described. Before a lumbar puncture is performed, optic fundi should be examined for evidence of increased intracranial pressure. If increased intracranial pressure is present, additional care must be utilized to prevent the possibility of cerebral herniation when CSF is removed. In most cases, CSF is removed from a needle that is inserted in the L3 to L4, L4 to L5 or L5 to S1 vertebral interspaces to ensure that the needle enters below the level of the conus medullaris of the spinal cord to minimize possible spinal cord injury from the procedure [PMID 3520526, PMID 22278331, ISBN 978-14162-9083].

Before the needle is inserted, the overlying skin must be thoroughly cleansed to remove the possibility of cutaneous bacterial flora contamination. Cutaneous or subcutaneous infection over the site of a lumbar puncture may require use of an alternative sampling site to remove the risk of possible introduction of infection into the spinal cord or brain [PMID 3520526, PMID 16871073, PMID 9168230]. After the needle has been inserted and before fluid is withdrawn, a manometer with a 3 way stopcock should be connected to measure the opening pressure. The normal opening pressure is 90-180 mm in adults when the patient is in a lateral position, but may be slightly higher when in a prone or sitting position [PMID 17101909, PMID 23064593]. The opening pressure may also be lower in older adults [PMID 23300737]. The closing pressure should be ~10-30 mm less than the opening pressure. Small, transient changes in the pressure are noted with coughing, straining or breathing [PMID 17101909]. Normal opening pressures are lower in infants and young children t4.6 [PMID 20818852, PMID 21907885]. These changes indicate the patency of the channels through which the CSF flows and variations are considered normal. The CSF pressure may be increased or decreased in a variety of disorders t4.7 [PMID 12870112, PMID 22278331].

t4.6	Normal range of CSF pressures
Age (months)	Pressure (mmH$_2$O)
0-1	10-14
1-24	20-70
25-72	40-100
Adult	90-180

t4.7	Causes of CSF pressure changes
Increased pressure	
Mass lesion (abscess, tumor, cerebral hemorrhage)	
Meningitis	
Cerebral edema	
Impairment of CSF absorption	
Thrombosis of venous sinuses	
Superior vena cava obstruction	
Hypo-osmolality	
Congestive heart failure	
Decreased pressure	
Spinal-subarachnoid block	
Dehydration	
Circulatory collapse	
CSF leakage	

If the opening pressure is normal, at least 20 mL of CSF can be removed without injury to the patient. If the opening pressure is >200 mm, no more than 2 mL of fluid should be removed to minimize the possibility of herniation. Lumbar puncture is a safe procedure when performed by an experienced practitioner utilizing standard methods and techniques [PMID 22278331, PMID 3520526]. Contraindications to performance of a lumbar puncture include infection of the skin or soft tissues overlying the site of puncture, coagulopathy or an intracranial space occupying brain lesion that results in a midline shift or increased pressure of the contents on the posterior fossa [PMID 3520526]. Use of alternative means of accessing CSF may be necessary, such as puncture at the cervical medullary junction in the C1 to C2 interspace when there is localized infection or a known spinal tumor. Cervical punctures have a higher risk of direct injury to the brain or vertebral artery. CSF may also be collected from catheters and shunts that are utilized for drainage of patients with communicating hydrocephalus or idiopathic intracranial hypertension [ISBN 978-141602-9083, PMID 12870112].

Careful thought should always be given to the types of specimens to be collected, as well as the volumes that will be necessary for performance of the desired assays. Before specimens are collected, any specimen that requires special handling or immediate processing should also be identified so that the sample may be processed to avoid degradation or morphologic changes to cells. Most CSF samples should undergo a minimum level of analysis that includes documentation of the opening pressure, cell counts and differentials in the 3rd tube collected, determination of glucose and protein concentrations and possible collection of tubes for culture, if clinically indicated. A serum glucose measurement should also be taken within an hour of the lumbar puncture so that the CSF serum:glucose ratio can be calculated. In addition to this standard analysis, the differential diagnostic considerations and patient profile should determine the choices of additional studies to be performed [ISBN 978-143770-9742, PMID 3520526, PMID 22278331, PMID 12870112]. As noted previously, most CSF examinations are performed to work up possible infections, tumor, suspected neuroimmunologic or demyelinating disorders, or hemorrhage t4.3.

The most common complication of lumbar puncture is headache occurring in 10%-25% of patients [PMID 22511093, PMID 20807248, PMID 20533959]. Other potential complications include brain herniation, bleeding, infection, backache, or nerve injury [PMID 22111091, PMID 22278331]. Bleeding may occur from trauma to blood vessels in the spinal canal, also termed traumatic tap. This will be manifested as blood in the spinal fluid and is usually minor and self limited. However, in patients who have coagulopathy, severe thrombocytopenia or who are receiving anticoagulants, the risk of bleeding is markedly increased and may cause a spinal subarachnoid hematoma or possible epidural or subdural bleeding [PMID 22111091, PMID 19775301]. Brain herniation in the presence of an elevated intracranial pressure is the most serious complication of lumbar puncture. Herniation is more likely to occur in at risk patients who have a pre-existing obstruction in the normal CSF pathways connecting the cranial compartment and the spinal compartment. This is most likely to occur with tumors and most patients will have evidence of increased intracranial pressure and possible papilledema of the optic fundi [PMID 22111091, PMID 11985377]. Herniation has been reported rarely in patients with meningitis, particularly bacterial meningitis [PMID 17712055]. If a marked fall in pressure occurs after removing 1-2 mm of CSF, cerebellar herniation or spinal cord compression above the puncture site may be suspected. At that time, no additional fluid should be removed.

Typically, CSF specimens are usually divided into 3-4 serially collected sterile tubes. Care should be taken to collect sufficient volumes of CSF for the testing desired t4.8.

t4.8 Volumes of CSF needed for testing

Test	Sample volume
Chemical analysis (including glucose & protein)	1-3 mL
Oligoclonal bands, myelin basic protein, IgG index,* angiotensin converting enzyme	0.5 mL per test
Bacterial Gram stain & culture	Minimum of 1 mL usually 3-5 mL
Viral polymerase chain reaction testing	1 mL per viral polymerase chain reaction test
Acid-fast bacteria smear & culture	5 mL
Cell count & differential	1-3 mL
Flow cytometry & cytopathology	Minimum of 5 mL, preferably 5-10 mL

*Measurement of an IgG index requires that a paired serum sample accompany the CSF specimen

Glass tubes should be avoided because of cell adhesion to the glass, which will affect cell counts and differential. The typical order of tube collection, as outlined in Chapter 2, will collect samples for all testing that may be necessary. Typically, the 1st tube collects a sample for chemistry and immunology studies, the 2nd tube for microbiologic studies and the 3rd tube for cell count and differential. Additional tubes for cytologic or other specialized studies may also be inserted at the 3rd or 4th positions. However, the clinical scenario and reason for the lumbar puncture should always be kept in mind, and the order of tubes may vary based on the clinical requirements for that specific patient. For example, in a staging lumbar puncture for acute lymphoblastic leukemia, the collection of adequate sample for cell count and differential as well as possible collection of additional materials for specialized testing, such as flow cytometric immunophenotyping, is the primary goal and collection of materials for microbiologic testing is usually not required. If malignancy is suspected and cytopathology and flow cytometry are desired, a minimum of 5 additional mL of CSF should be collected and more volume is often preferable. Tube 2 is usually collected for microbiologic studies. Because of concerns about contamination with skin flora, microbiologic studies should never be performed on the first tube collected. The volumes required for microbiologic studies are quite variable and, depending on the differential diagnostic considerations, up to 10-15 mL may need to be collected. Testing for neurological diseases by analysis of oligoclonal bands, myelin basic protein, immunoglobulin levels and angiotensin converting enzyme (ACE) requires 1-2 additional mL to be collected when a demyelinating or neuroimmunologic disorder is suspected in the initial chemistry tube. It is important that samples that address the most important differential diagnostic consideration should be collected initially. If there is gross hemorrhage (traumatic tap, bloody tap), then the initial tube is not suitable for chemistry or cell counts without comparison to a later tube collected when bleeding has lessened or abated to allow for correction of values due to peripheral blood contamination. Communication with the laboratory regarding testing volumes, the impact on peripheral blood contamination on testing and appropriate samples to collect to address the diagnostic concerns prior to performance of the lumbar puncture will ensure optimal collection and use of samples. All specimens should be delivered to the laboratory and

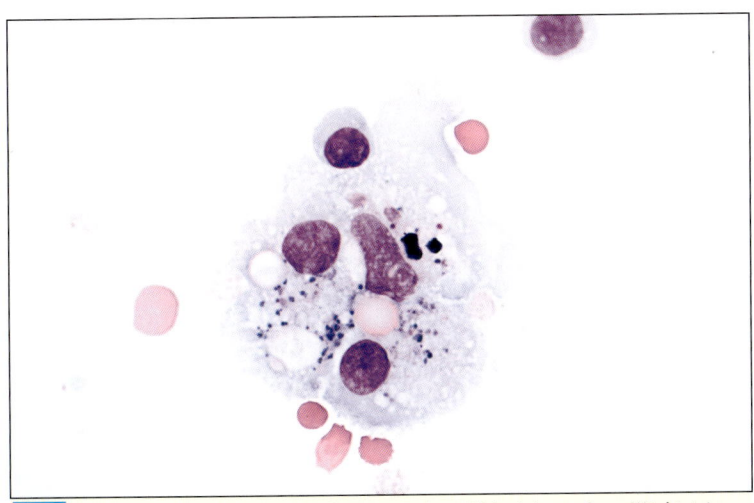

i4.1 Erythrophagocytosis in CSF macrophage in a patient with brain hemorrhage. Wright stain.

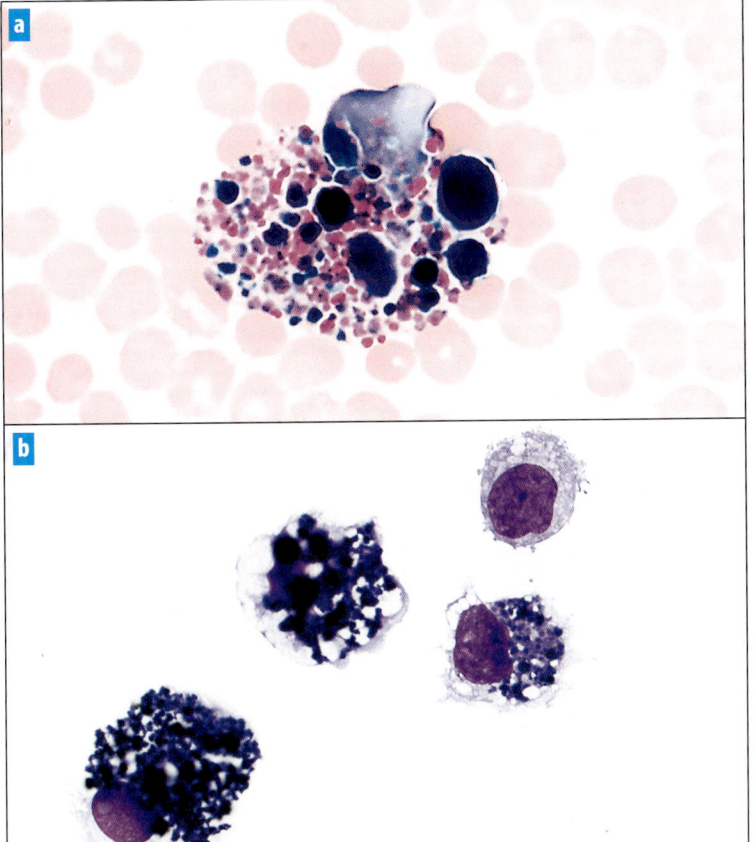

i4.2 **a** Macrophage containing hemosiderin. Wright stain.
b Multiple macrophages containing large & small granules of hemosiderin as identified by dark blue granules in a patient with a cerebral hemorrhage. Wright stain.

decrease between the 1st and 3rd collected tubes [PMID 23517256, PMID 12217474]. In a subarachnoid hemorrhage, the degree of hemorrhage will remain constant through all of the collected tubes [PMID 23517256, PMID 23067018]. A pale pink to yellow color (also termed xanthochromia) in the supernatant of centrifuge CSF, erythrophagocytosis i4.1 and evidence of hemosiderin laden macrophages i4.2a-b are all suggestive of subarachnoid hemorrhage. Frequently, the 3 tube test is utilized to distinguish between a subarachnoid hemorrhage and a traumatic tap. Blood counts are performed on 3 sequentially collected tubes of CSF. In a traumatic tap, the red cell count should diminish in each sample. In subarachnoid hemorrhage, the numbers of red cells will be expected to remain relatively constant [ISBN 978-143770-9742, PMID 12217474].

Gross examination

CSF is normally clear and colorless. In the presence of disease, the gross appearance of the fluid may change and the CSF may appear cloudy, turbid, bloody, viscous or clotted t4.9. In addition, it may show evidence of pigment or coloration. Turbidity or cloudiness begins to appear when leukocytes are >200 cells/µL or red cell counts exceed 400 cells/µL. The presence of microorganisms or increased protein levels can also lead to cloudy or turbid appearing CSF [PMID 22278331, PMID 12870112, PMID 11489408].

t4.9	Clinical significance of CSF gross appearance	
Gross appearance	**Cause**	**Major significance**
Crystal clear	Normal	None
Cloudy, turbid	RBCs	Hemorrhage (early, before RBC lysis)
		Traumatic tap
	WBCs	Meningitis
	Microorganisms	Meningitis
	Increased protein	Disorders that affect blood-brain barrier
		Production of IgG within central nervous system
Bloody	RBCs	Hemorrhage
Color (xanthochromia)	Hemoglobin	Old hemorrhage
		Lysed cells from traumatic tap
	Bilirubin	RBC breakdown
		Elevated serum bilirubin
	Carotene	Increased serum levels (dietary)
	Protein	See above
	Melanin	Metastatic malignant melanoma
Oily	X ray material	None
Viscous	Capsular polysaccharide	Cryptococcosis
	Mucus	Metastatic mucin producing carcinomas
	Liquid disc material	Needle injury to annulus fibrosus or ruptured disc
Fat globules	Fat	Fat embolism
Clot formation	Increased fibrinogen	Traumatic tap
		Subarachnoid block (Froin syndrome)
		Suppurative meningitis
		Tuberculous meningitis

RBC = red blood cell; WBC = white blood cell

processed quickly to minimize degradation or morphologic changes to the cells. CSF may be stored in the refrigerator for chemistry and immunology studies but refrigeration may impact sensitivity for microbiologic and morphologic analyses [ISBN 978-143770-9742, PMID 22278331].

A grossly traumatic tap occurs in ~10%-30% of lumbar punctures and some degree of bleeding may be seen in up to 70% of lumbar punctures [ISBN 978-143770-9742, PMID 20577138, PMID 12574013]. It is important to differentiate the red cells present from a traumatic tap from those due to an intracranial or intraspinal hemorrhage. In a traumatic tap, the presence of blood or hemorrhage usually will clear or

Pink to red colored CSF usually indicates the presence of blood, but red cells may be present in colorless CSF also [PMID 18572349]. Presence of blood in the CSF may have resulted from subarachnoid hemorrhage, intracerebral

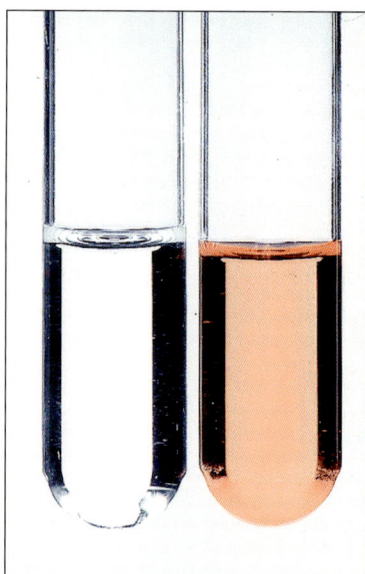
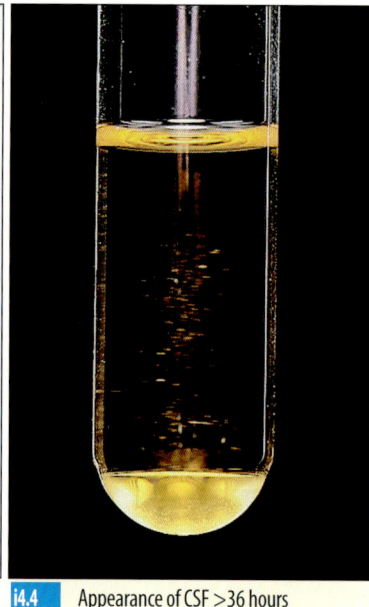

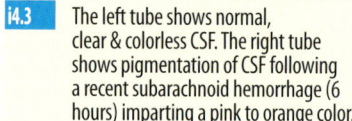

i4.3 The left tube shows normal, clear & colorless CSF. The right tube shows pigmentation of CSF following a recent subarachnoid hemorrhage (6 hours) imparting a pink to orange color.

i4.4 Appearance of CSF >36 hours after a subarachnoid hemorrhage demonstrating pigmentation of the CSF imparting a yellow color due to breakdown of blood components

hemorrhage, infarction or may arise due to a traumatic tap, as discussed above. Identification of decreasing red blood cell counts with the collection of subsequent tubes is suggestive of a traumatic tap [PMID 12217474, PMID 14759953]. However, identification of crenated red blood cells is not useful in differentiating a traumatic tap from pathologic bleeding [PMID 201417]. Frequently, immediate centrifugation of CSF will show clearing of the fluid with a traumatic tap but in a subarachnoid or other hemorrhage, centrifugation will leave a persistent pink or yellow tint (xanthochromia) due to the breakdown of hemoglobin, but this is not a sensitive predictor or differentiator of hemorrhage [PMID 15749414, PMID 18572349, PMID 14759953]. The lysis of red cells will begin within 1-2 hours, so it is important to process CSF specimens for red cell counts as soon as possible to prevent false positive detection of xanthochromia [PMID 11684714]. In addition, previous very bloody traumatic taps may result in coloration of the CSF in subsequent taps when repeated 2-5 days later. Clots may form in CSF where there has been extensive bleeding due to a traumatic tap. However, subarachnoid hemorrhage is usually not associated with clot formation. A variety of microorganisms, including bacteria, fungi and amoeba, can also cause cloudiness of the CSF [PMID 14524396, PMID 16545048, PMID 22278331]. Radiographic contrast material, fat globules or protein levels >150 mg/dL may also produce CSF cloudiness [PMID 11489408].

Usually CSF will have a viscosity that is similar to water. Increased viscosity of CSF may be seen in patients with metastatic mucin producing carcinomas, bacterial meningitis or has been described with release of material from a ruptured intravertebral disc into the CSF [PMID 20689477].

Pigmentation or coloration may also be noted in CSF in situations other than bleeding **t4.10** [PMID 14759953, PMID 1579414, PMID 18572349]. When hemorrhage has occurred, the fluid will have a slight pink or yellow coloration due to accumulation of pigmented compounds from the breakdown of hemoglobin

i4.3, **i4.4**. Other causes of CSF coloration include the presence of pigmented compounds, such as bilirubin or carotenes. CSF coloration may usually be identified by simple visual inspection of the CSF in front of a piece of white paper, but spectrophotometric analysis is a more sensitive method [PMID 11684714, PMID 18572349]. Because the breakdown of hemoglobin requires ~12 hours, the presence of CSF pigmentation without gross blood usually identifies a subarachnoid or intracerebral hemorrhage rather than a traumatic tap [PMID 11684714, PMID 15749414]. Typically, the CSF color changes following a hemorrhage will peak after 36-48 hours and will eventually disappear within 1 week to 10 days. Other pigments seen in the CSF include bilirubin, seen in cases with severe jaundice. Usually CSF will not show a change in color until the total plasma bilirubin reaches 10-50 mg/dL [PMID 20511372]. Patients with very high CSF protein levels (>150 mg/dL) due to bloody traumatic taps or pathologic states, such as spinal blockage, polyneuritis or meningitis, may also have some degree of pigmentation present. Pigmentation of the CSF may also occur in patients who have increased levels of vitamin A (hypervitaminosis A), melanin pigmentation from metastatic melanoma or rifampin antibiotic therapy. Artifactual coloration of the CSF may occur from red cell lysis caused by detergent contamination of the needle or collected tube or delay in CSF analysis for >1 hour without refrigeration of the sample [PMID 14759953, PMID 15749414, PMID 18572349].

t4.10 Causes of CSF pigmentation

Cause	CSF color
Bleeding due to subarachnoid & intracerebral hemorrhage, traumatic tap	Pink, orange, yellow
Jaundice, hyperbilirubinemia	Yellow
Elevated protein level (>150 mg/dL)	Yellow
Hypercarotenemia, hypervitaminosis A	Orange
Meningeal malignant melanoma	Brown
Rifampin therapy	Red-orange

Microscopic examination

Microscopic examination of CSF includes cell counts with a morphologic differential performed on stained smears. Cell counts are important data used for identification of traumatic taps by enumeration of contaminating red blood cell numbers. In addition, observation of increased white cell numbers, termed pleocytosis, is often associated with a variety of disease states. Pleocytosis may be graded as mild (5-50 WBCs/µL), moderate (51-200 WBCs/µL) or marked (>200 WBCs/µL). Because deterioration of cells and body fluid specimens begins within 1-2 hours, cell counts and differentials should be performed as soon as possible. Microscopic examination with appropriate staining will also help to identify infectious agents **i4.5a-c**, crystals, other particles **i4.6**, as well as cellular inclusions **i4.7** that may be seen in CSF [PMID 22278331, PMID 16545048].

4: Cerebrospinal Fluid

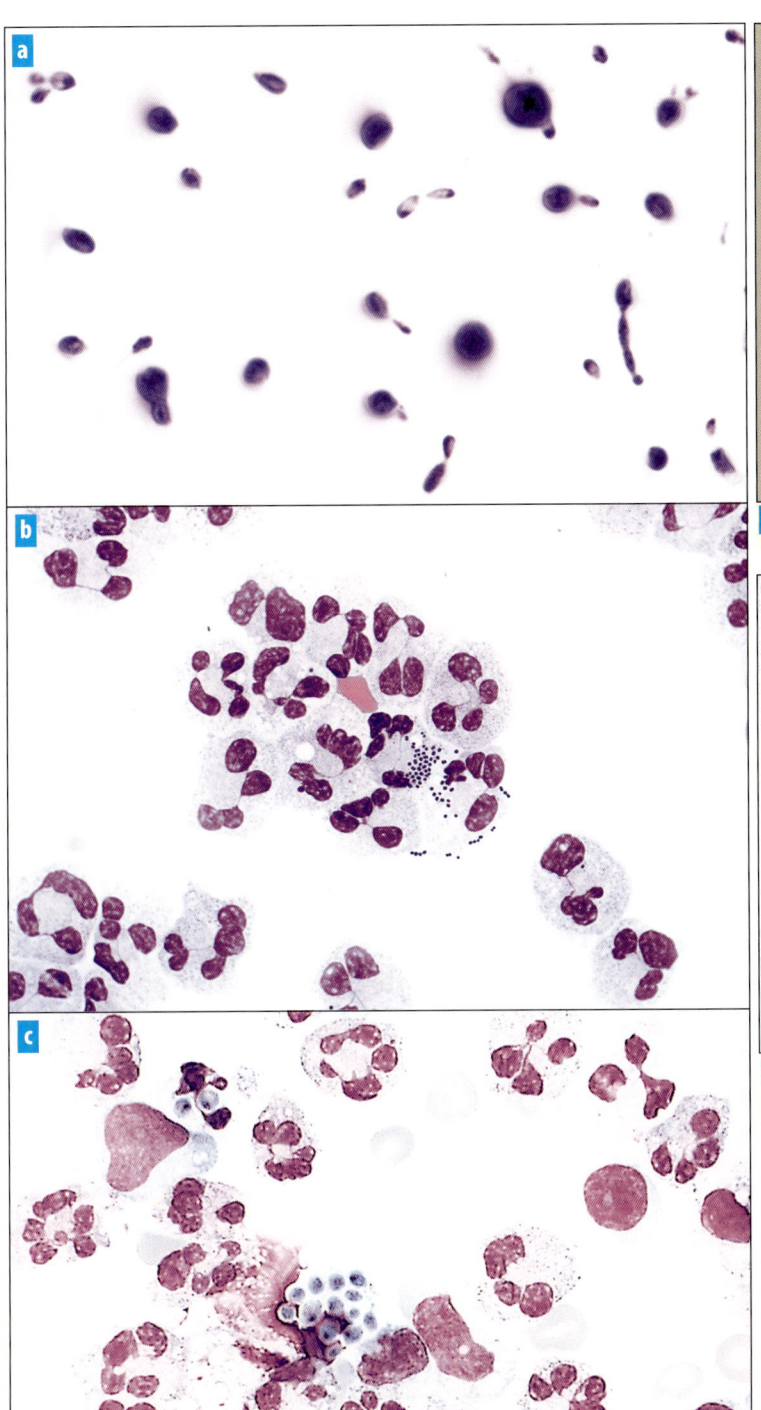

i4.5
a Multiple yeast forms showing linear & budding forms identified in a CSF. Wright stain.
b Patient with bacterial meningitis showing neutrophils ingesting many cocci on Wright stain
c Fungal meningitis with *Candida* yeast in CSF. Wright stain.

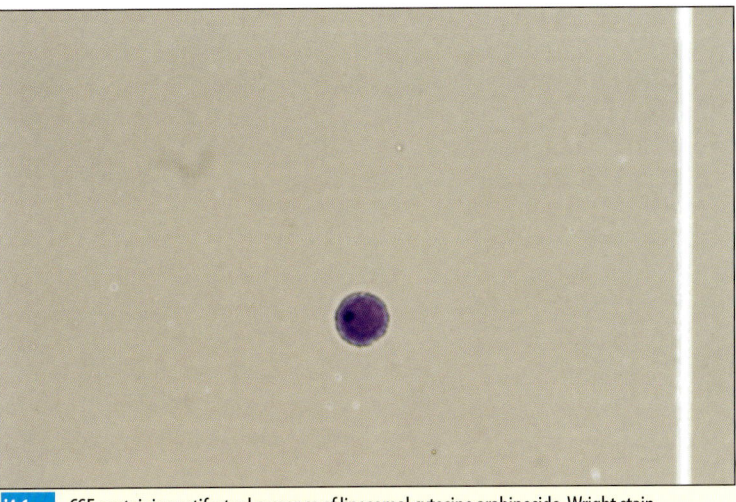

i4.6 CSF containing artifactual presence of liposomal cytosine arabinoside. Wright stain.

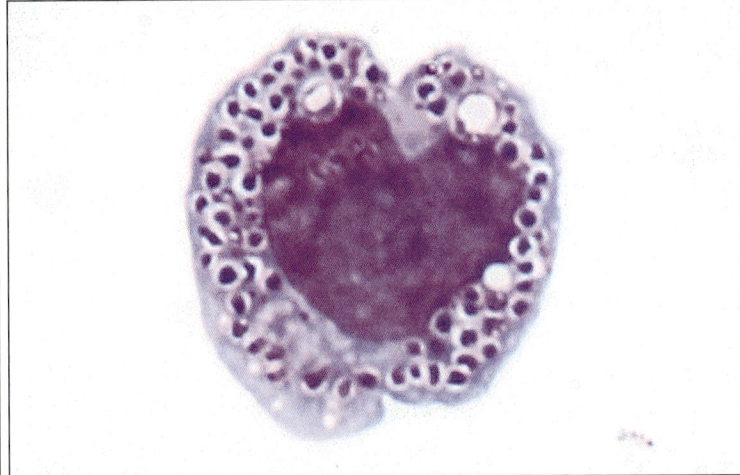

i4.7 Macrophage containing abnormal lysosomal storage products in a patient with Hunter-Hurler disease. Wright stain.

Cell counts

Traditionally, cell counts were performed using undiluted CSF using a manual counting chamber or hemocytometer. Because of the low cell counts present in most CSF samples, use of manual counts may be useful despite the limited precision of this methodology [PMID 21668655]. However, improvements in technology have allowed utilization of automated cell counts and differentials using CBC analyzers and specific analyzers for body fluids [PMID 23089709, PMID 20187854, PMID 15163317]. Limitations due to the low numbers of cells in obtaining accurate enumeration of white blood cells and red cells in CSF continues to be a challenge, and automated methods require careful adherence to the Clinical and Laboratory Standards Institute guidelines (CLSI approved guidelines H56-A, 2006). Automated counting methods also have been shown to be more reproducible and more rapidly obtained than manual counts [PMID 21668655, PMID 20187854], although low cell numbers and technical issues, such as use of red cell lysing agents, may adversely affect accuracy [PMID 20441472].

Care should be taken to mix the CSF specimen well to increase accuracy and reproducibility, but the coefficient of variation observed with manual counting techniques may exceed 50% and approach 15%-25% using automated methods [PMID 21668655, PMID 20187854]. If the CSF is grossly bloody or cloudy due to increased numbers of cells, dilution with saline may be necessary to allow for counting. Red cell numbers are also reported as they may help to identify a possible traumatic tap. Expected normal leukocyte counts will vary with the age of the patient. Leukocyte counts t4.11 range from 0-5 WBC/μL in adults, 0-30 WBC/μL in neonates, with a gradual decrease from neonatal levels to 0-10 WBC/μL in children 5 years of age to puberty. However, there is not good agreement on normal white blood cell reference ranges for children.

t4.11 Normal CSF differential cell count

Cells	Adults	Neonates
Total WBC count	0-5 WBC/μL	0-30 WBC/μL
Lymphocytes	40%-80%	5%-35%
Monocytes	15%-45%	50%-90%
Neutrophils	0%-6%	0%-8%*
Eosinophils	Rare	Rare
Neuroectodermal cells/ependymal cells	Very rare	Rare

Sedimentation or cytocentrifuge methods used & subject to variation. Data adapted with permission from Krieg AF, Kjeldsberg CR [ISBN 978-143770-9742].
*In high risk neonates without meningitis, the CSF may have >60% neutrophils; data from [PMID 2189977]

In normal CSF, RBCs should not be present. If numerous RBCs are present, one should suspect a traumatic tap, trauma, malignancy or hemorrhage. Usually, absolute red cell counts have limited diagnostic value but they may provide useful information about the degree of blood contamination in a traumatic tap and provide correction factors, which can be applied to other studies, such as correcting for true numbers of CSF leukocytes or protein levels when blood contamination is present. The measurements (WBC, RBC, protein) should all be performed on the same tube to allow for the corrections for blood contamination to have the most accuracy.

The correction formula is as follows:
$$WBC_{corr} = WBC_{obs} - WBC_{added}$$
where
$$WBC_{added} = WBC_{BLD} \times RBC_{CSF}/RBC_{BLD}$$

WBC_{corr} = corrected WBC count

WBC_{obs} = CSF leukocyte count

WBC_{added} = leukocytes added to CSF by traumatic tap

WBC_{BLD} = peripheral blood leukocyte count

RBC_{CSF} = CSF erythrocyte count

RBC_{BLD} = peripheral blood erythrocyte count

Similarly, corrections may be made for added total protein due to a traumatic tap as follows:
$$TP_{added} = [TP_{serum} \times (1 - HCT)] \times RBC_{CSF}/RBC_{BLD}$$

TP_{added} = total protein added to CSF by traumatic tap

TP_{serum} = total protein in serum

In general, these corrections amount to an increase of ~1 WBC per every 700 RBCs and 1 mg/dL protein for every 10,000 RBC/μL. These correction factors are accurate unless there is a very high peripheral blood white blood cell count (such as an acute leukemia, chronic leukemia or infection) or very low peripheral blood white cell counts. The accuracy of the correction factor is also impacted by the number of red cells. It is important that all clinical data, including peripheral blood WBC count, protein levels and underlying disease, be taken into account making clinical decisions based on corrected CSF data [ISBN 978-143770-9742].

If the CSF specimen is not examined promptly after collection, increased levels of leukocyte lysis may give a false impression of a low white cell count. Cell lysis is increased due to the hypotonicity and low concentration of proteins and lipids, which help to stabilize cell membranes of WBCs in CSF. Up to 40% of white cells may lyse after CSF is held for 2 hours at room temperature. Cell lysis may be significantly slowed by refrigeration. Neutrophils are the first cells to lyse, whereas lymphocytes and monocytes show slightly longer life spans [PMID 6477217].

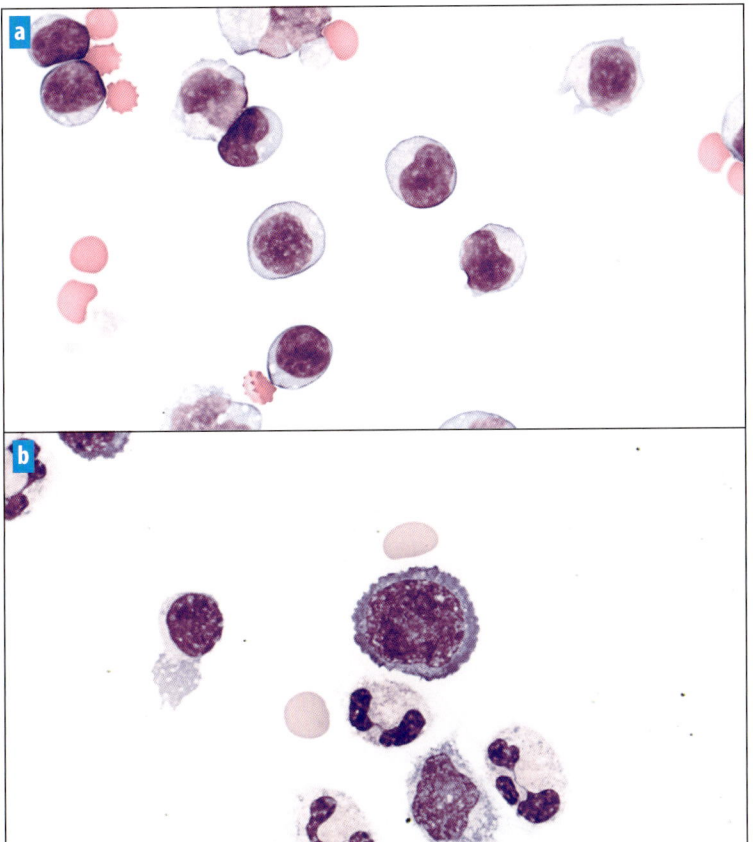

i4.8
a Lymphocytic & monocytic pleocytosis in a patient with viral meningitis showing increased numbers of small & reactive lymphocytes & monocytes. Wright stain.
b Neutrophilic pleocytosis in a patient with bacterial meningitis showing increased numbers of neutrophils with monocytes & lymphocytes. Wright stain.

t4.12	Causes of CSF lymphocytic pleocytosis
Meningitis	
Viral meningoencephalitis	
Bacterial meningitis (occasionally), early, uncommon organisms or partially treated	
Aseptic meningitis	
Tuberculous meningoencephalitis (mixed cell reaction)	
Syphilitic meningoencephalitis	
Leptospiral meningitis (often mixed cell reaction)	
Fungal meningitis (mixed cell reaction)	
Parasitic infectious (eg, trichinosis, cysticercosis, toxoplasmosis)	
Degenerative disorders	
Multiple sclerosis	
Guillain-Barré syndrome	
Subacute sclerosing	
Panencephalitis	
Drug abuse encephalitis	
Acute disseminated encephalomyelitis	
Other inflammatory conditions	
Polyneuritis	
Sarcoidosis of meninges	
Drug therapy	
CNS periarteritis	
Handl syndrome (headache with neurologic deficits & CSF lymphocytosis)	

t4.13	Cells in CSF & clinical significance
Type of cell	**Clinical significance**
Lymphocyte	Viral, tubercular, & fungal meningitis, bacterial meningitis (occasionally), multiple sclerosis
Neutrophil	Bacterial meningitis; early viral, tubercular, & fungal meningitis; intracranial hemorrhage; intrathecal injections; meningeal malignancy
Mixed cellular reaction (lymphocyte, neutrophil, monocyte)	Partially treated bacterial meningitis, chronic bacterial meningitis, cerebral abscess, tubercular meningitis, fungal meningitis, amebic meningitis
Eosinophil	Parasitic infections, allergic reactions, intracranial shunts
Macrophage	Chronic meningitis, treated bacterial meningitis, intrathecal injections, intracranial hemorrhage
Erythrophage (containing RBCs)	Hemorrhage (12 hrs-1 week)
Siderophage (containing hemosiderin)	Hemorrhage (2 days-2 months)
Hematoidinophage (containing hematin crystals)	Hemorrhage (>1 week-2 months)
Lipophage (containing fat)	Brain necrosis, infarct, anoxia, or trauma
Plasma cell	Subacute & chronic inflammatory reactions, multiple sclerosis
Malignant lymphoid cell	Lymphoma, leukemia
Blast	Acute myeloid leukemia, acute lymphoblastic leukemia/lymphoma
Other malignant cell	Primary brain tumor, metastatic tumor
Ependymal/choroid plexus cell	Trauma, surgery, ventricular shunts, neonate, intrathecal injections
Cartilage cells	Traumatic puncture
Bone marrow cells	Traumatic puncture
Primitive cell clusters (blastlike cells)	Intracranial hemorrhage in premature infant, neonate; possibly of germinal matrix origin

Differential count

A differential count should be performed on a stained smear made from the CSF. Frequently, the low number of cells present in CSF will require concentration of the CSF to allow for sufficient numbers of cells for analysis. Usually a differential count is performed on a cytocentrifuge preparation that has been stained with a Wright stain, although other stains, such as a Papanicolaou stain, may be useful in some circumstances (ie, large numbers of metastatic tumor cells). It is recommended that a stained smear be made and differential count performed even when the white blood cell count is within normal limits by automated counting. With normal white blood cell counts, 0.5 mL of normal CSF will yield ~30-50 cells by cytocentrifugation. Normal reference values for the leukocyte differential are presented in t4.11. Typically, lymphocytes and monocytes are the predominant cells observed. Neutrophils are not a common finding in normal CSF. Finding of eosinophils, ependymal cells, neuroectodermal cells or histiocytes is also quite unusual and may be an indication of disease, as discussed below [PMID 1583530, PMID 19185983].

Pleocytosis is the term given when increased numbers of white cells are present in a body fluid i4.8a-b. Pleocytosis is associated with various forms of infection, inflammation or possible malignancy. Depending on the predominant cell seen, in combination with the pleocytosis, specific disease processes may be indicated, as discussed further below t4.12, t4.13.

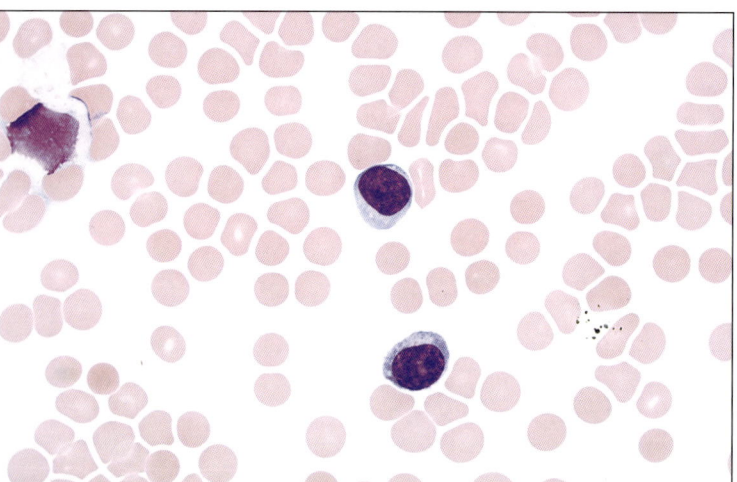

i4.9 Normal CSF usually shows very few cells; however, small lymphocytes & occasional monocytes may be seen. The large numbers of red cells in the background indicate the possibility of a traumatic tap. Wright stain.

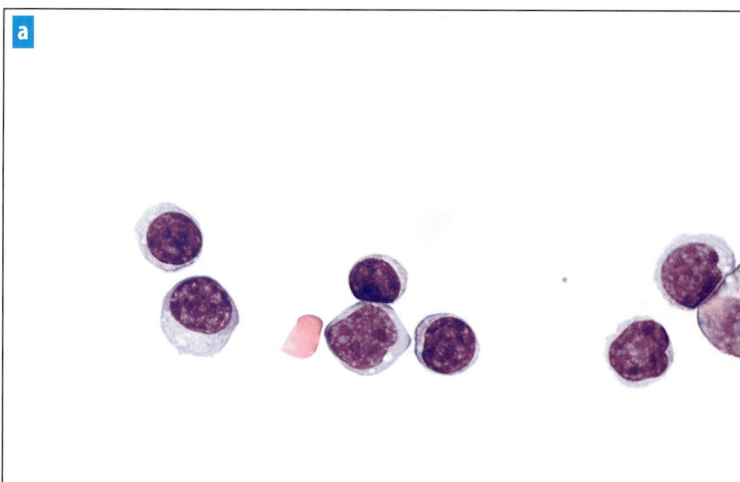

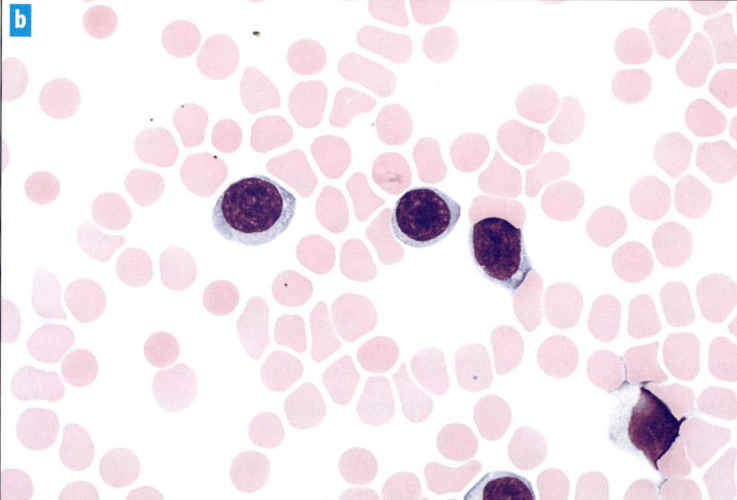

i4.10 **a** Small lymphocytes in CSF showing a mild range in cellular size & amount of cytoplasm with occasional plasmacytoid forms. Wright stain.
b Normal small to intermediate size lymphocytes present in CSF. The presence of red cells suggests the possibility of a traumatic tap. Some of these lymphocytes show activated appearing features with more abundant cytoplasm & larger nuclei with finer chromatin. Wright stain.

CSF normal cytology

A few red cells are frequently found in the CSF due to contamination by blood from a traumatic tap or minor injury to vessels during the lumbar puncture. This is particularly common in infants. The CSF normally contains a small number of lymphocytes and monocytes i4.9 [PMID 24275252]. The morphology of lymphocytes seen in the CSF is similar to that seen in the peripheral blood. ~75%-95% of the lymphocytes seen in the CSF are T cells [PMID 10353466, PMID 19046603]. There is often a spectrum of lymphocyte appearances including small or intermediate i4.10a-b and large or activated forms i4.11. In most cases where disease is not present, small lymphocytes should predominate.

The monocytes seen in CSF also appear similar to those seen in the blood. Monocytes may also develop into macrophages/histiocytes i4.12. Distinguishing monocytes from lymphocytes may be difficult, particularly in neonates in a cytocentrifuge preparation and the precision of automated counts is lower. Frequently in a cytocentrifuge slide, monocytes stick together i4.13 and may mimic neuroectodermal cells from the choroid plexus or ependymal cells. These collections of monocytes may also mimic tumor cells. In difficult cases, cytochemical staining (such as use of non-specific esterase stains) or use of flow cytometry or immunohistochemistry may help to distinguish monocytes from lymphocytes or tumor cells [PMID 19046603, PMID 17114955]. The ratio of lymphocytes to monocytes in adults is ~70:30. In young children and infants, the CSF tends to have a higher proportion of monocytes and monocytes may comprise up to 80% of the cells present and the proportion of monocytes may increase with acute infections [PMID 24275252, PMID 20441472, PMID 19046603, PMID 16121639, PMID 18630838, PMID 1583530].

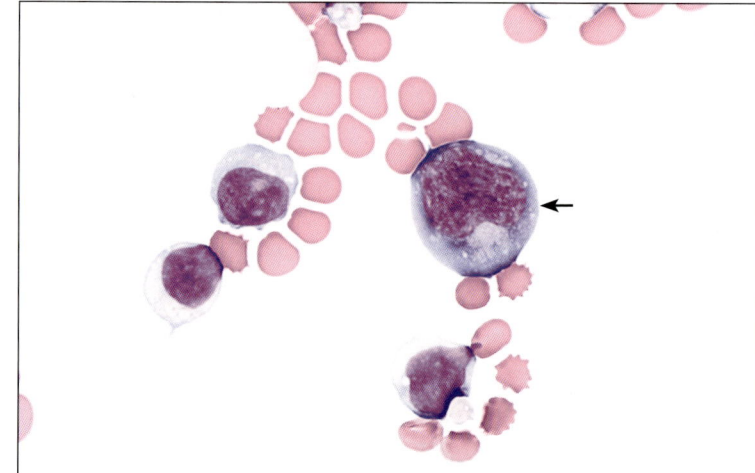

i4.11 Activated/immunoblastic lymphocyte identified in CSF in a patient with a viral disorder (arrow). Wright stain.

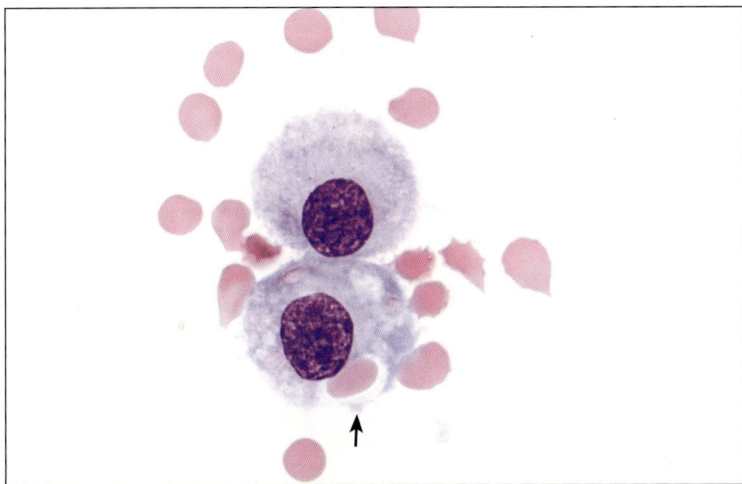

i4.12 Macrophages/histiocytes identified in a CSF showing characteristic abundant, somewhat granular cytoplasm & round to oval nuclear contours. The lower histiocyte also appears to have erythrophagocytosis. Wright stain.

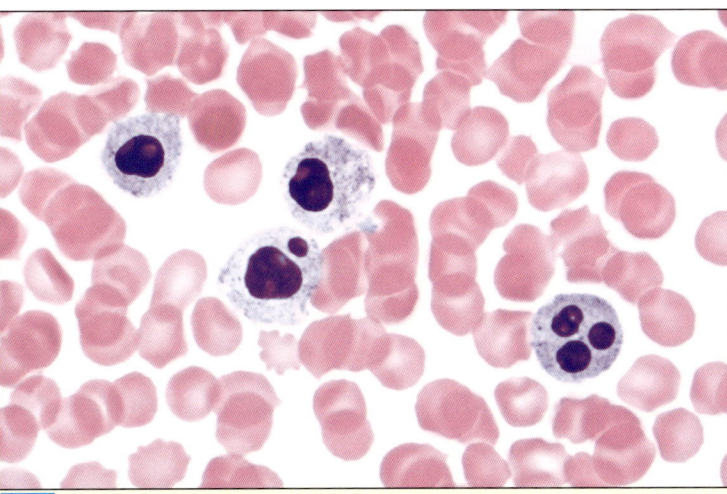

i4.14 Neutrophils in CSF showing degenerative changes, including nuclear condensation & fragmentation. Wright stain.

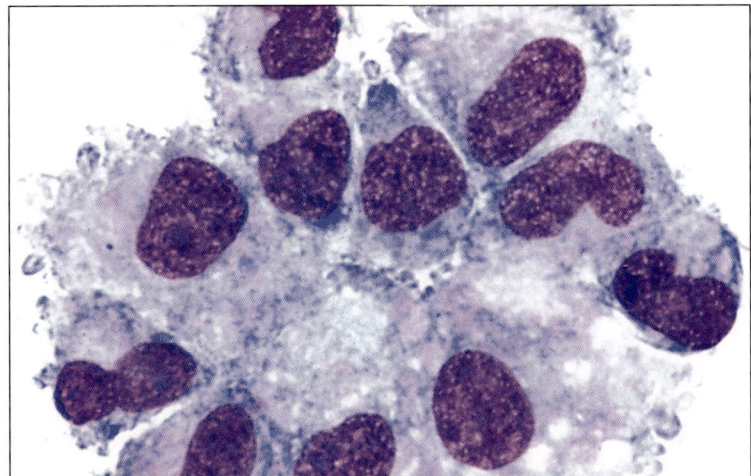

i4.13 Clump of monocytes in CSF mimicking the appearance of choroid plexus cells or malignant tumor. Wright stain.

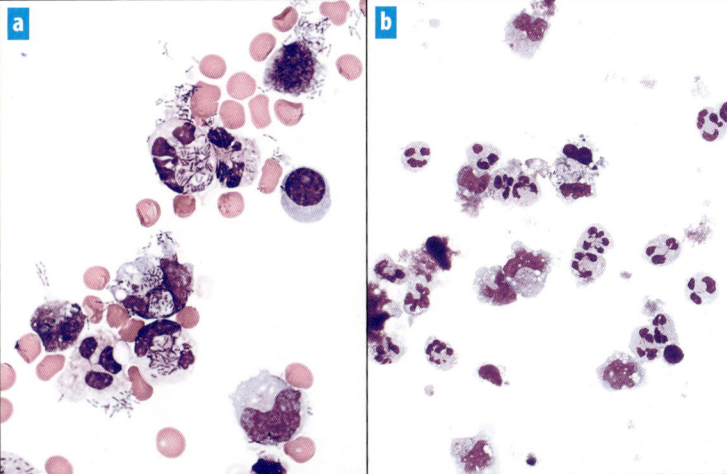

i4.15 **a** Neutrophil degeneration in a patient with bacterial meningitis. Note that the neutrophils have degeneration of nuclear & cytoplasmic features & contain numerous ingested bacilli. Wright stain.
b Neutrophilic degeneration in a patient with a shunt showing increased neutrophils with many degenerative features. Wright stain.

In normal CSF, neutrophils are usually only a small percentage of the cells [PMID 24275252, PMID 15163317]. It is thought that often neutrophils in normal (noninfectious) CSF may result from contamination by peripheral blood from the lumbar puncture procedure, thus increased numbers of neutrophils often reflects the degree of CSF blood contamination and the peripheral blood neutrophil count in normal CSF [PMID 12612231]. It should also be kept in mind that neutrophils are the cells which degenerate most rapidly in the CSF i4.14, and this is particularly true in cases of infection or inflammation from shunts i4.15a-b [PMID 3711287]. There is no general consensus regarding an upper limit of normal for neutrophils in CSF, particularly in children. It should be noted that up to 60% neutrophils have been reported in high risk neonates without attendant meningitis [PMID 2189977]. Correlation of the number of neutrophils in the CSF with that in the peripheral blood, as well as the number of red cells present, is important to determine whether the number of neutrophils present within the CSF is abnormal [PMID 18989240, PMID 12612231].

In addition to cells derived from the blood, normal brain cells i4.16 derived from the ventricular lining of the brain i4.17, ependymal cells or choroid plexus cells i4.18 may be occasionally seen in both normal and abnormal CSF preparations. These cells are more frequently found after ventricular or cisternal taps, but they may also be seen in some lumbar puncture specimens. Increased numbers of brain lining cells, which are frequently termed ventricular lining cells or neuroectodermal cells, are also seen following traumatic brain injury, brain surgery, ischemic infarction of the brain, imaging procedures and in some children with hydrocephalus and ventricular shunts. These cells are extremely uncommon in adults but may occasionally be seen in children with no apparent disease [PMID 7072664].

Histologic sections of the brain ependyma and choroid plexus show distinct morphologic differences between these structures. However, from a cytologic viewpoint it is difficult to differentiate between ependymal and

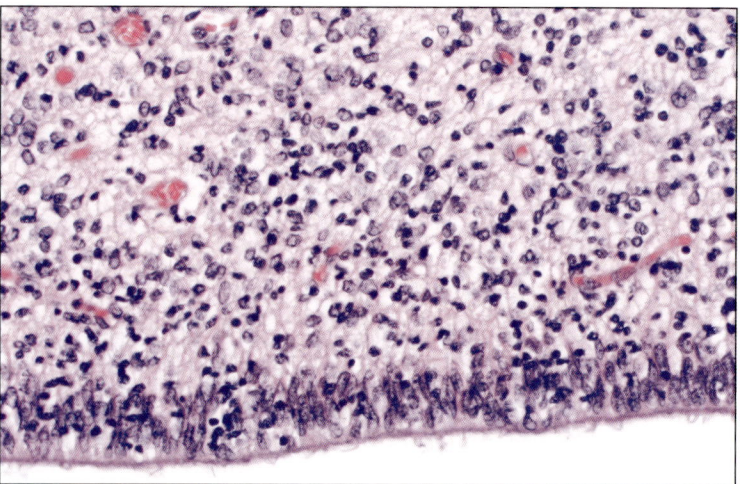

i4.16 Section of brain showing the lining cells & increased cellularity of the germinal matrix in a premature newborn. H&E stain.

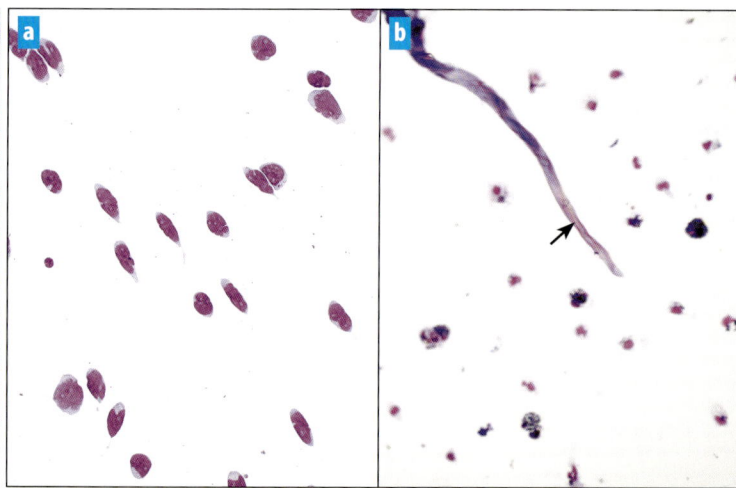

i4.19 **a** Many naked nuclei are present due to cytospin artifact. Wright stain.
b Cytospin preparation showing artifactual distortion of the cells & naked nuclei. In addition, a capillary (arrow) is present, which should not be confused with an organism. Wright stain.

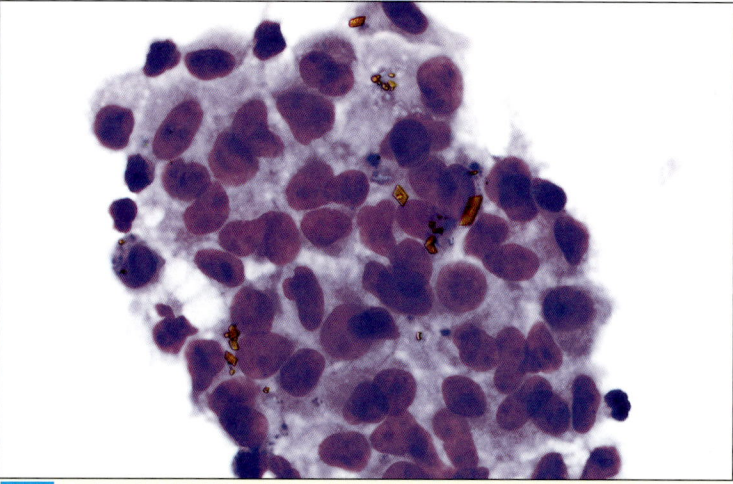

i4.17 Large clump of lining cells identified in CSF following trauma. Wright stain.

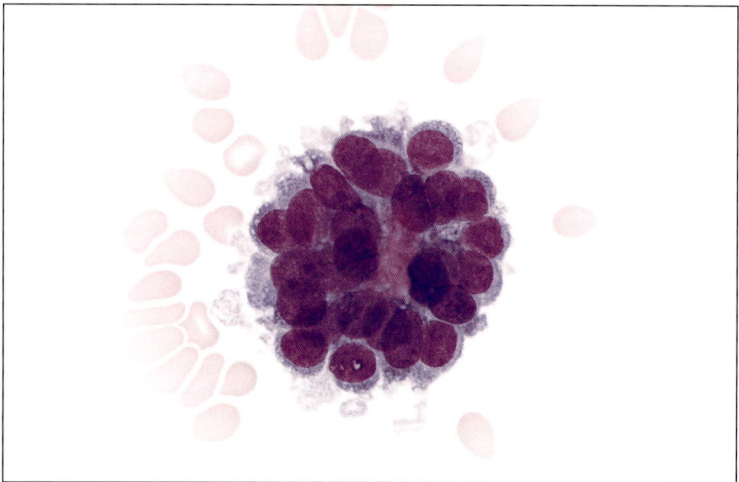

i4.18 Cluster of choroid plexus cells showing typical round nuclear contours & basophilic appearing cytoplasm. Wright stain.

choroid plexus cells in CSF preparations. It is thought that the majority of the lining cells seen in CSF preparations are choroid plexus cells. These cells may occur singly but are more often seen in papillary clusters or sheets i4.18. Choroid plexus cells have round to oval nuclei and are the size of small lymphocytes. The cytoplasm is moderate to abundant and gray-blue in color. The nuclear chromatin is delicate and finely granular and evenly distributed i4.18 but may appear dark and homogeneous. Nucleoli are not identified. The cytoplasmic borders may have vacuoles and occasionally cilia may be seen. In some cases, degeneration may cause the nucleus to appear pyknotic and eccentrically placed or may result in only naked nuclei i4.19a-b especially with cytocentrifugation. The main concern when these cells are present is possible malignancy [PMID 10561221]. In addition, children with choroid plexus papillomas that may result in hydrocephalus may present with increased numbers of benign appearing papillary clusters of choroid plexus cells [PMID 4419010, PMID 21701109]. As noted above, cytocentrifuge preparations of CSF may cause artifactual stickiness of lymphocytes and/or monocytes creating clusters, which should be distinguished from choroid plexus cells i4.13.

A variety of other cell types and noncellular elements may be seen in CSF t4.14. These include bone marrow cells, chondrocytes or cartilage cells, squamous epithelial cells, corpora amylacea, spindle cells, neurons and astrocytes. Occasionally, small fragments of muscle, fibrous tissue, adipose tissue or capillaries may be present. These findings are more common in infants and in patients who have vertebral abnormalities, including scoliosis, because of the difficulty of obtaining access to the CSF through the abnormal vertebral column. It is important to recognize these cells so that they may be distinguished from possible malignancy. Identification of these cells in CSF is nonspecific and nondiagnostic [PMID 2014779, PMID 268120, PMID 6942615].

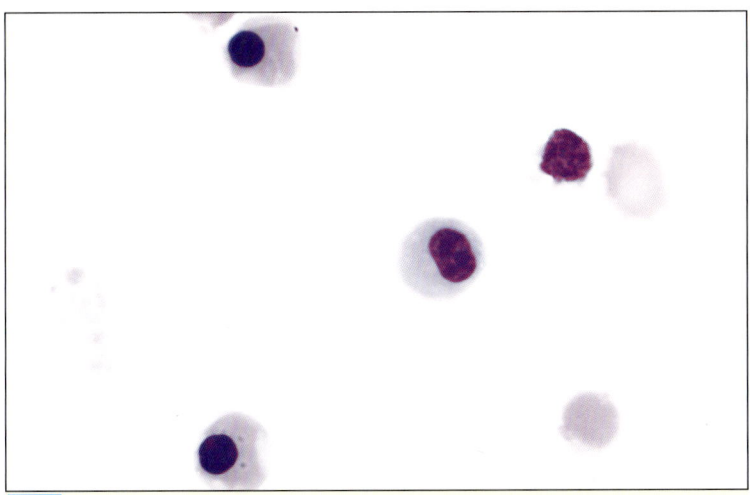

i4.20 Bone marrow cell contamination of CSF showing nucleated red cells & a myelocyte. Wright stain.

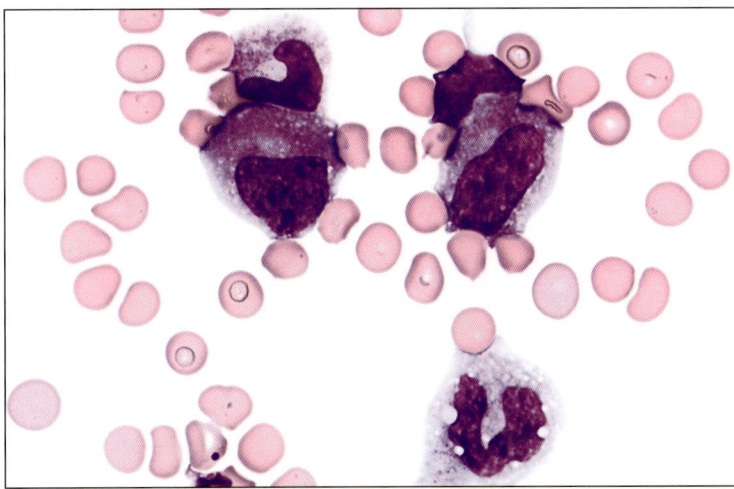

i4.21 Increased immature myeloid precursors due to bone marrow contamination of CSF, which could be worrisome for malignancy. Wright stain.

t4.14	Nondiagnostic cellular & noncellular elements that may be present in CSF specimens
Ependymal & choroid plexus cells	
Bone marrow cells	
Cartilage cells	
Squamous cells	
Erythrocytes & leukocytes (traumatic tap)	
Primitive cell clusters (blastlike cells, germinal matrix cells)	
Soft tissue elements from needle injury (adipose tissue, connective tissue, striated muscle, capillaries, nucleus pulposus)	
Corpora amylacea	
Respiratory epithelium, etc (from basilar skull fracture)	
Starch (from gloves)	
Radiographic contrast media	
Debris (dust particles, stain artifact, cellulose fibers, bacteria in contaminated stain)	

i4.22 **a** Chondrocyte (cartilage cell) in CSF. Wright stain. (Courtesy of J Cornbleet, MD) **b** Clump of chondrocytes (cartilage cells) in CSF. Papanicolau stain.

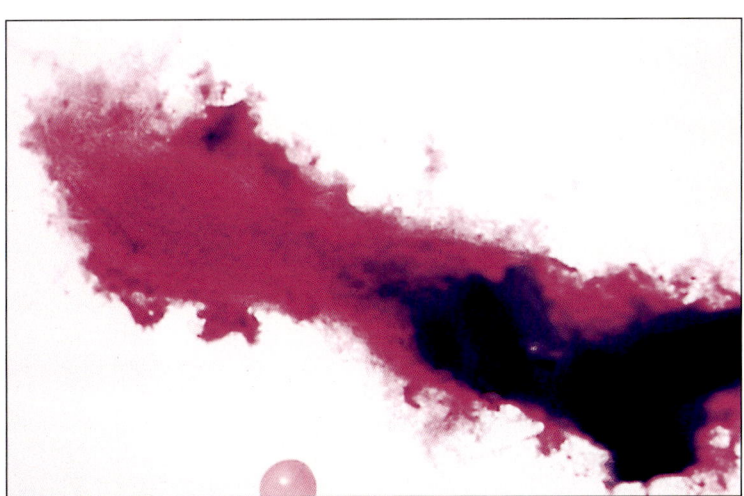

i4.23 Cartilage fragment in CSF. Wright stain. (Courtesy of J Cornbleet, MD)

The presence of bone marrow cells in the CSF is most commonly seen in infants and patients with difficult lumbar punctures or osteoporosis i4.20. Contamination by bone marrow cells occurs when the needle is pushed too far anteriorly and enters into the vertebral body. Megakaryocytes, in particular, may be mistaken for malignant cells. In addition, the immaturity of normal bone marrow may be mistaken for evidence of infection, leukemia or lymphoma i4.21. Bone marrow contamination may also occur from the needle scraping or entering the inferior or superior vertebral articular processes [PMID 2014779].

The presence of cartilage cells or chondrocytes in the CSF probably occurs from contamination when the needle nicks the intervertebral disc. Chondrocytes appear singly or in small clusters and often have a moderate amount of burgundy appearing cytoplasm in Wright stains or blue cytoplasm in Papanicolaou stains and a small pyknotic nucleus that is characteristically surrounded by a wide perinuclear clear zone i4.22a-b [PMID 2302041]. Although rare, the possibility of a chordoma should be considered in such cases. Occasionally, fragments of cartilage with similar burgundy coloration may be seen in the CSF i4.23. Mucinous or signet ring carcinomas involving the meninges may also exfoliate

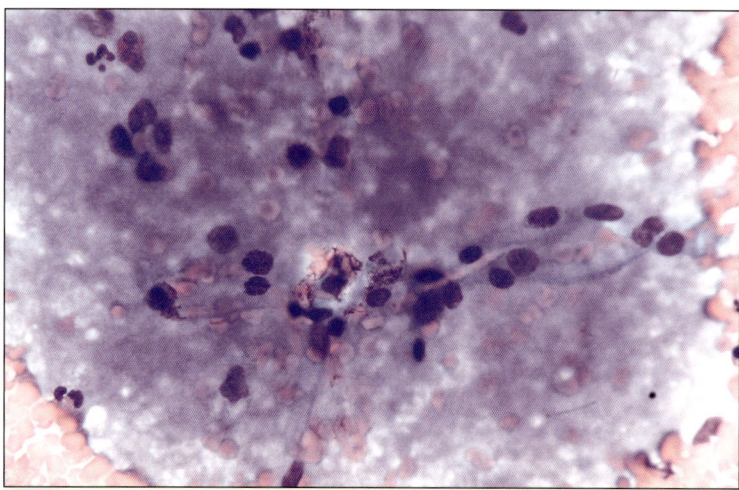

i4.24 Fragment of brain tissue present in CSF following trauma. Wright stain.

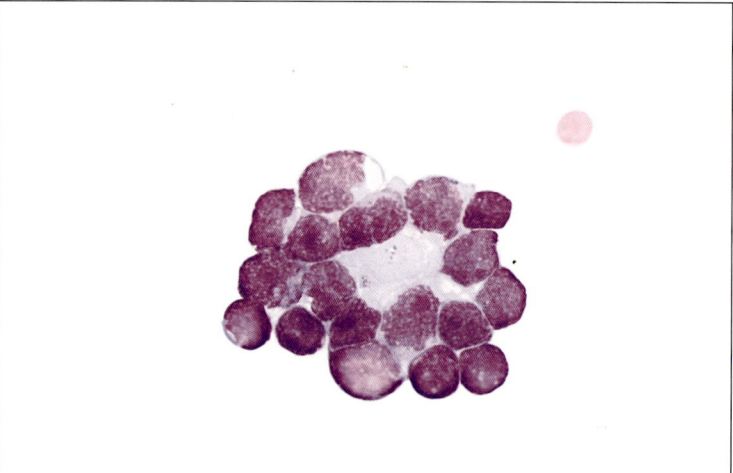

i4.25 Primitive cell cluster showing a grouping of immature appearing cells with fine chromatin identified in a neonate. Wright stain.

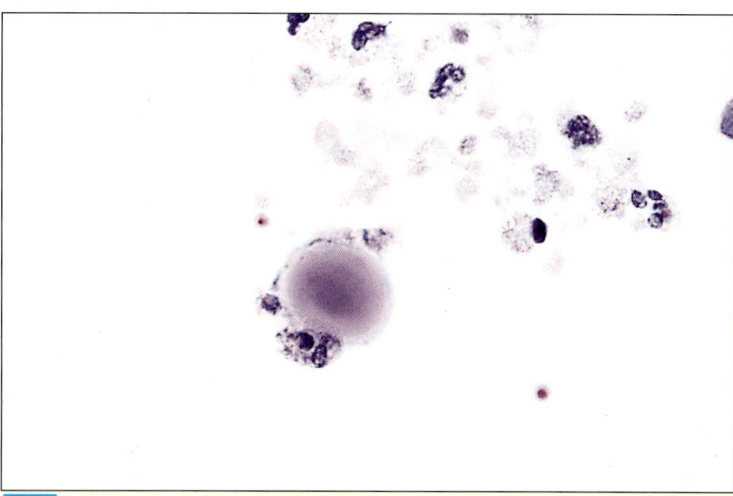

i4.26 Corpora amylacea in CSF. This shows the solid central staining pattern, which is characteristic. Wright stain. (Courtesy of SH Bigner, MD)

cells that look very similar to cartilage cells [PMID 14674086, PMID 24421850].

Squamous cells from the skin are occasionally encountered in CSF preparations and often contain bacteria. Squamous cell carcinoma cells from craniopharyngioma or splenoid sinus carcinomas may also be present and need to be differentiated from benign squamous cell contamination [PMID 6942615, PMID 24421850]. Primary brain tissue including neurons, astrocytes and glia cells may occasionally be seen when brain tissue is traversed during a ventricular puncture. Spindle shaped cells may also be present in clusters or may appear as clusters of bare nuclei. These are thought to originate from the arachnoid lining or astrocytes. Brain tissue fragments and primary brain cells may also be seen after intercranial surgery, intracerebral hemorrhage, cerebral trauma or in association with shunts i4.24. They may also be seen in some patients with encephalitis or multiple sclerosis [PMID 268120].

Blastlike cells or primitive germinal matrix cells, also known as undifferentiated leptomeningeal cells, may be seen in the CSF of neonates, especially with a history of birth trauma or prematurity. These cells have scant to moderate amounts of light basophilic cytoplasm and have blastlike nuclei with delicate chromatin and a single small nucleolus. They are often seen in clusters i4.25. These blastlike cells are most often seen in premature infants with subarachnoid or intraventricular hemorrhage and secondary hydrocephalus. They should be differentiated from choroid plexus or ependymal cells and malignant cells, such as lymphoblasts, neuroblastoma or medulloblastoma [PMID 9025871, PMID 8623760]. Germinal matrix cells originate from the subependymal cell layers of the brain, which are very prominent in newborns. As numerous small blood vessels permeate this area, it is a common site of hemorrhage and cellular exfoliation and vessels may occasionally be seen in CSF preparations i4.19b. This is hypothesized to be the mechanism underlying the sloughing of these cells into the CSF in premature infants [PMID 8623760].

Corpora amylacea are anuclear bodies formed of polysaccharides that form around the ventricles and pial surfaces of older individuals. They may be seen in the CSF of older patients and must be distinguished from possible infectious forms, such as yeast or cryptococci. Corpora amylacea stain homogenously or have a dark central core with concentric laminations i4.26 [PMID 216201]. This differs from the classic morphologic features seen with *Cryptococcus* where there is a refractile center and a surrounding capsule i4.27a or dense "starburst" appearance i4.27b. Both corpora amylacea and cryptococci will stain with periodic acid-Schiff (PAS), Alcian blue, and methenamine silver stains. Similarly, starch from rubber gloves may also be confused with cryptococcal organisms. Starch characteristically has a refractile angulated appearance and may have a Maltese cross configuration under polarized light, similar to what is seen in starch contamination in other fluids [PMID 7025539, PMID 1583530].

In basilar skull fractures, the meninges are torn, and structures from the sinuses may pass into the subarachnoid space and contaminate the CSF. Therefore, CSF may contain a mixture of cells, including ciliated columnar cells, mixed bacteria and other organisms from the sinuses [PMID 22655692].

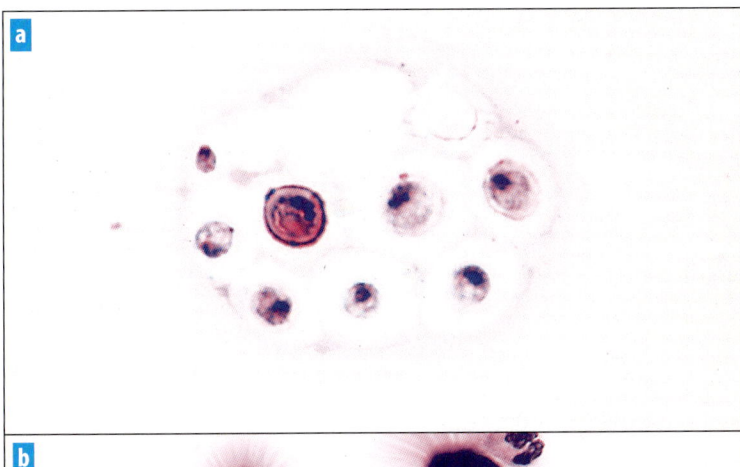

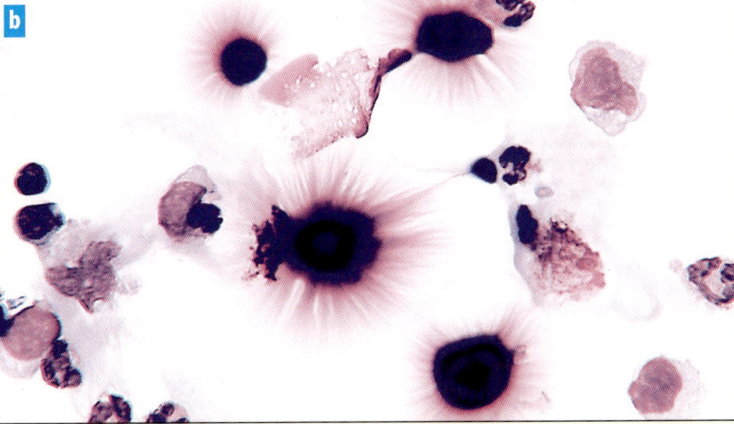

i4.27 **a** *Cryptococcus neoformans* in CSF in a patient who is immunosuppressed. This demonstrates the central organism which is surrounded by a halo. Wright stain.
b Starburstlike appearance of *Cryptococcus* in CSF. Wright stain. (Courtesy of J Cornbleet, MD)

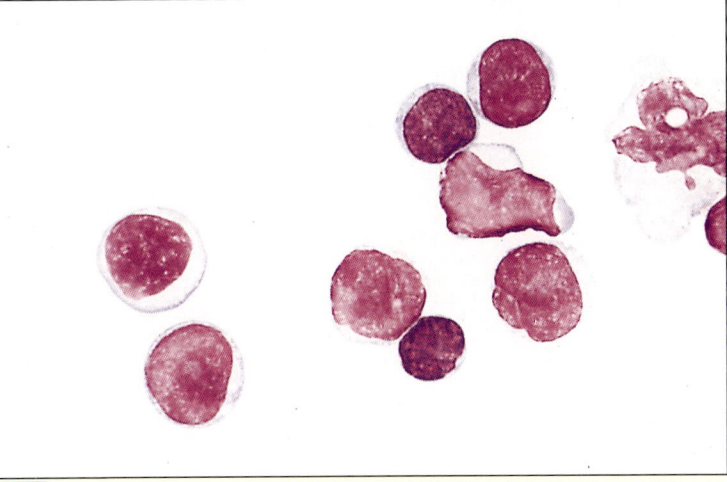

i4.28 Small lymphocytes & blastlike lymphocytes in the CSF of a newborn. Note the population of lymphoid cells with fine nuclear chromatin & scanty cytoplasm resembling lymphoblasts adjacent to more normal, mature appearing lymphocytes. Wright stain.

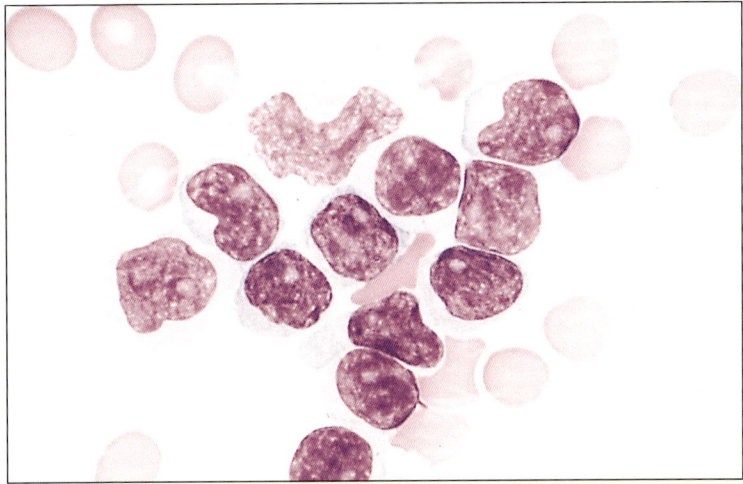

i4.29 Small lymphocytes with irregular nuclear contours in CSF. This is a common artifact, which may be seen in mature lymphocytes. Wright stain.

Abnormal cytology

Increased numbers of cells and a variety of nonintrinsic cells may be observed in the CSF and represent abnormal findings. A summary of the predominant cell types and clinical significance when found in CSF is presented in **t4.13**.

Lymphocytes in the CSF usually have a similar appearance to their counterparts in the blood. They may appear small or become transformed when exposed or activated by antigens. Thus, a spectrum of lymphoid cells may be seen including lymphocytes of varying sizes **i4.10a-b**, plasmacytoid lymphocytes, plasma cells or immunoblasts **i4.11** [PMID 16083828, PMID 11794481, PMID 7025539]. When lymphocytes become activated and display reactive changes, they may be difficult to distinguish from tumor cells. The stimulated, activated reactive or transformed lymphocyte is medium to large in size and has moderately abundant basophilic cytoplasm with moderately coarse chromatin. One or more nucleoli may be present **i4.11**. Occasionally, azurophilic granules may be seen in the cytoplasm. The cytoplasm is often moderately abundant. These reactive cells should not be referred to as "atypical" as this term is often used to describe possible malignant cells. These reactive lymphocytes are commonly seen in patients with viral meningitis and other inflammatory processes [PMID 6942615, PMID 1583530].

In comparison, lymphoblasts have immature, delicate chromatin and scant cytoplasm. Nucleoli may or may not be prominent. Blastlike lymphocytes may be seen in the normal CSF of newborns and should not be mistaken for leukemic cells **i4.28** [PMID 7072664]. One of the most helpful features in distinguishing between benign lymphoid pleocytosis and malignant cells is that the reactive process usually contains a mixture of small, large and transformed lymphocytes **i4.10, i4.11**. In contrast, malignant cells, either from lymphoma or lymphoblastic leukemia, tend to be more uniform in size and shape. The presence of irregular nuclear contours and nucleoli are not reliable features for distinguishing between benign lymphoid cells and malignant cells, and ancillary studies such as flow cytometry or molecular analysis may be required for definitive identification [PMID 16430456, PMID 17028920]. Cytocentrifuge artifact may induce considerable nuclear irregularities and may also emphasize the predominance of nucleoli, as well as making the nuclear chromatin appear somewhat fine **i4.29**. Frequently, lymphocytic pleocytosis is an expansion of lymphocytes [PMID 10353466, PMID 19046603]. A listing of the causes of CSF lymphocytic pleocytosis is presented in **t4.12**.

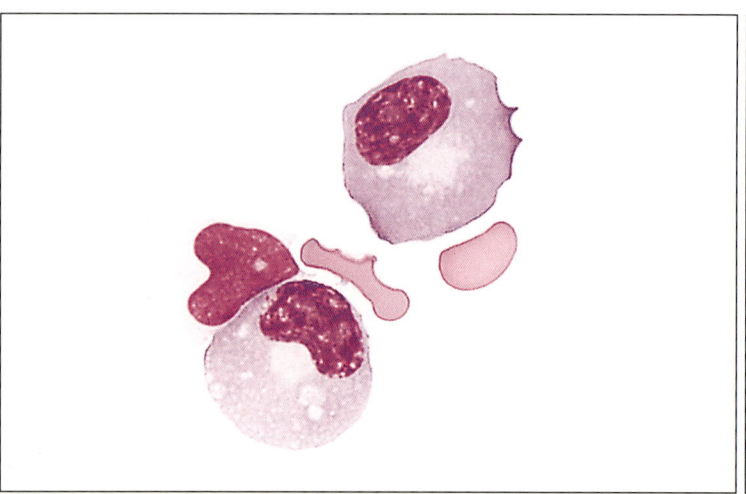

i4.30 Reactive plasma cells in CSF in a patient with Guillain-Barré syndrome. Wright stain.

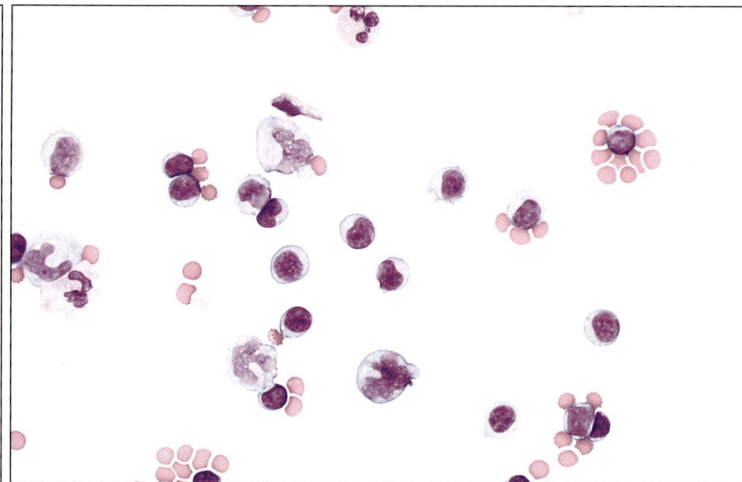

i4.31 Low power view of a patient with viral meningitis showing pleocytosis of small & activated lymphocytes with occasional monocytes. The relatively few red cells in the background suggest that this is a true lymphocytic pleocytosis and not due to peripheral blood contamination. Wright stain.

Plasma cells are not typically seen in CSF specimens from normal patients. The presence of plasma cells suggests an inflammatory process i4.30. Often, transitional forms between reactive lymphocytes and plasma cells, such as plasmacytoid lymphocytes may be present. Plasma cells are associated with a variety of inflammatory and infectious conditions t4.15 [PMID 6260507, PMID 11794481, PMID 7025539]. In some cases of multiple sclerosis, plasma cells may be the only cytologic abnormality noted [PMID 11213505].

t4.15	Causes of CSF plasmacytosis
Infectious causes	
Acute viral infections	
Parasitic CNS infections	
Syphilitic meningoencephalitis	
Tuberculous meningitis	
Other causes	
Multiple sclerosis	
Subacute sclerosing panencephalitis	
Guillain-Barré syndrome	
Sarcoidosis	

Monocytes, together with neutrophils and lymphocytes, may be present in a variety of disorders. Monocytic pleocytosis is often part of a mixed cell reaction where there are increased numbers of neutrophils, lymphocytes and plasma cells, as well as monocytes, reflecting migration of these cells into the CSF in response to release of inflammatory cytokines [PMID 9626995]. A pure monocytosis in the CSF is rarely seen. Usually, monocytes are not the predominant cell type seen [PMID 24275252, PMID 7025539, PMID 1583530]. Causes of CSF monocytic pleocytosis include meningitis, including tubercular or fungal meningitis, as well as rupture of a cerebral abscess t4.16 [PMID 3523200, PMID 6965948]. A mixed pattern without increased neutrophils is characteristic of viral i4.8a, i4.31 and syphilitic meningoencephalitis. Mononuclear phagocytes (histiocytes and macrophages) in CSF are probably derived from monocytes. These phagocytes may ingest red cells, leukocytes, microorganisms, pigment and lipids i4.1, i4.2a.

t4.16	Causes of CSF monocytic pleocytosis*
Meningitis	
Tuberculous meningitis	
Chronic meningitis	
Partially treated bacterial meningitis	
Syphilitic meningitis	
Viral meningitis	
Fungal meningitis	
Leptospiral meningitis	
Toxoplasma meningitis	
Amebic encephalomyelitis	
Other	
Rupture of brain abscess	
CNS hemorrhage	
Cerebral infarct	
Multiple sclerosis	
Reaction to foreign material (dyes, shunts)	
CNS malignancy	

Monocytic pleocytosis is usually associated with mixed cell reactions.

The material that is ingested may then be degraded or stored in the cytoplasm in the form of vacuoles i4.32. Frequently, these phagocytic cells are quite large in size and may be concerning for possible metastatic malignancy. Epithelioid histiocytes and multinucleated giant cells may also be

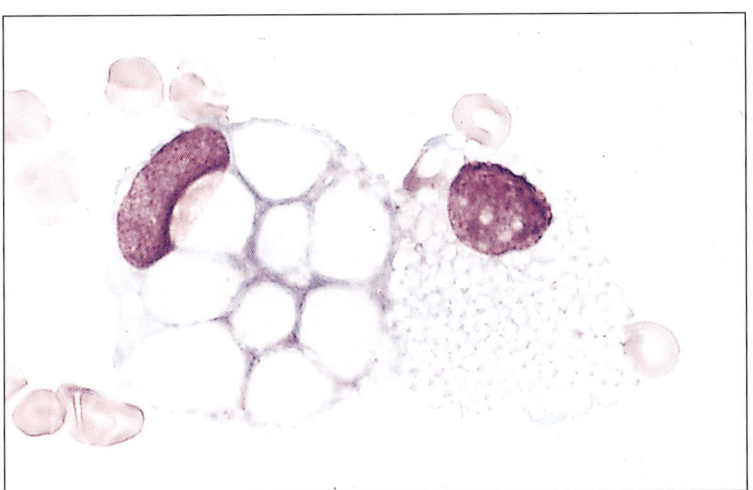

i4.32 Lipophage (with small vacuoles on right side) & macrophage with ghost red blood cells (larger vacuoles present on the left hand side) in a patient with cerebral infarct. Wright stain.

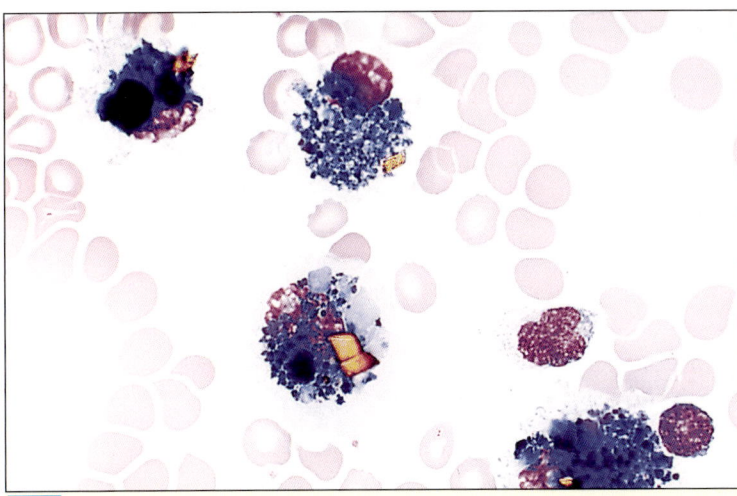

i4.34 Macrophage containing blue hemosiderin & hematin pigment (yellow crystals).

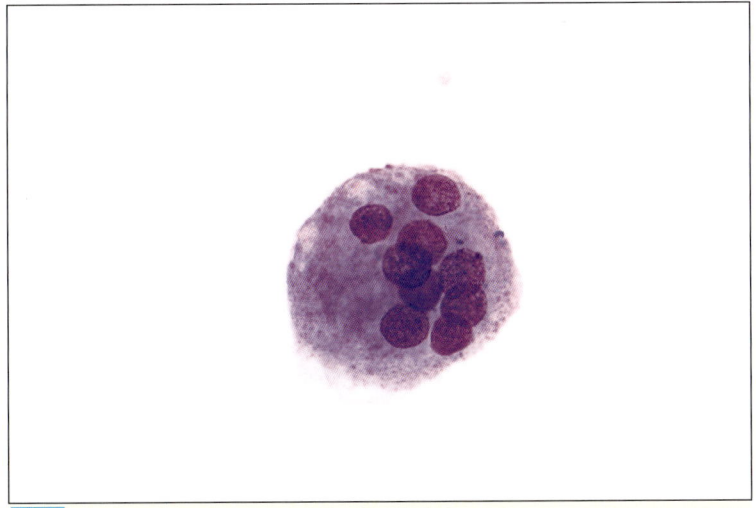

i4.33 Multinucleated histiocyte identified in the CSF. Wright stain.

present, particularly in granulomatous type disorders, such as tuberculosis and sarcoidosis **i4.33** [PMID 17636138].

Phagocytic cells are often prominent when hemorrhage occurs. Often, neutrophils and macrophages will increase with macrophages ingesting the red cells within a few hours **i4.1**. The phagocytized red cells are rapidly degraded and may appear as empty vacuoles in the cytoplasm of the macrophages. After ~4 days, hemosiderin is formed and is visualized as dark brown or black granules **i4.2a-b**. As degradation occurs, hematin pigment crystals **i4.34** may be formed. The presence of multiple siderophages is usually a reliable indication that hemorrhage has occurred. The presence of siderophages is not diagnostic of recent hemorrhage, as they may persist for several months after a hemorrhage has occurred [PMID 9025870]. Identification of a single cell with phagocytized red blood cells is also not an absolute indicator of hemorrhage [PMID 7025539, PMID 2014779]. Erythrophagocytosis may also occur from blood contamination from a recent (8-12 hours prior) CSF lumbar puncture. However, large numbers of macrophages with erythrophagocytosis and siderophages are strong morphologic evidence that a pathologic hemorrhage has occurred [PMID 9025870, PMID 1583530]. Similar cells with erythrophagocytosis may also be seen following traumatic birth, hydrocephalus or after CNS surgery [PMID 9025870]. The timing of events in the CSF following hemorrhage is summarized in **t4.17**.

t4.17	Changes in CSF following hemorrhage
Gross examination	
2-12 hours	Pink to orange pigmentation/coloration of CSF
12-24 hours	Yellow pigmentation/coloration of CSF (disappears in 2-4 weeks)
Microscopic examination	
2-24 hours	Erythrocytes, neutrophils (30%-60%), monocytes, macrophages, lymphocytes
12-48 hours	Macrophages, erythrophagocytosis, lymphocytes
48 hours	Vacuolated macrophages, erythrophagocytosis, siderophages (may persist for 2-8 weeks)
>1 week	Siderophages, macrophages with hematin crystals

Lipophages or foamy macrophages are macrophages that have ingested fat. They may be seen in the CSF following cerebral infarctions, brain abscesses or following some imaging procedures, such as myelography. Lipophages contain numerous small phagocytic vacuoles rather than the larger vacuoles seen in typical CSF macrophages **i4.32**. Foamy histiocytes in the CSF have also been observed with storage disorders such as Tay-Sachs disease and Hunter-Hurler syndrome **i4.7**. Clusters of histiocytes or macrophages or multinucleated giant cells may resemble tumor cells and have often been associated with cerebral shunts **i4.35** [PMID 1583530, PMID 10561221, PMID 7025539].

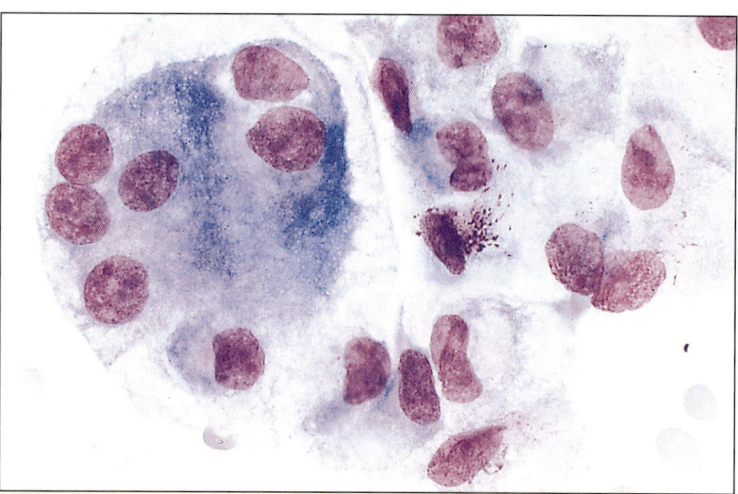

i4.35 Clusters of histiocytes resembling multinucleated giant cells or mesothelial cells in the CSF of a patient with a ventricular peritoneal shunt. Wright stain.

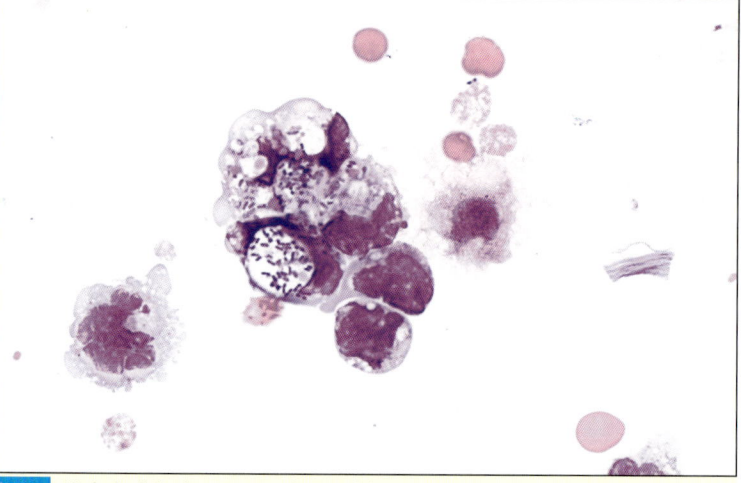

i4.36 Marked cellular degeneration of neutrophils & macrophages in a patient with bacterial meningitis. Note the ingested bacterial organisms in the degenerating cellular clump. Wright stain.

Neutrophils may be increased in a variety of infectious and noninfectious disorders of the CNS t4.18 [PMID 7025539, PMID 1583530, PMID 2411458].

t4.18 Causes of CSF neutrophilic pleocytosis

Meningitis
Bacterial meningitis
Early viral meningoencephalitis
Early tuberculous & mycotic meningitis
Amebic encephalomyelitis
Aseptic meningitis
Other infections
Cerebral abscess
Subdural empyema
HIV associated CMV radiculopathy
Other
CNS trauma or hemorrhage
Cerebral infarct
Primary brain tumor with tissue necrosis
Metastatic tumor in CSF
Spinal anesthesia or repeated lumbar punctures
Foreign material (drugs, dyes)
Following seizures

CMV = cytomegalovirus; HIV = human immunodeficiency virus

Often, the cytoplasmic granules of neutrophils are less prominent in CSF than in the blood. As noted previously, PMNs show rapid disintegration when left in CSF at room temperature. Frequently, the nuclei may show degeneration and fragmentation of the nuclei i4.14 [PMID 3711287]. In the presence of infection, neutrophils often show cytoplasmic vacuolation, loss of granules and blurring of nuclei i4.36 [PMID 1583530]. These degenerative features may make differential counts difficult. Neutrophilic pleocytosis is most commonly associated with bacterial meningitis, and in early stages, neutrophils may comprise >60% of the cells [PMID 16121639]. However, in some cases of viral meningitis, neutrophils may also be increased with gradual evolution to a lymphocytic pleocytosis within 2-3 days [PMID 20626298].

An absolute neutrophil count of >1,000 cells/µL has a high predictive value for bacterial meningitis in a meta-analysis of multiple studies particularly when combined with other features and laboratory tests such as CSF Gram stain, CSF protein, seizure or peripheral blood neutrophilia [PMID 22764093]. Persistence of neutrophils for >1 week may be seen with some noninfectious etiologies, such as infarction or tissue necrosis [PMID 4013654] or may indicate unusual organisms, such as fungal meningitis or meningitis due to *Brucellosis* or *Nocardia* [PMID 2277197].

Eosinophils are rarely seen in normal CSF. Increased numbers of eosinophils in the CSF have been associated with a variety of infectious and noninfectious disorders t4.19.

t4.19 Causes of CSF eosinophilic pleocytosis

Common causes
Parasitic infections
Fungal infections
Reaction to foreign material in CNS (drugs, shunts)
Acute polyneuritis
Idiopathic eosinophilic meningitis
Rare causes
Bacterial meningitis
Tuberculous meningoencephalitis
Viral meningitis
Rickettsial infection (Rocky Mountain spotted fever)
Leukemia, lymphoma
Myeloproliferative disorders
Primary brain tumors
Neurosarcoidosis

If there are ≥10% eosinophils in the CSF or an absolute count of ≥10 eosinophils/µL, the process is defined as an eosinophilic pleocytosis i4.37 [PMID 12637136]. Eosinophilic pleocytosis may also be seen in parasitic infections, fungal infections, allergic reaction to foreign material, such as drugs or shunts, as well as an idiopathic eosinophilic

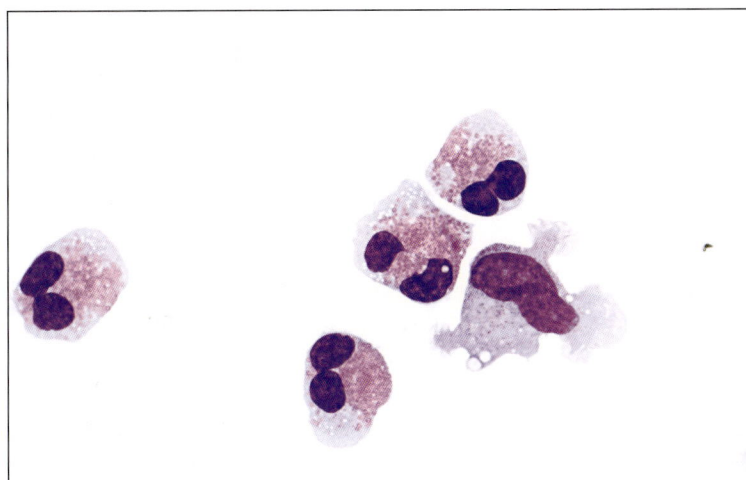

i4.37 Eosinophilia in the CSF of a patient with a shunt. Wright stain.

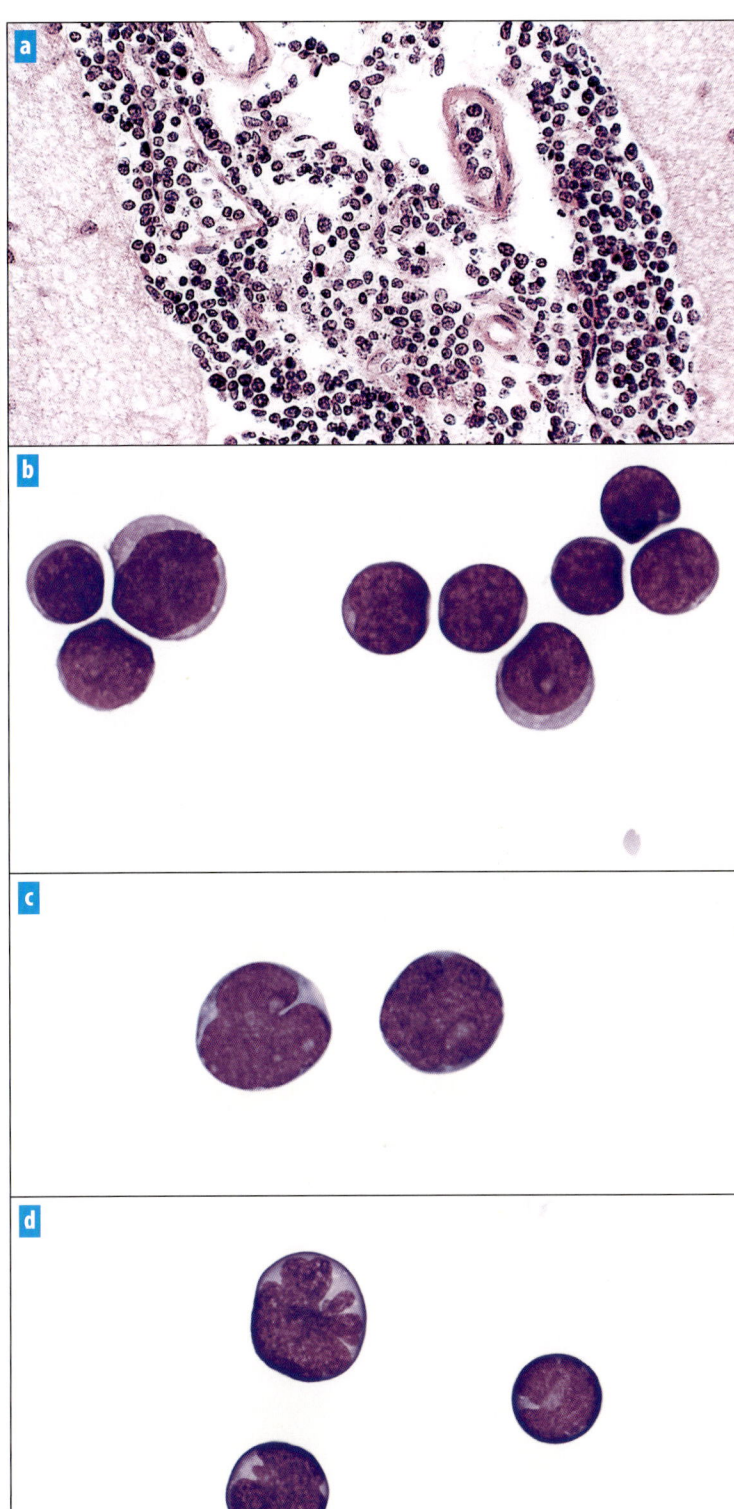

i4.38
a Leukemic meningitis. Meningeal infiltration by lymphoblasts in a patient with ALL. H&E stain
b Lymphoblasts in a patient with ALL showing variation in size & amount of chromatin. Most of the lymphoblasts show fine nuclear chromatin with very scanty to absent cytoplasm. Rare blasts (arrows) show slightly larger size with more abundant cytoplasm & more prominent nucleoli. Wright stain.
c Slightly higher power of lymphoblasts in a child with ALL showing the lack of significant amounts of cytoplasm & the fine nuclear chromatin with inconspicuous nucleoli. 1 blast shows mild nuclear irregularity. Wright stain.
d Lymphoblasts from a child with ALL showing more marked nuclear irregularity due to cytospin artifact. Note the relative lack of cytoplasm & the fine nuclear chromatin with inconspicuous nucleoli. Wright stain.

meningitis without evidence of a pathogen [PMID 12637136, PMID 14620646]. Frequently, eosinophilia of the CSF is mild (1%-4% eosinophils), but in children with malfunctioning shunts, it may be marked [PMID 22132920]. Basophils are not seen in normal CSF but may be seen in small numbers in inflammatory diseases, foreign body reactions, parasitic infections, convulsive disorders and in some cases of leukemia [PMID 12687751].

CSF analysis for malignancy

Examination of the CSF for tumor cells has moderate sensitivity but definitive identification of a tumor cell has high specificity for CNS or leptomeningeal involvement by tumor. The sensitivity of detection is highly tumor dependent, with the highest sensitivities being seen in patients with leukemias with relatively lower sensitivities for lymphomas, metastatic carcinomas and primary CNS malignancies. Sensitivities may be increased by using a method, such as CSF filtration or cytocentrifugation, to concentrate larger fluid volumes to increase detection of rare malignant cells [PMID 22523219, PMID 2425776]. Also serial punctures in patients where tumor is strongly suspected may help to increase the ability to detect tumor cells in CSF. Utilization of immunophenotyping or molecular techniques may also increase sensitivity for tumor cell detection, particularly when small numbers of tumor cells are present [PMID 7789240, PMID 15681484, PMID 23287431].

Acute leukemia

Any type of acute leukemia may involve the central nervous system, typically presenting as a leukemic meningitis **i4.38a** [PMID 10589079]. Patients may also have leukemic blasts in the central nervous system as a site of initial presentation or relapse before tumor cells is identified in either the peripheral blood or bone marrow [PMID 20605098]. Although morphologic features may be highly suggestive of blasts, usually additional methods including immunophenotyping by either immunocytochemical stains or flow cytometry are required for identification of blasts [PMID 15640938, PMID 22639108, PMID 23287431]. In addition to definitively identifying blasts, these studies are also helpful in identifying a cell of origin (eg, lymphoid vs myeloid vs monocytic). On the basis of cytomorphologic examination, the presence of a monotonous cellular population containing blastlike nuclei and scant cytoplasm is highly suspicious for involvement by leukemia [PMID 9180910, PMID 21761583]. Integration with clinical history and peripheral blood and bone marrow findings is also extremely important in helping to identify and subclassify the blasts in CSF [PMID 6947670]. It should be noted that cytocentrifugation may be associated with a variable degree of cellular distortion of both normal and leukemic cells. The process of cytocentrifugation may make normal reactive lymphocytes appear to have finer chromatin and more prominent nucleoli i4.28. However, reactive populations will tend to have a more heterogeneous population with ranges in cell size, chromatin features and amount of cytoplasm. Nucleoli may be present in both reactive and malignant cells. It should also be kept in mind that cellular degeneration occurs in both reactive and neoplastic populations, particularly if the CSF specimen is not examined immediately [PMID 21761583].

Involvement of the CNS by leukemia is more commonly observed in patients with acute lymphoblastic leukemia (ALL) than in acute myelogenous leukemia (AML). The morphologic features seen in the blasts often closely resemble those seen in the blood and bone marrow although cytocentrifugation may distort the morphology of the blasts causing them to appear larger, and have more cytoplasm or nuclear irregularities i4.38a-d [PMID 21761583, PMID 9180910]. Often, leukemic involvement of the CSF is associated with a relatively high CSF leukocyte count. However, it should be noted that patients with acute leukemia may have a nonspecific reactive pleocytosis or low numbers of leukocytes but definitive blasts [PMID 9180910, PMID 3459377]. In the past, when diagnosis of CNS involvement was predominantly based on cytomorphology, there was no uniform agreement on the definition of leukemic involvement. Most studies used white cell counts of 5-10 leukocytes/µL of CSF with unequivocal blasts identified morphologically. Utilization of more sensitive immunophenotypic methods, such as flow cytometry, has allowed identification of very small numbers of blasts with a high degree of certainty [PMID 7789240, PMID 15640938, PMID 23287431]. Several studies have suggested that the finding of even a small number of blasts in the CSF has a high probability of being associated with CNS relapse [PMID 12525508, PMID 16710032]. Use of directed antibody panels and flow cytometry will allow definite identification of even small numbers of blasts in a paucicellular specimen with a high degree of certainty. This approach is, of course, most easily applied when the subtype of leukemia is already known, as antibodies can be judiciously selected and applied to the small cell numbers. Although not as commonly used, cytochemical stains, such as myeloperoxidase staining, may also be useful in cases where flow cytometry was not obtained. In difficult cases, molecular analysis using polymerase chain reaction (PCR) may be useful, particularly with low level disease [PMID 15681484, PMID 12960693, PMID 23287431].

In patients with acute leukemia with extensive peripheral blood involvement, it is also extremely important to pay attention to the possibility of peripheral blood contamination of the CSF. Identification of red cells in the CSF suggests that there has been CSF contamination and the numbers of blasts identified in the peripheral blood must be compared to those present in the peripheral blood [PMID 6947666, PMID 12525508]. It is also possible that, by the occurrence of a traumatic tap, there has been iatrogenic introduction of blasts into the CNS. For this reason, most patients with any identification of CNS blasts will receive appropriate CNS prophylaxis and therapy [PMID 16710032, PMID 12525508]. There is also a possibility of contamination if bone marrow elements are present due to contamination from the vertebral bodies.

t4.20	Limited panel immunophenotyping for malignancy in CSF	
Lymphoid blasts	(B lymphoblasts) Dim CD45 TdT CD19 CD20 CD10 CD22 CD34	(T lymphoblasts) Dim CD45 TdT CD1a CD4 CD8 CD10
Myeloid blasts	Dim CD45 CD33 CD34 Myeloperoxidase CD117	
Non-Hodgkin lymphomas	(B non-Hodgkin lymphoma) CD20 κ λ CD5 CD10	(T non-Hodgkin lymphoma) CD3 CD4 CD8 CD30
Nonhematopoietic*	Keratins (eg, AE1,3) Neuroendocrine markers (synaptophysin, neuron specific enolase) HMB-45 for melanoma S100 Glial fibrillary acidic protein	

*Done by immunocytochemical methods only

ALL is the most commonly seen acute leukemia that involves the CSF. Examination of the CSF is an essential part of the workup and staging of any child or adult with ALL. In the CSF, lymphoblasts typically have a lacy or dispersed or occasionally finely granular chromatin that is evenly distributed i4.38b. Cytoplasm is scanty and often gray or basophilic i4.38b-d. Frequently, the blasts are slightly larger than accompanying benign lymphocytes. 1 or more nucleoli may be present, and these are often more prominent than seen in peripheral blood and bone marrow preparations due to cytocentrifuge artifact i4.38c. Nuclear contours are usually round and smooth but there may be nuclear indentations present i4.38b-c. It should be noted that viral infections and exposure of lymphocytes to chemotherapy might induce features in reactive lymphocytes that cause them to closely resemble blasts [PMID 21761583]. In this clinical situation, immunophenotyping is often essential in a directed fashion to distinguish between leukemic blasts and reactive lymphocytes [PMID 22025088]. An immunophenotypic panel must often be abbreviated due to the small number of cells. If an ALL is suspected or the known diagnosis, a limited panel utilizing 4-5 antibodies, as suggested in t4.20, may be utilized. If flow cytometry is not obtained, use of immunocytochemistry for TdT and B or T cell markers may also be useful. It is helpful to remember that most lymphocytes in a CSF pleocytosis will be T cells whereas the majority of childhood and adult ALLs will

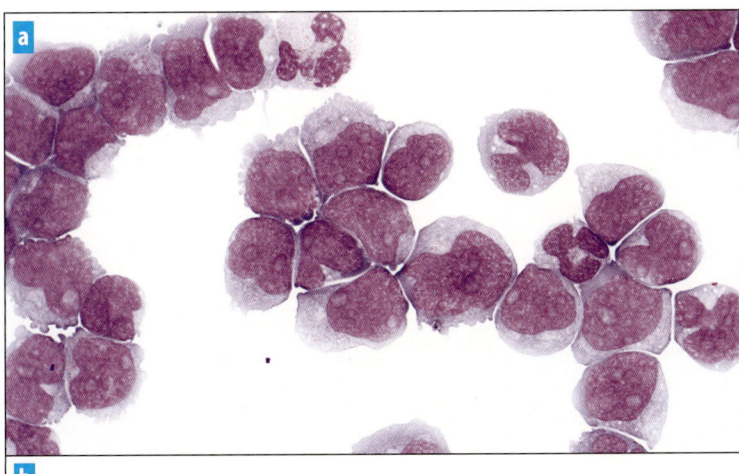
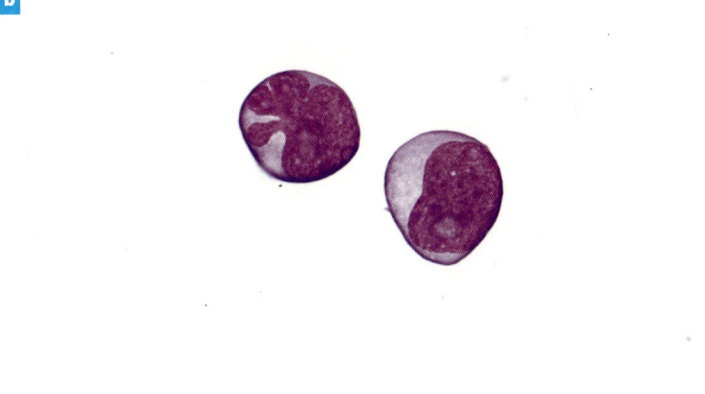
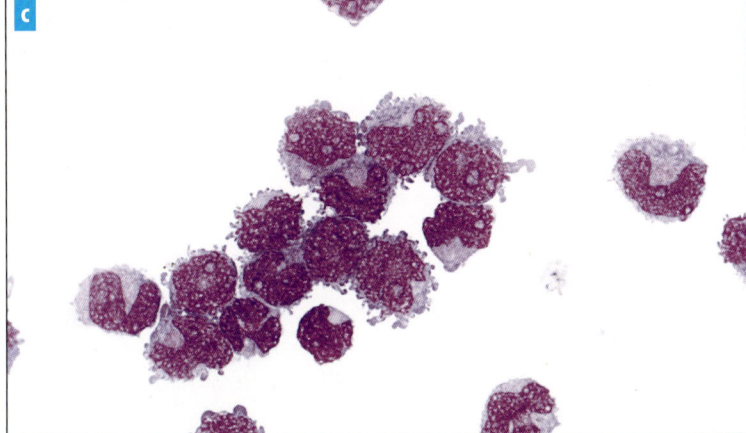

| i4.39 | a CSF from a patient with AML & central nervous system involvement showing increased numbers of large blasts with fine chromatin, relatively prominent nucleoli, irregular nuclear contours & moderate amounts of cytoplasm. Wright stain.
b Myeloblasts identified in the CSF of a patient with AML showing the oval to irregular nuclear contours, fine chromatin, prominent nucleolus & relatively abundant cytoplasm more characteristic of myeloid leukemias. Wright stain.
c Marked artifactual distortion of myeloblasts in a patient with AML. The relatively fragile nature of the blast causes nuclear & cytoplasmic fragility & may lead to significant artifact in cytospin preparations. Wright stain. |

be precursor B lymphoblasts. Distinguishing of T lymphoblasts may be somewhat more problematic, but judicious application of markers of immaturity (eg, CD1a, TdT, CD10 or coexpression of CD4 and CD8, CD34) is extremely helpful in identifying T lymphoblasts [PMID 3437410, PMID 3059292, PMID 15640938].

Involvement of the CNS by AML is less common but may be an initial site of relapse [PMID 15082912], or presentation [PMID 20605098]. CNS involvement by AML is associated with high peripheral blast counts, inversion of chromosome 16 and abnormalities of chromosome 11 [PMID 21692072]. Often

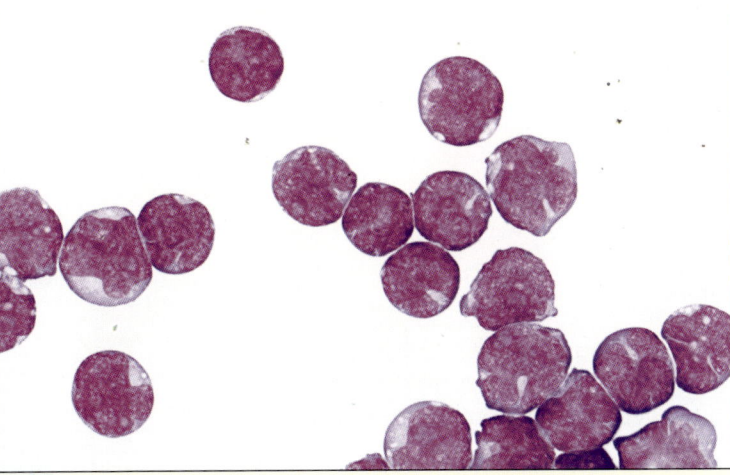

i4.40 Increased blasts in a patient with chronic myelogenous leukemia (CML) in myeloid blast crisis. The blasts have features of myeloblasts including large size, irregular nuclear contours, relatively prominent nucleoli & moderate amounts of cytoplasm. Wright stain.

the cytologic features of the blasts in AML are similar to those seen in the blood and bone marrow i4.39a-b, although distortion due to the blasts being present in fluid and cytospin artifact must be taken into account i4.39c. Typically, the blasts are quite large in size and have fine nuclear chromatin with multiple nucleoli. Often the blasts of AML will have more cytoplasm and nuclear irregularities than seen in ALL i4.39a-b [PMID 22639108]. Again, immunophenotypic analysis with careful attention to markers of immaturity (eg, CD34) is helpful [PMID 15640938, PMID 3437410]. It is extremely useful if the immunophenotype of the blasts involving the blood and/or bone marrow is known as that can allow a limited diagnostic panel to be performed by flow cytometry.

Chronic leukemias

Meningitis due to chronic leukemias, either chronic lymphocytic leukemia (CLL) or chronic myelogenous leukemia (CML), is relatively rare. CLL is the most common chronic leukemia to involve the central nervous system and is often associated with high white cell counts or prolymphocytic transformation [PMID 18446313, PMID 21769650]. CML involvement of the CNS in chronic phase is very unusual and more likely to involve the CNS in blast crisis i4.40 [PMID 15160941]. Because both CLL and CML are associated with very high peripheral blood white cell counts, the identification of neoplastic cells in the CSF must be distinguished from the more common finding of a traumatic tap introducing peripheral blood elements into the CSF. As in the acute leukemias, identification of CLL cells by flow cytometry is sensitive and specific. Identification of a monoclonal CD20 population that coexpresses CD5 with CD23 or CD200 expression is highly specific for CLL [PMID 11078802]. Unfortunately, there are no specific flow cytometry markers for CML involvement. In cases with suspected involvement, molecular or cytogenetic techniques to identify the BCL-ABL1 or Philadelphia chromosome may be of use [PMID 21881536].

Malignant lymphomas

Malignant lymphomas may infiltrate the meninges or involve the CNS directly. They may arise in the CNS or be secondary involvement from systemic disease [PMID 23670107,

4: Cerebrospinal Fluid

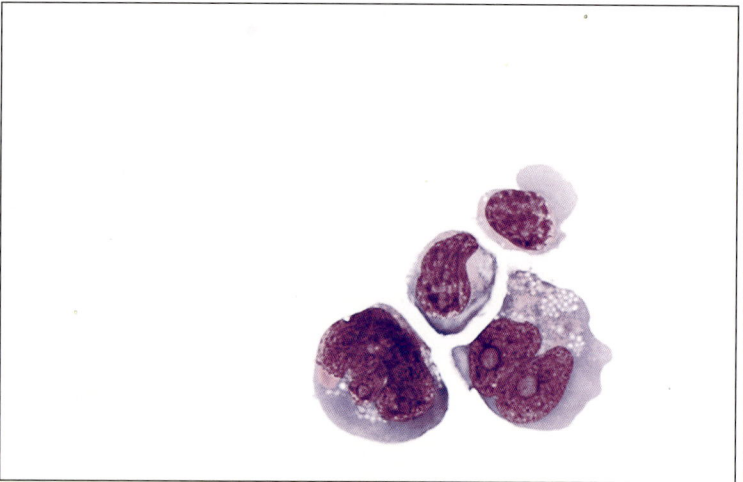

i4.41 Large neoplastic lymphoma cells identified in the CSF of a patient with peripheral T cell lymphoma (not otherwise specified). The neoplastic cells are large with abundant cytoplasm, prominent nucleoli & significant nuclear anaplasia. Wright stain.

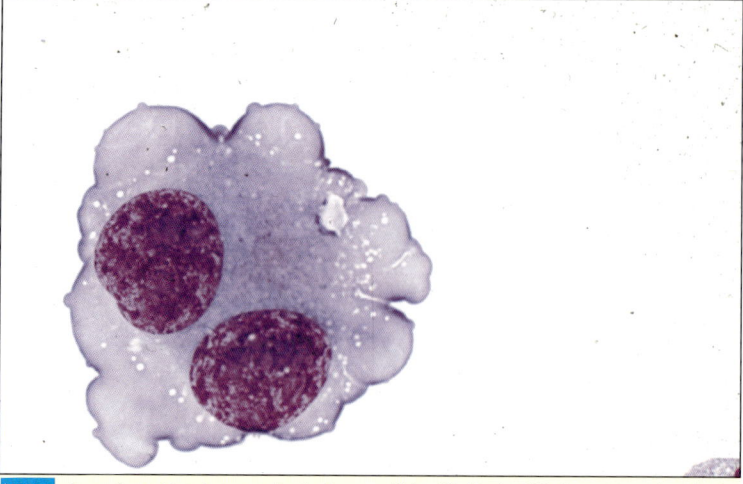

i4.43 A very large, binucleate neoplastic plasma cell identified in the CSF of a patient with multiple myeloma. Wright stain.

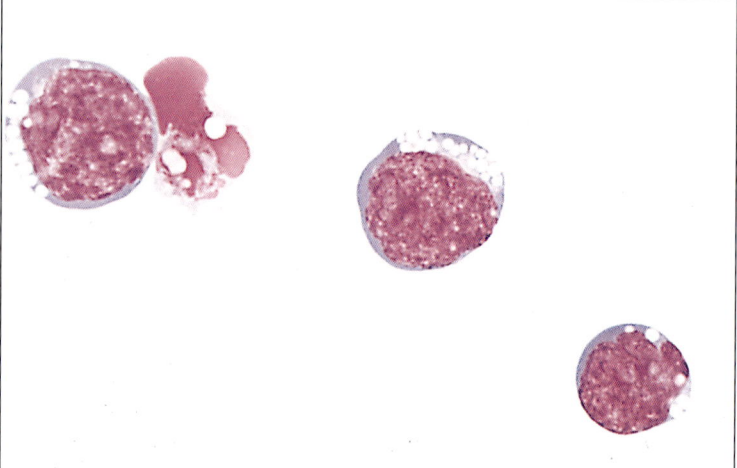

i4.42 Burkitt lymphoma with intermediate size & characteristic cytoplasmic vacuoles in the CSF of a patient with HIV/AIDS. Wright stain.

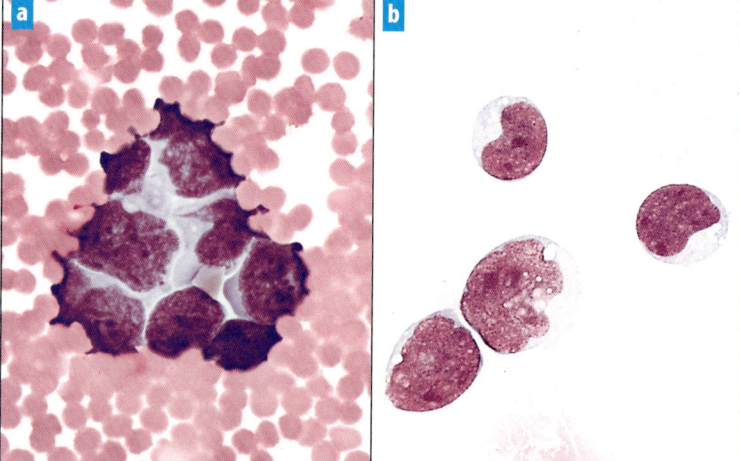

i4.44 **a** Cluster of medulloblastoma cells identified in the CSF of a child with a brain tumor. Wright stain
b Higher power of medulloblastoma cells in the CSF of a child. Wright stain.

[PMID 19660680, PMID 3710441]. In these cases, lymphoma cells may be identified in the CSF in a small number of cases [PMID 23319132]. The most commonly identified lymphomas in the CNS include Burkitt lymphoma in children, as well as lymphomas occurring in immunocompromised hosts. The immunosuppression associated lymphomas occur in patients with HIV infection, as well as patients with immunosuppressive therapy or older patients. In immunosuppressed or older patients, the most common subtype of lymphoma seen in the CNS is B cell large cell lymphoma. A small proportion of immunosuppressed patients may also have Burkitt lymphoma. There are also multiple reports of a variety of other lymphomas, including low grade lymphomas, T cell lymphomas and Hodgkin lymphoma, but these are extremely rare. Lymphoblastic lymphoma may also involve the CNS in a manner similar to ALL [PMID 19660680]. Often, the cytomorphologic features of the tumor cells in the CSF are highly indicative of the subtype of lymphoma and include enlarged cell size, nuclear atypia and anaplasia in large cell lymphomas **i4.41** or intermediate size with cytoplasmic vacuoles in Burkitt lymphoma **i4.42** [PMID 23319132, PMID 19660680, PMID 23287431]. In addition, judicious use of limited flow cytometric immunophenotyping or immunocytochemistry may be helpful in identification of a non-Hodgkin lymphoma [PMID 11078802, PMID 23319132, PMID 22025088, PMID 1971494]. Molecular testing, such as identification of T or B cell gene rearrangements, is also a highly sensitive method to identify CSF involvement by non-Hodgkin lymphoma [PMID 23287431].

Plasma cell myeloma may also involve the central nervous system and neoplastic plasma cells may be identified in spinal fluid **i4.43** [PMID 15101714]. However, it must be kept in mind that reactive plasmacytosis may also be seen in the CSF [PMID 7025539]. The possibility of a traumatic tap introducing bone marrow cells or the needle passing through a soft tissue plasmacytoma must also be considered. Identification of neoplastic plasma cells is often aided by immunophenotypic analysis by flow cytometry to demonstrate immunophenotypic aberrancies or clonality but may also be identified by using B cell gene rearrangements or cytogenetic FISH studies to identify myeloma specific abnormalities [PMID 15101714, PMID 20218151].

Primary CNS tumors

Primary CNS tumors are often located deep within the brain parenchyma and it is therefore not common for the tumor cells to be exfoliated into the CSF. However in children, medulloblastoma **i4.44a-b** and retinoblastoma are more

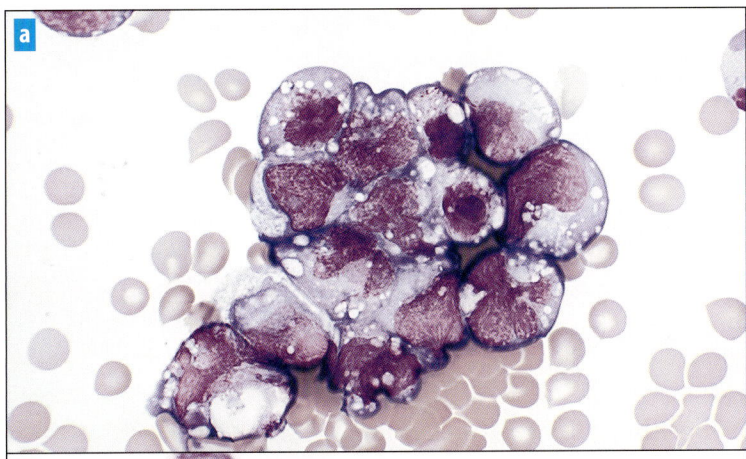
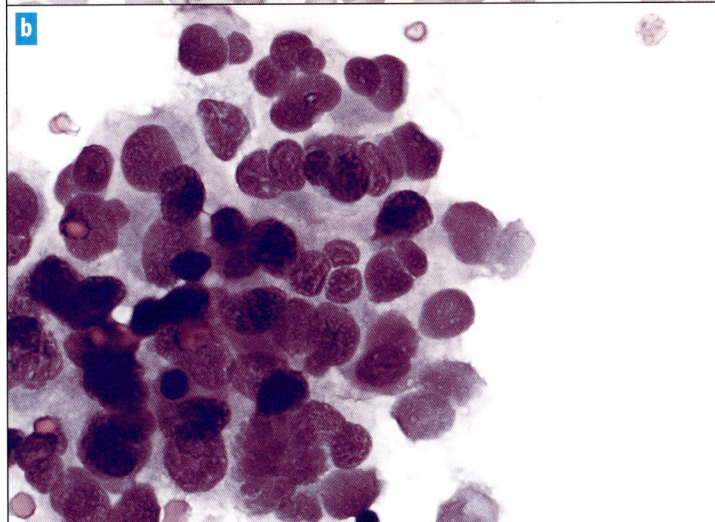
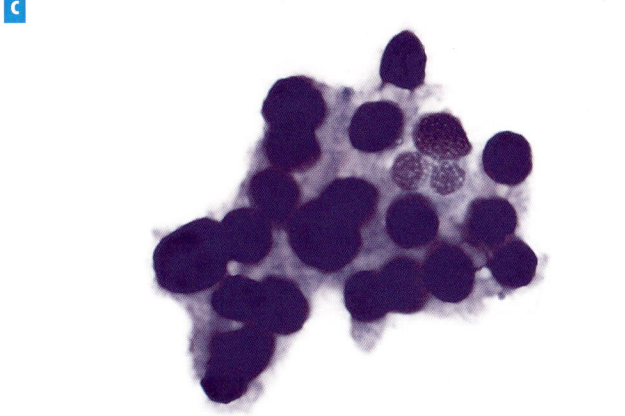

| i4.45 | a Cluster of tumor cells in the CSF from a patient with glioblastoma showing marked anaplasia. Wright stain.
b Cluster of tumor cells in the CSF from a patient with glioblastoma showing varying degrees of cellular hyperchromatism & cellular atypia. Wright stain.
c Cluster of cells in the CSF from a patient with glioblastoma showing marked hyperchromatism of the tumor cells. Wright stain.

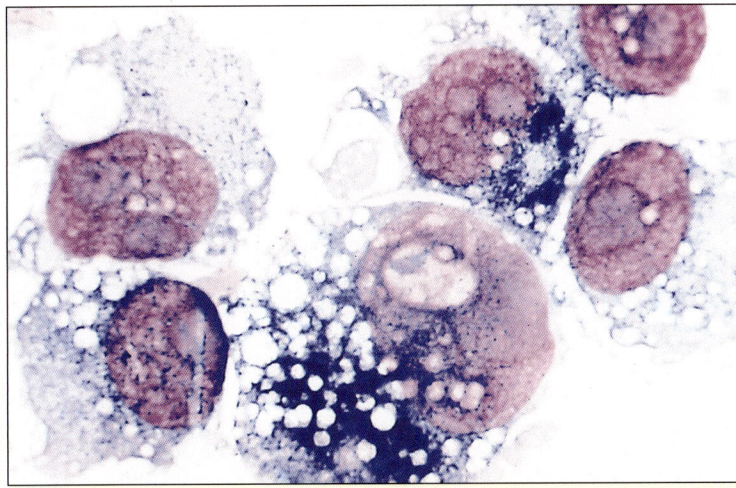

i4.46 Metastatic melanoma cells in a CSF demonstrating prominent nucleoli & atypical nuclear features with extensive deposition of melanin pigment in the cytoplasm. Wright stain.

likely to be seen. In adults, high grade glioblastomas i4.45a-c and ependymomas may also be seen. Much more rarely, other tumors such as chordomas and pinealoblastomas may be seen. The malignant cells are often easily identified by cytomorphology due to their large size and frankly neoplastic nuclear features, including abnormal chromatin i4.45b-c, prominent nucleoli and anaplasia i4.45a [PMID 7025539]. Careful correlation with clinical and radiologic features is often helpful in differentiating malignant cells from shedding of normal brain cells. Immunophenotypic analysis by immunocytochemical methods may also be helpful in identifying the type of CNS malignancy [PMID 3059292].

Metastatic malignancies

Metastatic disease of tumors involving other organs may also involve the central nervous system and be shed into the CSF. Typically these involve malignancies that have metastasized to the meningeal space [PMID 3656567, PMID 3228160]. Although relatively rare, melanoma i4.46 and carcinoma i4.47a-b may be identified in the CSF. In children, Wilms tumor, Ewing sarcoma, neuroblastoma i4.48 and embryonal rhabdomyosarcoma i4.49a-b may also metastasize to the meninges and CNS. Again, careful correlation with clinical features and use of immunocytochemical markers for the specific tumor type may help to identify the origin of the metastasis i4.47c [PMID 1971494, PMID 3245993, PMID 3059292]. However

4: Cerebrospinal Fluid

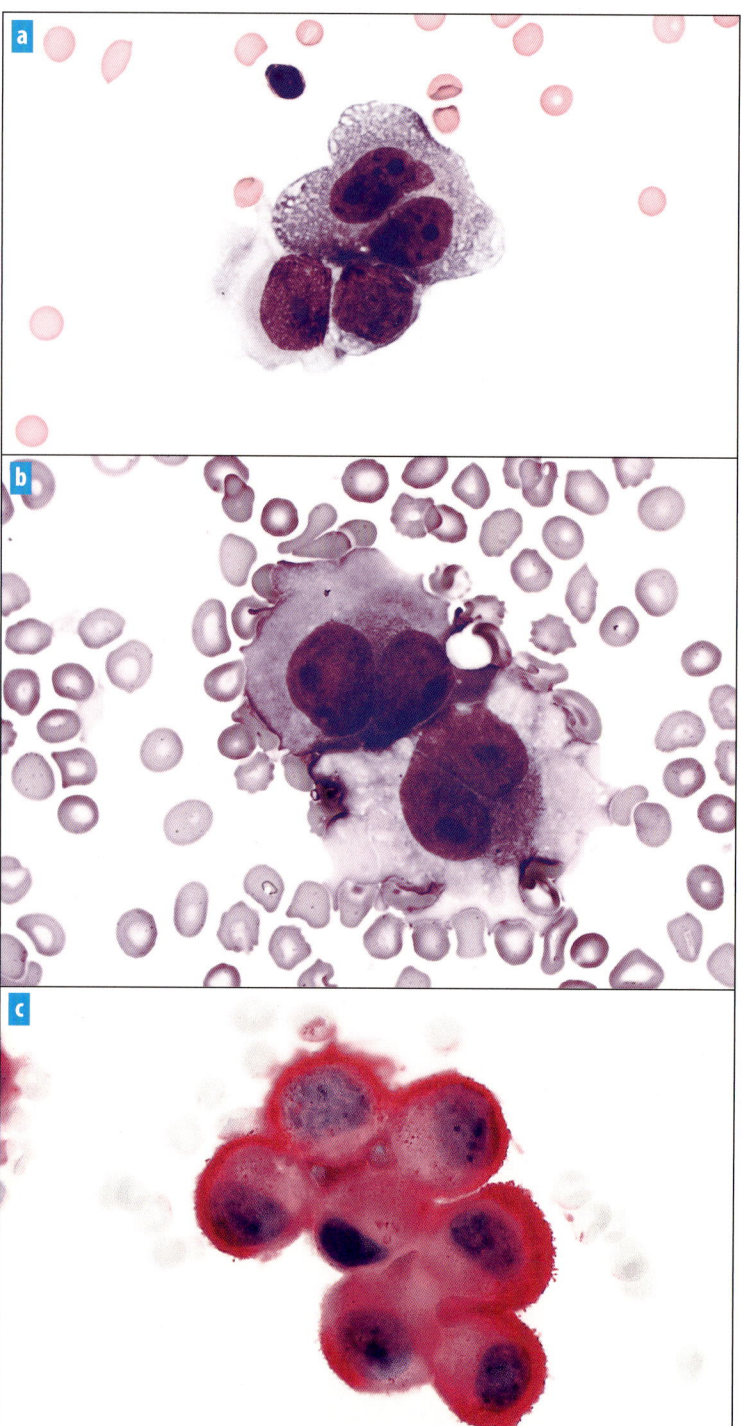

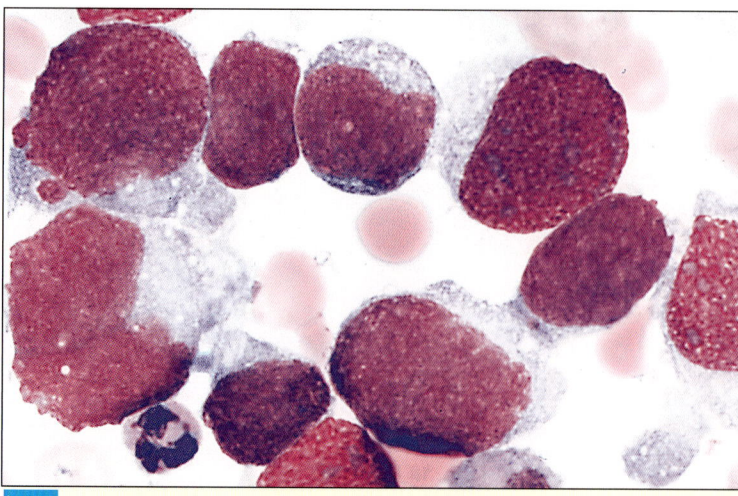

i4.48 Metastatic neuroblastoma cells in the CSF in a child. Note the extremely large size compared to the red cells and neutrophils. There are variable amounts of cytoplasm & dispersed nuclear chromatin with irregular nuclear contours. Wright stain.

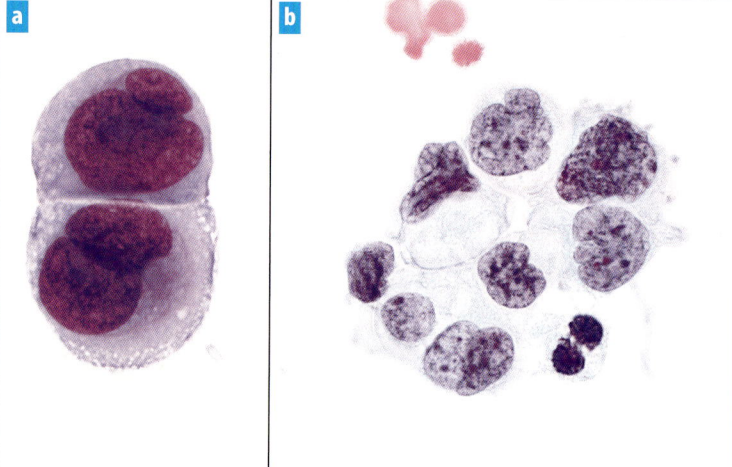

i4.49 **a** High power of metastatic rhabdomyosarcoma in the CSF. Wright stain.
b Metastatic embryonal rhabdomyosarcoma in the CSF of a child. Papanicolau stain.

i4.47 **a** Metastatic breast cancer in the CSF showing extremely large tumor cells with nuclear atypia & cytoplasmic vacuoles. Wright stain.
b Higher power of metastatic breast cancer in the CSF showing the large cell size & marked nuclear atypia. Wright stain.
c Keratin stain by immunocytochemical staining demonstrating keratin expression by carcinoma cells in CSF. Immunoalkaline phosphatase stain.

in ~10% of cases, with a primary presentation of meningeal carcinomatosis there may not be a known primary site. In these cases, careful workup with immunohistochemical stains to identify the cell type of origin can be extremely useful clinically and may aid in treatment decisions [PMID 3656567, PMID 3228160, PMID 3245993].

Chemical analysis

Total protein & albumin

The CSF normally contains <1% of the amount of protein present in plasma. The majority of CSF protein is derived mostly from plasma via ultrafiltration or pinocytosis but small quantities are synthesized intrathecally. The diffusional transfer of protein from plasma into the brain and CSF is a function of 4 properties:

1. the molecular radius of the protein
2. the charge of the protein
3. the plasma concentration of the protein
4. the functional state of the blood-CSF barrier

As such, prealbumin, albumin, and transferrin are the predominant proteins in the CSF.

The concentration of total protein in lumbar CSF is frequently cited as 15-45 mg/dL but the actual reference interval varies by age. Compared to older children and adults, neonates have a high concentration of CSF total protein and can be up to 400 mg/dL in premature infants and 130 mg/dL in infants born at term [PMID 10702528]. Concentrations decline in the first few weeks of life and approach those observed in adults by the end of the 1st year. In older adults, concentrations may be as high as 60 mg/dL. CSF total protein concentrations do not vary between genders.

Another variable is the analytical method used for measurement. Due to its low concentration, analytical methods for measuring total protein in CSF require greater analytical sensitivity than methods used for serum. The most commonly used methods to measure CSF total protein include pyrogallol red, benzethonium chloride, biuret, and modified reverse biuret. These methods do not detect all CSF proteins equally and so results can be disparate between methods.

A common cause of increased CSF total protein is the traumatic tap in which CSF is contaminated with blood. It has been reported that total protein will increase 1 mg/dL for every 1,000 RBCs/μL [PMID 11489408].

The measurement of CSF total protein is a sensitive but nonspecific indicator of CNS pathology and is usually performed to evaluate the integrity of the blood-CSF barrier. Inflammation caused by bacterial or viral meningitis increases the permeability of the blood-CSF barrier to plasma proteins as does high intracranial pressures that might result from traumatic brain injury, intracranial hemorrhage, or brain tumor. Elevation of the total protein concentration is the most frequent pathologic finding in the biochemical analysis of CSF.

Albumin, with a molecular weight of 69 kD, is synthesized in the liver and transported into the CSF. As an independent test, the measurement of albumin in CSF has little clinical utility. However, the ratio of the albumin concentration in the CSF vs the serum is relatively specific measurement of the integrity of the blood-CSF barrier. This CSF/serum albumin index is calculated as albumin$_{CSF}$ (mg/dL)/albumin$_{serum}$ (g/dL). A CSF/albumin index <9 is associated with an intact barrier. Values of 9-14 generally indicate mild impairment, 15-30 indicate moderate impairment, and values >30 represent severe impairment.

The CSF total protein concentration is nearly always increased (>150 mg/dL) in patients with bacterial meningitis. Increased CSF total protein is also seen in those with viral meningitis but to a lesser extent that with a bacterial cause [PMID 11489408]. Because CSF total protein can be increased due to a variety of causes, an elevated result taken in isolation has low specificity for any type of meningitis.

Glucose

The glucose concentration in CSF is maintained by both facilitated transport and simple diffusion from the blood, a process of equilibration that requires as many as 4 hours. Because the CSF glucose concentration is influenced by the concentration of glucose in the blood, the expected CSF glucose concentration from a fasting patient is 50-80 mg/dL (~60% of the blood concentration) [PMID 7882508]. In infants, the CSF:blood ratio is higher (>0.8) [PMID 7882508].

A variety of pathological conditions can alter the CSF glucose concentration. Abnormally low values are often observed in those with bacterial meningitis, mycobacterial, and fungal CNS infections. Other causes of low CSF glucose include chemical meningitis, inflammatory conditions, subarachnoid hemorrhage, and hypoglycemia [PMID 14524396]. The CSF glucose concentration is typically not decreased with most CNS infections of viral origin, although exceptions have been reported. An increased concentration of glucose in the CSF can occur due to hyperglycemia or a traumatic tap. There is no pathological process in the CNS that results in hyperglycorrhachia [PMID 14524396].

The correct interpretation of a CSF glucose concentration is not possible without knowledge of the blood glucose concentration. A patient with hyperglycemia may appear to have a normal CSF glucose concentration when it is, in fact, decreased. Similarly, a low CSF glucose value may be normal when obtained from a patient with hypoglycemia. Because of the equilibration delay, the timing of sample collections is important, particularly in individuals for whom CNS infection is of clinical concern.

The ability of CSF glucose to differentiation between septic and aseptic meningitis has been well studied. Decreased glucose results from increased anaerobic glycolysis in CNS tissue and white blood cells in addition to impaired transport from the blood [PMID 7882508]. In adults, the CSF glucose concentration is <40 mg/dL in ~50%-60% of patients and a CSF:blood ratio <0.4 is 80% sensitive and 98% specific for bacterial meningitis [PMID 8551828, PMID 15494903]. Due to the normally higher CSF:blood glucose ratio in infants, a higher cutoff (<0.6) is often used as a diagnostic threshold [PMID 15494903]. Overall, the clinical utility of the CSF glucose concentration is sufficiently sensitive and specific in individuals for whom the suspicion of aseptic meningitis is high. Further, values usually return to normal soon after therapy is initiated which supports the use of serial measurements in monitoring the effectiveness of treatment [PMID 7882508].

Lactate

Lactic acid is a carboxylic acid that can lose a proton from its carboxyl group, producing its conjugate base, lactate. Lactate is constantly produced from pyruvate via the enzyme lactate dehydrogenase under anaerobic conditions during normal metabolism and exercise. The concentration of lactate in the blood is usually 1-2 mmol/L but can rise dramatically during intense exercise.

The concentration of lactate in the CSF is a function of its synthesis in the CNS by glycolysis and is independent of blood lactate concentration. CSF lactate can increase as a result of hypoxia in inflamed CNS tissues, reduced blood flow as a result of cerebral edema, metabolic disorders of the respiratory chain, seizure, and malignancy [PMID 7882508, PMID 16243873]. Elevations are also observed with increased glucose metabolism by white blood cells and bacteria. As such, the measurement of lactate in the CSF has clinical utility as a test to help differentiate bacterial from viral meningitis.

Several studies have supported the hypothesis that CSF lactate is a more sensitive indicator of bacterial meningitis than either CSF protein or CSF glucose. 2 meta-analyses that included 25 and 33 studies both concluded that the diagnostic accuracy of CSF lactate was superior to that of CSF protein, CSF glucose, CSF:blood glucose ratio, and the CSF white blood cell count for differentiating bacterial from aseptic meningitis in adults and children [PMID 21194480, PMID 21382412]. Because of lack of assay standardization, the optimal cutoff concentration was wide and ranged from 2.1-4.4 mmol/L between the 2 studies. CSF lactate was less sensitive in those who had received antibiotics prior to sample collection. Because of its high negative likelihood ratio, lactate measurement was particularly useful for ruling out bacterial meningitis [PMID 21382412].

C reactive protein

C reactive protein (CRP) is a pentamer of nonglycosylated polypeptide subunits with a molecular weight of 120 kD. Because it is an acute phase reactant synthesized rapidly by the liver in response to inflammation, its measurement in CSF has been investigated as a marker of bacterial meningitis.

A meta-analysis of 24 studies that evaluated the performance of CRP in CSF reported sensitivities and specificities that ranged from 18%-100% and 75%-100%, respectively. The odds ratio was 241 (95% CI, 59-980) [PMID 9819187]. This same report concluded that a nonelevated CSF CRP value had a high negative predictive value (~98%) and could be relied upon to rule out bacterial meningitis. However, the routine use of CSF CRP in differentiating between bacterial and nonbacterial meningitis is not well established.

Immunoglobulins

Immunoglobulins in the CSF are present due to diffusion across the blood-CSF barrier or from intrathecal synthesis. Their detection and/or quantitation have been described for a variety of infectious and autoimmune diseases but the clinical utility of CSF immunoglobulin testing is best established for the assessment of multiple sclerosis.

Multiple sclerosis is a disease that results in the demyelination of brain and spinal cord white matter. The exact etiology of multiple sclerosis is unknown, but a body of research supports the concept that it is an immunologically mediated disease. The most common immunologic abnormality in individuals with multiple sclerosis is increased intrathecal synthesis of immunoglobulin G (IgG) in an oligoclonal pattern [PMID 11967640].

The IgG index and the oligoclonal band tests are 2 well established tests to evaluate intrathecal synthesis of IgG in the CNS. The IgG index is a quantitative indicator of intrathecal IgG synthesis and is determined from the IgG concentration in the CSF vs the serum. Because CSF IgG can be increased due to an impaired blood-CSF barrier it is necessary to correct the IgG index for that possibility. As such, the IgG index is calculated as (IgG_{CSF} [mg/dL] × $albumin_{serum}$ [g/dL])/($albumin_{CSF}$ [mg/dL] × IgG_{serum} [mg/dL]). An IgG index >0.70 is often used to indicate increased intrathecal IgG synthesis. It has a sensitivity of 60%-70% and a specificity of 92%-96% [PMID 14608891, PMID 15272896].

Oligoclonal bands are due to immunoglobulins generated by plasma cells specific to the CNS compartment. They appear early in the onset of multiple sclerosis and remain detectable throughout the course of disease, even during and after treatment [PMID 11967640]. The qualitative detection of oligoclonal bands in the CSF is ideally performed using isoelectric focusing (IEF) electrophoresis followed by immunodetection of IgG. Due to its high sensitivity (>95%) for multiple sclerosis, this method is considered the gold standard test for the detection of oligoclonal bands and is superior to older methods such as high resolution electrophoresis [PMID 15956157]. Importantly, oligoclonal bands are not specific to multiple sclerosis (specificity ~85%) and can also be observed in the CSF from patients with viral or bacterial meningoencephalitis, subacute sclerosing panencephalitis, neurosyphilis, Guillain-Barré syndrome, or meningeal carcinomatosis [PMID 11967640].

Proper interpretation of oligoclonal band testing requires paired CSF and serum samples that are analyzed in parallel. A positive result is one that demonstrates >2 unique oligoclonal bands in the CSF but no matching bands in the serum. There is no consensus regarding the number of unique bands that should be used to differentiate between a positive and a negative oligoclonal band test result. There is consensus regarding test interpretation and it is recommended that oligoclonal band test results be evaluated in terms of 5 classic patterns i4.50.

There are some special circumstances to consider when performing and/or interpreting oligoclonal band tests. First, a paired serum sample is required to accurately interpret patterns 2 through 5. If a paired serum sample is not available and there are no bands identified in the CSF, the presence of oligoclonal bands can still be excluded. Second, testing will sometimes reveal only a single unique band in the CSF for some patients. In one study, 33% (9/27) of patients with a single oligoclonal band developed an oligoclonal banding pattern at a later date [PMID 12682325]. Therefore, it is recommended that those with a single band undergo repeat testing if clinical suspicion for multiple sclerosis is high [PMID 15956157].

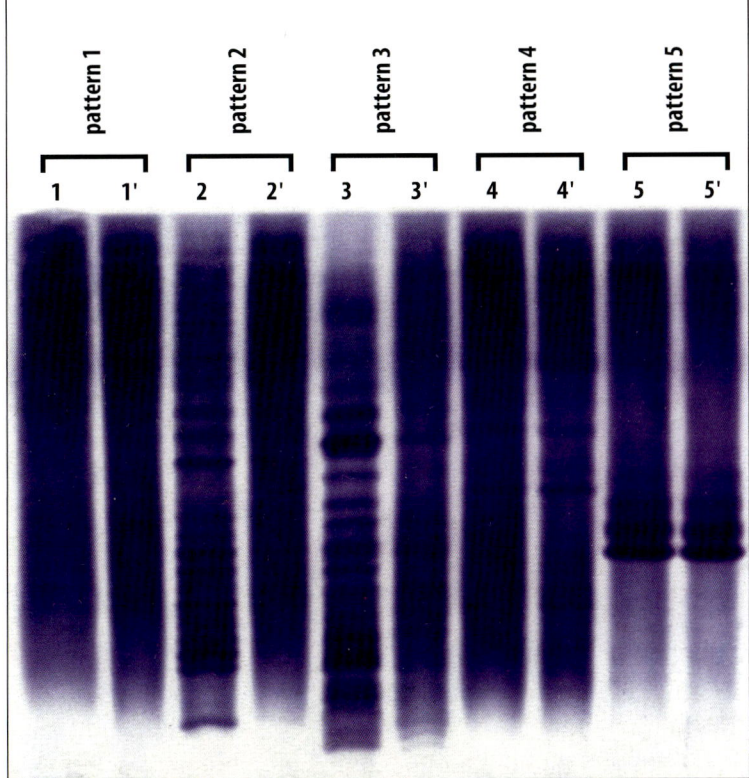

i4.50 Isoelectric focusing electrophoresis gel for the detection of oligoclonal bands in CSF. Note the 5 classic patterns that can be observed:
pattern 1: no bands in the CSF or serum, negative result
pattern 2: oligoclonal IgG bands in the CSF but not the serum, positive result and indicative of intrathecal IgG synthesis
pattern 3: oligoclonal IgG bands in the CSF and additional identical bands in the CSF and serum, positive result and indicative of intrathecal IgG synthesis
pattern 4: identical bands in the CSF and serum, negative result, indicative of a systemic immune reaction
pattern 5: monoclonal bands in the CSF and serum, negative result and indicative of the presence of a monoclonal IgG

Myelin basic protein

Myelin basic protein (MBP), an important component of the myelin sheath, was proposed as a marker for the diagnosis of multiple sclerosis >30 years ago. MBP accounts for ~1/3 of total CNS myelin protein. It is normally not detectable in CSF but MBP concentrations rise in response to neuronal damage [PMID 9532587]. Thus, similar to the IgG index and oligoclonal bands, MBP provides a nonspecific marker of CNS inflammation.

Despite the fact that its use was suggested decades ago, very few studies have evaluated the diagnostic accuracy of MBP in CSF as a biomarker for multiple sclerosis. The studies that have evaluated it have shown considerable variation in clinical performance leading to uncertainty regarding its clinical usefulness. In one study of 166 individuals (54 with multiple sclerosis), sensitivity and specificity were 62% and 71%, respectively [PMID 6171361], while in another study of 129 patients (84 with multiple sclerosis) these were 81% and 80%, respectively [PMID 10973861]. Notably, the concentration of MBP in CSF correlates weakly with clinical symptoms, which limits its usefulness as a monitoring test [PMID 9532587].

Transferrin

Transferrin is a 79.6 kD protein that is glycosylated with 2 N linked complex glycan chains which contain up to 8 sialic acid molecules. It is synthesized by the liver and functions as an iron transport protein. It is a β globulin because it migrates to the β region during protein electrophoresis. In contrast to most other plasma proteins, transferrin is actively transported into the CSF. There, neuraminidase results in the removal of the sialic acid molecules. Therefore, CSF contains 2 isoforms of transferrin: the fully sialated and the desialated variants. These are referred to as a β_1 and β_2 (tau) transferrin, respectively, due to the specific regions they migrate to during CSF protein electrophoresis. Because β_2 transferrin is unique to the CSF, its detection in fluids obtained from the nasal (rhinorrhea) or aural (otorhea) cavities can be used to diagnose CSF fistulas. Leakage of CSF into nasal or aural cavities may also be caused by trauma, intracranial surgical procedures, infection, hydrocephalus, congenital malformations, and neoplasms. A CSF fistula must be quickly differentiated from allergic rhinitis or infectious rhinosinusitis to prevent the subsequent development of meningitis.

Several electrophoretic methods have been used for the detection of serum β_2 transferrin. These include agarose gel electrophoresis, isoelectric focusing electrophoresis, immunofixation, and sodium dodecyl sulfate polyacrylamide gel electrophoresis combined with immunoblotting. Techniques that include immunochemical detection of β_2 transferrin are preferred due to increased analytical and clinical sensitivity. Several studies have demonstrated high sensitivity for the detection of CSF leaks [PMID 23023885, PMID 22483794, PMID 15608153]. False positive results can occur in individuals with glycosylation defects or alcohol dependence due to increased abundance of β_2 transferrin. Samples contaminated with blood have also been reported to reduce clinical specificity [PMID 23023885].

Bilirubin

A subarachnoid hemorrhage (SAH) is caused by spontaneous arterial bleeding into the subarachnoid space, usually from a cerebral aneurysm. For the vast majority of SAH patients, the diagnosis is confirmed by cranial computed tomography scanning. While the sensitivity of this radiologic test is very high (~97%), it fails to detect SAH in 2%-3% of affected patients [PMID 15749414]. The detection of CSF bilirubin formed from the degradation of hemoglobin has clinical utility for identifying individuals with a strong suspicion for SAH but for whom radiological evidence of the hemorrhage is lacking.

Following hemorrhage into the CSF, red blood cells undergo lysis and phagocytosis. The hemoglobin that is released from red blood cells is converted, in vivo, to bilirubin. Because the concentration of bilirubin in the CSF is too low to be accurately measured by traditional chemical methods, absorption spectrophotometry can be utilized to estimate the amount of bilirubin present.

This technique requires the absorbance of a CSF sample to be determined between wavelengths of 350-550 nm. CSF from an otherwise healthy individual shows

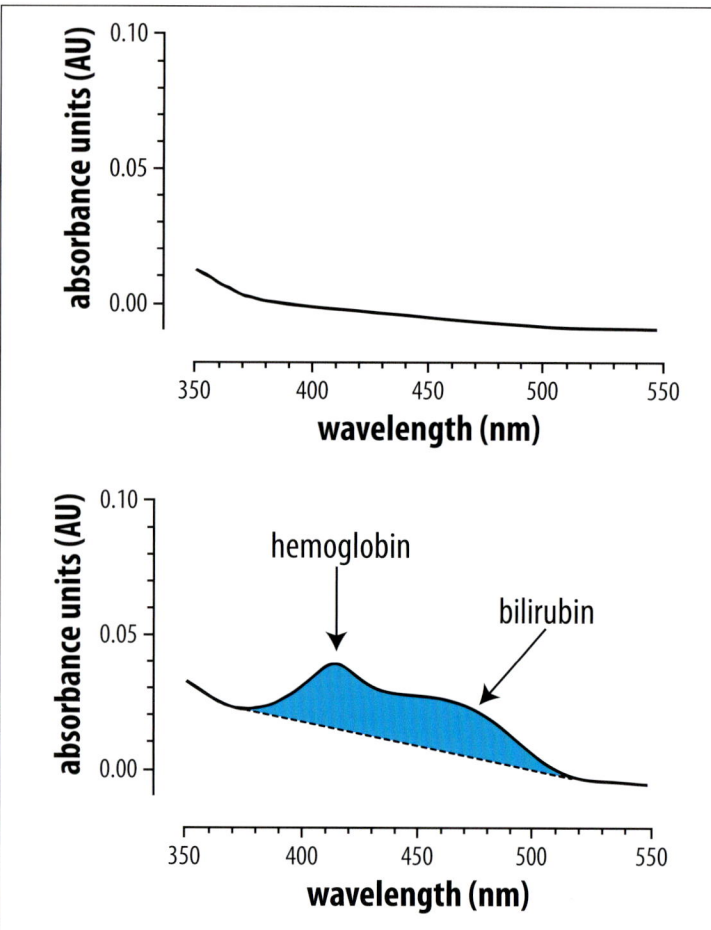

f4.2 Absorption spectrophotometry scans of CSF for determining the presence of bilirubin and hemoglobin in patients suspected of SAH

minimal absorption of light across these wavelengths and the resulting absorbance curves (wavelength vs absorbance) appear flat **f4.2**. CSF collected from an individual following a SAH will typically demonstrate the presence of hemoglobin and bilirubin, which absorb light maximally between 410-418 nm and 450-460 nm, respectively **f4.2**.

Following the scan, a baseline is drawn to form a tangent to the scan between 350-400 nm and 430-530 nm. The extent that the curve deviates from this baseline at 410-418 nm is proportional to the concentration of CSF hemoglobin. Similarly, the extent that the curve deviates from this baseline at 476 nm is proportional to the concentration of CSF bilirubin. Although bilirubin absorbs light maximally at 450 nm, guidelines recommend the use of 476 nm as this is where the absorption curves for hemoglobin and bilirubin are better separated **f4.2** [PMID 18482910].

The detection of CSF bilirubin by absorption spectrophotometry is sensitive but not specific. In 2 different studies that included 460 patients with suspected SAH (prevalence of 0.8%), sensitivity and negative predictive values were 100% but specificity and positive predictive values ranged from 75%-83% and 3.3-5.1%, respectively [PMID 15749414, PMID 16946154]. The low prevalence of SAH in patients tested accounts for the very low positive predictive value. The high sensitivity of the test makes it clinically useful to rule out SAH.

Because the intrathecal generation of bilirubin is time dependent, requiring 9-15 hours after the hemorrhage, false negative results can result from collecting CSF too early after the suspected bleed [PMID 18482910]. Hyperbilirubinemia can also lead to increased CSF bilirubin and so the measurement of bilirubin in a serum sample obtained along with the CSF is recommended. False negative results can occur in samples not protected from light, in samples with very large quantities of hemoglobin (the high hemoglobin peak suppresses the bilirubin peak), or if the CSF sample is obtained prior to 9 hours after the suspected bleed [PMID 18482910].

Adenosine deaminase

Adenosine deaminase (ADA) is an enzyme of the purine salvage pathway that irreversibly catalyzes the deamination of adenosine and deoxyadenosine nucleosides into inosine and deoxyinosine, respectively. ADA plays an important role in the proliferation, differentiation, and maturation of lymphocytes, and a deficiency of the enzyme leads to impaired lymphoid development and severe combined immunodeficiency disease [PMID 11091267]. Due to the stimulation of T cells by mycobacterial antigens, the measurement of ADA activity in CSF has clinical utility as rapid, noninvasive test of tuberculous meningitis.

A meta-analysis of 10 studies including 1,472 patients (283 with tuberculous meningitis), an elevated CSF ADA activity had a sensitivity of 79% and a specificity of 91% [PMID 20937176]. The authors concluded that a nonelevated result was insufficient to rule out tuberculous meningitis but that CSF ADA could help confirm that diagnosis.

ADA testing is not commonly performed in most clinical laboratories and there is not an agreed upon reference measurement method. Importantly, the cutoff used to identify tuberculous meningitis will influence the test's sensitivity and specificity. In areas where the incidence of tuberculosis is low, the test will have little value.

Tumor markers

There are several markers that are increased in the CSF of patients with primary and metastatic malignancy but the clinical utility of most of these is not well established. Those presented below have at least some established clinical utility is established.

α fetoprotein (AFP) is a 69 kD glycoprotein synthesized first by the fetal yolk sac and then by the fetal liver. AFP synthesis ceases shortly after birth, and serum concentrations fall rapidly thereafter. Increased concentrations of serum AFP are associated with intracranial germ cell tumors. These tumors account for only a small portion of germ cell tumors and are classified histologically as germinomatous and nongerminomatous germ cell tumors. Notably, AFP is not produced by germinomas, allowing AFP to be helpful in differentiating between the 2 tumor types. In 48 patients with intracranial germ cell tumor, serum and CSF AFP were correlated (detectable or not detectable in both) in 97% (47/48) paired samples. The 1 patient for whom CSF and serum AFP results did not agree had a nongerminomatous germ cell tumor (CSF was positive and serum was negative for AFP) [PMID 22547227]. These data suggest that an elevated concentration of AFP in either the CSF or serum is sufficient to classify a tumor as a nongerminomatous germ cell tumor.

Human chorionic gonadotropin (hCG) is a 45 kD glycoprotein normally produced by the placenta during pregnancy. Like AFP, serum concentrations of hCG are frequently detected in the serum and CSF of patients with intracranial germ cell tumors. Unlike AFP, however, only hCG is associated with germinomatous germ cell tumors [PMID 19841431]. When hCG is produced by an intracranial germ cell tumor, the concentration in the CSF tends to be greater than it is in the serum [PMID 19841431].

β_2 microglobulin is an 11.8 kD protein expressed on the cell membrane of all nucleated cells as a component of the MHC class I proteins. It is present in nearly all body fluids, and its small size results in it being easily filtered by the glomerulus. β_2 microglobulin in the serum is elevated in individuals with renal failure, inflammation, and neoplasms. Concentrations are quite elevated in those with lymphoproliferative disorders, particularly those of the B cell line.

The clinical usefulness of β_2 microglobulin in CSF has not been well established and few investigations have been published. It has been reported to be a sensitive but nonspecific marker for early diagnosis of CNS involvement in 6 adults with acute leukemia or lymphoma [PMID 1575009]. Other studies have reported that β_2 microglobulin in CSF is significantly higher in patients with CNS involvement of leukemia or lymphoma compared to those with leukemia or lymphoma that did not involve the CNS [PMID 6189578, PMID 6157089]. All of these studies were published >20 years ago and are limited by the small number of patients they included. The use of β_2 microglobulin in CSF remains investigational.

Carcinoembryonic antigen (CEA) is a glycoprotein with a molecular weight of 180 kD that is normally produced by fetal gastrointestinal tissue during development but not after birth. CEA can be synthesized by several adenocarcinomas such as gastrointestinal, breast, lung, ovarian, and pancreatic cancers. Its large mass prevents it from passing through the blood-CSF barrier, which limits is usefulness as a CSF tumor marker. However, evidence suggests that it is a good tumor marker for leptomeningeal carcinomatosis, a rare complication of cancer in which the disease spreads to the meninges and spinal cord. It occurs in ~5% of people with cancer and is usually fatal.

The measurement of CEA in the CSF as an adjunctive evaluation of leptomeningeal carcinomatosis has been described [PMID 3510343, PMID 20386641]. Relative to controls, CSF CEA concentrations are significantly higher in patients with leptomeningeal carcinomatosis than in those with malignancy but without CNS involvement or those with noncarcinomatous malignant lesions. These studies confirmed that elevated CEA concentrations in the CSF are quite specific for neoplasms.

Brain injury markers

S100B is a member of the S100 family of calcium binding proteins involved in signal transduction. S100B is found in glial cells of the nervous system, melanocytes, adipocytes, and chondrocytes. S100B is released in a variety of central nervous system disorders and can be considered as a surrogate marker of CNS injury. Its mechanism of release is uncertain, but it is likely due to release by damaged cells and/or secretion due to glial cell activation. It is first released into the extracellular space, enters the CSF, and passes through the arachnoid villi into the blood.

In patients with brain injury, increased concentrations of S100B protein in CSF have been correlated with the extent of the injury. Further, it have been shown to reliably predict outcomes in various clinical conditions, when measured against functional scores, symptoms, or measures of neuropsychological impairment [PMID 22145907]. In one study of 20 patients with traumatic brain injury, CSF S100B remained elevated for up to 3 days from injury and was highest in patients that died compared with those who survived [PMID 21368691]. Similarly, CSF S100B was elevated in serial CSF samples obtained from 10 children (peak concentration at 27 hours postinjury) who experienced traumatic brain injury compared to control patients without brain injury [PMID 11826241].

Like S100B, neuron specific enolase (NSE) has been extensively investigated as a marker of brain injury. NSE is the functionally active γ subunit of the glycolytic enzyme phosphopyruvate hydrolase. NSE is expressed by cells of the neuroendocrine system and by neural tissue. As such, its measurement in the serum is used clinically as a tumor marker and in the CSF as a marker of neuronal injury.

In a study of 20 patients with traumatic brain injury, CSF NSE was elevated for up to 3 days from injury and was highest in patients that died compared with those who survived [PMID 21368691]. In 10 children with traumatic brain injury, CSF NSE concentrations were significantly increased (peak concentration on day 1 postinjury) above those observed in control patients. In 5 children with inflicted injury, a second, higher NSE peak was observed following the initial peak and was sustained for up to 8 days suggesting delayed neuronal death in those patients [PMID 11826241].

CSF NSE has been significantly associated with the extent of the brain injury as well as with the degree of neurological and functional deficit due to the injury. In a study of 55 patients with brain injury, CSF NSE was significantly increased during the first 7 days relative to control patients. Further, a significant correlation was found between NSE and infarction volume and the degree of neurological and functional deficit [PMID 15921910].

Electrolytes and acid-base balance

There is no known clinical utility for the measurement of electrolytes or the assessment of acid-base balance in the CSF.

Sodium is the major electrolyte present in both the blood plasma and the CSF and the reference interval for both are similar (~136-145 mmol/L). However, due to differences in water content (~93% in plasma and ~99% in CSF), the absolute sodium concentration is slightly greater in plasma. Sodium in the CSF varies directly with its concentration in plasma.

The concentration of potassium in the CSF is tightly maintained (2.5-3.2 mmol/L) even when its concentration in plasma is altered. The CNS maintains strict regulation of potassium because extracellular potassium exerts depolarizing effects of neurons.

In contrast to sodium and potassium, CSF chloride is present at a higher concentration relative to the plasma (110-130 mmol/L). Changes in plasma chloride are quickly reflected in the CSF indicating passive transfer of this electrolyte between the 2 compartments.

1/2 of the total plasma calcium concentration is bound to protein or complexed to anions and the remaining 1/2 is unbound. CSF calcium approximates the later, diffusible fraction of plasma calcium and therefore its concentration is ~1/2 that of the plasma (1.05-1.35 vs 2.05-2.04 mmol/L, respectively). An active transport process regulates CSF calcium and so its concentration remains stable even when the plasma concentration varies.

Magnesium is the only cation with a CSF concentration that exceeds the plasma concentration (1.00-1.35 vs 0.66-1.07 mmol/L, respectively). Like calcium, CSF magnesium concentrations are not influenced by the plasma concentration, suggesting an active regulatory process.

Normally, the pH of the CSF is ~7.31, which is slightly less than that of arterial blood (7.41). The pCO_2 in the CSF ranges from 45-50 mm Hg and is slightly higher than in arterial blood (35-45 mm Hg). The bicarbonate concentration of CSF and arterial blood are similar (~23 mmol/L). The pH of CSF is quite stable, even when it changes dramatically in the blood. Mechanisms to regulate this stability include changes in respiratory rate, alterations in cerebral blood flow, the blood-CSF barrier being readily permeable to carbon dioxide but only slowly permeable to bicarbonate ion, and the intrinsic buffering capacity of CNS tissues.

Neurodegenerative disease markers

Alzheimer disease (AD) is a progressive neurodegenerative disease that leads to loss of memory and cognitive function. The detection and measurement of CSF markers associated with AD has been the subject of extensive research. While CSF biomarkers have been incorporated into the diagnostic criteria of AD for research purposes as supportive evidence for AD pathophysiology, none are in routine clinical use [PMID 17616482].

Pathologically, AD is characterized by amyloid plaques formed by fibrillar forms of β amyloid and neurofibrillary tangles formed by tau proteins. β amyloid is a peptide of 36-43 amino acids that is processed from the amyloid precursor protein, an integral membrane protein expressed in many tissues and concentrated in the synapses of neurons yet has an unknown function. Although β amyloid (1-40) is the most biologically abundant form of the protein, β amyloid (1-42) is more amyloidogenic and toxic and is prone to form amyloid plaques [PMID 23519967]. tau proteins are abundant in neurons of the CNS and are believed to stabilize microtubules, a function that is regulated by several different posttranslational modification steps, particularly phosphorylation. Abnormal hyperphosphorylation produces ptau protein, which dissociates from microtubules, leading to the formation of paired helical filaments that aggregate into neurofibrillary tangles [PMID 23519967].

Diagnostic criteria for AD are clinical and are based on the presence of an early and significant episodic memory impairment. Supportive features for research investigations include abnormal CSF concentrations of AD markers such as a low concentration of β amyloid (1-42), increased total tau or ptau concentration, or a combination of all 3 abnormal values [PMID 17616482].

Creutzfeldt-Jakob disease (CJD) is an incurable neurodegenerative disease of the CNS caused by an accumulation of self catalytically misfolded endogenous prion proteins. CJD is most often sporadic, but it can be inherited via mutations that cause protein misfolding or acquired through transmission by infected human tissues (or tissue extracts) or surgical procedures, or by ingestion of animal products that contain misfolded prion proteins.

Diagnosing CJD is complex and involves extensive clinical history and neurologic examinations including electroencephalographs, magnetic resonance imaging of the CNS, and exclusion of other possible causes of dementia. Several CSF markers have been investigated as markers of CJD including S100, NSE, tau protein, proteinase K resistant prion protein, and 14-3-3 protein [PMID 15304573]. Of these, 14-3-3 protein has produced the most consistent results in diagnosis of CJD.

The 14-3-3 protein belongs to a family of conserved regulatory proteins that are expressed in all eukaryotic cells. They can bind to several functionally diverse signaling proteins such as kinases, phosphatases, and transmembrane receptors. When detected in the CSF, the presence of 14-3-3 protein indicates substantial neuronal destruction. Increased CSF concentrations of 14-3-3 proteins have been described in patients with various forms of CJD. Testing for 14-3-3 protein is most often done qualitatively by Western blot but quantitative immunoassays are also available. The overall sensitivity and specificity of detectable 14-3-3 protein in the CSF in CJD are 85%-97% and 84%-97%, respectively [PMID 22710755]. In a study of 420 patients suspected of having a prion disease who were subsequently examined at autopsy, the 14-3-3 test had a sensitivity of 90% sensitivity but a specificity of only 40% [PMID 22843257]. The same study reported that measurement of tau protein was less sensitive but more specific (87% and 67%, respectively) than 14-3-3 protein. Neither protein is appropriate to use as a screening test and there is no established role for 14-3-3 measurement in the diagnosis of acquired or inherited CJD.

Microbiologic examination

The first line of interrogation for meningitis/meningoencephalitis involves the examination and profiling of the CSF. The tests performed on CSF that provide immediate information for meningitis include a total leukocyte count and differential, total protein, glucose, and (often undocumented) opening pressure. While the CSF profile is not always entirely specific for predicting a specific pathogen, it can typically guide the differential diagnosis and allow for cultures to be appropriately selected. Typically a bacterial culture and cytocentrifuged Gram stain are performed on all CSF specimens from patients suspicious of meningitis.

Blood cultures should be obtained in cases where bacterial meningitis is suspected, as they are often positive (pathogen dependent) and in some cases may provide the only definitive information as to the causative agent in the case of CSF culture negative/stain positive meningitis. CSF cultures will be positive in ~90% of meningitis caused by nonfastidious organisms. The CSF can be infected by a variety of bacteria, viruses, and parasites; for the sake of this text, only the most common or devastating pathogens among each group will be discussed t4.21.

t4.21 Pathogens in meningitis/meningoencephalitis

Bacteria	Haemophilus influenzae
	Neisseria meningitidis
	Streptococcus pneumoniae
	Streptococcus agalactiae (group B)
	Enterobacteriaceae (eg, Escherichia coli, Klebsiella, Enterobacter, Citrobacter)
	Listeria monocytogenes
	Aerobic Gram– rods (eg, Acinetobacter & Pseudomonas)
Mycobacterium	Mycobacterium tuberculosis
Spirochetes	Borrelia burgdorferi
	Treponema pallidum
Fungi	Cryptococcus species
	Candida species
	Aspergillus species
	"Black yeasts" (eg, Exophiala, Hortea, Aureobasidium, Sporothrix)
	Endemic mycoses (eg, Histoplasma, Coccidioides, Blastomyces)
	Contaminants to sterile infectibles (poorly defined)
Viruses	Enteroviruses (echovirus, coxsackievirus, poliovirus, numbered enteroviruses)
	Arthropod borne viruses (eg, West Nile virus, Powassan virus)
	Herpesviridae (eg, herpes simplex virus type 2, varicella zoster virus)
	Other (lymphocytic choriomeningitis virus, adenovirus, mumps virus)
Free living amoebae	Acanthamoeba species
	Naegleria fowleri
	Balamuthia mandrillaris
Parasites	Angiostrongylus cantonensis
	Gnathostoma spinigerum
	Toxocara species
	Taenia solium
	Baylisascaris procyonis
	Unusual trematode complications (eg, Paragonimus, Schistosoma)

Bacterial meningitis

The diagnosis of bacterial meningitis is the most compelling reason for examining the cerebrospinal fluid. Appropriate collection and microbiologic examination is essential for every patient in whom the clinical findings suggest even the slightest possibility of bacterial meningitis. The major reasons for this are as follows:

- untreated bacterial meningitis is a lethal disease capable of rapid progression
- early diagnosis and treatment with appropriate antibiotics is often curative; even a slight delay may result in a permanent CNS deficiency
- the selection of adequate antimicrobials depends on a knowledge of the specific causative agent

Historically the 3 most common agents of bacterial meningitis worldwide were *Neisseria meningitidis*, *Streptococcus pneumoniae*, and *Haemophilus influenzae* type B (HiB); accounting for up to 77% of cases in 1986 [PMID 20610819]. Intense vaccination efforts were aimed at eradicating these pathogens, with HiB having the first vaccine used in many countries worldwide. In 1995 a followup study showed dramatic reduction of HiB meningitis, while *N meningitidis* and *S pneumoniae* rates remained unchanged for all age groups [PMID 20610819]. Vaccination with a heptavalent vaccine against *N meningitidis* has similarly led to a dramatic reduction in meningitis; however a more comprehensive tetravalent vaccine was released in 2005, for which the impact has not been established [PMID 20610819]. Recent data suggests that *S pneumoniae* remains the leading cause of bacterial meningitis in the United States (~61%), with many meningitis cases caused by serogroups included in the 23-valent vaccine. It is unclear why the vaccine does not provide convincing protection against meningeal disease; however this may explain why *S pneumoniae* remains the most common pathogen in several vaccine compliant countries [PMID 23141619].

Streptococcus agalactiae group B (GBS) is a significant cause of neonatal meningitis, particularly in children <3 months of age. Acquisition occurs during passage of the baby through the birth canal of a mother who is colonized with GBS. In the United States, specific guidelines have been designed to screen mothers in the 35th week of pregnancy and to treat GBS colonized women with penicillin-G during delivery. This practice has reduced neonatal meningitis due to GBS by 80%.

Listeria monocytogenes is the causative agent of ~2% of bacterial meningitis and is a concern mainly for the elderly and perinates [PMID 20610819]. The incidence has gone down in recent years thanks to better food handling practices aimed at reducing the contamination of ready to eat food. This likely accounts for a reduction in perinatal meningitis attributed to *Listeria*.

Gram– bacilli from the Enterobacteriaceae are also significant causes of neonatal meningitis. *E coli* is typically associated with early onset neonatal meningitis (within the 1st week of life), while late onset meningitis is typically associated with *E coli* as well as *Klebsiella*, *Citrobacter*, and *Enterobacter* [PMID 20610819]. Nosocomial meningitis of any age group can involve aerobic nonfermenting Gram– rods such as *Acinetobacter baumannii* and *Pseudomonas aeruginosa* [PMID 20610819].

Mixed enteric flora of the human bowel can also be found in the CSF of immunocompromised patients. Organisms such as *Streptococcus bovis*, *Enterococcus* species, and members of the *Enterobacteriaciae* may be detected in the CSF in polymicrobial meningitis [PMID 14726461]. These infections should be treated aggressively to eradicate the bacteria, and the patient should also be tested for *Strongyloides stercoralis* by serology and stool ovum and parasite examination. During hyperinfection with *Strongyloides*, the larvae migrate through sterile sites in the body (such as the brain) and seed the tissue with enteric organisms that it inadvertently translocates from the human bowel [PMID 14726461].

For all bacterial causes of meningitis described above, a cytocentrifuged Gram stain or smear from centrifuged sediment in addition to culture of the CSF sediment (if specimen

4: Cerebrospinal Fluid

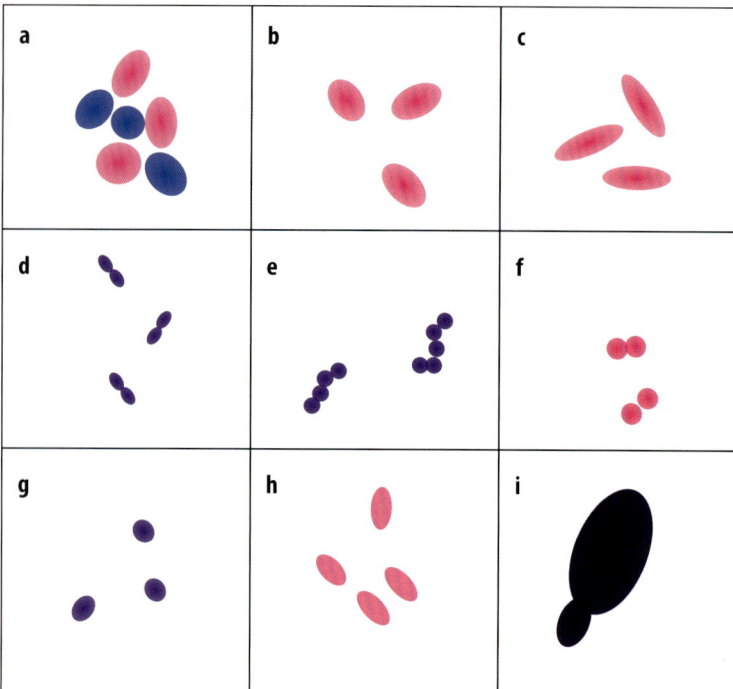

f4.3 Diagramatic representation characteristic of Gram stain morphologies of potential CSF pathogens. The following organisms are represented:
  a *Acinetobacter* species
  b *Escherichia coli*
  c *Pseudomonas aeruginosa*
  d *Streptococcus pneumoniae*
  e *Streptococcus agalactiae* (GBS)
  f *Neisseria meningitidis*
  g *Listeria monocytogenes*
  h *Haemophilus influenzae*
  i *Candida* species, budding form (may be very large, up to 8 µm in size)

volume is >1 mL) are the most common approaches to diagnosis (see Chapter 2). For specimens with very little volume, the culture should be performed with the entire specimen and a Gram stain should be sacrificed (with an accompanying explanation of the volume limitations). The Gram stain can be particularly helpful with these organisms, as the identification can often be predicted based on the uniqueness of the stain. For instance, *S pneumoniae* are lancet shaped Gram+ diplococci, *N meningitidis* are Gram– diplococci, *Haemophilus influenzae* are Gram– coccobacilli and *Listeria monocytogenes* are Gram+ coccobacilli. Enteric Gram– rods are plump Gram– rods in contrast to *Pseudomonas aeruginosa*, which are thin, long Gram– rods. *Acinetobacter baumannii* are characteristically large Gram variable coccobacilli. GBS are Gram+ cocci in chains, and cannot be predicted from their Gram stain, as most streptococci will show a similar staining pattern **f4.3**. In some cases, ingested bacteria may be seen in neutrophils or monocytes/macrophages during cytologic examination **i4.5b**, **i4.35**, **i4.51a-d** or in

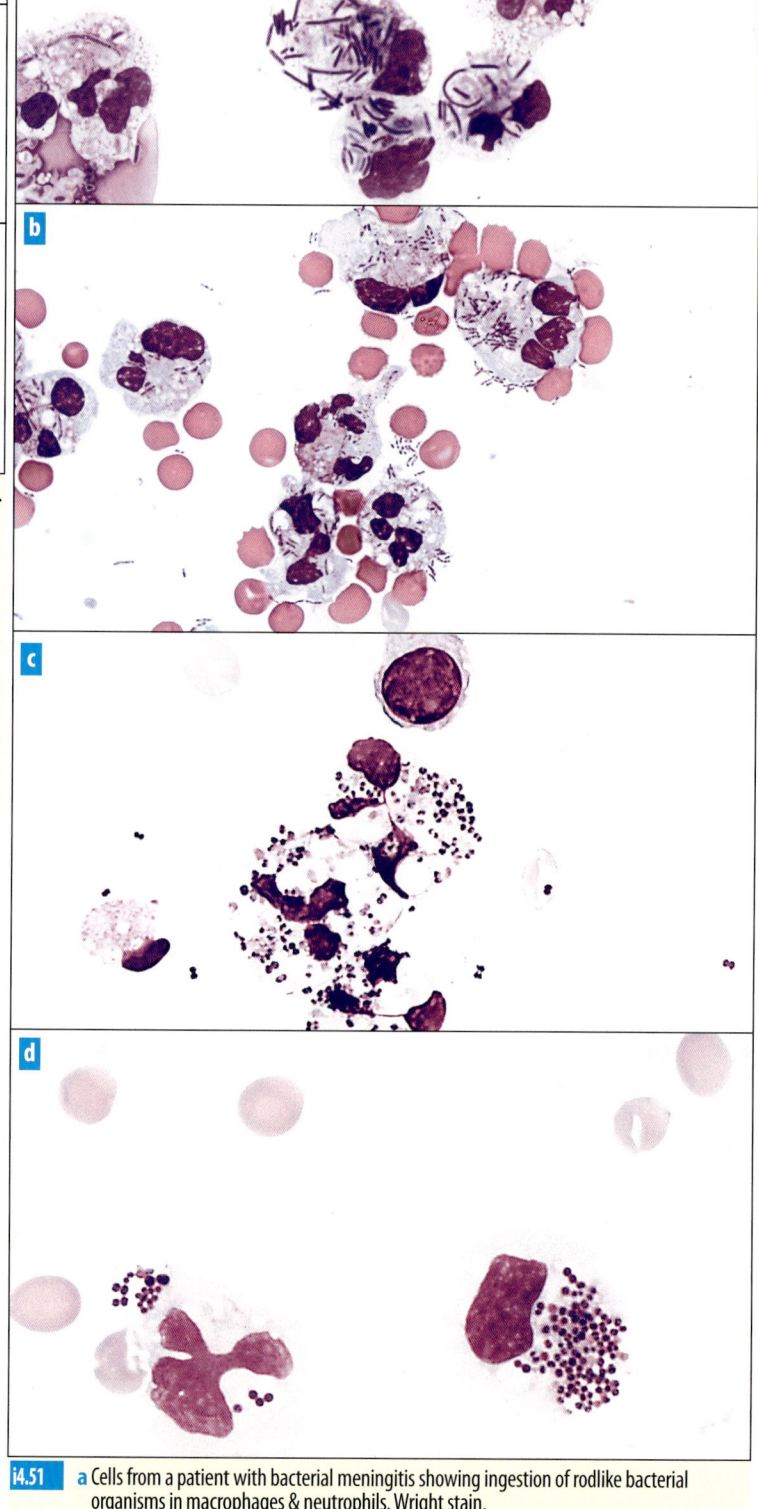

i4.51 **a** Cells from a patient with bacterial meningitis showing ingestion of rodlike bacterial organisms in macrophages & neutrophils. Wright stain.
b Case of bacterial meningitis showing ingestion of numerous bacilli by neutrophils & monocyte/macrophage cells in the CSF. Wright stain.
c Intracellular bacteria in the CSF of a patient with meningitis due to *Neisseria meningitidis*. Wright stain
d Intracellular bacteria in the CSF of a patient with meningitis due to *Streptococcus pneumoniae*. Wright stain.

4: Cerebrospinal Fluid

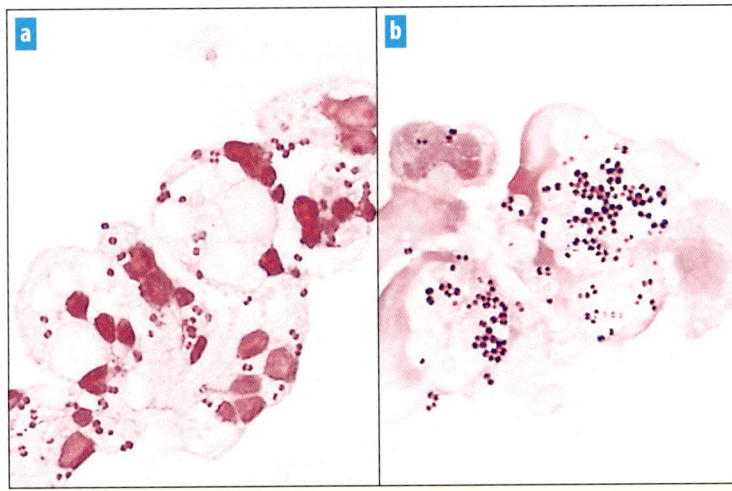

i4.52 a Many Gram− bacteria in CSF in a case of meningitis due to *Neisseria meningitidis*. Gram stain
b Many Gram+ bacteria in CSF in a case of meningitis due to *Streptococcus pneumoniae*. Gram stain

Viral meningitis

Aseptic meningitis is a term that is broadly used to describe a nonbacterial cause of meningitis. While these can be infectious and noninfectious in origin, the majority of aseptic meningitis cases are attributable to viral etiologies [PMID 17471037]. Though most cases of viral meningitis cannot be treated with antiviral drugs, detecting a viral agent can help guide supportive care and also can effectively rule out a bacterial etiology (particularly in the case of negative cultures and Gram stain). The CSF profile of typical viral meningitis is shown in **t4.22**. Of note, partially treated bacterial meningitis can resemble early viral meningitis when comparing the CSF profiles for the 2 clinical scenarios. This remains a diagnostic challenge, particularly in the case of patients that are transferred from an outpatient facility to an inpatient facility. These patients may not be conscious, or are otherwise unable to recall their antimicrobial treatments due to neurological dysfunction associated with their meningitis. A single universal laboratory profile for bacterial vs viral meningitis has not been established to date, and cumulative supportive evidence is the common approach to working through a differential diagnosis.

The most common etiologies of viral meningitis are listed in **t4.21**. Enteroviruses (poliovirus, echovirus, coxsackievirus, numbered enteroviruses) are the most frequently identified causes of viral meningitis, accounting for up to 90% of cases [PMID 18657719, PMID 17471037]. In most of these cases, the patients are <5 years of age [PMID 18657719]. Viral meningitis is most common during the summer months, and this can be predicted by the corresponding seasonality of enteroviruses. Nonenteroviral causes of meningitis are also seasonal, which compounds the summer bias of viral meningitis. Mosquito vectored viruses (arboviruses) such as West Nile virus (WNV), St Louis encephalitis (SLE), and La Crosse virus (LCV) are most common in the summer (reflecting peak insect populations and feeding activity) [PMID 18657719]. WNV causes aseptic meningitis in all age groups, whereas SLE and LCV each cause meningitis in children, but present as encephalitis in adults. Mumps virus is an uncommon in vaccine compliant countries, though a seasonal cause of viral meningitis. These infections typically cluster in late winter/early spring, and meningitis syndromes are more common in males [PMID 18657719].

Gram stained preparations **i4.52a-b**. All of the aforementioned organisms can be cultured readily on nonselective media such as Columbia blood agar or chocolate agar, with most organisms forming colonies in ~18-24 hours (if antimicrobial therapy was not initiated before CSF collection).

Despite the rapidity of growth for most bacteria associated with meningitis, rapid tests directly from the CSF were developed to lessen the diagnostic window for bacterial meningitis. The first of such tests were latex agglutination rapid assays. Despite their promising role in diagnosis, latex agglutination assays for *H influenzae*, *N meningitidis*, *S pneumoniae*, and GBS are all insensitive, and should not be used for the diagnosis of bacterial meningitis [PMID 20610819]. The *Streptococcus pneumoniae* antigen test for CSF however is a very sensitive and specific method for diagnosing pneumococcal meningitis. The assay is available in an immunochromatographic format and can be performed near point of care. One multisite study showed 99% sensitivity and specificity vs culture, essentially with 1/25th of the turnaround time [PMID 19191619]. To date, no analogous tests exist for meningococcus, GBS, or HiB.

t4.22 Typical CSF profiles for meningitis

	Normal	Bacterial	Fungal	Tuberculous	Viral	Amoebic (encephalitis)	Amoebic (meningoencephalitis)	Neurosyphilis
Glucose	40-85 mg/dL	Normal to decreased (≤40 mg/dL)	Low (<40 mg/dL)	Low (<40 mg/dL)	Normal (>40)	Normal to decreased (≤40 mg/dL)	Low (<40 mg/dL)	Normal to decreased (≤40 mg/dL)
Protein	15-45 mg/dL	Increased (>250 mg/dL)	Moderate/marked increase (25-500 mg/dL)	Moderate/marked increase (25-500 mg/dL)	Moderate increase (<100 mg/dL)	Increased (>250 mg/dL)	Increased (>250 mg/dL)	Increased (>250 mg/dL)
WBCs	0-5 cells/mm³	Increased (>500 cells/mm³)	Variable (>5 cells/mm³)	Variable (>5 cells/mm³)	Few (<100 cells/mm³)	Few (<100 cells/mm³)	Increased (>500 cells/mm³)	Variable (>5 cells/mm³)
Differential	60%-70% lymphocytes; 30% monocytes/macrophages	PMN predominance	Lymphocyte predominance	Lymphocyte predominance; PMNs may be elevated	Early: PMN predominance; Late: lymphocyte predominance	Lymphocyte predominance	PMN predominance	Lymphocyte predominance

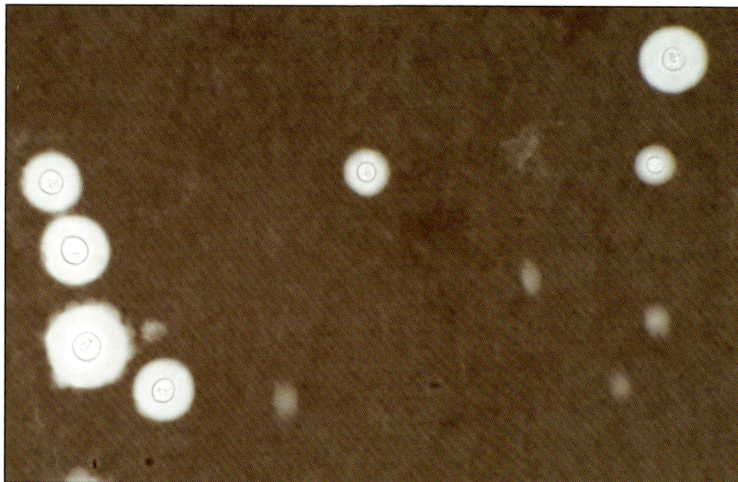

i4.53 India ink preparation demonstrating *Cryptococcus neoformans* at high magnification

Nonseasonal and unusual causes of viral meningitis include members of Herpesviridae. The 2 most common causes of herpesvirus meningitis are herpes simplex virus type 2 (HSV2) and varicella zoster virus (VZV) [PMID 18657719]. Meningitis with HSV2 and VZV can occur as a result of primary infection or reactivation of latent virus. Dissemination to the CNS can occur from hematogenous and neuronal routes [PMID 18657719]. HSV2 can cause recurrent meningitis in the absence of symptoms of genital herpes, but like genital HSV2 infections, recurrence can be controlled with suppressive antiviral therapy [PMID 18474734]. HSV2 meningitis can cause Mollaretlike meningitis in addition to generic aseptic meningitis [PMID 18474734]. The arenavirus lymphocytic choriomeningitis virus (LCMV) is a clinically and epidemiologically underappreciated cause of viral meningitis. The virus is acquired through inhalation or ingestion of rodent feces [PMID 18657719]. Individuals working in close contact with rodents, such as laboratory workers and pet shop employees, were traditionally considered at highest risk for infection.

Culture was once the standard modality for which viral meningitis was diagnosed (particularly for enteroviruses and herpes simplex virus which could be readily cultured in vitro); however molecular tests have largely replaced culture as the recommended diagnostic method for acute phase viral meningitis [PMID 18657719, PMID 15608000]. PCR is widely available for enteroviruses and has better sensitivity than culture in additional to faster turnaround times [PMID 17471037]. HSV2 detection by PCR is also recommended over culture in the acute phase of suspected viral meningitis [PMID 18657719]. Most arboviruses cannot be cultured routinely in the clinical laboratory and PCR is not readily available for many of these pathogens. Therefore intrathecal production of virus specific IgM antibody remains the standard diagnostic approach for these viruses [PMID 18657719]. When possible, PCR and CSF serology should be performed in cases of aseptic meningitis. This is particularly important as CSF collected in the early phase of infection (~5 days postinfection) may be positive by PCR and negative by serology, and the opposite may be true for later stage infections [PMID 15608000]. Retrospective diagnoses of arboviral meningitis can also be established by demonstrating IgG serocoversion between specimens collected at the onset of symptoms and 4-6 weeks after convalescence.

Fungal meningitis

The most common and frequently identified causes of fungal meningitis are caused by *Cryptococcus* species. Historically the India ink preparation was used for the detection of cryptococcal meningitis **i4.53**. Though this test is still used in many laboratories due to its excellent positive predictive value, the negative predictive value is unacceptably low, requiring additional interrogation through alternative testing modalities. A CSF Gram stain with cytocentrifugation (see Chapter 2) can also detect *Cryptococcus*; however the sensitivity of this stain is also not ideal. On Wright staining **i4.27** the yeast resembles mononuclear cells with a prominent halo or may appear as "sunburst" cells **i4.27a-b**. *Cryptococcus* can also be detected by the periodic acid-Schiff and methenamine silver stains. A CSF specimen that is cultured for bacterial etiologies may serendipitously recover *Cryptococcus*, though culture, and similar to India ink, has excellent positive predictive value but unacceptable negative predictive value.

Significant advances in the diagnosis of cryptococcal meningitis were achieved with the integration of latex slide agglutination for cryptococcal antigens in the CSF. Antigen detection assays have served as the recommended test modality for many years due to excellent specificity (99%) and sensitivity (97%) [PMID 1761681]. A positive test result in the CSF is typically indicative of active CNS disease, resulting in excellent positive predictive value. There are 4 serogroups of *Cryptococcus* (A, B, C & D) that are represented by 2 pathogenic species, *C neoformans* and *C gatti*. An important limitation of antigen detection is that not all serogroups of *Cryptococcus* are detected equally by each commercial kit. Latex agglutination is thought to detect each serogroup due to the polyclonal nature of the antibody preparation. The premier *Cryptococcus* antigen ELISA however does not readily detect serotype C&C like serotypes, whereas newer assays from IMMY can detect these serotypes [PMID 21697342, PMID 23114703].

Fungal meningitis caused by yeasts other than *Cryptococcus* are less frequently encountered, though often life threatening. *Candida albicans* can cause fungal meningitis and is becoming more common in HIV/AIDS patients but is particularly common in neonates and preterm neonates for whom the blood-brain barrier is significantly more permeable [PMID 8903210, PMID 12881799]. Patients undergoing neurosurgeries or with CSF leaks due to trauma or fistulas are also at risk of developing *Candida* meningitis **i4.5a-c** [PMID 8562739]. Culture and Gram stain are both standard diagnostic approaches for CSF specimens infected with *Candida*. In fact, *Candida* will typically grow in standard bacterial culture media and incubation temperatures (see Chapter 2).

Several "black yeasts" are also CSF-tropic, particularly of concern in immunocompromised patients. These fungi tend to be thermophilic (growth at 42°C) and form black yeast-like growth on solid media. Some examples of neurotropic fungi include *Exophiala dermatitidis*, *Exophiala jeanselmni*,

Sporothrix shenckii, *Hortea werneckii*, and *Aureobasidium pullans* [ISBN 978-1555816605].

Aspergillus (like *Candida*) is also a significant concern for HIV patients [PMID 8903210]. Cultures of CSF for *Aspergillus* are positive only 31% of the time, whereas detection of *Aspergillus* galactomannan antigen from the CSF is positive in 87% of cases in one meta-analysis [PMID 23178421]. The galactomannan antigen detection assay significantly reduces the turnaround time vs culture; however it is not FDA cleared for use on CSF specimens. Testing should be performed in a laboratory that has appropriately validated this specimen type (which will delay the turnaround time due to sending the specimen for testing off site).

Endemic dimorphic mycoses (existing in a yeast and mold phase) such as *Histoplasma* species, *Blastomyces dermatitidis*, and *Coccidioides immitis* are all geographically constrained, though clinically problematic agents of fungal meningitis. These infections are typically of concern in immunocompromised patients living in endemic regions or who harbor latent infections from past exposure in endemic regions. All of these organisms are difficult to recover in culture (particularly from CSF), and typically are best detected through the use of culture, stains, and serology.

Histoplasma capsulatum meningitis reportedly occurs in ~10% of cases following relapse of inadequately treated disseminated histoplasmosis [PMID 4015272]. Diagnosis of this fungal organism is difficult, even with appropriate cultures, serological markers, special stains, and urine antigen detection. Each method has poor sensitivity; therefore multiple methods should be used to maximize the diagnostic workup. Culture independent methods (urine antigen, serology) can also suffer from false positive results, and therefore positive results need to be interpreted carefully in the clinical context. These assays perform better in cases of disseminated histoplasmosis, rather than isolated CNS disease, where the organism may be shielded from the immune system and antigen likely will not concentrate distally in the urine [PMID 15736018]. While no consensus exists for the standardized approach to diagnosing *Histoplasma* CNS infections, at minimum the CSF should be cultured (>10 mL if possible), tested for antigen on a validated assay, and antibody detection by complement fixation should be performed [PMID 15736018]. The serum should also be tested for antibodies by complement fixation as well as antigen, to correlate with any positive CSF antibodies or antigen results that could be contamination from a traumatic tap [PMID 15736018]. Additionally, all patients with suspected Histoplasmosis should receive urine antigen testing.

C immitis, like *Histoplasma*, can be a significant life threatening disease when it involves the CNS. Before the introduction of amphotericin B, *Coccidioides* meningitis had a shockingly high case fatality rate. Despite amphotericin B, the morbidity associated with meningeal disease is still quite high [PMID 16323099]. The CSF profile resembles most fungal meningitides t4.22, but with very high levels of protein [PMID 16323099]. Diagnosing *Coccidioides* meningitis is typically achieved by visualization of spherules in biopsy tissue or cytology (staining with H&E, Wright stain or

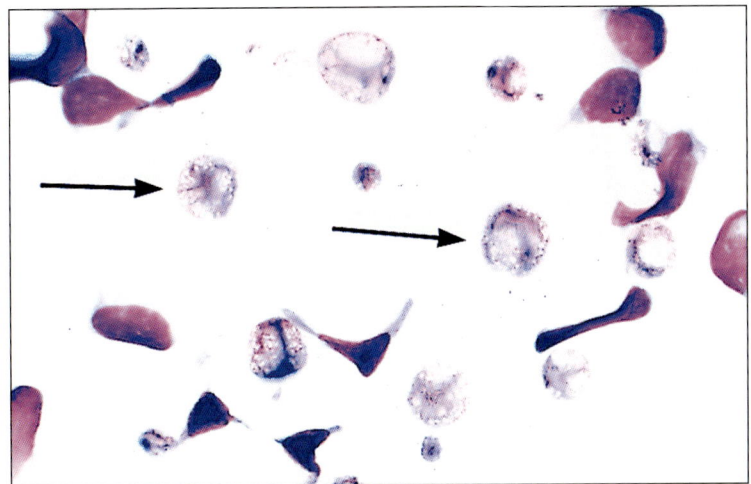

i4.54 *Coccidioides immitis* in the CSF with numerous immature spherules (arrows). Wright stain.

Grocott-Gomori methenamine-silver are commonly used) i4.54, culturing the organism from the CSF or tissue (very low yield), or through serological interrogation of the serum and CSF [PMID 18316002]. Acute infections are tested serologically using IgM detection methods such as immunodiffusion and/or ELISA, both of which provide qualitative results. Complement fixation provides total antibody response to the pathogen; however it provides a titer than can be used to predict severity of disease (dissemination) and/or response to therapy [PMID 18316002]. Any detection of *Coccidioides* specific antibodies in the CSF (particularly IgG) is considered evidence of *Coccidioides* meningitis [PMID 16323099]. As mentioned previously, testing of the serum in parallel is necessary to interpret the results of CSF antibody testing.

In 2013, a nationwide outbreak of fungal meningitis was described in the United States. In this outbreak, the causative organism was not one of the pathogens described above, but was identified as *Exserohilum rostratum* (a dematiaceous "black" mold) [PMID 23083312]. This organism is not CNS-tropic, and is considered an allergen rather than a pathogen. In the early phase of the outbreak, CSF specimens growing this organism were thought to be contaminated, either in the laboratory or during specimen collection. Eventually, contaminated methylprednisolone was identified as the source of the outbreak, originating form a compounding pharmacy [PMID 23083312]. Patients receiving injections in the epidural space were receiving large fungal burden in an otherwise immune privileged space, leading to catastrophic consequences including death [PMID 23083312]. While the organism implicated in this outbreak was a result of random environmental selection, it is paramount to report and consult on the presence of any mold growth in a CSF specimen regardless of its identity. In situations such as this, the importance of fungal CSF cultures cannot be overstated, as no other detection methods are universally employed. During this outbreak, use of the (1,3)-β-D-glucan detection assay was described for several cases involved in the early phase of the outbreak [PMID 23363831]. The assay is FDA cleared only for use on serum specimens and therefore there is no diagnostic cutoff established for CSF specimens (which may have lower concentrations of antigen that could be medically relevant) (1,3)-β-D-glucan is a component of many fungal cells walls that can be detected in serum, providing early evidence of invasive fungal infections. The specificity of the assay is important to consider however, as (1,3)-β-D-glucan can be found in surgical gauze, immunoglobulin preparations, and certain antibiotics [PMID 23621588]. Importantly, *Cryptococcus* will not be detected by this assay as the cell wall does not contain (1,3)-β-D-glucan, so cryptococcal antigen detection should be tested concurrently for suspected fungal meningitis [PMID 23621588].

Tuberculous meningitis

Tuberculous meningitis is a rare manifestation of disease caused by *Mycobacterium tuberculosis* (~1%); however it can kill or cause significant disabilities in over 1/2 of those infected [PMID 23972913]. Tuberculous meningitis can affect any patient with pulmonary TB, though cases are most common in those with HIV disease or very young children. In developing nations with high rates of HIV infection, tuberculous meningitis is a significant concern [PMID 23972913]. The bacillus Calmette-Guérin (BCG) vaccine has reduced the number of childhood tuberculous meningitis cases in addition to lowering the incidence of pulmonary TB [PMID 16616560]. Despite these prophylactic interventions, one of the greatest challenges in tuberculous meningitis is recognizing the symptoms early and achieving laboratory results to support the diagnosis. Early diagnosis and therapy are considered the most important factors in predicting clinical outcomes, with significant delays carrying often fatal results [PMID 13762229].

The CSF profile of tuberculous meningitis may resemble fungal meningitis **t4.22**. Given the high incidence of cryptococcal meningitis and tuberculous meningitis in areas with high HIV rates, this ambiguity can represent a significant clinical challenge. The standard laboratory approach to diagnosing tuberculous meningitis relies on stain and culture, despite their poor sensitivity. Ziehl-Neelsen staining (see Chapter 2) of large volumes of CSF provides, at best, 60% sensitivity [PMID 14715783]. Culture sensitivity is highly variable and depends largely on the volume of specimen cultured. The major limitation with culture is the diagnostic delay between culture and reporting (upwards of 4 weeks). These delays are not practical in cases of true tuberculous meningitis.

An alternative approach is to detect rRNA from *M tuberculosis* directly from the specimen using probe amplified detection (see Chapter 2). This test has poor sensitivity and as a result cannot exclude TB, but if positive can provide immediate results that can be used as an indication for treating with anti TB drugs. Of important consideration is the fact that the TB probe also detects other members of the TB complex of bacteria. However, given that CNS infections with other members of the TB complex are very rare, a positive probe result would likely indicate TB. PCR, though promising for diagnosing pulmonary TB, has not been established as a reliable and sensitive method for diagnosing tuberculous meningitis. Additional studies are required to optimize a PCR suitable for CSF testing.

Free living amoebic infections

So called "free living amoebae" are a group of genetically diverse eukaryotic protozoa that exist in nature in a wide variety of niches. Unlike the intestinal amoebae (eg, *Entamoeba histolytica*), which require a host for their life cycle, the free living amoebae are able to survive in the absence of a host, typically phagocytizing bacteria or other amoebae for nutrients. To date, 4 free living amoebae (*Acanthamoeba* species, *Naegleria fowleri*, *Balamuthia mandrillaris*, *Sappinia pedata*) have been shown to cause human disease, all capable of infecting the central nervous system. Environmental exposures are associated with free living amoeba infections, with each amoeba having unique risks for exposure. *Acanthamoeba* exists in tap water and almost all artificial water systems (including water towers, air conditioning units, dialysis machines, and hot tubs) and can be introduced to the eye through improper contact lens use and to the central nervous system through exposure of patients with impaired immune function [PMID 17428307]. *Balamuthia* is a soil organism, typically spread by wind/dust and is typically inhaled by the host. Like *Acanthamoeba*, the host must have immune dysfunction to become ill [PMID 17428307]. *Naegleria* can infect any individual; however the organism must be introduced into the nasal cavity with some amount of force for infection to ensue. Once in the nasal cavity, the trophozoite actively penetrates the cribriform plate and invades the brain [PMID 17428307]. These infections have been described in adolescent males partaking in water sports in warm bodies of water, individuals using neti pots with well water, and Muslims practicing ablution before prayer in which the water was contaminated [PMID 17428307, PMID 22919000, PMID 21291600].

All of these amoebae cause amoebic encephalitis except *Naegleria*, which causes a rapidly fatal meningoencephalitis. The CSF profile for these conditions can be variable, but often follow the pattern shown in **t4.22**. For each of these infections, the prognosis is poor, especially *Balamuthia* and *Naegleria*, for which few patients have ever survived [PMID 17428307]. Often the diagnosis is made postmortem from histopathologic sections of the brain (with PCR to ultimately

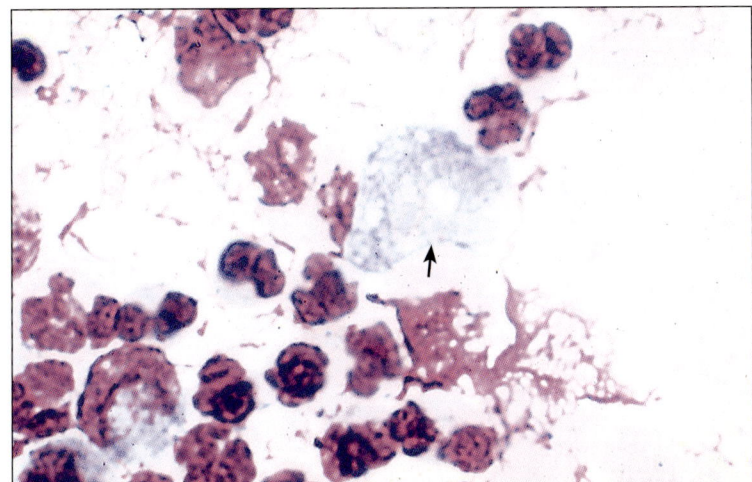

i4.55 Primary amoebic meningoencephalitis. A degenerating amoebic trophozoite is seen with sky blue cytoplasm (arrow). Wright stain. (Courtesy of JG dos Santos, MD)

identify the amoeba) but amoebae may rarely be visualized in the CSF i4.55. Cysts can be seen by H&E stain of brain tissue for both *Acanthamoeba* and *Balamuthia*, whereas *Naegleria* remains a trophozoite and may be in the CSF and brain tissue [PMID 17428307]. Though effective antimicrobial therapy is largely unproven, an additional challenge with treating these infections is the diagnostic delay encountered due to general unawareness of these pathogens.

CSF can be sent to the laboratory for stain (all 4 amoebae) and culture; however the yield is quite low from CSF for culture, and typically the cultures grow after the patient has expired. Culture for *Acanthamoeba* and *Naegleria* typically is achieved using a nonnutritive agar covered in *E coli* [PMID 17428307]. *Balamuthia* does not phagocytize or metabolize bacteria; therefore human brain cells in cell culture is required (clinically this is not a practical culture approach for most laboratories) [PMID 17428307]. Free living amoebae can be visualized in CSF with multiple stains or as a wet mount preparation [PMID 17428307]. The calcofluor white stain is simple to screen specimens, but lacks absolute specificity and is subject to artifacts. The Giemsa stain provides very good structural details of the amoebae, but is more challenging to interpret [PMID 17428307]. Inexperienced technologists could mistake white blood cells for *Naegleria* trophozoites, though the centrally located nucleolus of *Naegleria* should allow the 2 to be distinguished [PMID 17428307]. Ideally a combination of the 2 stains plus culture should be performed, though this may still only be marginally effective. PCR is available from the CDC, and though the test has excellent sensitivity and specificity, it is typically performed upon autopsy. If the laboratory is contacted to perform testing for pathogenic free living amoeba, the CDC should be contacted for guidance to ensure timely and appropriate specimen collection and testing occur. Experimental drugs are also available from the CDC for these infections on the basis of compassionate use.

Parasitic meningitis/meningoencephalitis

Eosinophilic meningoencephalitis (EM) and meningitis are often fatal clinical syndromes that can be caused by many different cestodes (tapeworms), trematodes (flukes), and nematodes (roundworms). Well documented causes of meningitis and/or EM are listed in t4.21. In the developed world, these infections are quite rare compared to bacterial and virus meningitis; however in the developing world these infections are more common and the true number of cases is likely underestimated due to resource limitations for testing and a lack of standardized reporting [PMID 19366917]. Most cases of parasite induced EM in the developed world occur in recent immigrants or return travelers; however, globalization and introduction of foreign host species has spread the distribution of some parasites into various parts of the developed world. In the United States for example, *Angiostrongylus cantonensis* is now considered endemic in states such as Florida, Louisiana, and Hawaii [PMID 19366917, PMID 23901374, PMID 23901371, PMID 21976573, PMID 19283982]. In Louisiana the worm exists primarily in the natural host snail, which is nonnative, while in Florida, the worm has infected native snails [PMID 23901374, PMID 19283982].

The diagnosis of helminthic meningitis is complicated, largely due to a lack of pathogen specific tests. The CSF profile is most notable for elevated eosinophils, typically reaching >10% of the total CSF leukocyte count [PMID 19366917]. This is typically a strong predictor of parasitic meningitis; however drug use/allergies, neoplasms, and other infections are capable of causing eosinophilic meningitis as well [PMID 19366917]. Of the parasites listed in t4.21, serological markers of infection are the current standard diagnostic methods. Though some of these infections are readily testable by serology at reference laboratories (eg, *Taenia solium*, *Schistosoma*, *Toxocara*), the majority cannot readily be tested for. The Centers for Disease Control and Prevention (CDC) can assist physicians in obtaining testing for organisms such as *Gnathostoma* and *Angiostrongylus*, and therefore prompt consultation should be sought when these infections are suspected. PCR assays have only recently been developed for these rare infections, and are not commercially available.

In rare cases, histopathologic analysis may reveal helminths within biopsied brain tissue. Genus level identification of these rare helminths by histologic analysis should only be performed by an expert clinical parasitologist. Consultation on histopathological specimens can be obtained in the United States by contacting the CDC's Division of Parasitic Diseases.

Neuroborreliosis

Lyme disease is a challenging infection to diagnose, and the disease is surrounded by controversy in both defining the true spectrum of symptoms, and the ideal way to test for the illness. A detailed review of Lyme disease can be found in Chapter 7. The diagnosis of neuroborreliosis

(CSF involvement of Lyme disease) employs a similar diagnostic algorithm as that described for serum testing in Chapter 7, where a total antibody ELISA or IFA test is performed as a screen, followed by IgM and/or IgG Western blot(s) using well defined interpretative criteria [PMID 7623762]. Demonstration of intrathecal production of Lyme antibodies is the preferred method for establishing a diagnosis of neuroborreliosis by the Infectious Disease Society of America (IDSA) [PMID 17029130]. Neuroborreliosis is best demonstrated in the laboratory with paired serum and CSF specimens, in which the titer of the CSF should be higher than the titer of the serum. As with any CSF antibody tests, the results can be confounded by serum contamination of the CSF during the collection. Care should be taken to examine the specimen for blood or evidence of a traumatic tap.

Neurosyphilis

Syphilis is a sexually transmitted disease caused by the spirochete *Treponema pallidum*. Like many other spirochetes, *T pallidum* cannot readily be cultured in the clinical laboratory and the diagnosis relies largely on serological markers. Syphilis is a systemic infection that can involve many organs; however the central nervous system is the greatest concern for syphilis complications. Neurosyphilis is a rare, though life threatening complication that once affected between 5-10 % of patients prior to the advent of penicillin therapy [PMID 13252075]. Successful treatment of early stages of syphilis largely prevents the development of neurosyphilis but despite standardized and successful treatment regimens, the clinical diagnosis of neurosyphilis remains a daunting challenge for physicians and laboratorians. One particular complication in the diagnostic process is that neurosyphilis can be symptomatic or asymptomatic. As a result of this challenge, the CDC has recommended that CSF examination be performed on all patients that display serological evidence of syphilis and neurological symptoms, or when serological titers of asymptomatic patients do not decline in response to appropriate therapy with benzyl penicillin-G [PMID 21160459]. Due to the success rate of treatment for primary syphilis and dramatic reduction of neurosyphilis, testing the CSF of asymptomatic patients has become controversial and difficult to achieve in most cases. On the contrary, patients with documented syphilis and neurological symptoms readily receive prompt CSF testing.

In advance of CSF testing, it is crucial that the patient's serum reflect a suspected case of syphilis that is consistent with the definition accepted by the local public health authority. This definition varies in different nations, as no universal criteria have been accepted. Historically a 2 tier test algorithm consisting of a nontreponemal screen followed by a treponemal specific test was used. In recent years, so called reverse algorithms have gained traction, which screen with a treponemal specific test, followed by a nontreponemal test for confirmation and subsequent confirmation of discrepant results with a second treponemal assay. For a detailed explanation of the methods, see the review by Binniker [PMID 22156894]. The use of either algorithm has become a controversial subject and is beyond the scope of this text, as the field is currently mixed in regards to which algorithm provides the most accurate results [PMID 22156894].

The interrogation of CSF involves a CSF profile that typically shows elevated leukocyte count and protein **t4.22** and a nontreponemal test for syphilis known as the CSF VDRL (venereal disease research lab) [PMID 20626434]. When the CSF profile reflects that of neurosyphilis and the CSF VDRL is reactive, neurosyphilis is likely. Importantly, the CSF VDRL cannot rule out neurosyphilis, as patients with documented neurosyphilis can test negative by CSF VDRL [PMID 20626434]. This is particularly problematic in immunocompromised patients, especially those with HIV/AIDS (the demographic with the highest incidence of syphilis).

Unlike serum testing via 2 tier testing, a treponemal specific test is not required to support the nontreponemal (VDRL) test result. If a physician chooses to perform treponemal specific testing on the CSF, the fluorescent treponemal antibody (FTA) is considered the most appropriate assay (in terms of sensitivity); however care must be taken when clinically interpreting this test, as the assay can be difficult and subjective for the laboratory to interpret [PMID 20626434]. These test limitations can result in positive results even in patients with normal CSF profiles (for which neurosyphilis is very unlikely). False positive results are most commonly explained by CSF samples that have serum contamination due to a traumatic tap (similar to concerns with diagnosing neuroborreliosis) [PMID 20626434]. However, the test can be positive without serum contamination in the absence of an abnormal CSF profile; a scenario that may simply reflect laboratory error or be otherwise unexplainable.

In the United States, neurosyphilis is a nationally notifiable disease, defined by the CDC with specific criteria. First the patient must have evidence of central nervous system infection with *T pallidum*. The patient must also have reactive serological tests for syphilis and a reactive CSF VDRL [2012 Case Definitions: Nationally Notifiable Conditions Infectious and Non-Infectious Case (2012). Atlanta, GA: Centers for Disease Control and Prevention].

Artifacts & pitfalls

- CSF analysis must be performed rapidly in order to ensure accurate testing, optimal morphologic examination & institution of proper therapy. Many cells degenerate when held in CSF & the ability to accurately do chemical analyses & perform cultures may be adversely impacted if samples are not handled correctly.

- Abnormal CSF results need to be interpreted with consideration of the possible impact due to collection of CSF or previous interventions. Traumatic or bloody taps may introduce increased numbers of cells & change the levels of chemical analytes measured within the CSF. The presence of shunts or previous procedures may also cause artifactual changes in the CSF.

- Although typical patterns of cellular infiltrates, glucose & protein may suggest possible etiologies for meningitis, there is significant overlap between the CSF profiles & definitive diagnosis often requires microbiologic, serologic or molecular testing.

- Because of significant artifact introduced by cytospinning or cellular concentration, normal cellular elements in the CSF may appear to be neoplastic. Careful correlation with clinical history, as well as judicious use of ancillary testing (immunophenotyping, molecular testing) may be necessary to definitively identify & characterize malignancies.

Key points

- Optimal & accurate test interpretation in CSF depends on collection of appropriate specimens with good turnaround time. Communication with the laboratory is essential to ensure appropriate testing of the small volumes that are collected in examination of cerebrospinal fluid.

- Complete evaluation of cerebrospinal fluid requires integration of clinical information, gross examination of the spinal fluid, microscopic examination, chemical analysis & microbiologic examination. Careful consideration of the differential diagnosis will determine the sequence of tubes collected for the testing & appropriate ordering of tests.

- CSF examination is essential for the workup & diagnosis of encephalitis, meningitis, multiple sclerosis, marrow syphilis, subarachnoid hemorrhage as well as identification of CNS involvement by a variety of malignancies.

- Ancillary testing may be extremely useful, particularly in identification of malignancies. However, the small numbers of cells present may require use of abbreviated immunophenotypic panels. Careful correlation with clinical history will allow targeted immunophenotyping by either flow cytometry or immunocytochemical staining. Correlation with clinical history is essential for optimal selection of an immunophenotypic panel and/or appropriate molecular testing.

References

PMID 10353466 Kleine TO, Albrecht J, Zöfel P [1999] Flow cytometry of cerebrospinal fluid (CSF) lymphocytes: alterations of blood/CSF ratios of lymphocyte subsets in inflammation disorders of human central nervous system (CNS). *Clin Chem Lab Med* 37(3):231-41

PMID 10561221 Gajjar A, Fouladi M, Walter AW et al [1999] Comparison of lumbar & shunt cerebrospinal fluid specimens for cytologic detection of leptomeningeal disease in pediatric patients with brain tumors. *J Clin Oncol* 17(6):1825-8

PMID 10589079 Sham RL, Phatak PD, Kouides PA et al [1999] Hematologic neoplasia & the central nervous system. *Am J Hematol* 62(4):234-8

PMID 10702528 Biou D, Benoist JF, Nguyen-Thi C et al [2000] Cerebrospinal fluid protein concentrations in children: age-related values in patients without disorders of the central nervous system. *Clin Chem* 46(3):399-403

PMID 10973861 Ohta M, Ohta K, Ma J et al [2000] Clinical & analytical evaluation of an enzyme immunoassay for myelin basic protein in cerebrospinal fluid. *Clin Chem* 46(9):1326-1330

PMID 11078802 Weisberger J, Wu CD, Liu Z et al [2000] Differential diagnosis of malignant lymphomas & related disorders by specific pattern of expression of immunophenotypic markers revealed by multiparameter flow cytometry (review). *Int J Oncol* 17(6):1165-77

PMID 11091267 Fischer A [2000] Severe combined immunodeficiencies (SCID). *Clin Exp Immunol* 122(2):143-149

PMID 11213505 Zeman D, Adam P, Kalistová H et al [2001] Cerebrospinal fluid cytologic findings in multiple sclerosis. A comparison between patient subgroups. *Acta Cytol* 45(1):51-9

PMID 11489408 Jerrard DA, Hanna JR, Schindelheim GL [2001] Cerebrospinal fluid. *J Emerg Med* 21(2):171-8

PMID 11684714 Cruickshank AM. [2001] ACP Best Practice No 166: CSF spectrophotometry in the diagnosis of subarachnoid haemorrhage. *J Clin Pathol* 54(11):827-30

PMID 11794481 Perini P, Calabrese M, Ranzato F et al [2001] Cerebrospinal fluid examination in the differential diagnosis of inflammatory myelopathies. *Neurol Sci* 22Suppl2:S65-8

PMID 11826241 Berger RP, Pierce MC, Wisniewski S R et al [2002] Neuron-specific enolase & S100B in cerebrospinal fluid after severe traumatic brain injury in infants & children. *Pediatrics* 109(2):E31

PMID 11967640 Correale J, de los Milagros Bassani Molinas,M [2002] Oligoclonal bands & antibody responses in multiple sclerosis. *J Neurol* 249(4):375-389

PMID 11985377 van Crevel H, Hijdra A, de Gans J [2002] Lumbar puncture & the risk of herniation: when should we first perform CT? *J Neurol* 249(2):129-37

PMID 12217474 Shaw KH, Edlow JA [2002] Distinguishing traumatic lumbar puncture from true subarachnoid hemorrhage. *J Emerg Med* 23(1):67-74

PMID 12525508 Bürger B, Zimmermann M, Mann G et al [2003] Diagnostic cerebrospinal fluid examination in children with acute lymphoblastic leukemia: significance of low leukocyte counts with blasts or traumatic lumbar puncture. *J Clin Oncol* 21(2):184-8

PMID 12574013 Shah KH, Richard KM, Nicholas S et al [2003] Incidence of traumatic lumbar puncture. *Acad Emerg Med* 10(2):151-4

PMID 12612231 Mazor SS, McNulty JE, Roosevelt GE [2003] Interpretation of traumatic lumbar punctures: who can go home? *Pediatrics* 111(3):525-8

PMID 12637136 Lo Re V 3rd, Gluckman SJ [2003] Eosinophilic meningitis. *Am J Med* 114(3):217-23

PMID 12682325 Davies G, Keir G, Thompson EJ et al [2003] The clinical significance of an intrathecal monoclonal immunoglobulin band: a follow-up study. *Neurology* 60(7):1163-1166

PMID 12687751 Fasipe F, Bestak M, Green NS [2003] Recurrent central nervous system acute lymphoblastic leukemia associated with cerebrospinal fluid eosinophilia & basophilia: a proposed cytokine-mediated mechanism. *Pediatr Hematol Oncol* 20(1):31-7

PMID 12870112 Roos KL [2003] Lumbar puncture. *Semin Neurol* 23(1):105-14

PMID 12881799 Moylett EH [2003] Neonatal *Candida* meningitis. *Semin Pediatr Infect Dis* 14(2):115-22

PMID 12960693 Scrideli CA, Queiroz RP, Takayanagui OM et al [2003] Polymerase chain reaction on cerebrospinal fluid cells in suspected leptomeningeal involvement in childhood acute lymphoblastic leukemia: comparison to cytomorphologic analysis. *Diagn Mol Pathol* 12(3):124-7

PMID 13252075 Clark EG, Danbolt N [1955] The Oslo study of the natural history of untreated syphilis; an epidemiologic investigation based on a restudy of the Boeck-Bruusgaard material; a review & appraisal. *J Chronic Dis* 2(3):311-44

PMID 13762229 Lincoln EM, Sordillo SUR, Davies PA [1960] Tuberculous meningitis in children. *J Pediatr* 57:807-23

PMID 14524396 Seehusen DA, Reeves MM, Fomin DA [2003] Cerebrospinal fluid analysis. *Am Fam Physician* 68(6):1103-8

PMID 14608891 Fortini AS, Sanders EL, Weinshenker BG et al [2003] Cerebrospinal fluid oligoclonal bands in the diagnosis of multiple sclerosis. Isoelectric focusing with IgG immunoblotting compared with high-resolution agarose gel electrophoresis & cerebrospinal fluid IgG index. *Am J Clin Pathol* 120(5):672-675

PMID 14620646 Hughes PA, Magnet AD, Fishbain JT [2003] Eosinophilic meningitis: a case series report & review of the literature. *Mil Med* 168(10):817-21

PMID 14674086 Glosová L, Dundr P, Effler J et al [2003] Gallbladder carcinoma cells in cerebrospinal fluid as the first manifestation of a tumor. A case report. *Acta Cytol* 47(6):1087-90

PMID 14715783 Thwaites GE, Chau TT, Farrar JJ [2004] Improving the bacteriological diagnosis of tuberculous meningitis. *J Clin Microbiol* 42:378-79

PMID 14726461 Keiser PB, Nutman TB [2004] *Strongyloides stercoralis* in the mmunocompromised Population. *Clin Microbiol Rev* 17(1):208-17

PMID 14759953 Graves P, Sidman R [2004] Xanthochromia is not pathognomonic for subarachnoid hemorrhage. *Acad Emerg Med* 11(2):131-5

PMID 15082912 Bae SH, Ryoo HM, Cho HS et al [2004] Meningeal relapse in a patient with acute promyelocytic leukemia: a case report & review of the literature. *J Korean Med Sci* 19(2):311-4

PMID 15101714 Fassas AB, Ward S, Muwalla F et al [2004] Myeloma of the central nervous system: strong association with unfavorable chromosomal abnormalities & other high risk disease features. *Leuk Lymphoma* 45(2):291-300

PMID 15160941 Leis JF, Stepan DE, Curtin PT et al [2004] Central nervous system failure in patients with chronic myelogenous leukemia lymphoid blast crisis & Philadelphia chromosome positive acute lymphoblastic leukemia treated with imatinib (STI-571). *Leuk Lymphoma* 45(4):695-8

PMID 15163317 Mahieu S, Vertessen F, Van der Planken M [2004] Evaluation of ADVIA 120 CSF assay (Bayer) vs chamber counting of cerebrospinal fluid specimens. *Clin Lab Hematol* 26(3):15-9

PMID 15272896 Bourahoui A, De Seze J, Guttierez R et al [2004] CSF isoelectrofocusing in a large cohort of MS & other neurological diseases. *Eur J Neurol* 11(8):525-529

PMID 15304573 Castellani RJ, Colucci M, Xie Z et al [2004] Sensitivity of 14-3-3 protein test varies in subtypes of sporadic Creutzfeldt-Jakob disease. *Neurology* 63(3):436-442

PMID 15494903 Tunkel AR, Hartman BJ, Kaplan SL et al [2004] Practice guidelines for the management of bacterial meningitis. *Clin Infect Dis* 39(9):1267-1284

PMID 15608000 Davies NW, Brown LJ, Gonde J et al [2005] Factors influencing PCR detection of viruses in cerebrospinal fluid of patients with suspected CNS infections. *J Neurol Neurosurg Psychiatry* 76(1):82-7

PMID 15608153 Papadea C, Schlosser RJ [2005] Rapid method for β2-transferrin in cerebrospinal fluid leakage using an automated immunofixation electrophoresis system. *Clin Chem* 51(2):464-470

PMID 15640938 Babusíková O, Zelezníková T [2004] The value of multiparameter flow cytometry of cerebrospinal fluid involved by leukemia/lymphoma cells. *Neoplasma* 51(5):345-51

PMID 15681484 Pine SR, Yin C, Matloub YH et al [2005] Detection of central nervous system leukemia in children with acute lymphoblastic leukemia by real-time polymerase chain reaction. *J Mol Diagn* 7(1):127-32

PMID 15736018 Wheat LJ, Musial CE, Jenny-Avital E [2005] Diagnosis & management of central nervous system histoplasmosis. *Clin Infect Dis* 40(6):844-52

PMID 15749414 Wood MJ, Dimeski G, Nowitzke AM [2005] CSF spectrophotometry in the diagnosis & exclusion of spontaneous subarachnoid haemorrhage. *J Clin Neurosci* 12(2):142-6

PMID 1575009 Hansen PB, Kjeldsen L, Dalhoff K et al [1992] Cerebrospinal fluid β-2-microglobulin in adult patients with acute leukemia or lymphoma: a useful marker in early diagnosis & monitoring of CNS-involvement. *Acta Neurologica Scandinavica* 85(3):224-227

PMID 1583530 Bigner SH [1992] Cerebrospinal fluid (CSF) cytology: current status & diagnostic applications. *J Neuropathol Exp Neurol* 51(3):235-45

PMID 15921910 Selakovic V, Raicevic R, Radenovic L [2005] The increase of neuron-specific enolase in cerebrospinal fluid & plasma as a marker of neuronal damage in patients with acute brain infarction. *J Clin Neurosci* 12(5):542-547

PMID 15956157 Freedman MS, Thompson EJ, Deisenhammer F et al [2005] Recommended standard of cerebrospinal fluid analysis in the diagnosis of multiple sclerosis: a consensus statement. *Arch Neurol* 62(6):865-870

PMID 16083828 Shenkier TN [2005] Unusual variants of primary central nervous system lymphoma. *Hematol Oncol Clin North Am* 19(4):651-64, vi

PMID 16121639 Strik H, Luthe H, Nagel I et al [2005] Automated cerebrospinal fluid cytology: limitations & reasonable applications. *Anal Quant Cytol Histol* 27(3):167-73

PMID 16243873 Chow SL, Rooney ZJ, Cleary MA et al [2005] The significance of elevated CSF lactate. *Arch Dis Child* 90(11):1188-1189

PMID 16323099 Johnson RH, Einstein HE [2006] Coccidioidal meningitis. *Clin Infect Dis* 42(1):103-107. Epub 2005 Nov 29

PMID 16430456 Nückel H, Novotny JR, Noppeney R et al [2006] Detection of malignant hematopoietic cells in the cerebrospinal fluid by conventional cytology & flow cytometry. *Clin Lab Hematol* 28(1):22-9

PMID 16545048 Lawrence RH [2005] The role of lumbar puncture as a diagnostic tool in 2005. *Crit Care Resusc* 7(3):213-20

PMID 16616560 Trunz BB, Fine PEM, Dye C [2006] Effect of BCG vaccination on childhood tuberculous meningitis & miliary tuberculosis worldwide: a meta-analysis & assessment of cost-effectiveness. *Lancet* 367:1173-80

PMID 16710032 Dutch Childhood Oncology Group, te Loo DM, Kamps WA et al [2006] Prognostic significance of blasts in the cerebrospinal fluid without pleiocytosis or a traumatic lumbar puncture in children with acute lymphoblastic leukemia: experience of the Dutch Childhood Oncology Group. *J Clin Oncol* 24(15):2332-6

PMID 16871073 Baer ET [2006] Post-dural puncture bacterial meningitis. *Anesthesiology* 105(2):381-93

PMID 16946154 Perry JJ, Sivilotti MLA, Stiell IG et al [2006] Should spectrophotometry be used to identify xanthochromia in the cerebrospinal fluid of alert patients suspected of having subarachnoid hemorrhage? *Stroke* 37(10):2467-2472

PMID 17028920 Rosanda C, Gambini C, Carlini B et al [2006] Diagnostic identification of malignant cells in the cerebrospinal fluid by tumor-specific qRT-PCR. *Clin Exp Metastasis* 23(3-4):223-6

PMID 17029130 Wormser GP, Dattwyler RJ, Shapiro ED et al [2006] The clinical assessment, treatment, & prevention of lyme disease, human granulocytic anaplasmosis, & babesiosis: clinical practice guidelines by the Infectious Diseases Society of America. *Clin Infect Dis* 43(9):1089-134

PMID 17101909 Whiteley W, Al-Shahi R, Warlow CP et al [2006] CSF opening pressure: reference interval & the effect of body mass index. *Neurology* 67(9):1690-1

PMID 17114955 Etzell JE, Keet C, McDonald W et al [2006] Medulloblastoma simulating acute myeloid leukemia: case report with a review of "myeloid antigen" expression in nonhematopoietic tissues & tumors. *J Pediatr Hematol Oncol* 28(11):703-10

PMID 17428307 Visvesvara GS, Moura H, Schuster F [2007] Pathogenic & opportunistic free-living amoebae: *Acanthamoeba* species., *Balamuthia mandrillaris, Naegleria fowleri,* & *Sappinia diploidea*. *FEMS Immunol Med Microbiol* 50(1):1-26

PMID 17471037 Lee BE, Davies HD [2007] Aseptic meningitis. *Curr Opin Infect Dis* 20(3):272-7

PMID 17616482 Dubois B, Feldman HH, Jacova C et al [2007] Research criteria for the diagnosis of Alzheimer disease: revising the NINCDS-ADRDA criteria. *Lancet Neurol* 6(8):734-746

PMID 1761681 Gade W, Hinnefeld SW, Babcock LS et al [1991] Comparison of the PREMIER cryptococcal antigen enzyme immunoassay & the latex agglutination assay for detection of cryptococcal antigens. *J Clin Microbiol* 29(8):1616-9

PMID 17636138 Joseph FG, Scolding NJ [2007] Sarcoidosis of the nervous system. *Pract Neurol* 7(4):234-44

PMID 17712055 Joffe AR [2007] Lumbar puncture & brain herniation in acute bacterial meningitis: a review. *J Intensive Care Med* 22(4):194-207

PMID 18040800 Persidsky Y, Ramirez SH, Haorah J [2006] Blood-brain barrier: structural components & function under physiologic & pathologic conditions. *J Neuroimmune Pharmacol* 1(3):223-36

PMID 18316002 Parish JM, Blair JE [2008] coccidioidomycosis. *Mayo Clin Proc* 83(3):343-48; quiz 348-9

PMID 18446313 Hanse MC, Van't Veer MB, van Lom K et al [2008] Incidence of central nervous system involvement in chronic lymphocytic leukemia & outcome to treatment. *J Neurol* 255(6):828-30

PMID 18474734 Berger JR, Houff S [2008] Neurological complications of herpes simplex virus type 2 infection. *Arch Neurol* 65(5):596-600

PMID 18482910 Cruickshank A, Auld P, Beetham R et al [2008] Revised national guidelines for analysis of cerebrospinal fluid for bilirubin in suspected subarachnoid haemorrhage. *Ann Clin Biochem* 45(Pt 3):238-244

PMID 18572349 Arora S, Swadron SP, Dissanayake V [2010] Evaluating the sensitivity of visual xanthochromia in patients with subarachnoid hemorrhage. *J Emerg Med* 39(1):13-6

PMID 18630838 Heller T, Nagel I, Ehrlich B et al [2008] Automated cerebrospinal fluid cytology. *Anal Quant Cytol Histol* 30(3):139-44

PMID 18657719 Irani DN [2008] Aseptic meningitis & viral myelitis. *Neurol Clin* 26(3):635-55, vii-viii

PMID 18989240 Greenberg RG, Smith PB, Cotten CM et al [2008] Traumatic lumbar punctures in neonates: test performance of the cerebrospinal fluid white blood cell count. *Pediatr Infect Dis J* 27(12):1047-51

PMID 19046603 Ichiyama T, Kajimoto M, Matsushige T et al [2009] Mononuclear cell subpopulations in CSF & blood of children with bacterial meningitis. *J Infect* 58(1):28-31

PMID 19185983 Regeniter A, Kuhle J, Mehling M et al [2009] A modern approach to CSF analysis: pathophysiology, clinical application, proof of concept & laboratory reporting. *Clin Neurol Neurosurg* 111(4):313-8

PMID 19191619 Moïsi JC, Saha SK, Falade AG et al [2009] Enhanced diagnosis of pneumococcal meningitis with use of the Binax NOW immunochromatographic test of *Streptococcus pneumo*niae antigen: a multisite study. *Clin Infect Dis* 48Suppl2:S49-56

PMID 19283982 Diaz JH [2008] Helminthic eosinophilic meningitis: emerging zoonotic diseases in the South. *J La State Med Soc* 160(6):333-42

PMID 19366917 Graeff-Teixeira C, da Silva AC, Yoshimura K [2009] Update on eosinophilic meningoencephalitis & its clinical relevance. *Clin Microbiol Rev* 22(2):322-48

PMID 19410151 Rekate HL [2009] A contemporary definition & classification of hydrocephalus. *Semin Pediatr Neurol* 16(1):9-15

PMID 19660680 Pui CH, Thiel E [2009] Central nervous system disease in hematologic malignancies: historical perspective & practical applications. *Semin Oncol* 36(4Suppl2):S2-S16

PMID 19664713 Abbott NJ, Patabendige AA, Dolman DE et al [2010] Structure & function of the blood-brain barrier. *Neurobiol Dis* 37(1):13-25

PMID 1971494 Hovestadt A, Henzen-Logmans SC, Vecht CJ et al [1990] Immunohistochemical analysis of the cerebrospinal fluid for carcinomatous & lymphomatous leptomeningitis. *Br J Cancer* 62(4):653-654

PMID 19775301 van Veen JJ, Nokes TJ, Makris M [2010] The risk of spinal hematoma following neuraxial anaesthesia or lumbar puncture in thrombocytopenic individuals. *Br J Hematol* 148(1):15-25

PMID 19841431 Fujimaki, T [2009] Central nervous system germ cell tumors: classification, clinical features, & treatment with a historical overview. *J Child Neurol* 24(11):1439-1445

PMID 201417 Veuger AJ, Kortbeek LH, Booij AC [1977] Siderophages in differentiation of blood in cerebrospinal fluid. *Clin Neurol Neurosurg* 80(1):46-56

PMID 2014779 Craver RD, Carson TH [1991] Hematopoietic elements in cerebrospinal fluid in children. *Am J Clin Pathol* 95(4):532-5

PMID 20187854 de Jonge R, Brouwer R, de Graaf MT et al [2010] Evaluation of the new body fluid mode on the Sysmex XE-5000 for counting leukocytes & erythrocytes in cerebrospinal fluid & other body fluids. *Clin Chem Lab Med* 48(5):665-74

PMID 20218151 Al-Sobhi E, Osoba AO, Karar A et al [2009] Multiple myeloma of the central nervous system: a clinicopathological review. *East Mediterr Health J* 15(6):1570-9

PMID 20386641 Kang SJ, Kim KS, Ha YS et al [2010] Diagnostic value of cerebrospinal fluid level of carcinoembryonic antigen in patients with leptomeningeal carcinomatous metastasis *J Clin Neurol* 6(1):33-37

PMID 20435061 Oreskovic D, Klarica M [2010] The formation of cerebrospinal fluid: nearly a hundred years of interpretations & misinterpretations. *Brain Res Rev* 64(2):241-62

PMID 20441472 Kleine TO, Nebe CT, Löwer C et al [2010] Evaluation of cell counting & leukocyte differentiation in cerebrospinal fluid controls using hematology analyzers by the German Society for Clinical Chemistry & Laboratory Medicine. *Clin Chem Lab Med* 48(6):839-48

PMID 20511371 Griffiths MJ, Chow E, Panting MD et al [2010] Comparison of original (2003) & revised (2008) national guidelines for reporting of cerebrospinal fluid spectrophotometric scanning for suspected subarachnoid haemorrhage against patient outcome. *Ann Clin Biochem* 47(Pt4):375-7

PMID 20533959 Bezov D, Ashina S, Lipton R [2010] Post-dural puncture headache: part II prevention, management, & prognosis. *Headache* 50(9):1482-98

PMID 20577138 Pappano D [2010] "Traumatic Tap" proportion in pediatric lumbar puncture. *Pediatr Emerg Care* 26(7):487-9

PMID 20605098 Cheng H, Yang Y, Dai W et al [2010] Acute leukemia presenting with blasts first found in the cerebrospinal fluid but not in the peripheral blood. *J Clin Neurosci* 17(10):1252-5

PMID 20610819 Brouwer MC, Tunkel AR, van de Beek D [2010] Epidemiology, diagnosis, & antimicrobial treatment of acute bacterial meningitis. *Clin Microbiol Rev* 23(3):467-92

PMID 20626298 Makis A, Shipway D, Hatzimichael E et al [2010] Cytokine & adhesion molecule expression evolves between the neutrophilic & lymphocytic phases of viral meningitis. *J Interferon Cytokine Res* 30(9):661-5

PMID 20626434 Ghanem KG [2010] REVIEW: Neurosyphilis: a historical perspective & review. *CNS Neurosci Ther* 16(5):e157-68

PMID 20689477 Yetkin F, Kayabas U, Ersoy Y et al [2010] Cerebrospinal fluid viscosity: a novel diagnostic measure for acute meningitis. *South Med J* 103(9):892-5

PMID 20807248 Bezov D, Lipton R, Ashina S [2010] Post-dural puncture headache: part I diagnosis, epidemiology, etiology, & pathophysiology. *Headache* 50(7):1144-52

PMID 20818852 Avery RA, Shah SS, Licht DJ et al [2010] Reference range for cerebrospinal fluid opening pressure in children. *N Engl J Med* 363(9):891-3

PMID 20937176 Xu HB, Jiang RH, Li L et al [2010] Diagnostic value of adenosine deaminase in cerebrospinal fluid for tuberculous meningitis: a meta-analysis. *Int J Tuberc Lung Dis* 14(11):1382-1387

PMID 21160459 Workowski KA, Berman S, Centers for Disease Control & Prevention (CDC) [2010] Sexually transmitted diseases treatment guidelines, 2010. *MMWR Recomm Rep.* 59(RR-12):1-110

PMID 21194480 Huy NT, Thao NTH, Diep DTN et al [2010] Cerebrospinal fluid lactate concentration to distinguish bacterial from aseptic meningitis: a systemic review & meta-analysis. *Crit Car* 14(6):R240

PMID 21291600 Shakoor S, Beg MA, Mahmood SF et al [2011] Primary amebic meningoencephalitis caused by *Naegleria fowleri*, Karachi, Pakistan. *Emerg Infect Dis* 17(2):258-61

PMID 21368691 Böhmer AE, Oses JP, Schmidt AP et al [2011] Neuron-specific enolase, S100B, & glial fibrillary acidic protein levels as outcome predictors in patients with severe traumatic brain injury. *Neurosurgery* 68(6):1624-30- discussion 1630-1

PMID 21382412 Sakushima K, Hayashino Y, Kawaguchi T et al [2011] Diagnostic accuracy of cerebrospinal fluid lactate for differentiating bacterial meningitis from aseptic meningitis: a meta-analysis. *J Infect* 62(4):255-262

PMID 216201 Preissig SH, Buhaug J [1978] Corpora amylacea in cerebrospinal fluid. A source of possible diagnostic error. *Acta Cytol* 22(6):511-4

PMID 21668655 Zimmermann M, Ruprecht K, Kainzinger F et al [2011] Automated vs manual cerebrospinal fluid cell counts: a work & cost analysis comparing the Sysmex XE-5000 & the Fuchs-Rosenthal manual counting chamber. *Int J Lab Hematol* 33(6):629-37

PMID 21692072 Shihadeh F, Reed V, Faderl S et al [2012] Cytogenetic profile of patients with acute myeloid leukemia & central nervous system disease. *Cancer* 118(1):112-7

PMID 21697342 Percival A, Thorkildson P, Kozel TR [2011] Monoclonal antibodies specific for immunorecessive epitopes of glucuronoxylomannan, the major capsular polysaccharide of *Cryptococcus neoformans*, reduce serotype bias in an immunoassay for cryptococcal antigen. *Clin Vaccine Immunol* 18(8):1292-6

PMID 21701109 Anei R, Hayashi Y, Hiroshima S et al [2011] Hydrocephalus due to diffuse villous hyperplasia of the choroid plexus. *Neurol Med Chir* 51(6):437-41

PMID 21761583 Perske C, Nagel I, Nagel H et al [2011] CSF cytology—the ongoing dilemma to distinguish neoplastic & inflammatory lymphocytes. *Diagn Cytopathol* 39(8):621-6

PMID 21769650 Moazzam AA, Drappatz J, Kim RY et al [2012] Chronic lymphocytic leukemia with central nervous system involvement: report of 2 cases with a comprehensive literature review. *J Neuro Oncol* 106(1):185-200

PMID 21881536 Yeung DT, Parker WT, Branford S [2011] Molecular methods in diagnosis & monitoring of hematological malignancies. *Pathology* 43(6):566-79

PMID 2189977 Rodriguez AF, Kaplan SL, Mason EO Jr [1990] Cerebrospinal fluid values in the very low birth weight infant. *J Pediatr* 116(6):971-4

PMID 21907885 Lee MW, Vedanarayanan VV [2011] Cerebrospinal fluid opening pressure in children: experience in a controlled setting. *Pediatr Neurol* 45(4):238-40

PMID 21928018 Oi S [2011] Classification of hydrocephalus: critical analysis of classification categories & advantages of "multi-categorical hydrocephalus classification" (Mc HC). *Childs Nerv Syst* 27(10):1523-33

PMID 21976573 Hochberg NS, Blackburn BG, Park SY et al [2011] Eosinophilic meningitis attributable to *Angiostrongylus cantonensis* infection in Hawaii: clinical characteristics & potential exposures. *Am J Trop Med Hyg* 85(4):685-90

PMID 22025088 Ahluwalia MS, Wallace PK, Peereboom DM [2012] Flow cytometry as a diagnostic tool in lymphomatous or leukemic meningitis: ready for prime time? *Cancer* 118(7):1747-53

PMID 22100360 Sakka L, Coll G, Chazal J [2011] Anatomy & physiology of cerebrospinal fluid. *Eur Ann Otorhinolaryngol Head Neck Dis* 128(6):309-16

PMID 22111091 Cooper N [2011] Lumbar puncture. *Acute Med* 10(4):188-93

PMID 22132920 Fulkerson DH, Sivaganesan A, Hill JD et al [2011] Progression of cerebrospinal fluid cell count & differential over a treatment course of shunt infection. *J Neurosurg Pediatr* 8(6):613-9

PMID 22145907 Michetti F, Corvino V, Geloso MC et al [2012] The S100B protein in biological fluids: more than a lifelong biomarker of brain distress. *J Neurochem* 120(5):644-659

PMID 22278331 Wright BL, Lai JT, Sinclair AJ [2012] Cerebrospinal fluid & lumbar puncture: a practical review. *J Neurol* 259(8):1530-45

PMID 22483794 Lescuyer P, Auer L, Converset V et al [2012] Comparison of gel-based methods for the detection of cerebrospinal fluid rhinorrhea. *Clin Chim Acta* 413(13-14):1145-1150

PMID 22511093 Alstadhaug KB, Odeh F, Baloch FK et al [2012] Post-lumbar puncture headache. *Tidsskr Nor Laegeforen* 132(7):818-21

PMID 22523219 Huppmann AR, Rheingold SR, Bailey LC et al [2012] Detection of leukemic lymphoblasts in CSF is instrument-dependent. *Am J Clin Pathol* 137(5):795-9

PMID 22547227 Qaddoumi I, Sane M, Li S et al [2012] Diagnostic utility & correlation of tumor markers in the serum & cerebrospinal fluid of children with intracranial germ cell tumors. *Child's Nerv Sys* 28(7):1017-1024

PMID 22639108 Crespo-Solis E, López-Karpovitch X, Higuera J et al [2012] Diagnosis of acute leukemia in cerebrospinal fluid (CSF-acute leukemia). *Curr Oncol Rep* 14(5):369-78

PMID 22655692 Ziu M, Savage JG, Jimenez DF [2012] Diagnosis & treatment of cerebrospinal fluid rhinorrhea following accidental traumatic anterior skull base fractures. *Neurosurg Focus* 32(6):E3

PMID 22710755 Puoti G, Bizzi A, Forloni G et al [2012] Sporadic human prion diseases: molecular insights & diagnosis. *Lancet Neurol* 11(7):618-628

PMID 22764093 Nigrovic LE, Malley R, Kuppermann N [2012] Meta-analysis of bacterial meningitis score validation studies. *Arch Dis Child* 97(9):799-805

PMID 2277197 Peacock JE Jr [1990] Persistent neutrophilic meningitis. *Infect Dis Clin North Am* 4(4):747-67

PMID 22843257 Hamlin C, Puoti G, Berri S et al [2012] A comparison of tau & 14-3-3 protein in the diagnosis of Creutzfeldt-Jakob disease. *Neurology* 79(6):547-552

PMID 22919000 Yoder JS, Straif-Bourgeois S, Roy SL et al [2012] Primary amebic meningoencephalitis deaths associated with sinus irrigation using contaminated tap water. *Clin Infect Dis* 55(9):e79-85

PMID 2302041 Chen KT, Moseley D [1990] Cartilage cells in cerebrospinal fluid. *Arch Pathol Lab Med* 114(2):212

PMID 23023885 McCudden CR, Senior BA, Hainsworth S et al [2013] Evaluation of high resolution gel β(2)-transferrin for detection of cerebrospinal fluid leak. *Clin Chem Lab Med* 51(2):311-315

PMID 23064593 Schwartz KM, Luetmer PH, Hunt CH et al [2013] Position-related variability of CSF opening pressure measurements. *AJNR Am J Neuroradio* 34(4):904-7

PMID 23067018 Ward MF, Bonomo JB, Adeoye O et al [2012] Cost-effectiveness of diagnostic strategies for evaluation of suspected subarachnoid hemorrhage in the emergency department. *Acad Emerg Med* 19(10):1134-44

PMID 23083312 Kauffman CA, Pappas PG, Patterson TF [2013] Fungal infections associated with contaminated methylprednisolone injections. *N Engl J Med* 368(26):2495-500

PMID 23089709 Fleming C, Brouwer R, Lindemans J et al [2012] Validation of the body fluid module on the new Sysmex XN-1000 for counting blood cells in cerebrospinal fluid & other body fluids. *Clin Chem Lab Med* 50(10):1791-8

PMID 23114703 Hansen J, Slechta ES, Gates-Hollingsworth MA et al [2013] Large-scale evaluation of the immuno-mycologics lateral flow & enzyme-linked immunoassays for detection of cryptococcal antigen in serum & cerebrospinal fluid. *Clin Vaccine Immunol* 20(1):52-5

PMID 23141619 McIntyre PB, O'Brien KL, Greenwood B et al [2012] Effect of vaccines on bacterial meningitis worldwide. *Lancet* 380(9854):1703-11

PMID 23178421 Antinori S, Corbellino M, Meroni L et al [2013] *Aspergillus* meningitis: a rare clinical manifestation of central nervous system aspergillosis. Case report & review of 92 cases. *J Infect* 66(3):218-38

PMID 23215851 Symss NP, Oi S [2013] Theories of cerebrospinal fluid dynamics & hydrocephalus: historical trend. *J Neurosurg Pediatr* 11(2):170-7

PMID 23287431 Galati D, Di Noto R, Del Vecchio L [2013] Diagnostic strategies to investigate cerebrospinal fluid involvement in hematological malignancies. *Leuk Res* 37(3):231-7

PMID 23300737 Fleischman D, Berdahl JP, Zaydlarova J et al [2012] Cerebrospinal fluid pressure decreases with older age. *PLoS One* 7(12):e52664

PMID 23319132 Scott BJ, Douglas VC, Tihan T et al [2013] A systematic approach to the diagnosis of suspected central nervous system lymphoma. *JAMA Neurol* 70(3):311-9

PMID 23363831 Lyons JL, Roos KL, Marr KA et al [2013] Cerebrospinal fluid (1,3)-β-D-glucan detection as an aid for diagnosis of iatrogenic fungal meningitis. *J Clin Microbiol* 51(4):1285-7

PMID 23517256 Czuczman AD, Thomas LE, Boulanger AB et al [2013] Interpreting red blood cells in lumbar puncture: distinguishing true subarachnoid hemorrhage from traumatic tap. *Acad Emerg Med* 20(3):247-56

PMID 23519967 Kang JH, Korecka M, Toledo JB et al [2013] Clinical utility & analytical challenges in measurement of cerebrospinal fluid amyloid-β(1-42) & τ proteins as Alzheimer disease biomarkers. *Clin Chem* 59(6):903-916

PMID 23621588 Perfect JR [2013] Fungal diagnosis: how do we do it & can we do better? *Curr Med Res Opin* 29Suppl4:3-11

PMID 23670107 Korfel A, Schlegel U [2013] Diagnosis & treatment of primary CNS lymphoma. *Nat Rev Neurol* 9(6):317-27

PMID 23832074 Preuss M, Hoffmann KT, Reiss-Zimmermann M et al [2013] Updated physiology & pathophysiology of CSF circulation—the pulsatile vector theory. *Childs Nerv Syst* 29(10):1811-25

PMID 23901371 Wallace GD [2013] The discovery of humans in Hawai'i infected with *Angiostrongylus cantonensis*, & early epidemiological findings. *Hawaii J Med Public Health* 72(6Suppl2):5

PMID 23901374 Teem JL, Qvarnstrom Y, Bishop HS et al [2013] The occurrence of the rat lungworm, *Angiostrongylus cantonensis*, in nonindigenous snails in the Gulf of Mexico region of the United States. *Hawaii J Med Public Health*. 72(6Suppl2):11-4

PMID 23972913 Thwaites GE, van Toorn R, Schoeman J [2013] Tuberculous meningitis: more questions, still too few answers. *Lancet Neurol* 12(10):999-1010

PMID 2411458 Schumann GB, Crisman LG [1985] Cerebrospinal fluid cytopathology. *Clin Lab Med* 5(2):275-302

PMID 2425776 Davey DD, Foucar K, Giller R [1986] Millipore filter vs cytocentrifuge for detection of childhood central nervous system leukemia. *Arch Pathol Lab Med* 110(8):705-8

PMID 24275252 Bremell D, Mattsson N, Wallin F et al [2014] Automated cerebrospinal fluid cell count - New reference ranges & evaluation of its clinical use in central nervous system infections. *Clin Biochem* 47(1-2):25-30

PMID 24421850 Bae YS, Cheong JW, Chang WS et al [2013] Diagnostic accuracy of cerebrospinal fluid (CSF) cytology in metastatic tumors: an analysis of consecutive CSF samples. *Korean J Pathol* 47(6):563-8

PMID 268120 Mathios AJ, Nielsen SL, Barrett D et al [1977] Cerebrospinal fluid cytomorphology identification of benign cells originating in the central nervous system. *Acta Cytol* 21(3):403-12

PMID 3059292 Weston CL, Glantz MJ, Connor JR [2011] Detection of cancer cells in the cerebrospinal fluid: current methods & future directions. *Fluids Barriers CNS* 8:14

PMID 3228160 Lombardi G, Zustovich F, Farina P et al [2011] Neoplastic meningitis from solid tumors: new diagnostic & therapeutic approaches. *Oncologist* 16(8):1175-1188

PMID 3245993 Subirá D, Serrano C, Castañón S et al [2012] Role of flow cytometry immunophenotyping in the diagnosis of leptomeningeal carcinomatosis. *Neuro Oncol* 14(1):43-52

PMID 3437410 van Dongen JJM, Lhermitte L, Böttcher S et al [2012] EuroFlow antibody panels for standardized n-dimensional flow cytometric immunophenotyping of normal, reactive & malignant leukocytes. *Leukemia* 26(9):1908-1975

PMID 3459377 McIntosh S, Ritchey AK [1986] Diagnostic problems in cerebrospinal fluid of children with lymphoid malignancies. *Am J Pediatr Hematol Oncol* 8(1):28-31

PMID 3510343 Klee GG, Tallman RD, Goellner JR et al [1986] Elevation of carcinoembryonic antigen in cerebrospinal fluid among patients with meningeal carcinomatosis. *Mayo Clin* 61(1):9-13

PMID 3520526 Gorelick PB, Biller J [1986] Lumbar puncture. Technique, indications, & complications. *Postgrad Med* 79(8):257-68

PMID 3523200 Lyons RW, Andriole VT [1986] Fungal infections of the CNS. *Neurol Clin.* 4(1):159-70

PMID 3656567 Le Rhun E, Taillibert S, Chamberlain MC [2013] Carcinomatous meningitis: leptomeningeal metastases in solid tumors. *Surg Neurol Int* 4(Suppl4):S265-S288

PMID 3710441 Grisariu S, Avni B, Batchelor TT et al [2010] Neurolymphomatosis: an International Primary CNS Lymphoma Collaborative Group report. *Blood* 115(24):5005-5011

PMID 3711287 Steele RW, Marmer DJ, O'Brien MD et al [1986] Leukocyte survival in cerebrospinal fluid. *J Clin Microbiol* 23(5):965-6

PMID 4013654 De Reuck J, De Coster W, Vander Eecken H [1985] Cerebrospinal fluid cytology in acute ischaemic stroke. *Acta Neurol Belg* 85(3):133-6

PMID 4015272 Wheat J, French M, Batteiger B et a1 [1985] Cerebrospinal fluid *Histoplasma* antibodies in central nervous system histoplasmosis. *Arch Intern Med* 145:1237-1240

PMID 4419010 Wilkins RH, Odom GL [1974] Ependymal-choroidal cells in cerebrospinal fluid. Increased incidence in hydrocephalic infants. *J Neurosurg* 41(5):555-60

PMID 6157089 Mavlight GM, Stuckey SE, Cabanillas FF et al [1980] Diagnosis of leukemia or lymphoma in the central nervous system by β 2-microglobulin determination. *New Engl J Med* 303(13):718-722

PMID 6171361 Gerson B, Cohen SR, Gerson I et al [1981] Myelin basic protein, oligoclonal bands, & IgG in cerebrospinal fluid as indicators of multiple sclerosis. *Clin Chem* 27(12):1974-1977

PMID 6189578 Koch TR, Lichtenfeld KM, Wiernik PH [1983] Detection of central nervous system metastasis with cerebrospinal fluid β-2-microglobulin. *Cancer* 52(1):101-104

PMID 6260507 Pelc S, De Maertelaere E, Denolin-Reubens R [1981] CSF cytology of acute viral meningitis & meningoencephalitis. *Eur Neurol* 20(2):95-102

PMID 6477217 Chow G, Schmidley JW [1984] Lysis of erythrocytes & leukocytes in traumatic lumbar punctures. *Arch Neurol* 41(10):1084-5

PMID 6942615 Takeda M, King DE, Choi HY et al [1981] Diagnostic pitfalls in cerebrospinal fluid cytology. *Acta Cytol* 25(3):245-50

PMID 6947666 Rohlfing MB, Barton TK, Bigner SH et al [1981] Contamination of cerebrospinal fluid specimens with hematogenous blasts in patients with leukemia. *Acta Cytol* 25(6):611-5

PMID 6947670 Borowitz M, Bigner SH, Johnston WW [1981] Diagnostic problems in the cytologic evaluation of cerebrospinal fluid for lymphoma & leukemia. *Acta Cytol* 25(6):665-74

PMID 6965948 Cassleman ES, Hasso AN, Ashwal S et al [1980] Computed tomography of tuberculous meningitis in infants & children. *J Comput Assist Tomogr* 4(2):211-6

PMID 7025539 Bigner SH, Jonston WW [1981] The cytopathology of cerebrospinal fluid. I. Nonneoplastic conditions, lymphoma & leukemia. *Acta Cytol* 25(4):345-53

PMID 7072664 Pappu LD, Purohit DM, Levkoff AH et al [1982] CSF cytology in the neonate. *Am J Dis Child* 136(4):297-8

PMID 7623762 Centers for Disease Control & Prevention (CDC) [1995] Recommendations for test performance & interpretation from the Second National Conference on Serologic Diagnosis of Lyme Disease. *MMWR Morb Mortal Wkly Rep* 44(31):590-1

PMID 7789240 Tani E, Costa I, Svedmyr E et al [1995] Diagnosis of lymphoma, leukemia, & metastatic tumor involvement of the cerebrospinal fluid by cytology & immunocytochemistry. *Diagn Cytopathol* 12(1):14-22

PMID 7882508 Watson MA, Scott MG [1995] Clinical utility of biochemical analysis of cerebrospinal fluid. *Clin Chem* 41(3):343-360

PMID 8551828 Tunkel AR, Scheld WM [1995] Acute bacterial meningitis. *Lancet* 346(8991-8992):1675-1680

PMID 8562739 Nguyen MH, Yu VL [1995] Meningitis caused by *Candida* species: an emerging problem in neurosurgical patients. *Clin Infect Dis* 21(2):323-7

PMID 8623760 Jaffey PB, Varma SK, DeMay RM et al [1996] Blastlike cells in the cerebrospinal fluid of young infants: further characterization of clinical setting, morphology & origin. *Am J Clin Pathol* 105(5):544-7

PMID 8903210 Ampel NM [1996] Emerging disease issues & fungal pathogens associated with HIV infection. *Emerg Infect Dis* 2(2):109-16

PMID 9025870 Craver RD [1996] The cytology of cerebrospinal fluid associated with neonatal intraventricular hemorrhage. *Pediatr Pathol Lab Med* 16(5):713-9

PMID 9025871 Fernandes SP, Penchansky L [1996] Tumor like clusters of immature cells in cerebrospinal fluid of infants. *Pediatr Pathol Lab Med* 16(5):721-9

PMID 9168230 Simsa J [1997] How to reduce the risk for contamination of the central nervous system by spinal needles. *Reg Anesth* 22(3):297

PMID 9180910 Goldsby RE, Morgan JG, Egger MJ et al [1997] Lymphoblast morphology in predicting leukemic meningeal relapse with low chamber count & lymphoblasts. *Med Pediatr Oncol* 29(2):98-102

PMID 9532587 Whitaker JN [1998] Myelin basic protein in cerebrospinal fluid & other body fluids. *Multiple Sclerosis* 4(1):16-21

PMID 9626995 Lahrtz F, Piali L, Spanaus KS et al [1998] Chemokines & chemotaxis of leukocytes in infectious meningitis. *J Neuroimmunol* 85(1):33-43

PMID 9819187 Gerdes LU, Jørgensen PE, Nexø E et al [1998] C-reactive protein & bacterial meningitis: a meta-analysis. *Scand J Clin Lab Invest* 58(5):383-393

ISBN 978-141602-9083 Morrison BM [2009] Physiology of cerebrospinal fluid secretion, recirculation, & resorption. In: Irani DN ed. *Cerebrospinal Fluid in Clinical Practice*. Elsevier Saunders, p11-17

ISBN 978-141602-9083 Turtzo LC [2009] Cerebrospinal fluid acquisition & analysis in modern clinical practice. In: Irani DN ed. *Cerebrospinal Fluid in Clinical Practice*. Elsevier Saunders, p55-62

ISBN 978-143770-9742 Karcher DS, McPherson RA [2011] Cerebrospinal, synovial, serous body fluids, and alternative specimens. In: McPherson RA, Pincus MR, ed. *Henry's Clinical Diagnosis & Management by Laboratory Methods*, 22e. Elsevier Saunders, p480-508

ISBN 978-155581-6605 Larone DH [2011] *Medically Important Fungi*, 5e. ASM Press

Case Definitions: Nationally Notifiable Conditions Infectious & Non-Infectious Case [2012] Centers for Disease Control & Prevention

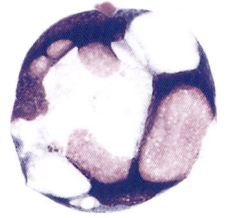

Kjeldsberg CR, Grenache DG, Couturier MR, Cohen MB

Pleural & Pericardial Fluid
Chapter 5

Anatomy & pathophysiology

The pleura (Greek: side, rib) consists of a thin, serous membrane that envelops the lung as well as the chest wall, diaphragm, and mediastinum. The 2 layers are contiguous, and the space between them forms the pleural cavity, which is lined by a single layer of mesothelial cells (the mesothelium). The outer layer, the parietal pleura, is adherent to the chest wall, and the inner layer, the visceral pleura, invests the lung except at the hili where vessels, bronchi, and nerves enter the lung. Normally, the 2 layers of pleura are in apposition, separated only by a small amount of fluid that facilitates movement of the 2 membranes against each other. The pleural cavity, therefore, is not a true cavity but only becomes so in the presence of disease that causes the accumulation of fluid therein. [Light 2007]

Similar to the pleural cavity, the pericardial (Greek: around the heart) cavity is only a potential cavity formed by 2 serous membranes that are closely apposed to each other (one lining the heart [visceral pericardium] and the other lining the inside of the pericardium [parietal pericardium]) and separated by small amounts of serous fluid. This fluid allows the heart to move easily during contraction and relaxation. Following injury or the onset of disease, more fluid may accumulate within the cavity, causing a separation between the visceral and parietal pericardia.

The accumulation of fluid within the pleural or pericardial cavities is called an effusion, and fluids that accumulate in pleural or pericardial cavities are referred to as serous effusions. The aspiration of pleural fluid is called thoracentesis. A thoracentesis is indicated for any undiagnosed pleural effusion. In addition to its diagnostic uses, thoracentesis may have therapeutic benefit to relieve dyspnea (shortness of breath) caused by large effusions.

Pleural fluid is normally produced by the parietal pleura and absorbed by the visceral pleura. The fluid is formed by filtration of plasma through the capillary endothelium, and its presence is dependent on the hydrostatic pressure in capillaries, plasma osmotic pressure, lymphatic resorption, and permeability of capillaries. Fluid is reabsorbed by lymphatic vessels and venules in the visceral pleura. Changes in the rate of production or removal of fluid can explain the accumulation of fluid.

A pleural effusion develops from an imbalance or disruption in the homeostatic forces that control movement of fluid across pleural membranes t5.1. A pleural effusion develops when the amount of fluid that enters the pleural cavity exceeds the amount that can be removed (via the lymphatics). Thus, pleural effusions can result from increased pleural fluid formation, decreased lymphatic resorption from the pleural cavity, or a combination of these factors. Pleural effusions are typically diagnosed by physical exam and chest radiography.

t5.1	Pathophysiologic factors in fluid formation & associated disorders
Increased hydrostatic pressure: congestive heart failure	
Decreased oncotic pressure: nephrotic syndrome	
Increased capillary permeability: infection	
Decreased lymphatic drainage: malignancy	
Increased negative pressure in pleural cavity: bronchial obstruction, atelectasis	
Rupture of a blood vessel: trauma	

>90% of pleural effusions are caused by congestive heart failure (CHF), cirrhosis of the liver, pleural and/or pulmonary infection, malignancy, or pulmonary emboli t5.2. Sometimes, several factors play a role in the etiology of pleural effusions. CHF or chronic kidney disease (CKD) may change the hydrostatic and osmotic forces across the pleura and cause an effusion that is an ultrafiltrate of plasma. Such an effusion is called a transudate. A localized disease, such as bronchopneumonia, is associated with increased permeability of the capillaries in the pleura and causes an effusion rich in leukocytes and serum proteins, and sometimes microorganisms. Such an effusion is called an exudate.

t5.2 Causes of pleural effusions
Transudates
Atelectasis
Cirrhosis
Congestive heart failure
Nephrotic syndrome
Peritoneal dialysis
Postsurgery
Superior vena cava obstruction
Exudates
Infections
Bacterial pneumonia, lung abscess, empyema
Fungal
Parasitic
Viral
Tuberculosis
Neoplastic disease
Metastatic malignancy: carcinoma, sarcoma
Primary intrathoracic malignancy: carcinoma of the lung, mesothelioma
Lymphoma and leukemia
Pulmonary embolization and/or infarction
Rheumatologic diseases
Rheumatoid arthritis
Systemic lupus erythematosus
Gastrointestinal disease
Abscess: subphrenic, hepatic
Esophageal rupture
Pancreatitis
Myocardial infarction
Trauma
Hemothorax
Chylothorax
Chylous effusion
Trauma
Malignancy: carcinoma, lymphoma
Tuberculosis

t5.3 Causes of pericardial effusions
Infections
Viral pericarditis
Bacterial pericarditis
Tuberculous pericarditis
Fungal pericarditis
Cardiovascular disease
Congestive heart failure
Myocardial infarction
Postinfarction syndrome
Cardiac rupture
Aortic dissection
Neoplastic disease
Metastatic carcinoma, sarcoma
Mesothelioma
Lymphoma, leukemia
Trauma
Metabolic
Uremia
Myxedema
Rheumatologic disease
Coagulation disorder: anticoagulant therapy

Accumulation of fluid in the pericardial cavity (pericardial effusion) is most frequently caused by damage to the lining of the cavity associated with changes in the permeability of the membranes due to infection (pericarditis), malignancy, or metabolic injury (eg, CKD leading to uremia) t5.3. The procedure of aspiration of pericardial fluid is called pericardiocentesis. In acute pericarditis, a fibrinous exudate interferes with pericardial venous and lymphatic drainage and predisposes the patient to effusion.

The major infectious agents responsible for pericarditis and pericardial effusion are viruses, especially the Coxsackie and echoviruses. Purulent bacterial and tuberculous effusions are less common. CKD is commonly associated with pericardial effusion. Significant effusion is often associated with the postinfarction syndrome (Dressler syndrome). Cardiac rupture or acute aortic dissection rapidly produces a bloody effusion and cardiac tamponade. Metastatic tumors and, rarely, primary tumors of the pericardium (mesothelioma) are often associated with large effusions. Lung and breast carcinomas, together with lymphoma and leukemia, are the most common causes of secondary malignant pericardial effusions. Traumatic pericardial effusions caused by stab wounds or crush injuries frequently result in cardiac tamponade, which is often fatal.

Specimen collection

A thoracentesis is indicated for any undiagnosed pleural effusion or for therapeutic reasons when fluid causes significant dyspnea. Position papers of the American College of Physicians & the American Thoracic Society have summarized the general application, safety, efficacy, and cost of diagnostic thoracentesis [PMID 4051357, PMID 2751171].

The procedure of thoracentesis consists of inserting a needle, under local anesthetic, into the pleural cavity and aspirating fluid. The specimen should be collected in heparinized tubes to avoid clotting, particularly if bloody. For a cell count an EDTA tube should be used. Aliquots for aerobic and anaerobic bacterial cultures are best inoculated into blood culture media at the bedside. When malignancy, mycobacterial infection or fungal infection is suspected, at least 100 mL should be submitted.

If cytologic examination cannot be performed immediately, the specimen should be refrigerated. Reasonable morphologic features will be maintained for 48-72 hours at refrigerator temperature. For determination of pleural fluid pH, the sample should be collected anaerobically, in a heparinized syringe, and sent to the laboratory. Finally, venous blood should be obtained for total protein, LD, cholesterol, and possibly bilirubin for comparison with pleural fluid.

A diagnostic thoracentesis is generally a safe and low risk procedure, and serious complications are uncommon. Complications of thoracentesis include pneumothorax, hemothorax, reexpansion pulmonary edema, and rarely air embolism. Leakage of air into the pleural space through the needle is the most common cause of pneumothorax. Hemothorax may be caused by trauma to the intercostal blood vessels. It is estimated that ~2% of all pleural infections are due to contamination of the pleural space at the time of thoracentesis. Removal of >1,000 mL of pleural fluid at any one time may result in pulmonary edema or severe hypotension. A thoracentesis may be contraindicated in a severe coagulopathy or with severe thrombocytopenia.

Pleural biopsy

A biopsy of the pleura is indicated in patients with an exudative pleural effusion of undetermined origin. A pleural biopsy may especially be useful in the diagnosis of malignancy, eg, mesothelioma, or tuberculosis. If tuberculosis pleuritis is considered, a portion of the pleural biopsy specimen should be cultured for *Mycobacteria*. The identification of granulomas in the biopsy usually suggests tuberculosis, but fungal disease, sarcoidosis, and rheumatoid pleuritis should also be considered.

Transudates & exudates

Effusions of pleural and pericardial (as well as peritoneal) cavities have classically been divided into transudates and exudates t5.4 [PMID 4642731]. In general, transudates indicate fluid that has accumulated because of a systemic disease. The effusion is usually bilateral. A common disorder associated with transudates is CHF. Exudates are usually associated with localized disorders involving the pleural surfaces such as inflammatory conditions, malignancy, or infection. CHF and cirrhosis of the liver cause most transudative pleural effusions, while cancer, pneumonia, and pulmonary emboli cause most exudative pleural effusions.

t5.4 Pleural fluid laboratory differentiation of transudates & exudates

	Transudate	Exudate
Appearance	Clear, pale yellow	Cloudy, turbid, purulent or bloody
Specific gravity	<1.015	>1.015
Pleural fluid protein:serum protein ratio	<0.5	>0.5
Pleural fluid LD	<2/3 of the upper reference limit for serum LD	>2/3 of the upper reference limit for serum LD
Pleural fluid:serum LD ratio	<0.6	>0.6
Pleural fluid: serum bilirubin ratio	<0.6	>0.6
Pleural fluid cholesterol	<45 mg/dL	>45 mg/dL
Pleural fluid:serum cholesterol ratio	<0.3	>0.3
Cells	Few	Many

The main usefulness in defining a pleural effusion as a transudate or an exudate is to determine which effusions need further laboratory (or other) evaluation. If the effusion is a transudate, usually no further diagnostic procedures are needed. If the effusion is an exudate, more extensive diagnostic procedures are indicated to determine the cause of the effusion. Although transudates and exudates frequently differ in such characteristics as color, appearance (clear vs cloudy or bloody), and cell count, these assessments are unreliable in establishing which type of effusion is present.

The most reliable tests for differentiating between the transudates and exudates are the simultaneous analysis of pleural fluid and serum for total protein and lactate dehydrogenase (LD) concentration (Light criteria). In transudates, the ratio of pleural fluid total protein to serum total protein is <0.5, while the corresponding LD ratio is <0.6. Exudates have corresponding ratios higher than 0.5 and 0.6, respectively. It has also been suggested that transudates have LD activity that is >2/3 of the upper reference limit for serum LD activity t5.4 [PMID 12075059, PMID 9713637].

Using the results of simultaneous testing of serum and pleural fluid protein and LD activity, together with those of a good clinical history and physical examination, an accurate determination of exudates vs transudates should be possible in >90% of patients with effusions.

Cholesterol levels in pleural effusions have been recommended in differentiating exudates from transudates. A pleural fluid cholesterol level <45 mg/dL is usually associated with transudates, while >45 mg/dL is usually associated with exudates. In addition, a pleural cholesterol:serum cholesterol ratio (P:S CHOL) of <0.3 is usually associated with transudates, and a ratio of >0.3 is usually associated with exudates. Pleural fluid cholesterol levels and serum cholesterol levels correlate in patients with exudative lesions but not in patients with transudates. It is thought that elevated levels of pleural fluid cholesterol are related to increased permeability of the pleural capillaries. These cholesterol tests may have greater sensitivity and specificity than the previously recommended tests of protein ratio and LD ratio.

None of these tests are 100% effective in separating transudates from exudates. The Light criteria misclassify ~25% of transudates as exudates, and most of these patients are on diuretics [PMID 11403751]. Inaccuracies in separating transudates from exudates are common when the measured biochemical values are close to the cutoff values. Cholesterol and/or bilirubin concentration values may be useful when the protein and LD activity in the pleural fluid are equivocal. The reader is referred to the sections on chemical analysis for a more detailed discussion of these test parameters.

When the specimen is classified as an exudate, other studies are necessary to define the disease process further. Gram staining, staining for acid-fast organisms, cultures, and counterimmunoelectrophoresis may be indicated if an infection is suspected. Cytologic tests and biopsy may be diagnostic in cases of a suspected malignant condition.

The 4 leading causes of pleural effusions in order of incidence are congestive heart failure, malignancy, pneumonia and pulmonary embolism. Congestive heart failure and cirrhosis cause most transudative effusions, and malignancy, bacterial and viral pneumonia and pulmonary embolism cause most exudative effusions.

Recommended tests

To minimize unnecessary laboratory studies it is important to have a clear differential diagnosis in mind [PMID 18195577]. The results of laboratory studies should always be correlated with the clinical findings and results of other studies to arrive at an accurate diagnosis.

The purposes of laboratory testing of serous effusions are
- to differentiate transudates from exudates
- to differentiate malignant from nonmalignant effusions in patients with exudative effusions
- to diagnose specific causes of a serous effusions, eg, infection

A similar mindset is applicable to pericardial effusions although the focus is often more focused on the etiology (2 and 3, above) rather than determining the nature of the serous effusion, ie, transudative vs exudative [PMID 9149572]. t5.4 lists tests useful in differentiating transudates from exudates and t5.5 lists the most useful laboratory tests in most patients and tests useful in selected patients.

Gross examination

The initial step in the investigation of pleural & pericardial effusions is the gross examination, which can play an important role in determining the pathogenesis of the effusion t5.6. Transudates are usually clear and pale yellow, and do not clot. Exudates are cloudy to purulent, and often clot while standing because of the presence of the serum protein fibrinogen. Exudative fluid usually contains large numbers of leukocytes and elevated protein content. Occasionally, exudates may be straw colored, similar to transudates. A cloudy, purulent fluid is usually associated with an infectious process. The presence of clearly visible pus is diagnostic of empyema. Anaerobic bacterial infection of the pleura may produce a feculent odor. A green white, turbid fluid may be seen with rheumatoid pleuritis.

t5.5 Laboratory tests in pleural effusion

Useful in most patients
Gross examination
Pleural fluid and serum protein ratio
Pleural fluid and serum LD ratio
Cytology
Stains and cultures for microorganisms

Useful in selected patients
PCR for select microorganisms
pH
Lipid analysis
Immunologic studies
Pleural fluid cholesterol
Adenosine deaminase
Amylase
Pleural fluid and serum bilirubin ratio Immunohistochemistry/flow cytometry
Pleural biopsy

Limited usefulness
Leukocyte count and differential
RBC count
Pleural fluid glucose
Tumor markers
Complement, rheumatoid factor, ANA

t5.6 Pleural fluid gross appearance & clinical significance

Appearance	Significance
Transudates	
Clear straw colored	Further analysis usually not necessary
Exudates*	
Cloudy, purulent	Infectious process, empyema
Red tinged to bloody	If not traumatic tap: malignancy, pulmonary infarction, trauma
Green white, turbid	Rheumatoid pleuritis
Milky white or yellow bloody	Chylous effusion
Milky or green, metallic sheen	Pseudochylous (chyliform) effusion
Viscous, hemorrhagic or clear	Mesothelioma
Anchovy paste color "chocolate sauce"	Rupture of amebic liver abscess

*Some exudates may appear clear and straw colored

Hemorrhagic fluid may be present because of a traumatic tap, malignancy, pulmonary infarction, rupture of an aortic aneurysm, chest trauma, pancreatitis, or tuberculosis. Metastatic adenocarcinoma is sometimes associated with mucoid, bloodstained fluid. Blood tinged fluid may also be seen in transudates, and only 1-2 mL of peripheral blood in 1,000 mL of pleural fluid will produce a blood tinged appearance. A traumatic tap must be distinguished from other sources of blood in the pleural fluid. In a traumatic tap, the blood is usually not distributed consistently and gradually clears as aspiration proceeds. A hematocrit should be obtained on bloody fluids. A pleural fluid hematocrit >1% is usually associated with malignancy, pulmonary embolus, or chest trauma. A hematocrit level >50% of that of the peripheral blood is associated with a true hemothorax, as may be seen in chest injuries.

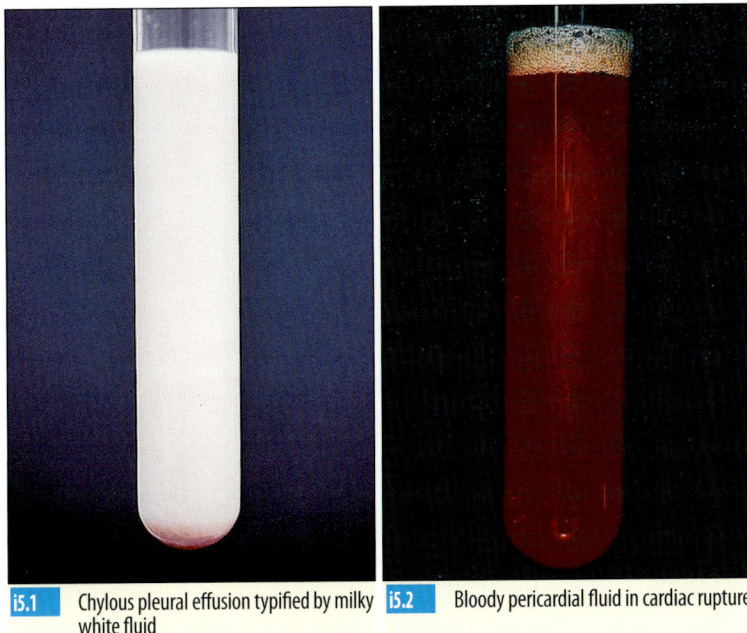

| i5.1 | Chylous pleural effusion typified by milky white fluid | i5.2 | Bloody pericardial fluid in cardiac rupture |

needs to consider empyema and chylothorax in addition to pseudochylothorax. As previously discussed, in empyema centrifugation results in a clear supernatant.

Normally, only a small amount of clear, pale yellow fluid is present in the pericardial cavity. A pericardial effusion due to infection or malignancy usually has a turbid appearance. Blood streaked, cloudy fluid is frequently caused by tumors and tuberculosis. A bloody effusion is seen in cardiac rupture or puncture i5.2. Renal failure with uremia is usually associated with clear, straw colored fluid. A milky fluid may be seen when damage to the lymphatic system has occurred.

Cell count

Leukocyte counts have limited value in separating transudates from exudates. It is primarily useful in cases of infection, ie, an elevated white blood cell count with increased numbers of PMNs in bacterial disease. Neutrophilia may also be seen in pulmonary infarction, pancreatitis, early tuberculosis, and subphrenic abscess. A predominance of lymphocytes is often seen in tuberculosis, viral infection, malignancy, true chylothorax, rheumatoid pleuritis and uremic effusions.

When the pleural fluid is turbid, milky, and/or bloody, the specimen should be centrifuged and the supernatant examined. If the turbidity clears with centrifugation, it was most likely due to an increased number of cells or debris. However, if the turbidity persists after centrifugation, the patient most likely has a chylothorax or a pseudochylothorax. Chylous and so called pseudochylous effusions are typified by milky white pleural fluid i5.1. However, the classic milky white appearance may be present in <50% of cases of chylous effusions. It may be yellow or green and turbid, or even bloody. Following trauma, the chylous is frequently bloody, which may mask the milky appearance of chylothorax. Following centrifugation, fluid from a chylothorax remains opaque, whereas the milky fluid of empyema becomes clear.

A true chylothorax is rare and results from leakage of the thoracic duct, which is most commonly caused by a malignancy such as lymphoma or carcinoma. In rare cases, it may be the presenting sign of a malignant lymphoma. The 2nd leading cause of chylothorax is trauma, especially associated with cardiovascular surgery. The 3rd most common cause of chylothorax is idiopathic, including most cases of congenital chylothorax. Chylothorax is the most common form of pleural effusion encountered in the newborn. The origin of congenital chylothorax is unknown.

A pseudochylous effusion does not result from disruption of the thoracic duct but is associated with chronic effusions (usually several years) as seen in rheumatoid pleuritis and tuberculosis. Pseudochylothorax is much less common than chylothorax. When turbid or milky pleural fluid is present in a patient with longstanding pleural effusion, one

Microscopic examination

An examination of the cells present in pleural or pericardial fluids and a differential cell count should be performed on a stained smear made by cytocentrifugation or other methods. Morphologically, the cytocentrifuge preparation is usually superior to a push smear. For routine clinical laboratory evaluation, a Romanowsky (Wright stain) stain and a Pap stain should be utilized (Romanowsky stain is especially useful in hematologic malignancies). The Pap stain provides superior nuclear detail and is better for the identification of squamous cells as in squamous cell carcinoma. Cell blocks may be a useful addition when a malignancy is suspected, especially for immunohistochemical studies, eg, keratin expression. A higher rate of recovery of tumor cells has been demonstrated in specimens examined with a combination of smear and cell block techniques. However, since the majority of effusions are benign, the routine use of cell blocks may not be a cost effective method of detecting malignancy. Cell blocks should only be used if initial cytologic preparations are suspicious or if clinical history indicates a likelihood of malignancy.

The cell types encountered in pleural, pericardial, as well as peritoneal fluids are granulocytes (polymorphonuclear leukocytes [PMNs], eosinophils, and basophils), lymphocytes, plasma cells, mononuclear phagocytes (monocytes, histiocytes and macrophages), mesothelial cells, and malignant cells.

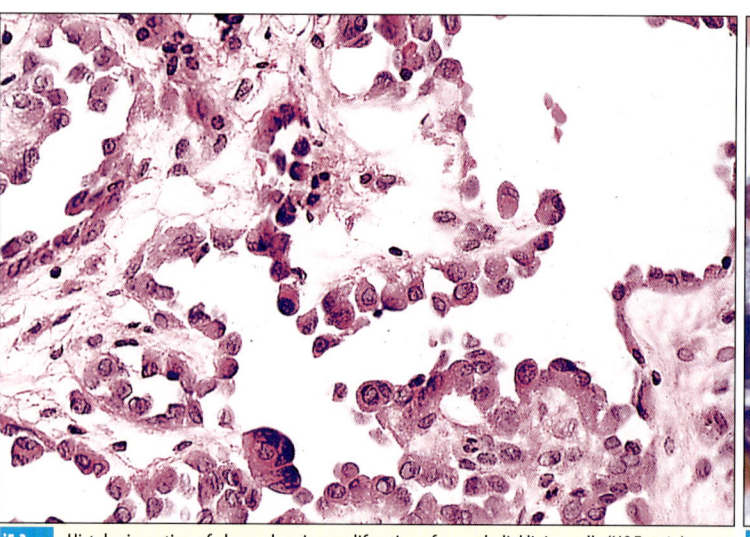

i5.3 Histologic section of pleura showing proliferation of mesothelial lining cells (H&E stain)

i5.5 Higher power view of mesothelial cells with basophilic cytoplasm. Vacuoles are often seen in the cytoplasm.

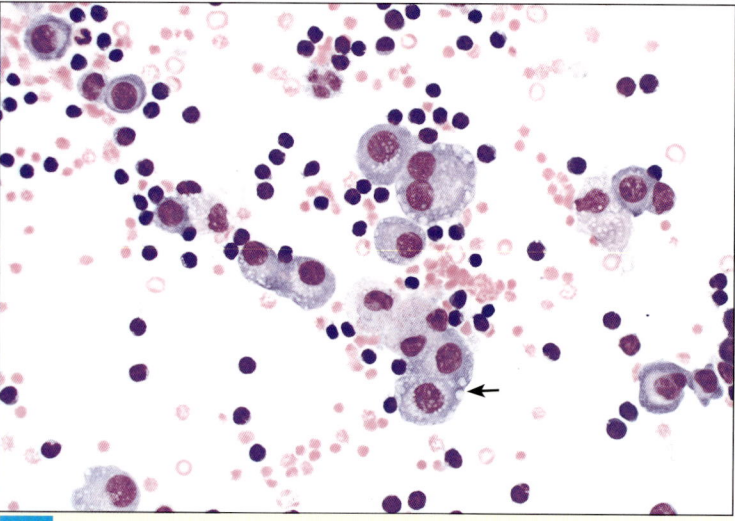

i5.4 Low power view of many mesothelial cells (arrow) & small lymphocytes

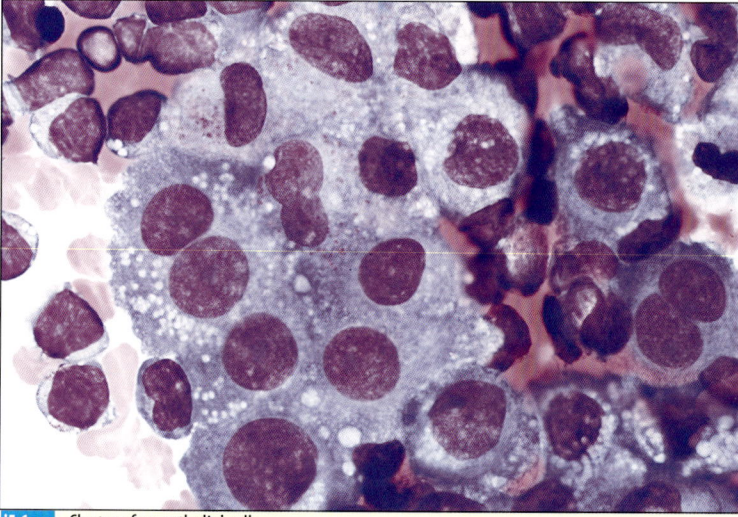

i5.6 Cluster of mesothelial cells

Mesothelial cells form the lining of pleural, pericardial, and peritoneal cavities i5.3. Because of their variable appearance, they frequently cause difficulty in the microscopic examination and may be mistaken for malignant cells. It is essential to become familiar with the wide range of appearances seen in benign mesothelial cells in order to separate out reactive and proliferative mesothelial changes from malignancy, both primary and metastatic i5.4-i5.17.

During inflammatory processes, mesothelial cells undergo proliferation and often desquamate into the serous fluid. These cells are notoriously pleomorphic. They may occur singly, in flat sheets, or rarely in 3 dimensional clusters that may have a spherical or papillary appearance. The cells are large and measure from 15-25 μm in air dried specimens. With alcohol fixation, the mesothelial cells are smaller, measuring from 10-14 μm in diameter. They may, however, be smaller or considerably larger than the measurements given. The cytoplasm is usually abundant but may be scanty, is light gray to deep blue, and may have a perinuclear zonal pallor i5.17. Cytoplasmic vacuoles of variable size may be seen i5.5, i5.10. The nucleus is round to oval and occupies

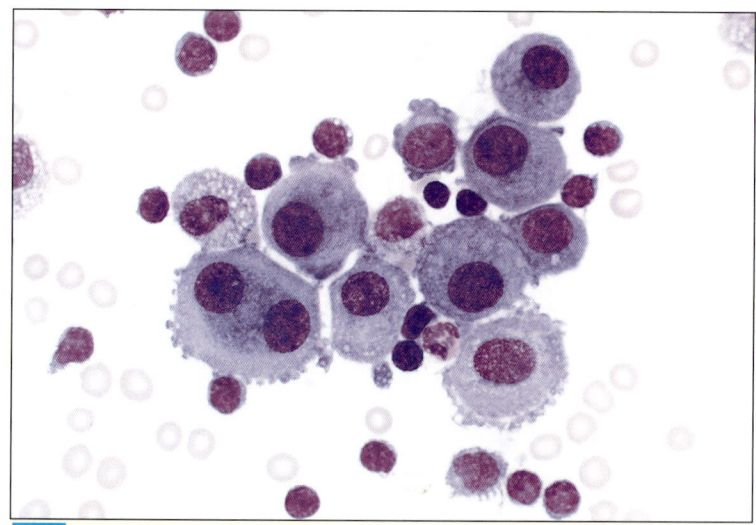

i5.7 Mesothelial cells of varying sizes

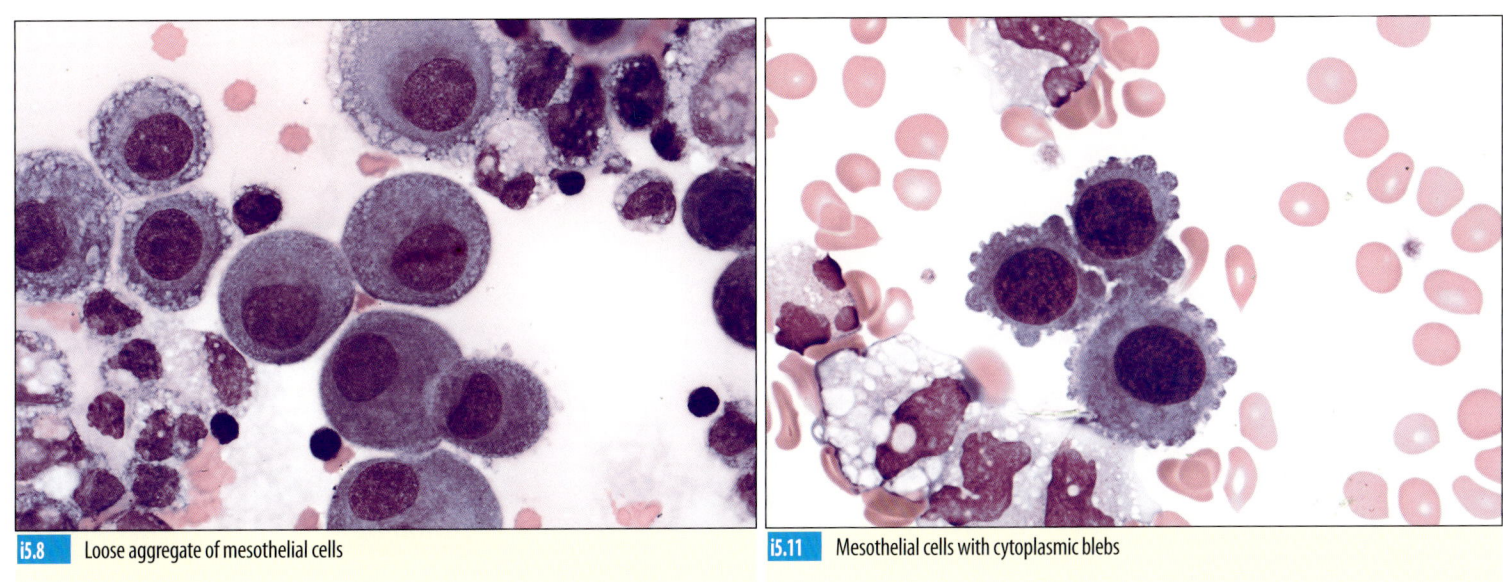

i5.8 Loose aggregate of mesothelial cells

i5.11 Mesothelial cells with cytoplasmic blebs

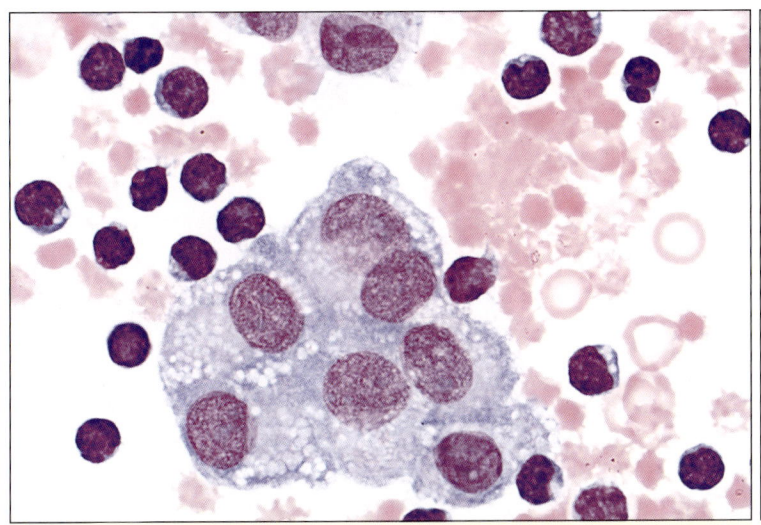

i5.9 Cluster of mesothelial cells having an orderly mosaic appearance

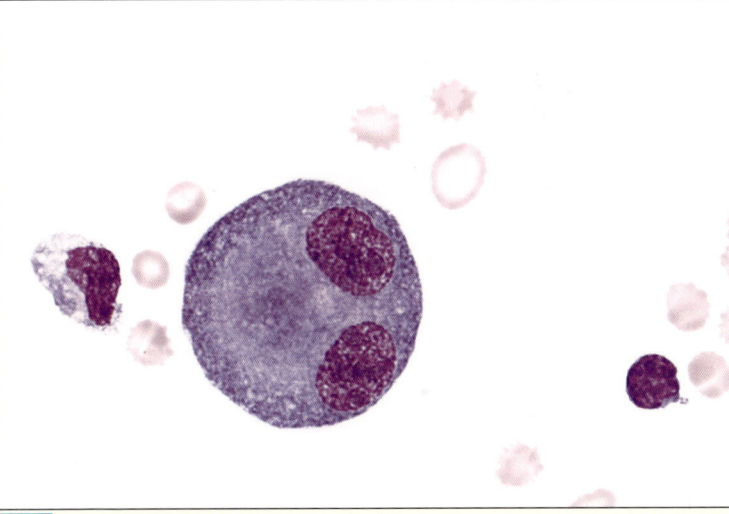

i5.12 A binucleate mesothelial cell

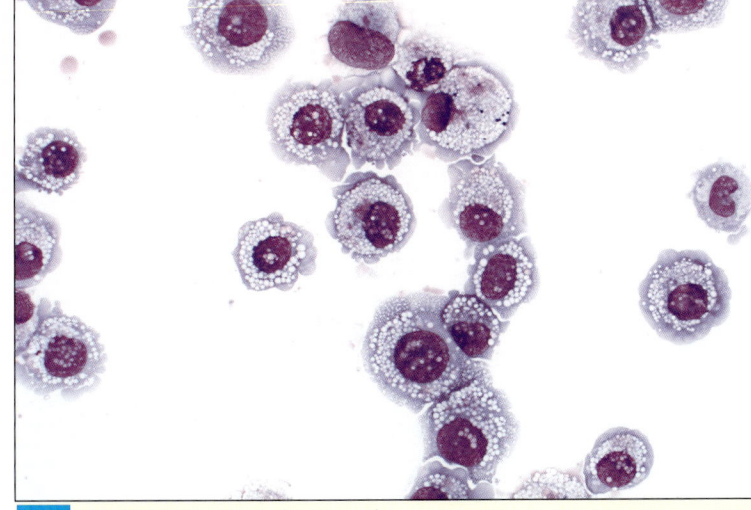

i5.10 Mesothelial cells with cytoplasmic vacuoles

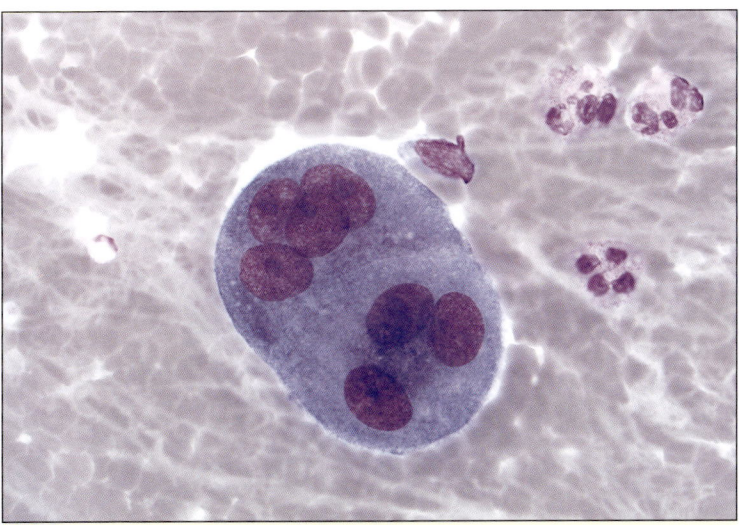

i5.13 2 multinucleated mesothelial cells connected to each other

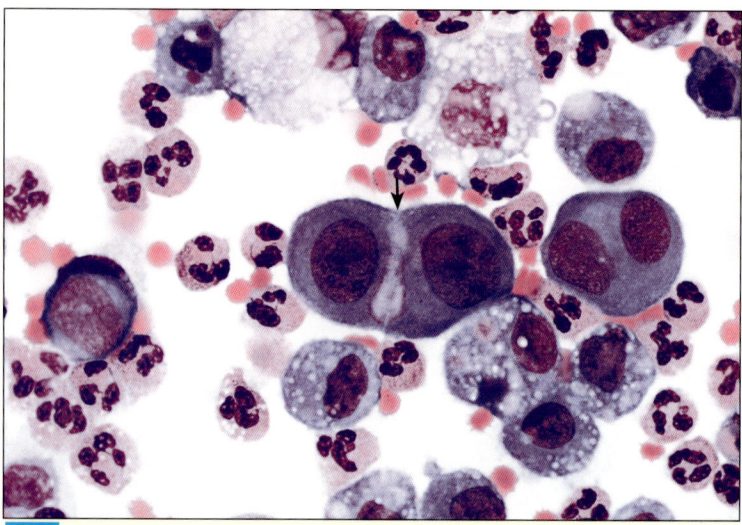
i5.14 2 mesothelial cells articulate with each other with a cleft or clear space ("window") between the cells

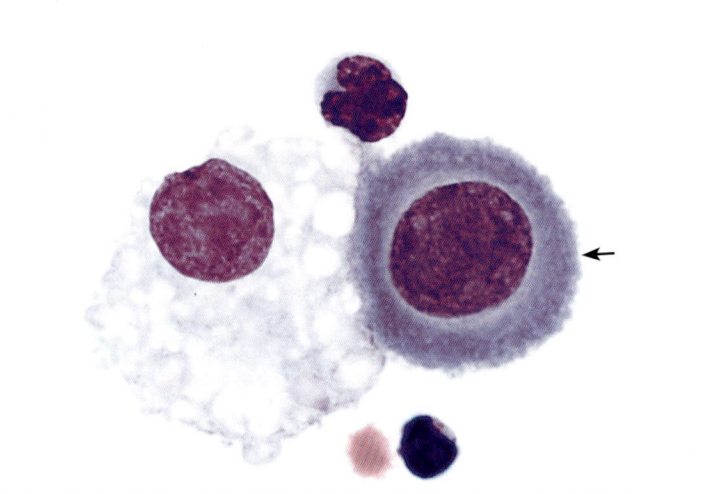
i5.17 A mesothelial cell (arrow) & a macrophage with vacuoles representing phagocytosed "ghost" red blood cells

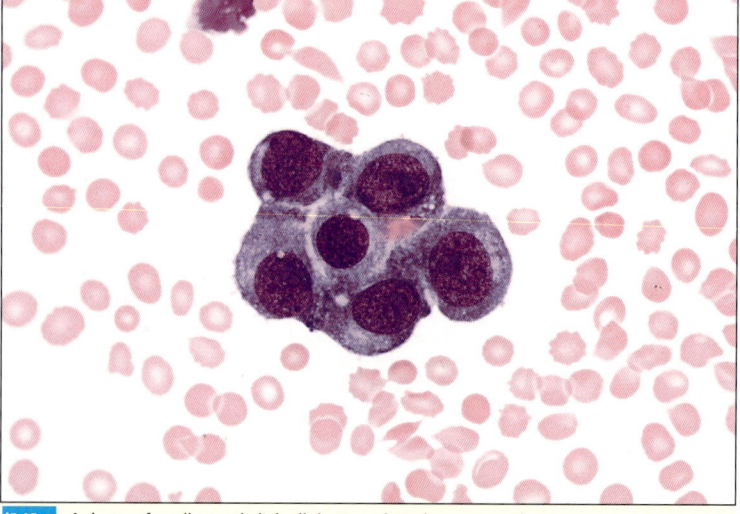
i5.15 A cluster of small mesothelial cells having relatively scant cytoplasm

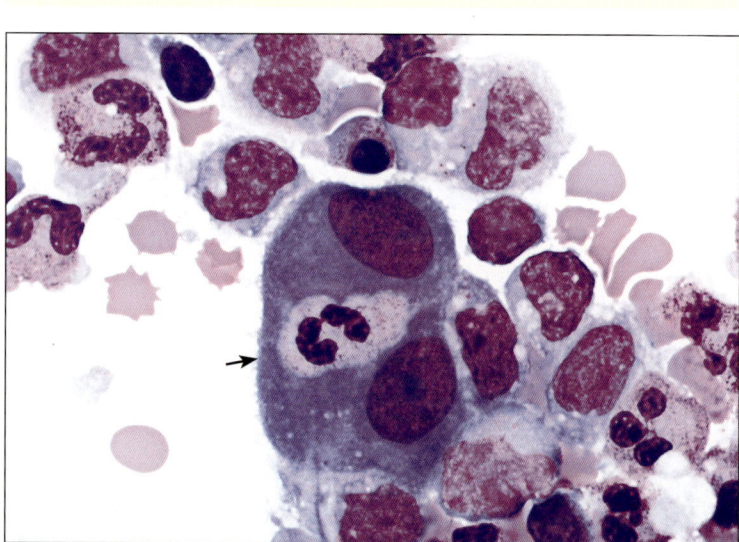
i5.16 A binucleate mesothelial cell having phagocytosed a PMN (arrow)

~1/3-1/2 the cell's diameter. The nuclear contour is usually smooth and regular, but may be irregular. The chromatin is stippled, dark purple, and uniformly distributed. 1-3 spherical nucleoli may be seen. Some mesothelial cells may resemble large plasma cells.

Various attempts have been made to classify the mesothelial cells according to their appearance and terms such as reactive, activated, hyperplastic, proliferative, and atypical are used. Unfortunately, there is no general agreement on the definition of these terms and since they are usually not meaningful clinically, their use should be avoided. The term proliferative and hyperplastic mesothelial cells usually refers to clusters of mesothelial cells, typically with moderate to scant cytoplasm and hyperchromatic nuclei. The term reactive mesothelial cells usually refers to cells with slightly irregular nuclei and prominent nucleoli. The term typical mesothelial cells usually refer to cells that resemble malignant cells and that the cytopathologist cannot always exclude from malignancy. So called atypical mesothelial cells may be particularly associated with liver cirrhosis, irradiation, connective tissue disorders, foreign bodies, neoplasms, infarction, and chronic inflammation of long duration. Mesothelial cells may be multinucleated, occasionally containing 20 or more nuclei i5.13. At times they may form glandlike structures.

Mesothelial cells, when they appear in clumps, are usually in loose aggregates and often are connected to each other in a characteristic manner i5.6, i5.9. The cell borders are often "squared off" with clefts or clear spaces ("windows") between the cells i5.14. Sometimes the cytoplasm of one cell appears to be clasping (embracing) another cell. One may also see large sheets of mesothelial cells having an orderly mosaic appearance i5.9. When cells have multilayered formation or 3 dimensional spheroidal arrangements, they are more likely to be malignant. These types of arrangements are usually better appreciated with a Papanicolaou stain.

Clumps of mesothelial cells may be distinguished from malignant cells by comparing their appearance within the clump and with other more readily identified mesothelial cells in the same smear thereby recognizing the "family similarity." The uniform regular arrangement of the mesothelial cell usually indicates a benign origin. Benign mesothelial cell nuclei usually have a smooth nuclear outline and evenly distributed fine chromatin. The nucleoli may be large and prominent, but they are usually uniform in size and shape. In contrast, malignant cells frequently show nuclear outline irregularities together with irregular chromatin disbursement and nucleoli of varying size and shape t5.7.

t5.7 Morphologic features helpful in distinguishing benign mesothelial cells from adenocarcinoma cells		
Microscopic appearance	Mesothelial cells	Adenocarcinoma cells
"2nd cell" population	Absent	Present
Cell clumps	Borders between cells are usually angular or "squared" off, often with clear spaces between cell ("windows")	Borders between cells are often obscure; cytoplasm and vacuoles often join or coalesce
3 dimensional aggregates	Uncommon	Common
Cells	Rounded	Columnar
Cell borders	Ruffled, lacy	Distinct, sharp
Cytoplasm	2 tone Glycogen	Homogeneous Mucin
Increased N:C ratio	Usually absent	Usually present
Nucleus	Central	Eccentric
Nuclear outline	Usually smooth	Often irregular
Hyperchromasia	Usually present	Variable
Nuclear molding	Usually absent	May be present
Nucleoli	When present usually small	May be large and angulated
Immunohistochemistry*	Calretinin+, WT1+	Ber-EP4+, B72-3+, CD15+

Mesothelioma vs adenocarcinoma

Sometimes it may be impossible to differentiate mesothelial cells from malignant cells. In such cases, immunohistochemistry and flow cytometry may be helpful. Mitoses may be present in benign mesothelial cells and in malignant cells, and are of little diagnostic significance except when obviously abnormal. Difficulties in the distinction of mesothelial cells from malignant cells may particularly occur in smears that are technically not well prepared. When the cell concentration, for example, is high or bloody, there is an increased tendency for clumping of the cells and such cells are frequently overstained. In such cases, the specimen must be diluted to obtain optimal morphology. When only a thick overstained preparation is available, the examination should be made by reviewing cells at the periphery of the smear where the staining reaction is not as dark.

Degenerative mesothelial cells may show pyknosis and karyorrhexis, and they may contain peculiar cytoplasmic inclusions of varying colors. Degenerative changes may also be seen in the form of ground glass appearance to the cytoplasm and a coarse, motley, salamilike nuclear chromatin pattern. In longstanding effusions, the cytoplasm of the mesothelial cells may be filled with vacuoles that sometimes fuse and push the nucleus against the cell membrane producing a signet ringlike appearance. It is important not to mistake these degenerating cells for metastatic adenocarcinoma cells. Mesothelial cells may show evidence of phagocytosis i5.16. Mesothelial cells also frequently show a morphologic transformation characterized by loss of basophilia and development of foamy vacuolation, which produces a morphologic appearance indistinguishable from macrophages. Mesothelial cells may transform into macrophages and it is common to see various morphologic intermediate forms between mesothelial cells and macrophages. It is generally of no clinical significance to differentiate mesothelial cells from macrophages.

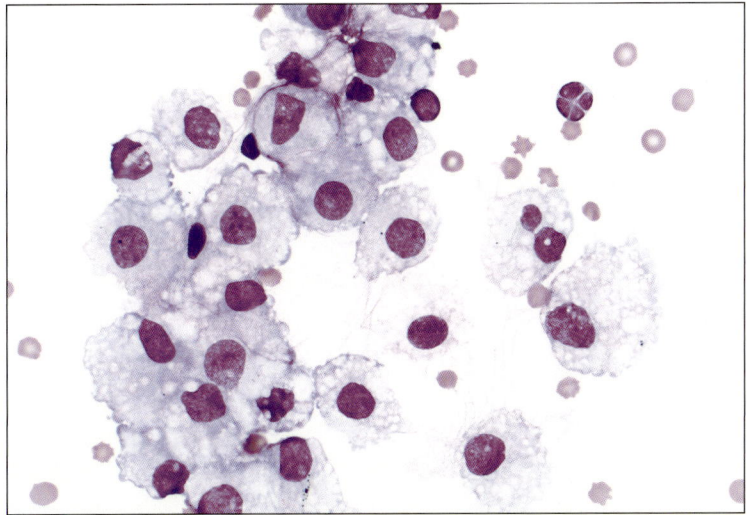

i5.18 Multiple macrophages

Mesothelial cells are seen in variable numbers in most effusions and are increased with pneumonia, pulmonary infarction, and malignant disorders. In tuberculous pleurisy, or when heavy concentrations of pyogenic organisms are present within the serous cavities, mesothelial cells are characteristically scarce. This is probably due to a fibrinous exudate covering the mesothelial lining of the cavity. Unusually small numbers of mesothelial cells may also be seen in patients in whom a sclerosing agent has been used as treatment for recurring malignant effusions and in patients with rheumatoid pleuritis.

Mononuclear phagocytes (monocytes, histiocytes, and macrophages) are usually seen in variable numbers in pleural, pericardial, and peritoneal effusions i5.18-i5.23. Since both histiocytes and mesothelial cells may be transformed into macrophages, the distinction between them is not always obvious. The terms macrophage and histiocyte are used synonymously in this book although some authors distinguish between them by defining the macrophages as those that show evidence of phagocytosis. Macrophages vary in size and have a diameter of 15-25 µm. The cytoplasm is pale gray, cloudy, and frequently vacuolated. The nuclei may be bean shaped, lobular, ovoid, or round. Sometimes large (up to 50 µm) macrophages may be seen. So called signet ring cells are formed when the small vacuoles fuse forming one or 2 large vacuoles that flatten the nucleus against the side of the cell membrane i5.21,. Signet ring cell is a descriptive term and may be seen often in benign and malignant cells.

A variety of names have been given to the macrophages depending on the material they have phagocytosed. If the term lipophage is used, then phagocytosed free lipid material is present in tiny phagocytic vacuoles. When digestion

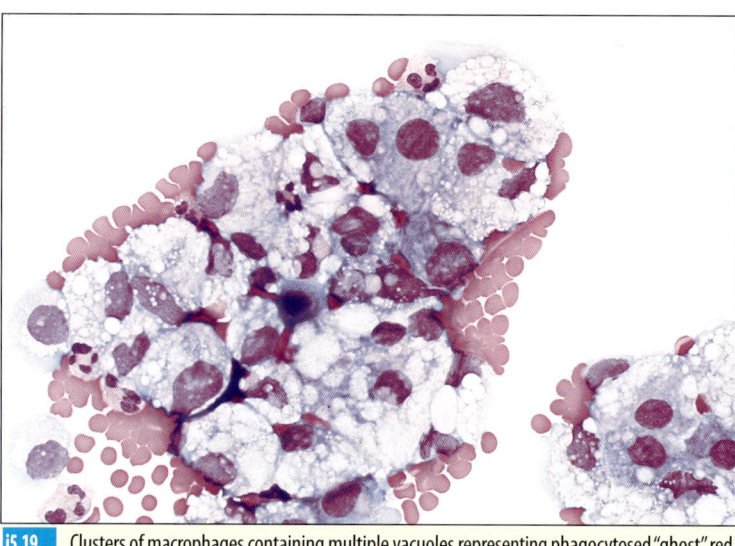

i5.19 Clusters of macrophages containing multiple vacuoles representing phagocytosed "ghost" red blood cells

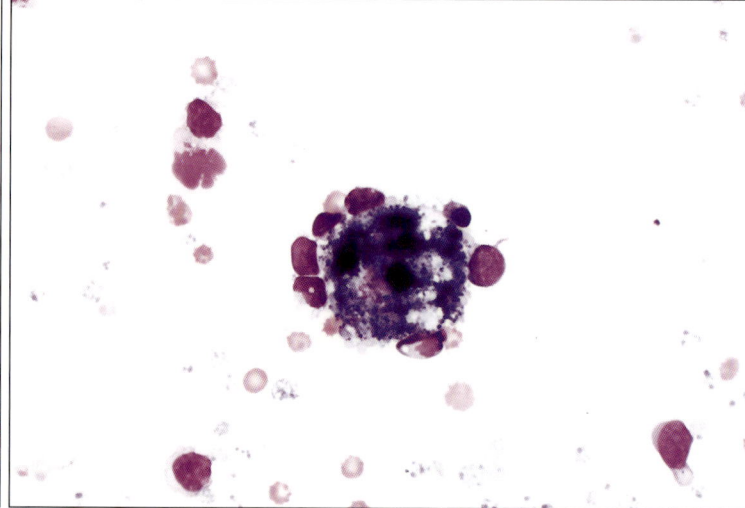

i5.22 A macrophage containing hemosiderin pigment

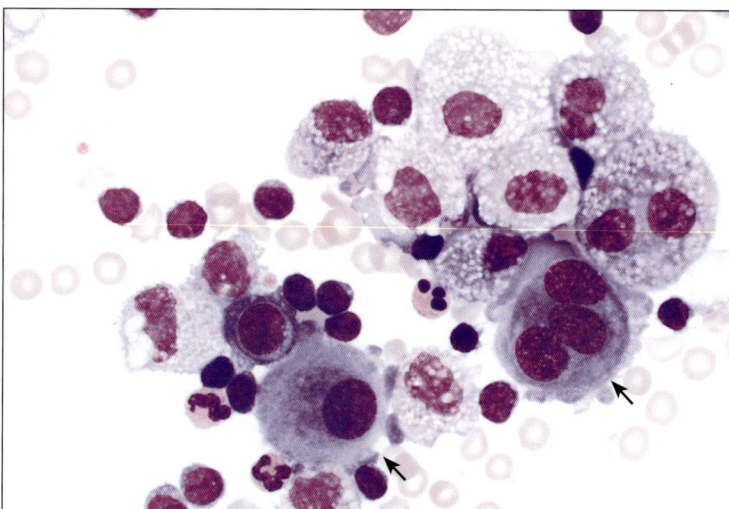

i5.20 Mesothelial cells (arrows) & macrophages

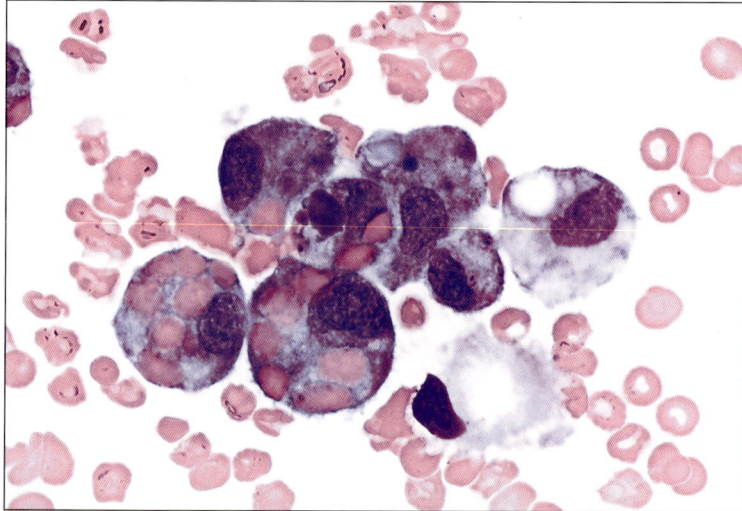

i5.23 Macrophages having phagocytosed multiple red blood cells

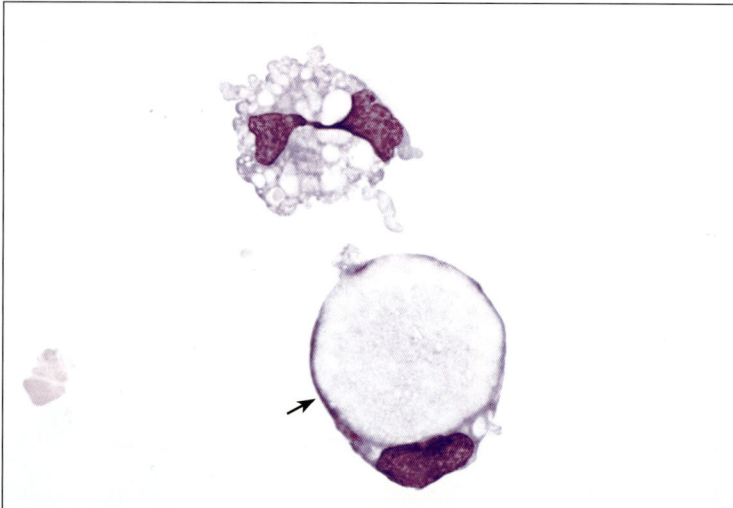

i5.21 A "signet ring" macrophage (arrow)

of the phagocytosed neutrophil occurs, the remnants may be seen in the form of purple granules or pigment. An erythrophage is a macrophage that contains phagocytosed red blood cells i5.23. As red blood cells break down, hemosiderin pigment is seen within the macrophage and the term siderophage is used i5.22. The hemosiderin appears as darkly stained blue black granules in air dried smears. Crystalline hematin pigment may also be present. It is important not to mistake ingested and digested cellular products within the macrophage for intracellular organisms. Bacteria and yeast that may be present in macrophages and neutrophils characteristically have a regular shape. Yeast may have a capsule with a small clear zone around each individual organism. Macrophages may also contain bile pigment that may appear black or yellow and carbon that is black.

Lymphocytes are seen in variable numbers in most serous effusions i5.24-i5.28. They may be small, medium, or large in size, and they may exhibit reactive (transformed) changes. It is important to be aware of the various

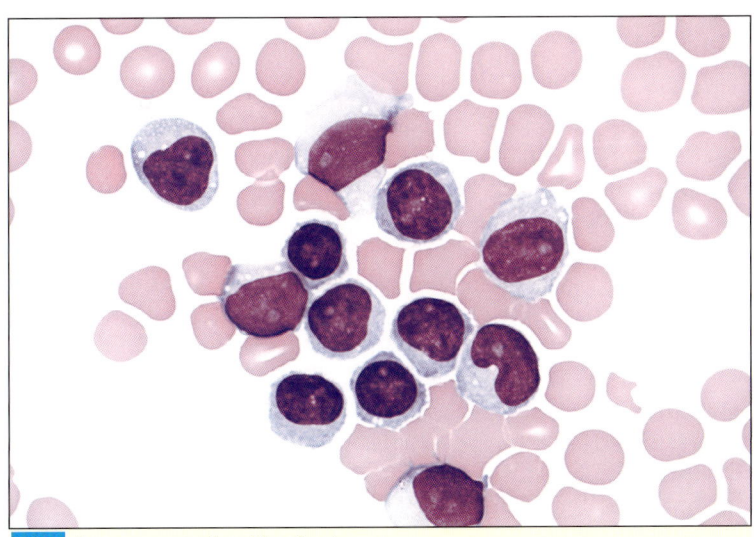

i5.24 Loose aggregate of small lymphocytes

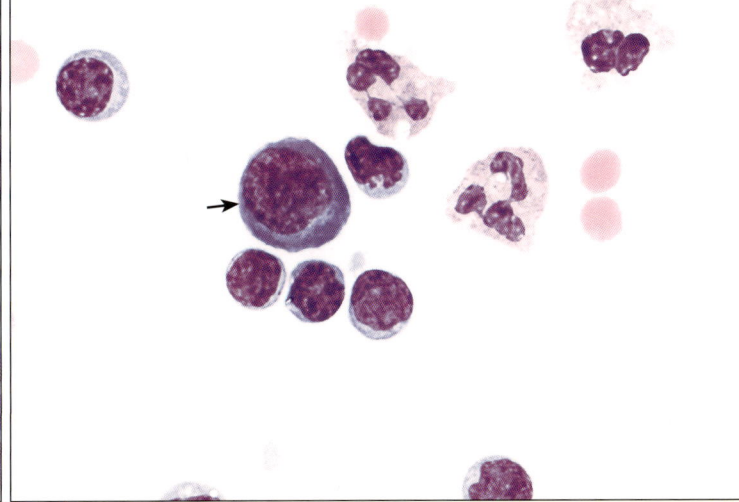

i5.26 An immunoblast (arrow)

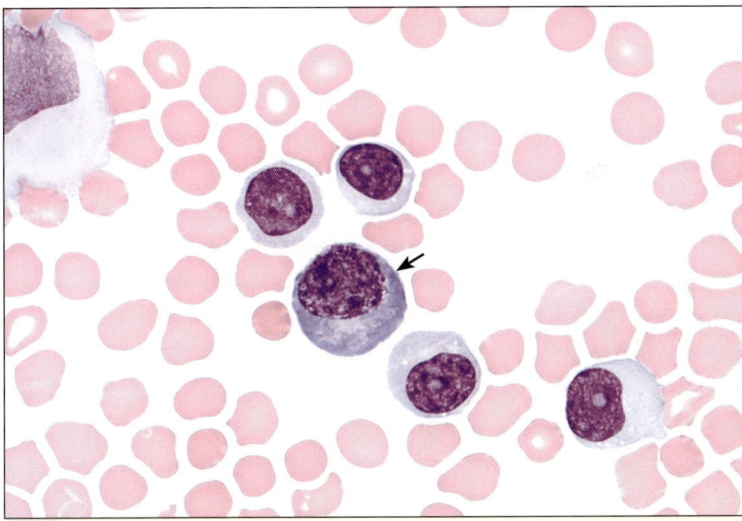

i5.25 A transformed, activated plasmacytoid lymphocyte (arrow)

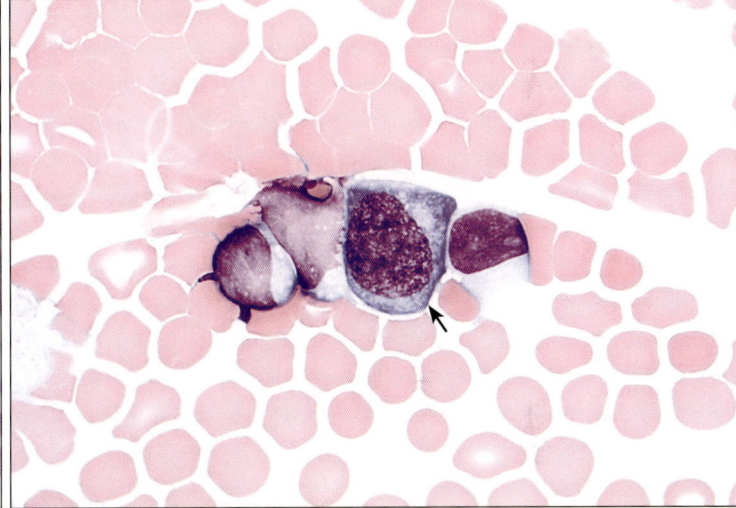

i5.27 An immunoblast (arrow)

morphologic features that lymphocytes have as they morphologically transform in response to many stimuli. Such lymphocytes may have an immature appearance, suggesting lymphoblastic leukemia or lymphoma if they represent the predominant cell type. Lymphocytic nucleoli are often more prominent in effusions than in peripheral blood and the nuclei may be cleaved. The irregularity of the nuclear contours that is sometimes seen is often caused by centrifugation during the concentration process, and therefore caution should be used in morphologic evaluation . A variable number of transformed or reactive lymphocytes may be present. These are large lymphocytes with abundant deep blue cytoplasm and often with several prominent nucleoli i5.26-i5.27. Mitoses are fairly common in the transformed lymphoid cells and they should not be mistaken for evidence of malignancy. In difficult cases, flow cytometric analysis may be very helpful.

Tuberculosis and malignant effusions frequently show a predominance of small lymphocytes. In tuberculosis, the fluid characteristically shows lymphocytosis and only a few

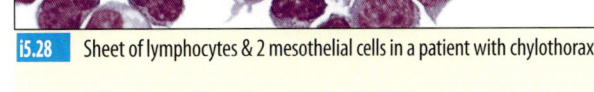

i5.28 Sheet of lymphocytes & 2 mesothelial cells in a patient with chylothorax

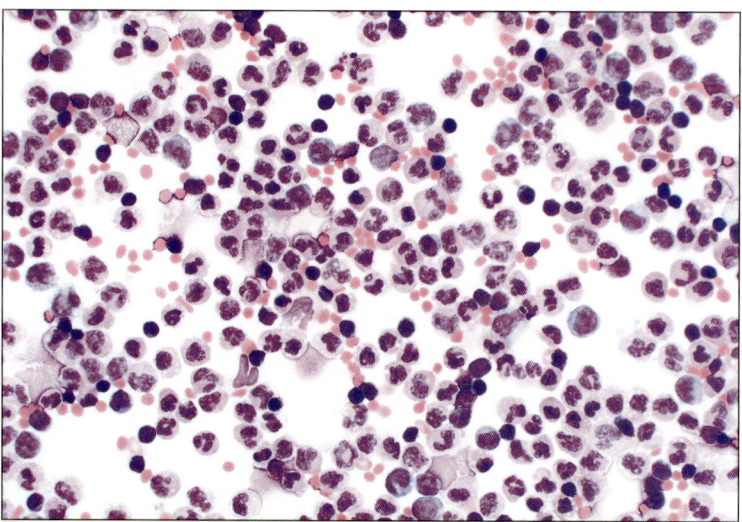

i5.29 Numerous PMNs in a patient with bacterial pneumonia

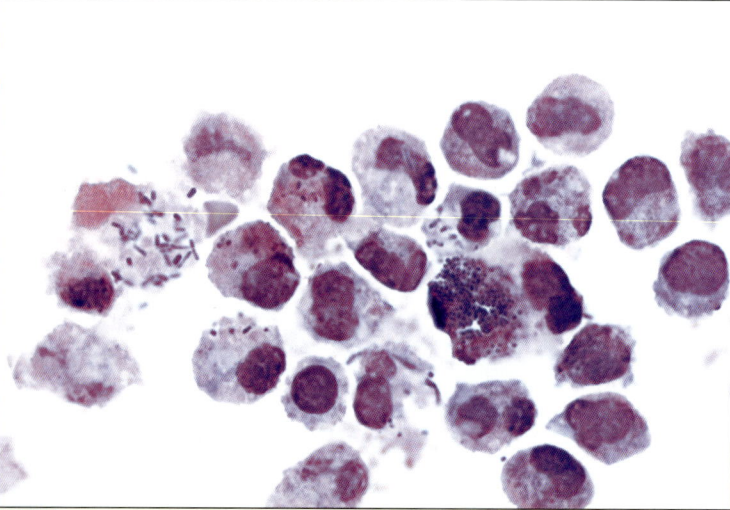

i5.30 Degenerating PMNs with intracellular bacteria

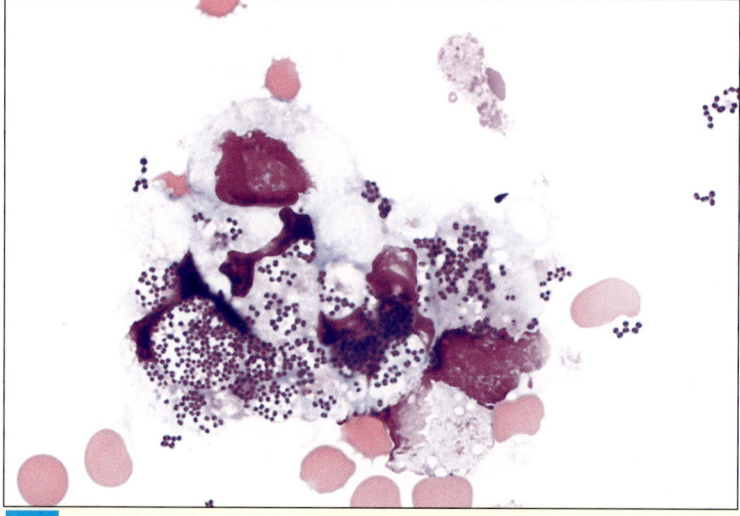

i5.31 Multiple intracellular & extracellular cocci in a patient with pneumonia

mesothelial cells. However, the absence of lymphocytosis does not rule out the diagnosis of tuberculosis or malignant effusions. In non-Hodgkin B cell lymphomas, the malignant lymphocytes are generally uniform or monotonous in size, shape, and staining characteristics. This is in contrast to benign, inflammatory lymphocytosis in which there is usually a mixture of different types of lymphocytes, which may appear polymorphous. However, in many T cell lymphomas, like anaplastic large cell lymphoma, the cells may be very pleomorphic. Lymphocytic pleural effusions may also be associated with leakage of the thoracic duct (chylothorax). In such patients, the lymphocytes are usually small and uniform i5.28. A lesser degree of lymphocytosis may be seen in CHF and cirrhosis.

Immunophenotypic studies have shown that the majority of lymphoid cells in reactive effusions are T cells with the CD4:CD8 ratio being somewhat higher than that reported for the peripheral blood. Phenotypic analysis of pleural fluid lymphocytes is probably not helpful in distinguishing tuberculosis from other nonmalignant effusions. It has been observed that B cells could represent up to ~35% of cells in benign cases and as few as ~5% in a case of malignant B cell effusions. This suggests that the relative numbers of T cells and B cells alone may not be adequate to differentiate benign from malignant effusions. The presence of a monoclonal B cell population, however, is usually associated with a malignant lymphoma.

Plasma cells may be seen in fluid specimens of patients with rheumatoid arthritis, malignant disorders, tuberculosis, and other conditions associated with lymphocytosis.

Neutrophils may differ in appearance in serous fluids i5.29. They may appear more or less identical to those seen in the blood or may be difficult to recognize as PMNs. In longstanding effusions, the granules may be decreased in number or lost. The nuclei may appear as densely stained spherical fragments and may be mistaken for nucleated RBCs. Occasionally, the cytoplasm may have a blue color so that the PMNs resemble lymphocytes. In effusions, due to infection, the PMNs may show evidence of degeneration in the form of vacuolation, loss of granules, and blurring of the nuclei i5.30-i5.31.

Gram stains are useful in detection and identification of bacteria i5.32-i5.33. *Echinococcus* from a ruptured hydatid cyst is clear without staining i5.34.

It is debatable how valuable the differential leukocyte count is in the differential diagnosis. The number of PMNs present in different effusions may vary but a predominance of PMNs suggests bacterial pneumonia, pulmonary infarction, or pancreatitis. Serous fluid neutrophilia is usually the initial cell reaction to these conditions. Later, a predominance of mononuclear cells and mesothelial cells may be noted.

Eosinophilic pleural effusion has been defined as an effusion in which there are >10% eosinophils i5.35. Pleural fluid eosinophilia may occur in a wide array of disorders including infections, neoplasms, pulmonary infarction, connective tissue disorders, and hypersensitivity states, in association with parasites and in pneumothorax. When peripheral blood eosinophilia is also present, one should consider the possibility of hydatid disease, Löffler syndrome, periarteritis nodosa, trauma, or Hodgkin lymphoma. Pleural fluid eosinophilia is thus not a helpful

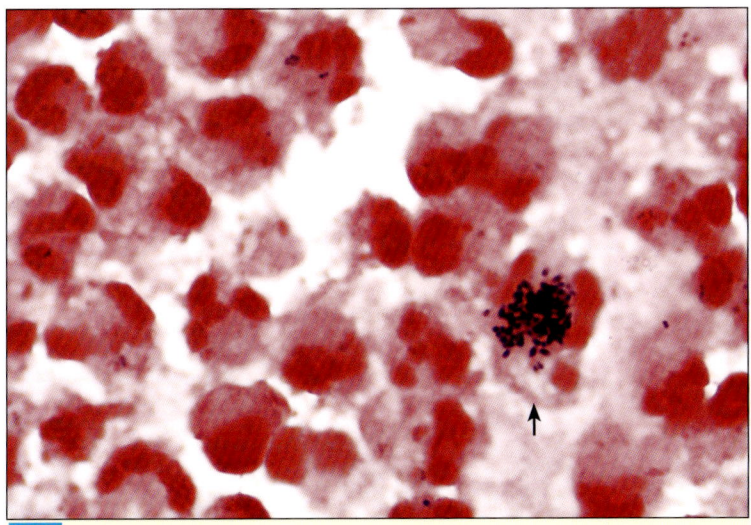

i5.32 Gram+ bacteria (arrow)

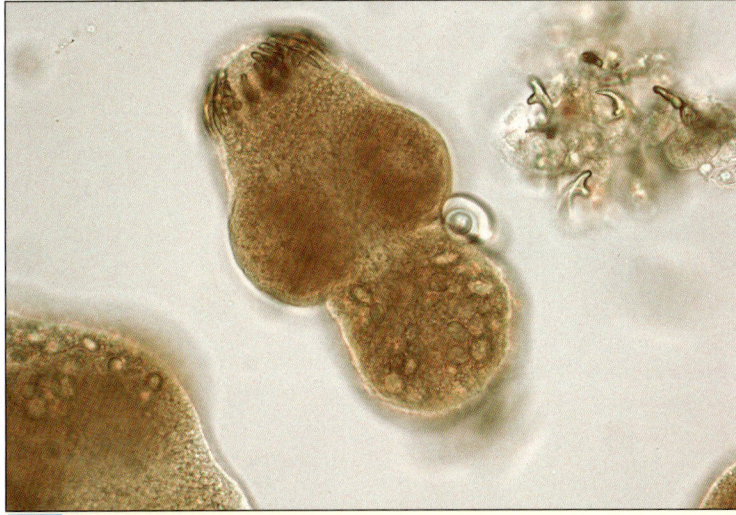

i5.34 *Echinococcus* organisms in pleural fluid

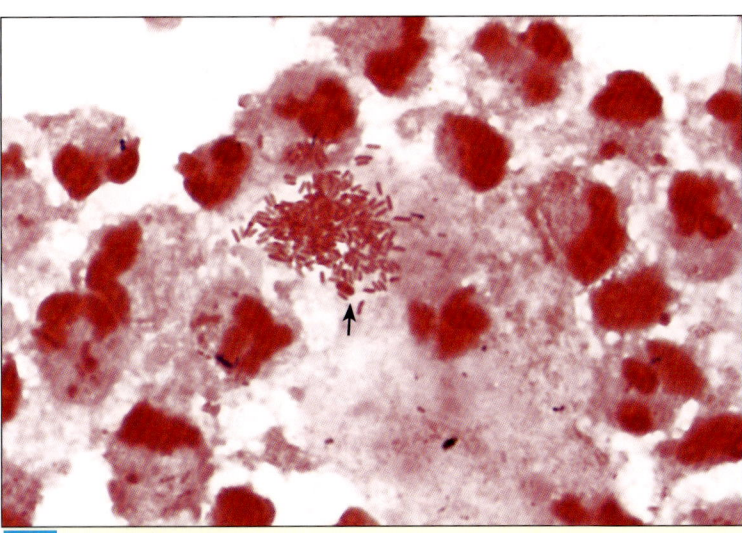

i5.33 Gram− bacteria (arrow)

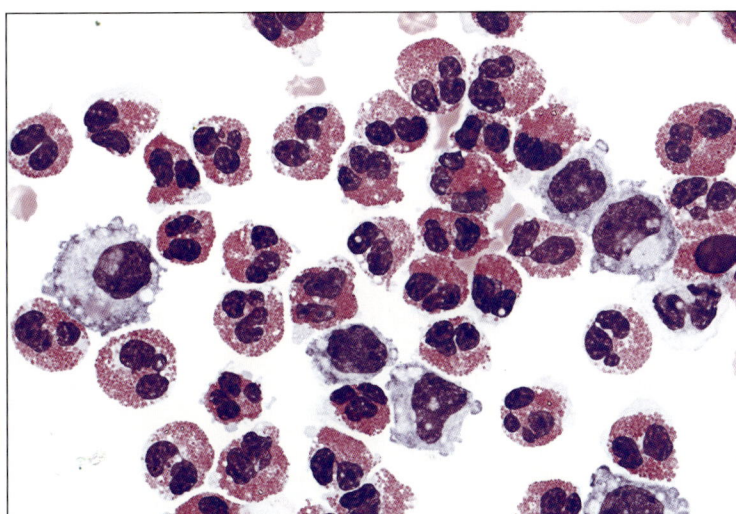

i5.35 Pleural eosinophilia from patient with pneumothorax

diagnostic finding. It may, however, be a marker for a more favorable immune or inflammatory response to pleural disease [PMID 8915232]. Charcot-Leyden crystals have been described in eosinophilic pleural effusions.

Mast cells and basophils often accompany eosinophils, and 5%-10% may be seen in pleural fluid eosinophilia.

Lupus erythematosus (LE) cell formation has been reported in pleural, pericardial, and peritoneal fluids i5.36. Serous fluids allowed to stand at room temperature may have more LE cells than the same fluid examined shortly after it was aspirated which indicates that LE cells are formed in vitro and in vivo. So called "tart cells," which are cells morphologically similar to LE cells, are more frequently seen in serous fluids. They represent small macrophages that have phagocytosed a nonhomogenized nucleus of another cell. The phagocytosed nuclear material in an LE cell is smooth and homogeneous.

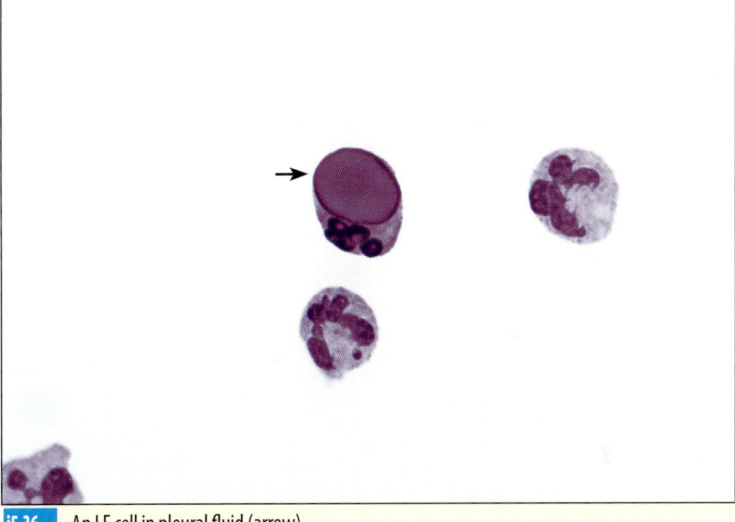

i5.36 An LE cell in pleural fluid (arrow)

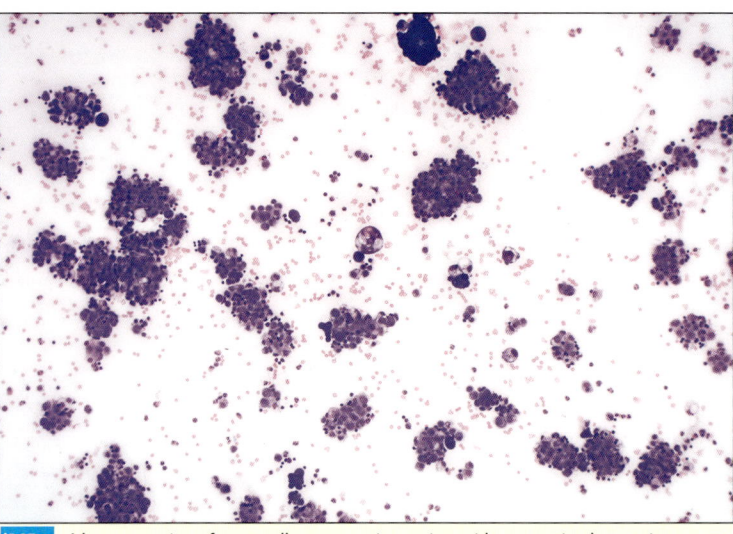
i5.37 A low power view of tumor cell aggregates in a patient with metastatic adenocarcinoma

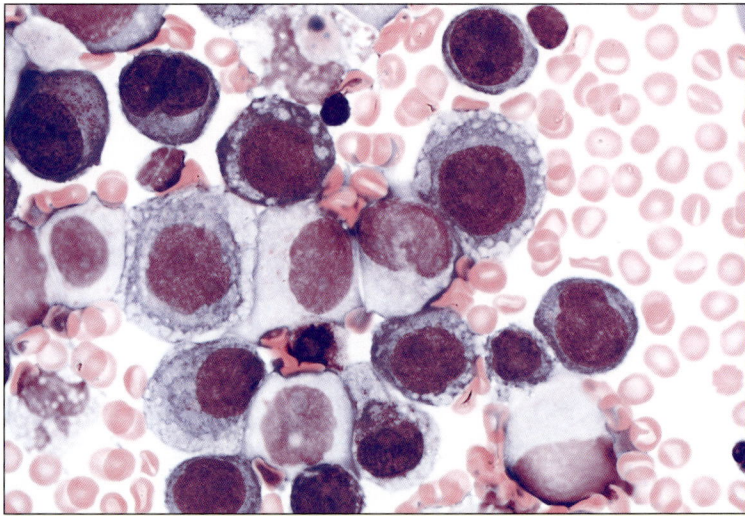
i5.39 High power view of metastatic breast carcinoma cells

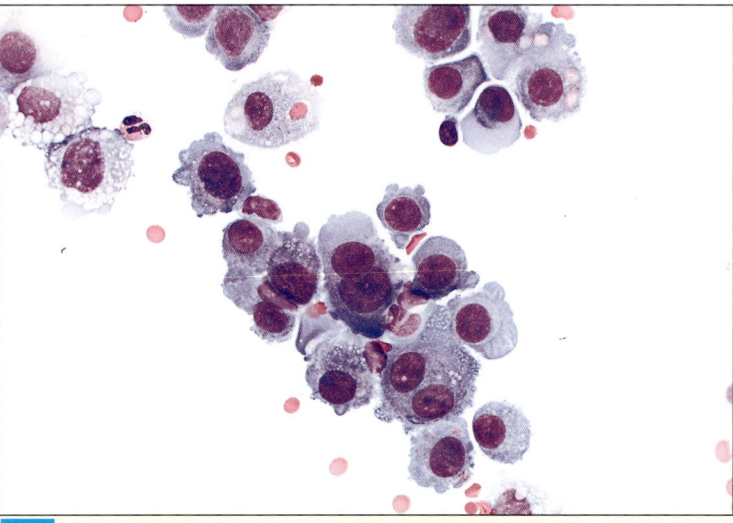
i5.38 Cluster of metastatic breast carcinoma cells resembling mesothelial cells

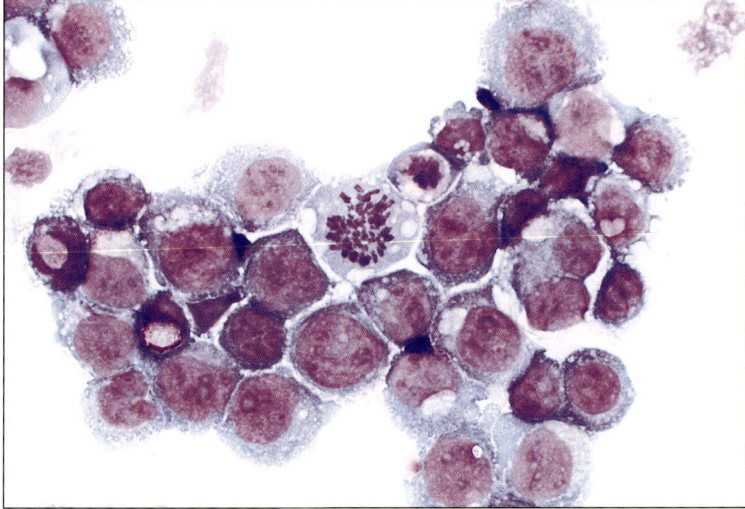
i5.40 Metastatic breast carcinoma with an abnormal mitotic figure

Megakaryocytes and immature myeloid cells may be seen in pleural fluid associated with myeloproliferative disorders. It is important not to mistake these cells for metastatic carcinoma, malignant mesothelioma, or lymphomas.

Malignant cells from a variety of neoplasms may be encountered in pleural and pericardial cavities, and microscopic examination for malignant cells may be the most important part of the examination of an undiagnosed exudative fluid i5.37-i5.68. A more detailed description of various malignant conditions is found under the section "Clinical considerations."

As mentioned earlier, when performing the microscopic examination it is important to be aware that a variety of artifacts and cellular changes may be present in serous fluid specimens. The cytocentrifuge instrument is generally excellent for concentrating the cells on the slide. There are, however, frequently various cellular distortions caused by the spinning process i5.70-i5.71.

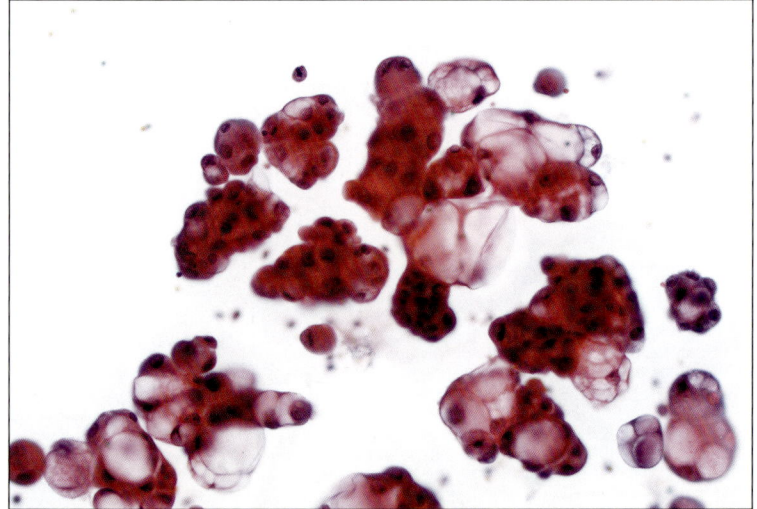
i5.41 Metastatic breast adenocarcinoma. Papanicolaou stain.

5: Pleural & Pericardial Fluids

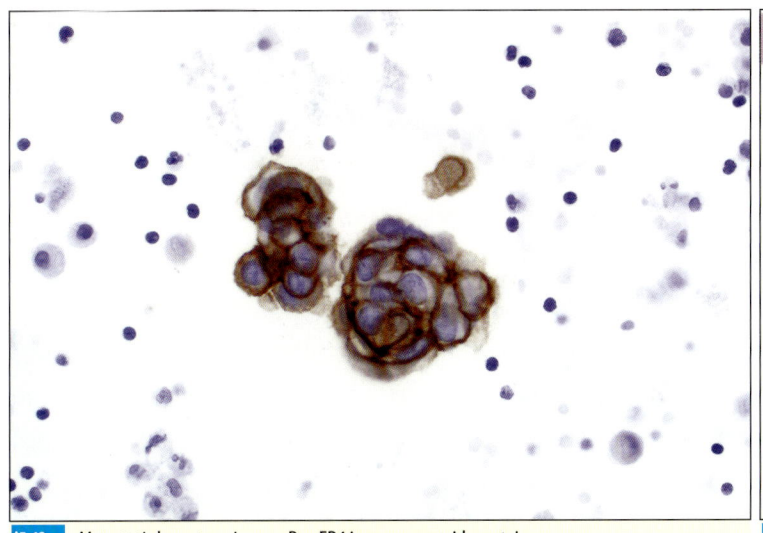

i5.42 Metastatic breast carcinoma. Ber-EP4 immunoperoxidase stain.

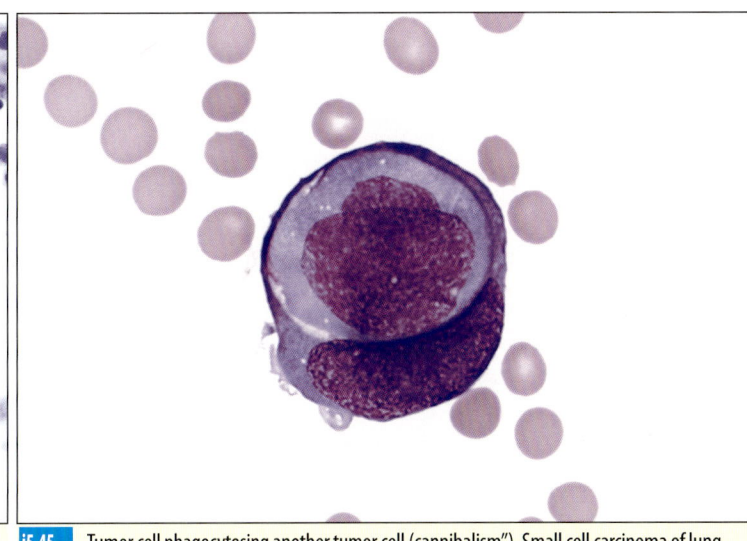

i5.45 Tumor cell phagocytosing another tumor cell ("cannibalism"). Small cell carcinoma of lung.

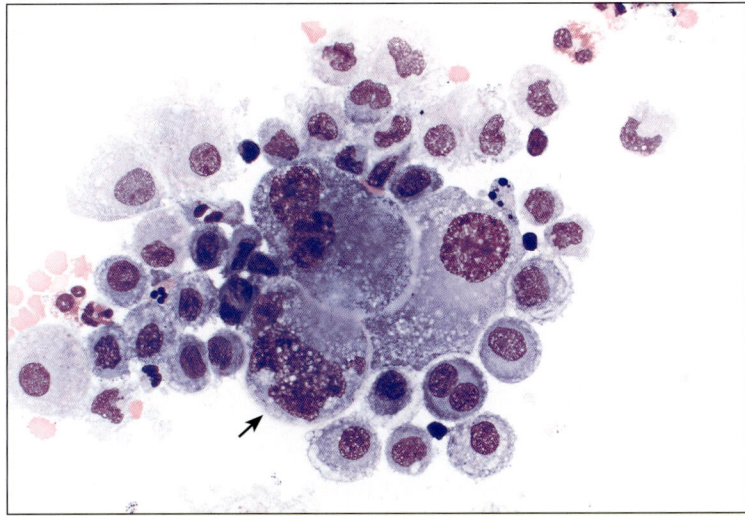

i5.43 Metastatic lung carcinoma cells (arrow) surrounded by mesothelial cells & macrophages

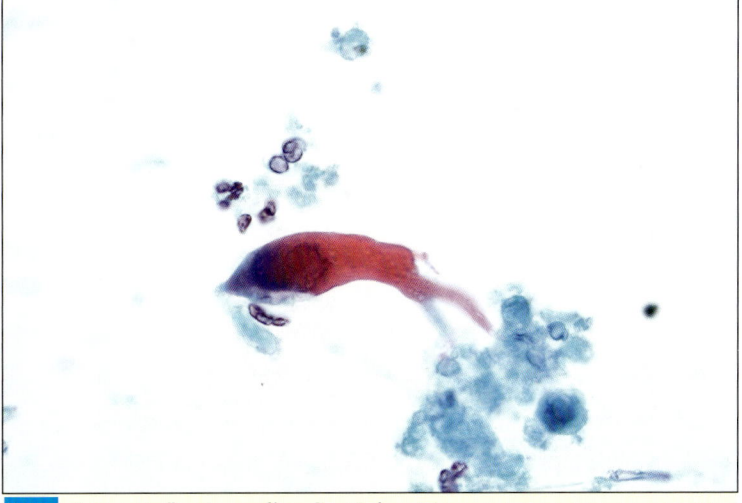

i5.46 Squamous cell carcinoma of lung. Papanicolaou stain.

i5.44 Typical arrangement of small cell carcinoma of lung showing molding of nuclei (arrow)

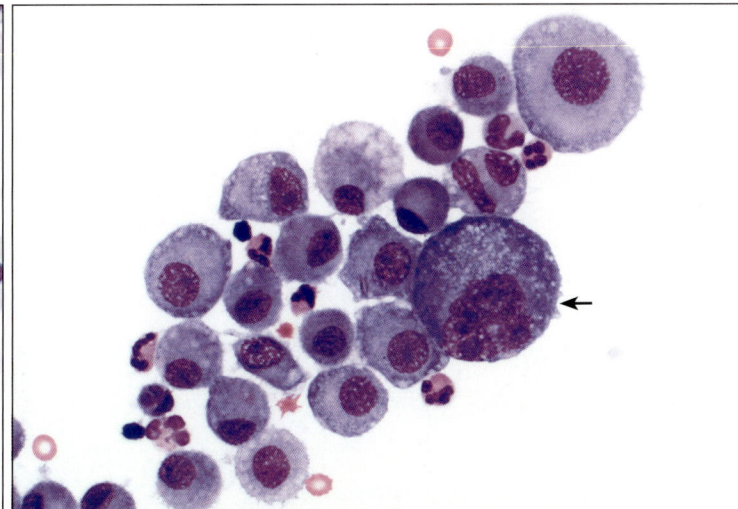

i5.47 Metastatic carcinoma of unknown primary (arrow)

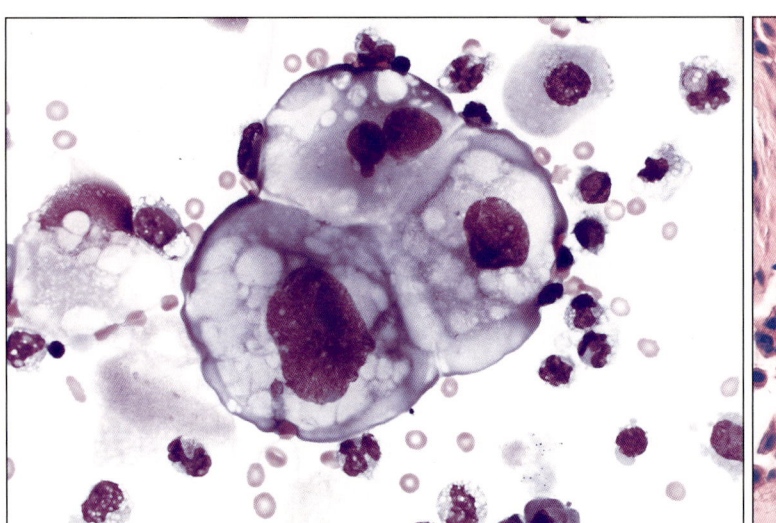
i5.48 Giant tumor cells in metastatic adenocarcinoma

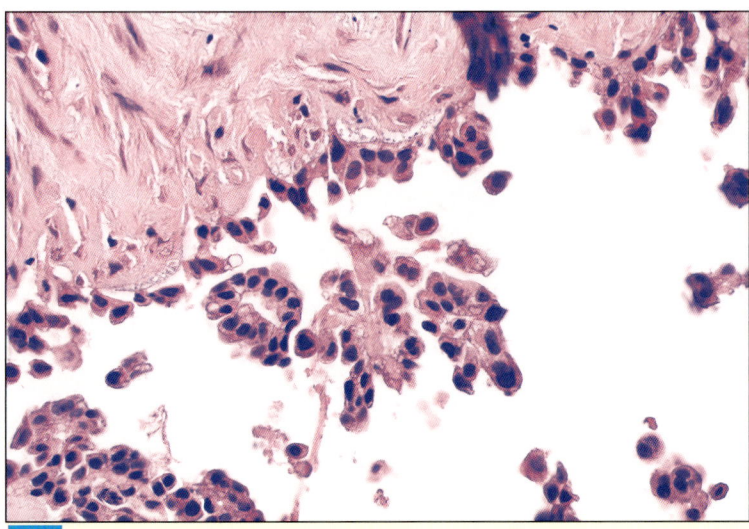
i5.51 Malignant mesothelial cells. Cell block (H&E stain).

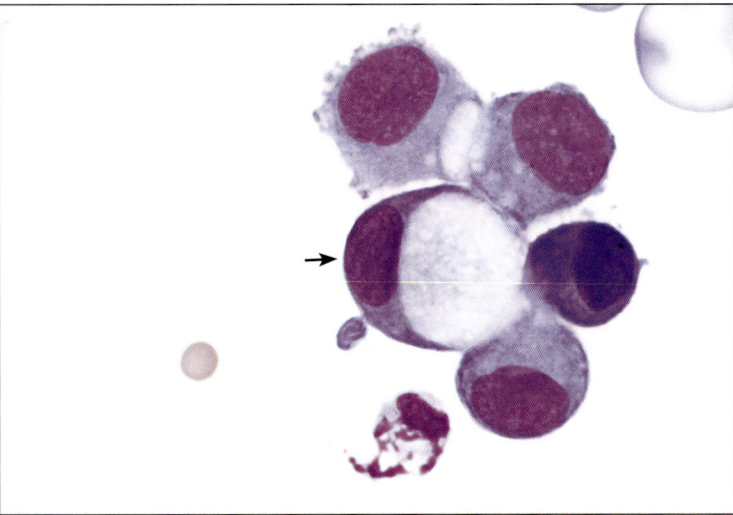
i5.49 Metastatic carcinoma of unknown primary with a "signet ring" tumor cell (arrow)

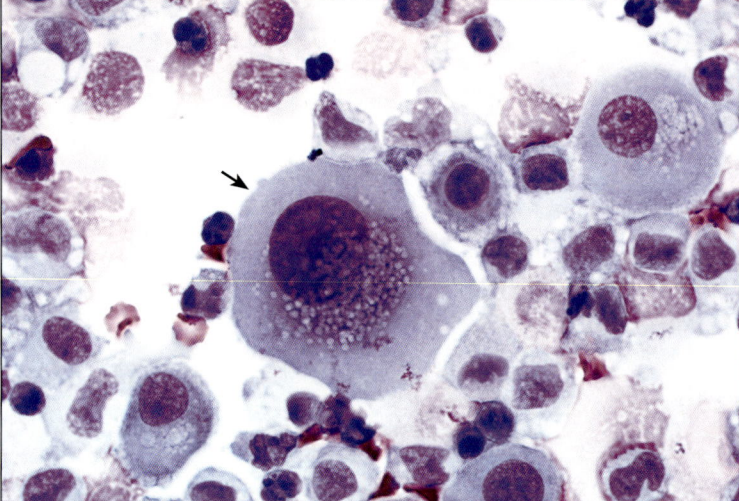
i5.52 A large malignant mesothelial cell (arrow)

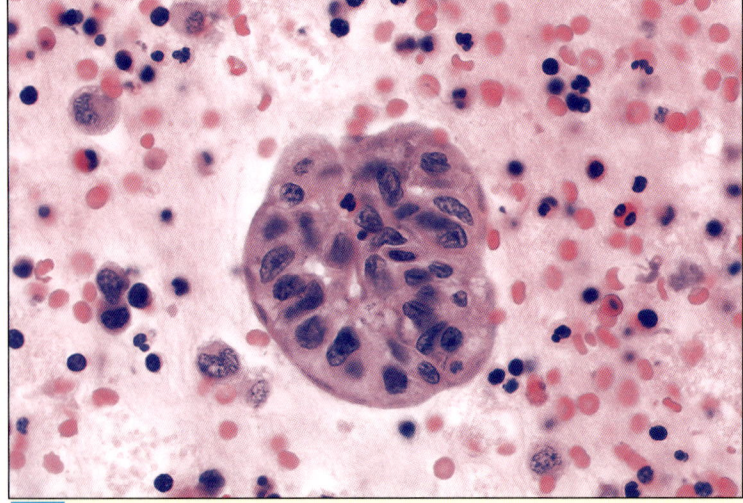
i5.50 Metastatic adenocarcinoma. Cell block (H&E stain).

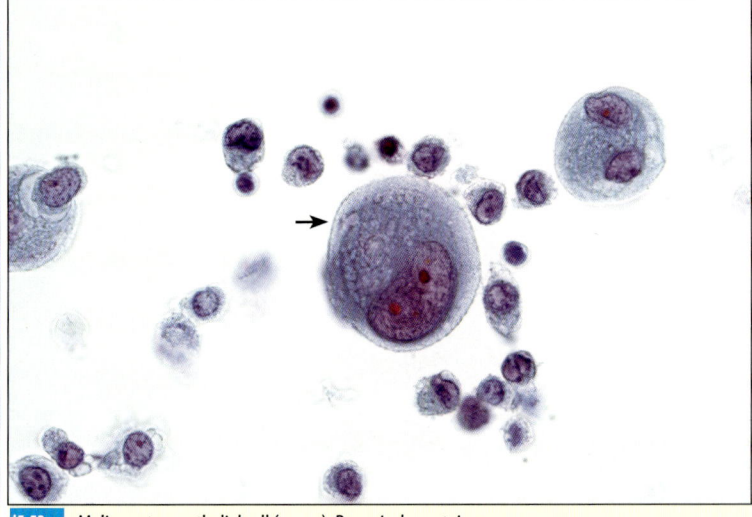
i5.53 Malignant mesothelial cell (arrow). Papanicolaou stain.

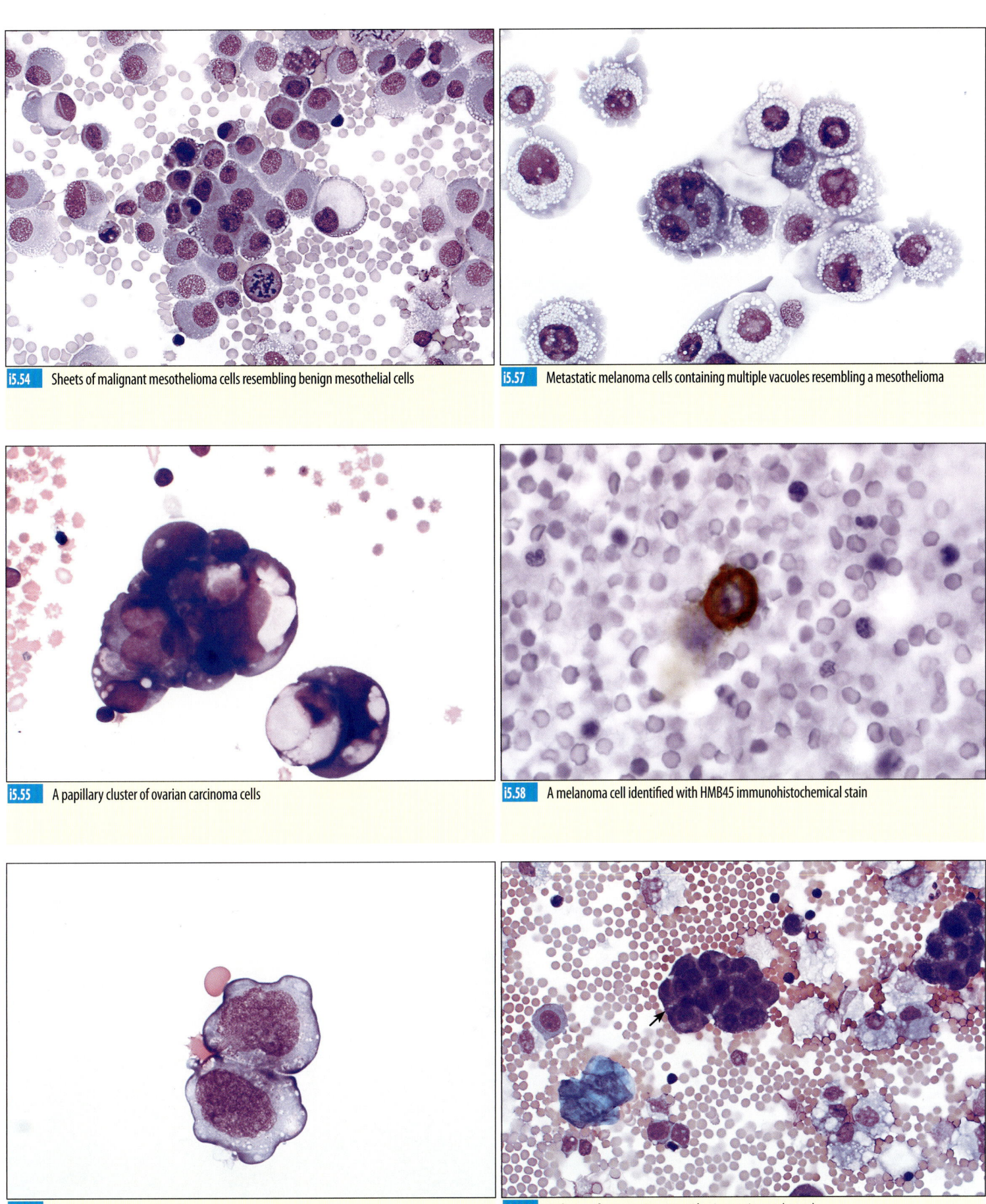

i5.54 Sheets of malignant mesothelioma cells resembling benign mesothelial cells

i5.57 Metastatic melanoma cells containing multiple vacuoles resembling a mesothelioma

i5.55 A papillary cluster of ovarian carcinoma cells

i5.58 A melanoma cell identified with HMB45 immunohistochemical stain

i5.56 Metastatic esophageal carcinoma

i5.59 A cluster of metastatic neuroendocrine carcinoma (arrow)

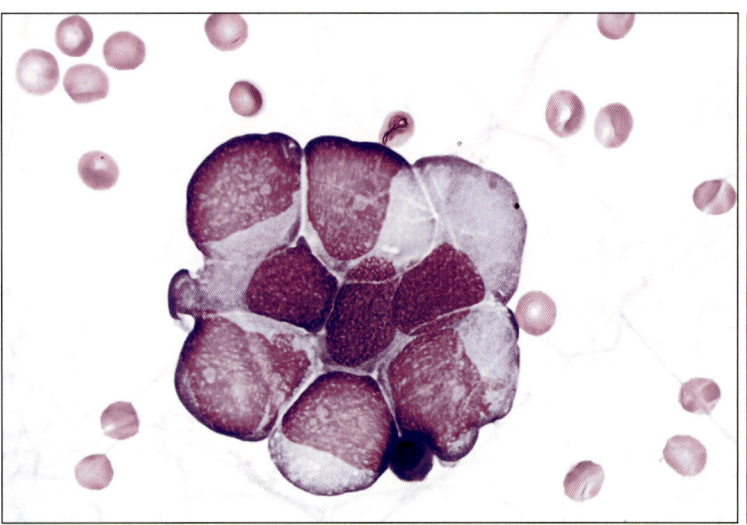
i5.60 A cluster of metastatic prostate carcinoma cells

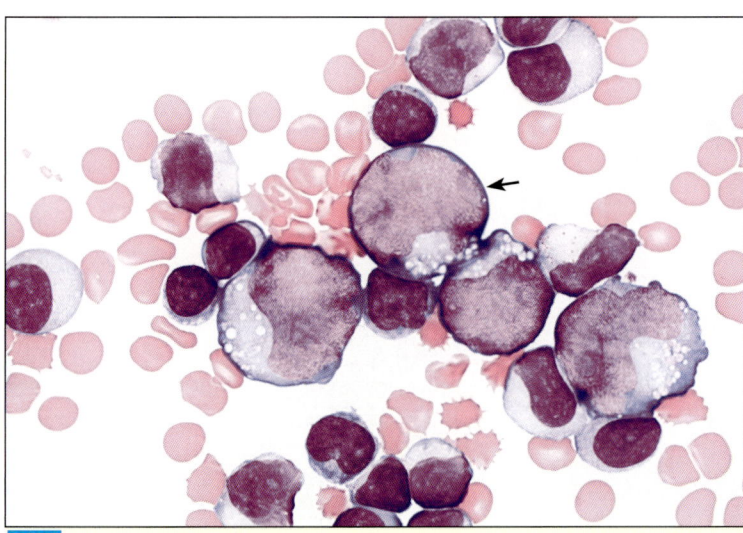
i5.63 Higher power view of non-Hodgkin large cell lymphoma (arrow)

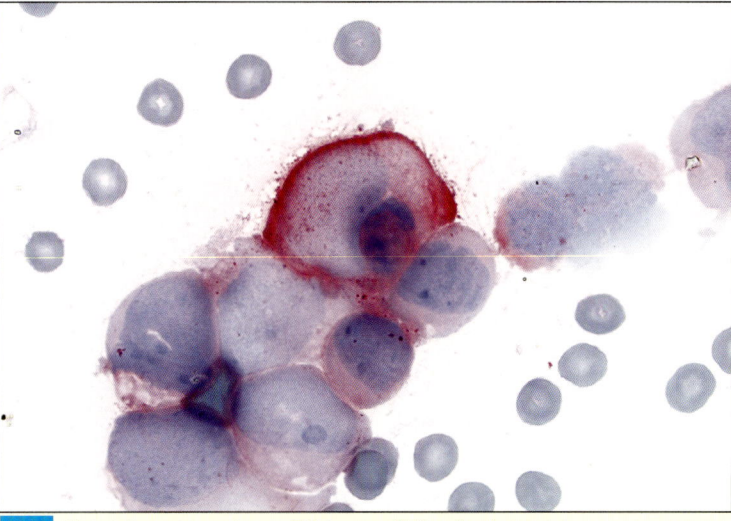
i5.61 Metastatic prostate carcinoma. EMA immunoalkaline phosphatase stain.

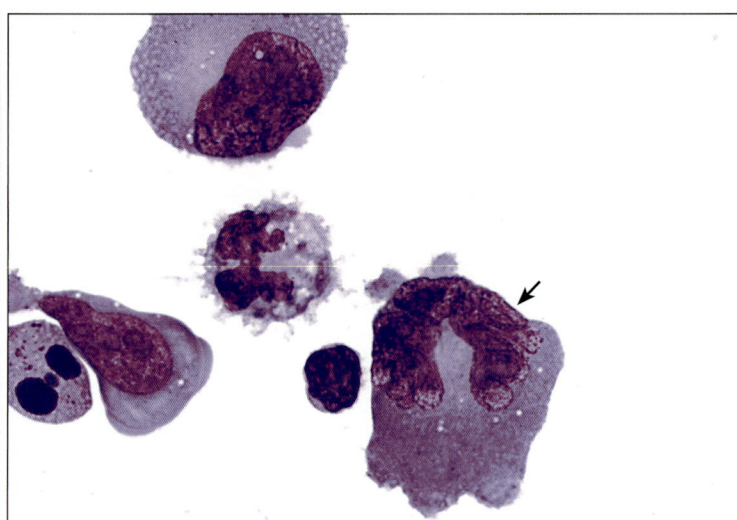
i5.64 Anaplastic large cell lymphoma "hallmark" cell (arrow)

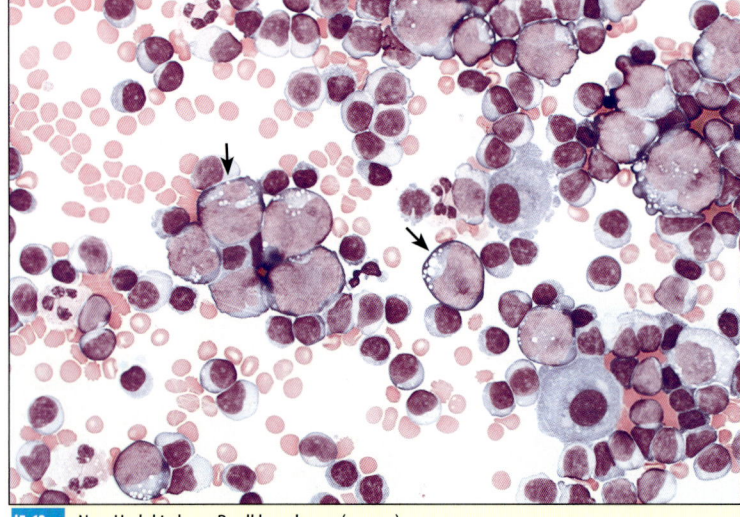
i5.62 Non-Hodgkin large B cell lymphoma (arrows)

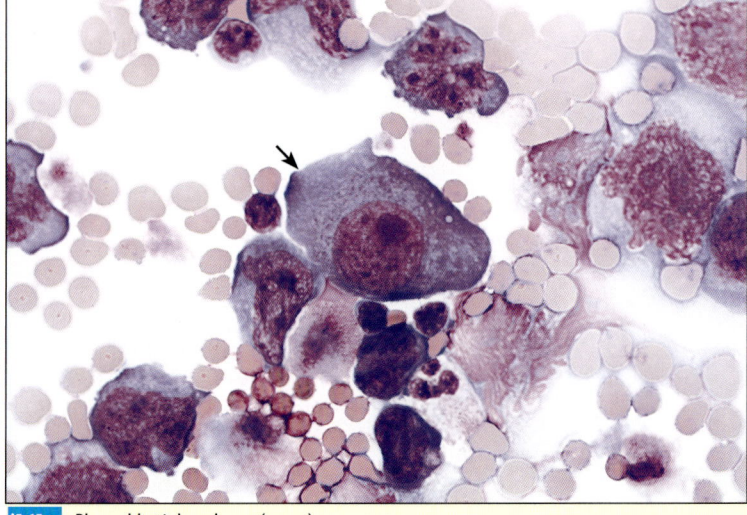
i5.65 Plasmablastic lymphoma (arrow)

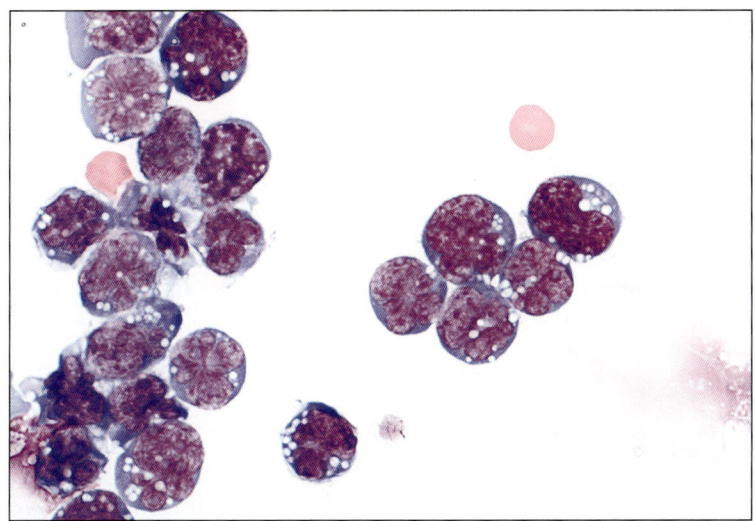
i5.66 Burkitt lymphoma with the characteristic vacuolated blue cytoplasm

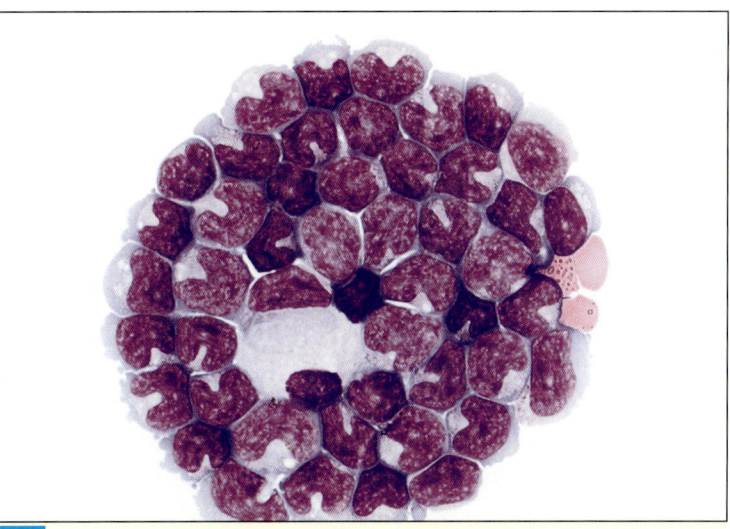
i5.69 Cytocentrifuge spinning artifact in a patient with chylothorax. The lymphocytes are clustered together & have irregular nuclear contours.

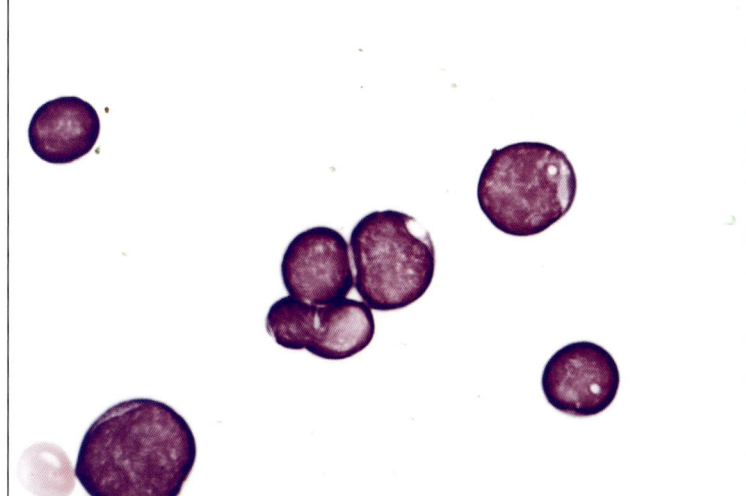
i5.67 Lymphoblastic lymphoma cells having the characteristic scant cytoplasm & delicate nuclear chromatin pattern

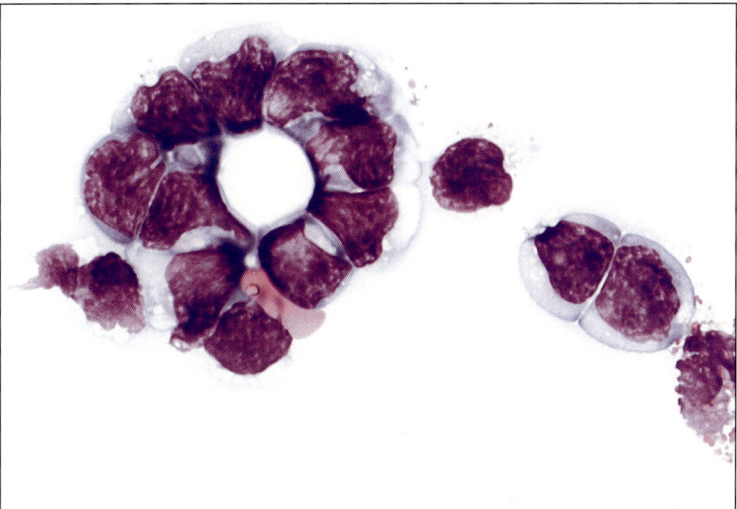
i5.70 Cytocentrifuge spinning artifact of benign lymphocytes producing a pseudorosette or ductlike structure

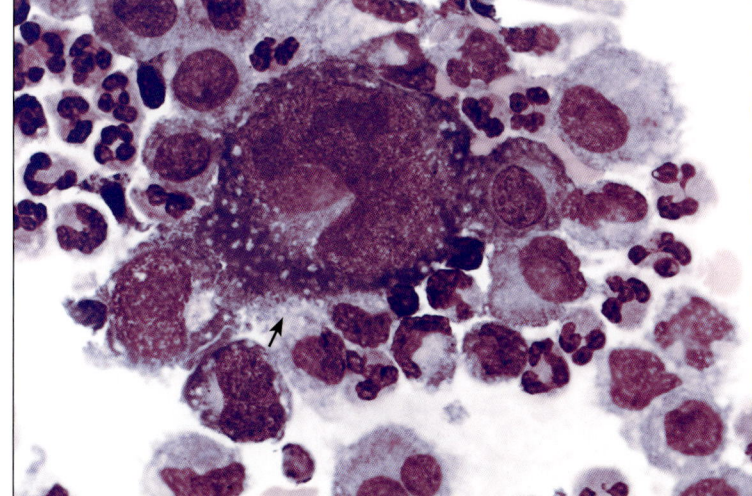
i5.68 A large Reed-Sternberg cell (arrow) in Hodgkin lymphoma

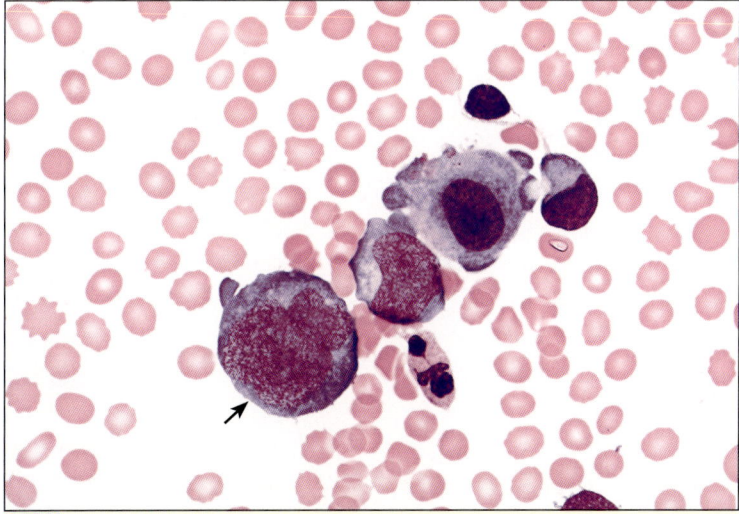
i5.71 In longstanding effusions the tumor cells often enlarge, become distorted, swollen & vacuolated. Here a myeloblast has become larger than a mesothelial cell (arrow).

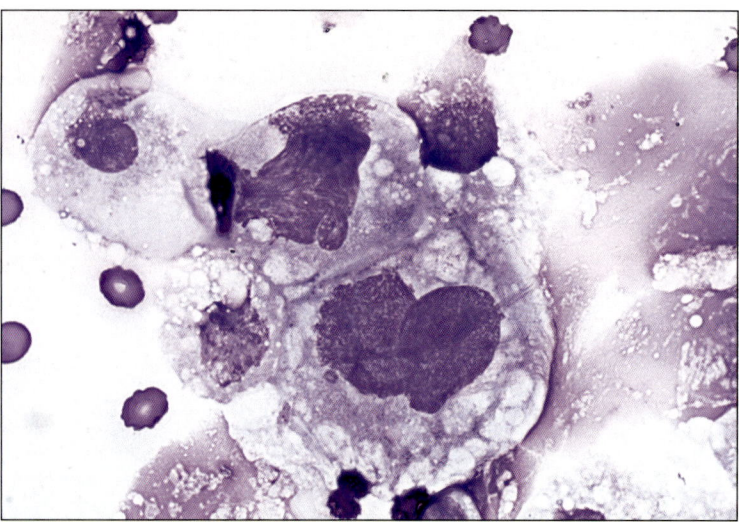

i5.72 Degenerative changes seen in malignant cells in a longstanding effusion

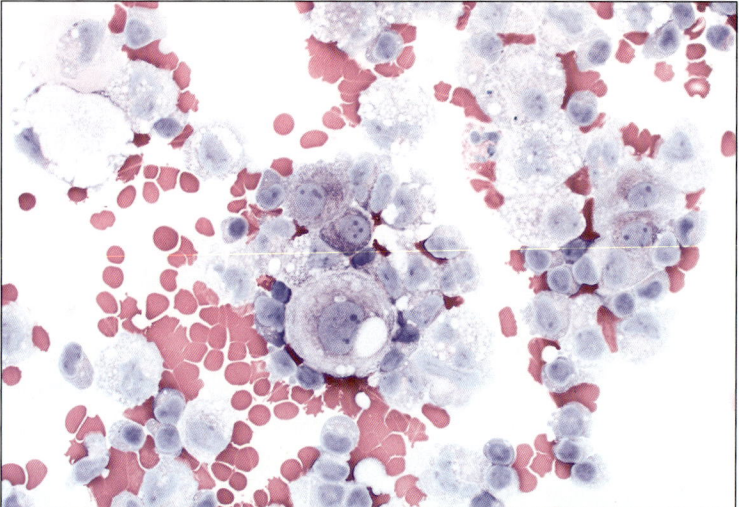

i5.73 Unsatisfactory Wright-Giemsa stain because the buffer was too acidic. Note the orange red color of the red blood cells & the washed out appearance of the macrophages, mesothelial cells & the lymphocytes.

Degenerative changes in cell morphology are frequently seen in longstanding effusions i5.72. It is important that the quality of the Wright-Giemsa stain be excellent i5.73. When the cell concentration is too heavy, the cells are often overstained and there is a tendency for the cells to cluster.

Clinical considerations

The cause of pleural transudates that are frequently bilateral and result from hydrodynamic imbalance is usually diagnosed easily as congestive heart failure, chronic kidney disease, cirrhosis, or malnutrition. In the disorders associated with transudates, microscopic examination reveals few cells that are mainly macrophages, mesothelial cells, and a variable number of lymphocytes.

Unilateral pleural effusion, particularly on the right side, may occur when disease develops below the diaphragm as in cirrhosis with ascites, subdiaphragmatic abscess, hepatic abscess, acute pancreatitis, and tumors.

Pleural effusions are common during the first few days after abdominal surgery but usually resolve spontaneously. In the majority of postoperative cases, they are associated with atelectasis, the presence of peritoneal fluid, or irritation of the diaphragm. Pleural effusion (transudate) is a common occurrence during the first 24 hours after childbirth. However, in the absence of any signs of cardiopulmonary disorders, no therapy is indicated.

A parapneumonic effusion is a pleural effusion associated with bacterial pneumonia, lung abscess, or bronchiectasis. The term empyema is used for those parapneumonic effusions of which the pleural fluid culture is positive and viscous. Exudative effusions are seen in ~50% of all patients with bacterial pneumonia. The pleural leukocyte count ranges from 5,000-25,000/mL with a predominance of neutrophils. When a pyogenic organism is present, the neutrophils frequently degenerate into pus cells that are easily broken down resulting in numerous basket cells consisting of spread out nuclear material. Microorganisms are sometimes easily identified in the smear preparations i5.30-i5.33.

Tuberculous pleuritis in contrast to parenchymal tuberculosis often presents as an acute illness involving younger patients. The effusions are usually unilateral, straw colored, or occasionally serosanguineous. Microscopic examination of pleural fluid reveals leukocytosis with usually >50% small lymphocytes. In some patients, polymorphonuclear leukocytes (PMNs) may predominate initially. Another characteristic feature of tuberculous pleurisy is the paucity of mesothelial cells because the serosal surface becomes covered by fibrin and granulation tissue. Thus, the presence of a substantial number of mesothelial cells would be most unusual in tuberculosis. Rarely, in longstanding cases (after several years), so called "cholesterol effusion," or pseudochylothorax, may be observed. Microscopic examination of this fluid frequently shows cholesterol crystals. Both pleural fluid and sputum should be cultured for mycobacteria when tuberculous pleuritis is suspected. A pleural biopsy may be helpful in establishing the diagnosis of tuberculous pleuritis. In general, the combination of biopsy and fluid examination improves the diagnostic sensitivity.

Pleural effusions due to viral infection have not been well studied, and the incidence, therefore, is not known. In general, the pleural effusions associated with viral infections are usually small and the microscopic examination of the fluid reveals a predominance of lymphocytes, mesothelial cells, and macrophages. In herpes simplex and cytomegalovirus (CMV) infections, transformed lymphoid cells in pleural effusions may contain intranuclear inclusions and multinucleated giant cells may be present. Immunocytologic studies using a monoclonal antibody against the virus may be helpful in the diagnosis.

Pulmonary embolism is one of the more common causes of pleural effusions, and occurs in ~50% of patients [PMID 1247347]. It is likely that many of the patients with undiagnosed pleural effusions have pulmonary embolization. When associated with pulmonary infarction, the effusions are usually small serosanguineous exudates. Unfortunately, the fluid usually reveals no specific diagnostic features and the results of both the gross and microscopic examinations are variable. In >1/2 of the effusions, the fluid is bloody and initially shows a predominance of PMNs. Later, lymphocytes and macrophages predominate. Thus, the presence of clear pleural fluid does not exclude the possibility of pulmonary embolism.

Persistent exudative effusions containing >80% lymphocytes have been described following coronary bypass grafting [PMID 3259069]. Postpericardiotomy syndrome should, therefore, be considered in postcoronary artery bypass grafting patients with lymphocytic exudative pleural effusions.

Pleural effusions may be seen in patients with rheumatoid arthritis [PMID 6066230]. The pleural effusion usually appears when the disease has been present for several years but occasionally the effusion may precede the development of arthritis. Examination of the pleural fluid often shows a markedly decreased glucose concentration and a low pH. The fluid is pale yellow or green white and may be turbid or pseudochylous. Microscopic examination in many but not all patients reveals a unique picture that is thought to be pathognomonic of rheumatoid disease [PMID 5676332]. A characteristic triad of elongated macrophages, giant multinucleated macrophages, and granular material has been described. The macrophages are thought to have exfoliated from granulomatous inflammation of the pleura and the amorphous granular material is formed as the macrophages undergo necrosis and disintegrate. The amorphous granular necrotic background material sometimes may be so abundant that it may be the dominant feature. In addition, variable numbers of PMNs and lymphocytes are present. Mesothelial cells are usually markedly decreased or absent in specimens that show these morphologic features.

Pleural effusions have been described in 16% of patients with systemic lupus erythematosus (SLE) [PMID 13223169, PMID 6605838]. The effusions are usually small and bilateral. Rarely, the pleural effusion may be the first clinical manifestation of SLE. The fluid is usually yellow or pseudosanguineous and microscopic examination reveals predominantly PMNs with a variable number of lymphocytes. LE cells may be seen in pleural fluid of patients with lupus pleuritis. The most useful test, however, for making the diagnosis of lupus pleuritis is determination of the antinuclear antibody (ANA) level in the pleural fluid. Microscopic examination usually shows a predominance of lymphocytes with a variable number of PMNs, macrophages, and mesothelial cells. Transformed lymphoid cells are frequently seen and when plentiful may sometimes suggest the diagnosis of non-Hodgkin lymphoma.

A pleural effusion is seen in ~10% of patients with acute pancreatitis [PMID 4872925]. It is usually found in the left pleural cavity but may be bilateral. The fluid is usually serosanguineous exudate made up predominantly of PMNs. The fluid amylase level is at least twice as high as the serum level.

Pleural and pericardial effusions may be seen in uremia and in patients undergoing longterm dialysis. The pleural effusion in such cases is usually unilateral, serosanguineous, or hemorrhagic and contains a predominance of lymphocytes. The fluid is usually an exudate [PMID 1115470, PMID 1115469]. Bacterial pericarditis is characterized by a leukocytosis (>1,000/mL) with a predominance of PMNs. Similar findings may be observed in patients with viral pericarditis and postmyocardial infarction syndrome.

Malignant disorders

Malignant disease is one of the most common causes of pleural and pericardial effusions t5.8. Therefore, the most important part of the laboratory investigation is the cytologic examination of the effusion for malignant cells. Pleural effusions develop in ~50% of patients who have disseminated lung and breast cancer. Lung cancer is the leading cause of malignant pleural effusion and is most commonly adenocarcinoma followed by small cell carcinoma i5.43-i5.46. The 2nd most common cause of malignant pleural effusion is breast carcinoma i5.38-i5.42. Effusions are also common in patients with malignant lymphoma i5.62-i5.68, malignant mesothelioma i5.51-i5.54, ovarian carcinoma i5.55, gastrointestinal carcinoma i5.56, and less commonly with sarcoma. A true chylous effusion is often associated with lymphoma.

t5.8	Malignant neoplasms associated with pleural effusion	
Men	**Women**	**Children**
Lung	Breast	Hematopoietic
Colorectal	Lung	Wilms tumor
Pancreas	Ovary	Neuroblastoma
Lymphoma	Lymphoma	
Hepatocellular	Colorectal	
Mesothelioma	Uterus	

In determining the site of the primary tumor, it is helpful to consider the side of the pleural effusion (right or left pleural cavity) and the patient's sex. Of malignant effusions originating from lung, breast, or ovarian tumors, 90% are ipsilateral to the primary tumor and pleural metastases from primary sites other than lung usually indicate tertiary spread from liver metastases. Carcinoma or lymphoma is the most likely cause of bilateral effusions in the absence of congestive heart failure.

Malignant neoplasms produce pleural effusions through a number of different mechanisms and it should not be expected that all effusions in cases of cancer will contain malignant cells [PMID 7047062]. The neoplasm may cause lymphatic and capillary obstruction resulting in reduced absorption of fluid and protein. In addition, malignant cells may produce chemical mediators that increase capillary permeability. Neoplastic lesions may also cause endobronchial obstruction with pneumonia or atelectasis. Occasionally, the tumor erodes a blood vessel causing hemothorax. A massive bloody effusion in the absence of trauma is almost always caused by a malignant disorder.

Pleural effusions in patients with malignancies may not be directly related to a neoplasm within the thorax. A number of patients with malignant disease have hypoproteinemia due to malnourishment and this may be associated with transudative effusions. Patients with malignancies also have an increased incidence of pneumonia and pulmonary embolus, both of which may cause pleural effusions.

Malignant effusions are usually exudates. The leukocyte count is variable and often shows a predominance of lymphocytes but many neutrophils may also be present. Frequently, many mesothelial cells are seen sometimes outnumbering the malignant cells. The number of malignant cells found in effusions that are associated with malignant neoplasms varies greatly. Bilateral effusions are often associated with obstruction of lymphatic vessels. When this occurs, a cytologic study of the effusion often reveals no malignant cells. In contrast, many malignant cells may be seen where there are free growing tumor cells within the fluid and in the adjacent pleura. Exfoliation of solid tumors implants into the pleura is associated with a moderate number of tumor cells.

When a malignant effusion is suspected, a fluid specimen should always be sent to the cytology laboratory for examination. Cytologic analysis of pleural fluid is diagnostic of malignancies in ~60% of all patients with subsequently documented pleural malignancies. In lung and breast carcinoma, this may increase to 70% or 80%. The smear prepared as part of the routine examination of the pleural fluid in the clinical laboratory should also be carefully examined for malignant cells. In general, the greater number of methods that are employed to detect malignant cells the better the chances for arriving at the correct diagnosis.

Unfortunately, there is no single microscopic feature that is diagnostic of malignancy. Many cytology textbooks will describe features such as large cell size, high nuclear:cytoplasmic ratio, nuclear hyperchromasia with irregularities of the chromatin pattern, large nucleoli, and increase mitotic activity as being characteristic of malignancy. Some of these criteria, however, may be misleading in the microscopic examination of serous effusions. Benign mesothelial cells and benign transformed/reactive lymphocytes may have several features suggesting malignancy and some malignant cells may have few of the criteria previously described. For example, cells in adenocarcinoma may have abundant cytoplasm; cells from oat cell carcinoma and lymphoma are not large; and cells from adenocarcinoma and oat cell carcinoma may not have hyperchromatic nuclei. Furthermore, a higher mitotic rate may be seen in benign transformed lymphocytes than in malignant cells. As described earlier, mesothelial cells are particularly troublesome since they may, and often do, resemble malignant cells.

In separating mesothelial cells from malignant cells, it is useful to define a "2nd cell" population that is distinctly (although often subtly so) different from the spectrum of changes in the mesothelial cell population t5.7. Carcinoma cells frequently aggregate in clumps or cell balls, and sometimes show glandlike formation. These clumps of cells are best seen when the smear is scanned under low power. Tumor cell balls are mainly seen in metastatic breast and ovarian carcinoma but may also be seen in lung and gastrointestinal tract carcinomas. Mesothelial cells can also form cell balls. Malignant cells usually look "foreign" and different from cells encountered in benign fluids. The malignant cells may be monomorphic (similar in size and shape) or pleomorphic (variable in size and shape). The cells may be found singly, in sheets, and in acinar or papillary formation. They may be small or larger than normal mesothelial cells. The nuclear:cytoplasmic ratio is usually increased but this depends on the degree of maturation and the nature of the primary tumor. In mucus or keratin producing malignancies, the cytoplasm is often abundant. The cytoplasm may be basophilic or vacuolated and may contain mucus. Abnormal mitotic figures may be seen although they are typically rare.

Most malignant serous effusions are caused by metastatic adenocarcinoma. Of the primary lung carcinomas, adenocarcinoma is the most common cell type to involve the pleura because of its peripheral location. Tumors of this type may be associated with multiple round cell aggregates with or without giant vacuoles. In addition, the tumor cells may be isolated and bizarre and monstrous forms may be seen. Increased nuclear/cytoplasmic ratios, irregular nuclear borders, large nucleoli, sharply defined cytoplasmic borders, and 3 dimensional aggregates are useful cytologic criteria to distinguish adenocarcinoma from benign conditions in pleural effusions.

Small cell carcinoma of the lung has a characteristic cell structure i5.44. Cells of this type resemble large lymphocytes but are larger (~20 μm). The nuclear chromatin is fine, resembling lymphoblasts and the nucleoli are usually indistinct. The cytoplasm is scant and the cells are often seen in small groups with the nuclei showing molding or a mosaic pattern. When occurring as single or separated cells, they may be difficult to distinguish from lymphoma, lymphoblastic leukemia, or neuroblastoma (and similar, so called, small, round blue cell tumors).

Pleural effusions are ultimately seen in ~50% of patients with breast carcinoma with 50%-80% of the effusions being ipsilateral to the primary tumor and ~10% bilateral i5.38-i5.42 [PMID 6170424, PMID 6261936]. Neoplastic cells in pleural effusions associated with metastatic breast carcinoma are particularly abundant with infiltrating duct carcinoma. The tumor cells are often seen as tight round clumps or cell balls. The individual cancer cells are often relatively small and fairly uniform in size and shape and resemble mesothelial cells. The absence of intercellular "windows" and the definition of a "2nd cell" population may be particularly useful in identification. The distinction between breast carcinoma cells and mesothelial cells may be extremely difficult especially when the malignant cells occur singly. Immunohistochemistry studies may be helpful in distinguishing between malignant cells and mesothelial cells using a panel of antibodies.

The incidence of pleural effusion in non-Hodgkin lymphomas is reported to be between 5%-20% [PMID 3548191]. When an adequate number of malignant cells are present and when the observer is familiar with the variable appearance of benign, transformed (reactive) lymphocytes, it is usually not difficult to make a diagnosis of lymphoma i5.63-i5.67. Problems may arise, however, in differentiating between a CLL/small lymphocytic lymphoma and a benign lymphocyte rich effusion. Large cell lymphomas may sometimes be difficult to distinguish from an undifferentiated carcinoma. The use of immunohistochemistry and flow cytometry is important for making a correct diagnosis in such cases.

Pleural effusions in Hodgkin lymphoma are much less common than with non-Hodgkin lymphoma and are characterized by a mixed cell population consisting of benign appearing small lymphocytes, and variable number of plasma cells, eosinophils, and neutrophils. The diagnosis of Hodgkin lymphoma may be difficult unless one can find diagnostic Reed-Sternberg (RS) cells i5.68.

In malignant mesothelioma, a pleural effusion is almost always present. The fluid is characteristically viscous or gelatinous resembling synovial fluid. Clumps of atypical mesothelial cells are seen but it may be difficult to differentiate between reactive and malignant mesothelial cells i5.51-i5.54. Similarly, it may be difficult to distinguish between malignant mesothelioma and adenocarcinoma. Immunohistochemistry may be helpful in separating these entities, using a panel of antibodies.

Neuroblastoma cells in serous effusions have morphologic features similar to small cell carcinoma but show less nuclear molding. Occasional rosettelike formations may be seen. In children, it is important to distinguish neuroblastoma cells from non-Hodgkin lymphoma, particularly lymphoblastic lymphoma, since the treatment is very different. Immunohistochemistry studies and flow cytometry are helpful in such cases.

Malignant melanoma may metastasize to pleural and pericardial (and peritoneal) cavities. The cells may resemble mesothelial cells and therefore difficult to recognize as malignant i5.57-i5.58. The presence of melanin pigment is a useful feature in the diagnosis of melanoma but is often difficult to identify. The melanin pigment stains black with Romanowsky stain and golden brown in a Pap stain, and may also be present within macrophages that have phagocytosed the melanin. Melanin pigment should be distinguished from hemosiderin pigment within macrophages. In amelanotic melanomas, immunohistochemistry is usually necessary to make a definitive diagnosis.

The identification of metastatic sarcomas is often problematic because such tumor cells tend to round up whether they are round cell or spindle cell neoplasms. The most useful feature is the recognition, at low power, of a distinct population of cells in the background of mesothelial cells and inflammatory cells. The clinical history is often the key tipoff, and immunohistochemistry is usually required to make a definitive diagnosis.

Correct identification of malignant neoplastic cells in pericardial fluid is usually straightforward. In a study of pericardial fluid specimens from 72 patients with malignant pericardial effusions, 80% of the neoplasms were epithelial and 20% were nonepithelial [PMID 6933801]. The most common tumors involving this anatomic site are lung and breast carcinomas. As in pleural effusions, metastatic lung adenocarcinoma is characterized by pleomorphic nuclei and prominent nucleoli, whereas metastatic breast carcinoma is characterized by uniform tumor cells often forming clusters (balls). An interesting observation has been the paucity of reactive cells such as lymphocytes and histiocytes in specimens that contained tumor cells. This is in contrast to the abundant inflammatory cells and mesothelial cells in the majority of negative specimens. The pericardial effusions associated with malignant cells are usually bloody whereas bloody fluid was present in only a small number of tumor negative pericardial effusions. Blood may also be seen in the pericardial cavity as a result of an aortic aneurysm or aortic dissection, trauma, rupture of the heart, myocardial infarction, or an association with coagulation defects.

Chemical analysis

Total protein & lactate dehydrogenase

As described previously it is necessary to discriminate between an exudative and a transudative effusion. The former requires additional testing to identify the cause while the diagnosis of the latter can usually be determined by clinical presentation. Exudates are characterized by the presence of high molecular weight proteins which transudates lack. As such, the measurement of total protein and/or albumin in pleural fluid is often performed. However, these measurements are usually of little clinical value unless they are paired with other tests to calculate specific ratios.

The criteria of Light and colleagues are frequently used for differentiating an exudate from a transudate [PMID 4642731]. Exudates are characterized by the presence of high molecular weight proteins which transudates lack. Therefore, a fluid to serum ratio of total protein that is >0.5, a fluid to serum ratio of lactate dehydrogenase (LD) >0.6, or a fluid LD activity that is >2/3 of the upper reference limit for serum LD supports the diagnosis of an exudate t5.4. Light criteria are 98% sensitive in identifying exudates but they lack specificity as only 77% of transudates are identified correctly [PMID 8339626, PMID 23508114].

The use of the serum to pleural fluid albumin gradient (serum albumin minus pleural fluid albumin) has been demonstrated to improve the specificity of Light criteria in patients with transudative pleural effusions due to heart failure [PMID 23508114]. The measurement of natriuretic peptides such as NT-proBNP and BNP have also been used to correctly identify 90% of pleural transudates misclassified by Light criteria with NT-proBNP having greater utility than BNP [PMID 19363209]. It has been recommended that NT-proBNP be measured in pleural fluid whenever a suspected cardiac effusion meets the exudative criteria [PMID 20573057]. However, because serum NT-proBNP is elevated in heart failure its measurement in pleural fluid may have no added value.

Glucose

Normally, the glucose concentration in pleural fluid is equivalent to its concentration in the blood. All transudates and most exudates will have a glucose concentration >60 mg/dL. Concentrations less than this suggest the presence of tuberculosis, malignant disease, rheumatoid disease, or a complicated parapneumonic effusion or empyema. Rare causes of decreased glucose concentrations in pleural fluid include paragonimiasis, hemothorax, Churg-Strauss syndrome, and lupus pleuritis [PMID 18195577].

Glucose measurements should be performed as quickly as possible, ideally within 4 hours of sample collection [PMID 20573057]. However, one study demonstrated that pleural fluid glucose concentrations were not significantly affected by a 24 hour delay in analysis [PMID 18556632].

Pericardial glucose concentrations do not have any demonstrated clinical utility [PMID 9149572].

pH

The pH of pleural fluid is normally 7.64, which is slightly higher than the pH of blood due to a bicarbonate gradient between the 2 compartments. Pleural fluid pH and glucose often track each other so fluids with a low glucose concentration often have a decreased pH [PMID 16623208]. Pleural fluid pH is clinically useful to determine if a parapneumonic effusion should be drained. Thresholds to initiate drainage have been reported for a pH <7.10-7.30 but because no single value is definitive, pleural fluid pH must be used in conjunction with clinical judgment. A pH value greater than the cutoff supports medical management of the effusion. A metaanalysis of 7 studies that reported results for pleural fluid pH, glucose, and LD indicated that low pH (7.21-7.29) had the highest diagnostic accuracy for identifying effusions requiring drainage [PMID 7767510].

Pleural fluid pH may also have utility for determining prognosis in patients with malignant effusions. In one study of 60 patients with malignant effusions, 20 had a pleural fluid pH <7.30 and had a significantly greater initial positive cytology rate, a shorter mean survival, and a poorer response to pleurodesis [PMID 3341671]. Similarly, a study of 125 patients with metastatic pleural carcinoma reported significantly shorter survival in patients with a pleural fluid pH <7.20 and pleural fluid glucose <60 mg/dL [PMID 8222811]. In contrast, a metaanalysis of 433 patients concluded that pleural fluid pH testing offered only modest information for identifying patients who are likely to die within 3 months of pleurodesis [PMID 12796164].

The measurement of pleural fluid pH is particularly prone to preanalytical sources of error, particularly due to its exposure to atmospheric air, which will significantly increase pH [PMID 18556632]. Pleural fluid samples must be collected anaerobically and the pH determined using a blood gas analyzer within 1 hour of collection [PMID 18556632]. The use of a pH meter or pH paper will produce inaccurate results and must not be used [PMID 9824016]. Guidelines from the American College of Chest Physicians emphasize that the use of a blood gas analyzer for pleural fluid pH measurements is the preferred method for categorizing and managing parapneumonic effusions [PMID 11035692].

Pericardial pH measurements do not have any demonstrated clinical utility [PMID 9149572].

Lipids

Because chyle contains chylomicrons and a high concentration of triglyceride, the measurement of triglyceride in pleural fluid can help differentiate a chylous effusion from a nonchylous effusion. A concentration >110 mg/dL is the consensus cutoff for identifying a chylous effusion [CLSI C49-A 2007] but this cutoff is only ~85% sensitive [PMID 19181646]. Lipoprotein electrophoresis is considered to be the gold standard test for identifying chylomicrons in pleural fluid and should be performed when the triglyceride concentration is between 50-110 mg/dL or if it is <50 mg/dL and there is strong clinical suspicion of a chylous effusion [CLSI C49-A 2007]. Because a pseudochylous effusion (see below) can also have elevated triglyceride, the concentration of cholesterol in the fluid should also be determined as it will be low in a chylous effusion but elevated in a pseudochylous effusion [PMID 12728146].

Chronic exudative effusions that persist for months to years can result in a pseudochylous effusion. Due to a high lipid content of cholesterol crystals or lecithin-globulin complexes, the fluid has a milky white appearance yet does not contain chylomicrons. In contrast to chylous effusions, pseudochylous effusions usually have a triglyceride concentration <110 mg/dL with a cholesterol concentration >200 mg/dL and do not contain chylomicrons [PMID 12728146].

When Light criteria are equivocal the measurement of cholesterol in the effusion can help to differentiate a transudate from an exudate, which are expected to have low and high cholesterol concentrations, respectively. Cholesterol cutoffs for this differentiation have been reported to be 45 mg/dL and 60 mg/dL but a metaanalysis of 8 studies that included a total of 1,448 patients determined the optimal cutoff to be 45 mg/dL [PMID 9106577]. Using Light criteria with cholesterol maintained the high sensitivity of Light criteria (100%) but improved its specificity to 95% [PMID 7587426].

Pericardial cholesterol concentrations do not have any demonstrated clinical utility [PMID 9149572].

Adenosine deaminase

Adenosine deaminase (ADA) is an enzyme of the purine salvage pathway that irreversibly catalyzes the deamination of adenosine and deoxyadenosine nucleosides into inosine and deoxyinosine, respectively. ADA plays an important role in the proliferation, differentiation, and maturation of lymphocytes and a deficiency of the enzyme leads to impaired lymphoid development and severe combined immunodeficiency disease [PMID 11091267]. Due to the stimulation of T cells by mycobacterial antigens, the measurement of ADA activity in pleural fluid has clinical utility as a rapid, noninvasive test of tuberculous pleuritis and pericarditis [PMID 22579767, PMID 18344697].

In one study of 2,104 patients with pleural effusion (10.5% due to extrapulmonary tuberculosis), a pleural fluid ADA result >35 U/L was 93% sensitive and 90% specific for the diagnosis of tuberculous pleuritis [PMID 20816597]. In the absence of tuberculous pleuritis, pleural fluid ADA is most often elevated in empyema, malignancy (especially lymphoma), rheumatoid arthritis, systemic lupus erythematosus and infections such as brucellosis and Q fever [PMID 20392619].

ADA in pericardial fluid has not been well studied. One study of 212 patients with pericardial effusions (151 due to tuberculosis) reported that an ADA cutoff of >40 U/L produced a sensitivity of 87% and a specificity of 89% for identifying tuberculous pericarditis [PMID 17121764]. Another study of 48 patients with pericardial effusions (9 due to tuberculosis) reported sensitivity and specificity to be 89% and 72%, respectively at the same cutoff [PMID 17625694]. A recent study conducted in an area of high TB incidence, using IFN-γ and PCR as adjunct diagnostic measures, showed no utility of ADA testing in diagnosing tuberculous pericarditis [PMID 23945888].

ADA testing is not commonly performed in most clinical laboratories and there is no agreed upon reference measurement method. Importantly, the cutoff used to identify tuberculous pleuritis or pericarditis will influence the test's sensitivity and specificity. In areas where the incidence of tuberculosis is low the test will have little value.

Amylase

The activity of amylase in pleural fluid may be useful in the evaluation of an exudative effusion. Activity may be increased in a variety of conditions, most commonly in pleural malignancy, pancreatitis, pneumonia, tuberculosis, cirrhosis, and esophageal rupture [PMID 12728146]. Amylase activities are considered elevated when they exceed the upper serum reference value or are considerably higher (usually 1.5-2.0× the upper limit) than those of a simultaneously analyzed serum specimen.

The routine measurement of pleural fluid amylase activity is usually not clinically indicated because it does not identify the source of the effusion. In one study of 379 patients with pleural effusions of various causes, the measurement of amylase was not diagnostically informative nor was it cost effective [PMID 11176736]. The same study recommended amylase testing only when the pretest probability of pancreatic disease or esophageal rupture is high.

Increased pleural fluid amylase activity is nearly always present following esophageal rupture. The amylase in these cases is salivary in origin since this amylase rich fluid enters the pleural space through the esophageal defect. Verification of the salivary origin of the increased amylase activity is possible by measuring amylase isoenzymes, either electrophoretically or by selective inhibition of the salivary gland component [PMID 5027585].

Tumor markers

Several tumor markers have been investigated as potential biomarkers to help distinguish malignant from benign effusions, most notably carcinoembryonic antigen (CEA), cancer antigen 125 (CA125), cancer antigen 15-3 (CA15-3), cancer antigen 19-9 (CA19-9), CK19 fragments (CYFRA 21-1), and soluble mesothelin related peptides (SMRP). Unfortunately, reports on these and other tumor markers have been largely disappointing due to overall poor sensitivity and specificity [PMID 15115678].

A study of 416 patients with pleural effusions (58% of which were malignant) evaluated the performance of CEA, CA125, CA15-3 and CYFRA 21-1 to detect malignancy. Using cutoffs that were selected to achieve a specificity of 100%, the sensitivities of the single markers were all ≤30%. Combination testing (any marker above the cutoff) produced a sensitivity of 54% [PMID 15596670].

Another study that evaluated the performance of CEA and CA19-9 in 198 pleural fluid effusions (51% malignant) reported sensitivities of 52% and 35%, respectively, for all malignancies at a specificity ≥95% [PMID 20529669]. Sensitivities were greatest in those with lung cancer (81% and 54%, respectively) and in all marker secreting tumors (75% and 50%, respectively). The authors wisely advised that the use of pleural fluid tumor markers should include simultaneous measurement of the same marker in serum.

More promising results have been observed for SMRP and its potential utility in the diagnosis of malignant pleural mesothelioma. Mesothelin is a cell surface glycoprotein involved in cell adhesion and signaling that is expressed by normal mesothelial cells but is overexpressed in some cancers including mesothelioma. Mesothelin can be cleaved from the cell membrane producing SMRP. The measurement of SMRP in pleural fluid may offer advantages over its measurement in serum.

In a study of 166 patients with pleural effusions being investigated for possible malignancy, 24 were diagnosed with mesothelioma and had SMRP results that were 0.9 fold and 6.6 fold higher compared to those with metastatic carcinomas and benign effusions, respectively [PMID 19299498]. At a cutoff of 20 nM, SMRP had a sensitivity of 71% and a specificity of 90%. Notably, SMRP concentrations diagnosed mesothelioma more reliably than cytologic examination (71% vs 35%). Similar results were reported in a study of 192 patients with pleural effusions (52 with mesothelioma). Sensitivity and specificity were 67% and 98%, respectively at the same 20 nM cutoff [PMID 17356060]. These results suggest that pleural fluid SMRP provides added diagnostic value and may enhance the use of conventional cytology.

Complement, rheumatoid factor & antinuclear antibody

Pleural effusions are common in individuals with connective tissue diseases and are the most common intrathoracic manifestation of rheumatoid arthritis [PMID 8325082]. Pleural fluid concentrations of complement C4 are frequently low (<4 mg/dL) in patients with rheumatoid arthritis, presumably due to complement conversion to immune complexes [PMID 6981226]. Guidelines from the British Thoracic Society recommend the measurement of complement C4 in pleural effusions when suspicion is high for a connective tissue disease related cause, but the strength of this recommendation is low (grade C) [PMID 12728146].

Rheumatoid factor can be measured in pleural fluid and its detection strongly suggests a rheumatoid origin of the pleural effusion [PMID 16765714]. A titer of >1:320 is often observed. However, its measurement is of questionable value because the concentration of rheumatoid factor in pleural fluid usually reflects the concentration observed in the serum [PMID 22448326].

The detection of antinuclear antibodies (ANA) in pleural fluid is of little diagnostic value beyond their detection in the serum. However, testing may be useful due to the test's high negative predictive value. In patients with systemic lupus erythematosus and a pleural effusion of uncertain origin, a negative ANA result essentially rules out SLE as the cause of the effusion [PMID 17283581].

Microbiologic examination

A parapneumonic effusion is one associated with bacterial pneumonia or lung abscess. The fluid may be turbid or clear and may be sterile. It may resolve without complications following appropriate antibiotic therapy. Conversely, the fluid may be frankly purulent (empyema) and loculate in the pleural space. These more complicated cases usually have a pleural fluid pH <7.00 and/or a glucose level <40 mg/dL (see the sections "Glucose" and "pH") [PMID 7424940]. Although each case should be individualized, the treatment for empyema usually consists of immediate and complete drainage of the pleural space by use of a chest tube, as well as by vigorous administration of antibiotics selected on the basis of both aerobic and anaerobic cultures and antimicrobial susceptibility testing.

Although a vast array of microbes have been recovered from the pleural space, the most common organisms are *Streptococcus* species, *Staphylococcus aureus*, enteric Gram– bacilli, and anaerobic bacteria [PMID 10516908]. The era of antimicrobial therapy has produced marked changes in the microbiology of empyema. *Streptococcus pneumoniae*, once the predominant pathogen, only accounts for 10% of pleural infections (this may also be a result of vaccine efficacy) [PMID 9363140]. Marked increases have been seen for both *Staphylococcus aureus* and various Gram– bacilli including *Haemophilus influenzae*, *Klebsiella pneumoniae*, and *Pseudomonas aeruginosa* [PMID 10516908]. There is also a high incidence of pleural infections with anaerobic bacteria, particularly in patient populations at risk of aspiration [PMID 4131173, PMID 7316625]. The epidemiology of organisms recovered from pleural fluid (importantly) cannot be considered static, as evidence in comparison of 2 studies performed over 40 years apart. In the older study, anaerobes alone were identified in 23 of 83 cases (35%) of pleural infection, and anaerobic plus aerobic bacteria were identified in an additional 34 cases (41%) [PMID 4131173]. The predominant bacteria, in order of prevalence, were *Staphylococcus aureus*, *Fusobacterium nucleatum*, *Prevotella melaninogenicus*, *Bacteroides fragilis*, *Clostridium* species, *Escherichia coli*, and *Pseudomonas aeruginosa*. In a recent study of 315 pleural specimens, *Streptococcus* accounted for 33% of cultured isolates with the anginosus group accounting for 17% of these streptococci [PMID 22982641]. Gram+ anaerobic cocci accounted for 17%, while the *Enterobacteriaciae* and *Pseudomonas* accounted for only 8% and 4% respectively (anaerobic Gram– rods were rarely encountered) [PMID 22982641]. Both of these studies illustrate the need for careful specimen transport and processing to ensure recovery of anaerobic bacteria, since the relative rates of anaerobic infections seem constant despite the changing distribution of genera. Institutions with expertise in anaerobic microbiology would therefore be more likely to report higher rates of anaerobic infections of the pleural space. The aerobic actinomycetes *Nocardia* and *Streptomyces* are also opportunistic pathogens (particularly in immunocompromised hosts) that can cause pneumonia and subsequent empyema in well established infections [PMID 3062727]. These organisms are typically slow growing and require additional resources in terms of optimal growth media and identification methods.

Atypical pneumonias may be caused by various bacteria, viruses, and fungi. Bacteria such as *Mycoplasma pneumoniae*, *Legionella pneumophilia*, *Francisella tularensis*, *Brucella* species, *Bacillus anthracis*, *Chlamydophila psittici*, and *Coxiella burnetti*; fungi such as *Histoplasma capsulatum* and *Coccidioides immitis*; and viruses such as influenza A&B, adenovirus, parainfluenza 1-3, respiratory syncytial virus, human metapnemovirus, and coronaviruses are also responsible for atypical pneumonias [PMID 18986277]. In contrast to parapneumonic infections, the pleural fluid in atypical pneumonias usually resolves spontaneously. The pH and glucose levels are not low, and the fluid shows a predominance of lymphocytes [PMID 3062725]. One important distinction with these pathogens (particularly the bacteria and fungi) is that they are generally more fastidious than the conventional causes of empyema. In fact, organisms such as *C burnetti*, *C psittici*, and *M pneumoniae* are considered "nonculturable" in most clinical laboratories. As a result, these organisms can be interrogated by serological assays or (if available) molecular methodologies such as real time PCR (see Chapter 2) should be performed directly from the pleural fluid specimen. These tests are typically only available in reference laboratories, which will increase the time to result, therefore reaffirming the importance of empiric antimicrobial therapy for atypical pneumonias.

Bacterial/mycobacterial stains (eg, Gram stain, acid-fast stain) and culture are fundamental to any body fluid examination and this is true for both pleural and pericardial specimens. Specimens should be collected in sterile transport tubes and/or directly inoculated in blood culture bottles at bedside if possible. All specimens should be transported immediately to the laboratory at room temperature for bacterial culture. The reliability of stains depends primarily on the microscopic competence and experience of the laboratory scientist as well as the preparation method of the stain itself. Sensitivity can be significantly increased with inclusion of a cytocentrifugation step in advance of staining (see Chapter 2). In addition to a Gram stain, acridine orange may be used to increase sensitivity and enhance detection of bacteria, specifically in turbid specimens that are not amenable to centrifugation and not easily visualized with Gram stain [PMID 3358655]. This stain requires a fluorescent microscope for visualization, and may not be available in smaller microbiology laboratories. Culture should include nonselective solid media for both aerobic and anaerobic organisms, a blood bottle inoculation for increased sensitivity, and special liquid media for acid-fast bacilli (see Chapter 2). The culture yield is best for blood bottle cultures, and should take priority to solid media if volume restrictions exist [PMID 21459855, PMID 10385010].

In tuberculous effusions the direct staining for acid-fast bacilli is positive in <10% of cases, [PMID 6788249] and cultures are positive, on average, only 31.5% of the time [PMID 4988357]. The accuracy can be improved by obtaining multiple cultures, concentrating large volumes of fluid, and using liquid culture media [PMID 4630686]. The culture of pleural biopsy specimens gives the highest percent of positive results than any other single procedure [PMID 6788249, PMID 4988357]. A pleural biopsy for histologic study is usually positive in >50% of cases and has the distinct advantage that the examination can be completed in a relatively short period of time [PMID 6788249]. The demonstration of a granuloma in pleural tissue is highly suggestive of tuberculosis (TB), although other disorders including sarcoidosis, rheumatoid pleuritis, and fungal diseases may also stimulate granulomatous pleuritis. Nevertheless, patients with granulomatous lesions have TB in ~95% of cases [PMID 4988357]. These biopsy specimens should be stained and carefully searched for acid-fast organisms whether a granuloma is present or not and repeat biopsies may be required. When these various approaches are combined, up to 95% of cases are accurately identified [PMID 4988357]. Detection of M tuberculosis by DNA probe may also be considered from pleural fluid; however this assay cannot be reliably performed on bloody specimens and the specimen type is not FDA approved; prior consultation with the microbiology laboratory is imperative.

Additional tests to aid in determination of tuberculous effusions include adenosine deaminase (ADA) and interferon-γ (IFN-γ) levels. ADA has been used historically as a marker of tuberculous effusion with reasonable sensitivity and specificity in both HIV infected patients and uninfected patients [PMID 22474483]. However, these performance characteristics are dramatically affected by the cutoff established by the performing laboratory as well as the population prevalence of TB. In regions of low incidence of TB, the test has little value [PMID 3653300]. Furthermore, there are several medical conditions that can be attributed to increased ADA including Q fever, brucellosis, lung cancer, lymphoma, empyema, rheumatoid arthritis, and systemic lupus erythematosus [PMID 19672657]. IFN-γ levels can also contribute to the diagnosis of tuberculous effusion, with similar caveats of ADA testing. The cutoff established by the laboratory as well as the local prevalence of TB can negatively affect the specificity and sensitivity of IFN-γ for predicting a tuberculous effusion, and correspondingly the cutoffs published in many studies to date have been variable (with studies conducted in regions with dramatically different TB prevalence) [PMID 3653300, PMID 20473171]. Importantly, the newer IFN-γ release assays used worldwide on blood specimens for aiding in the diagnosis of tuberculosis do not perform well from pleural fluid, as the assay relies on adequate cellularity and subsequent stimulation in vitro with antigen; IFN-γ levels are of greater utility [PMID 19386693].

The less common (but nonetheless important) diseases of the pleura include fungi and parasites. In fungal disease, inclusion of appropriate cultures is paramount for accurate diagnosis, and specimens should be maintained at room temperature for optimal yield from these cultures. The calcofluor white stain can be helpful in the early detection of fungal elements; however, the stain can be challenging to read in purulent specimens and also requires a fluorescent microscope with appropriate filters. In cases of cryptococcal pleuritis, the measurement of cryptococcal antigen can aid in diagnosis; however, this is not an FDA approved specimen for commercially available assays, therefore this specimen type requires appropriate validation by the performing laboratory [PMID 6992663].

3 parasites are commonly associated with the pleural space: *Entamoeba histolytica*, *Echinococcus granulosus*, and *Paragonimus westermanni*. Pleuropulmonary involvement with *Entamoeba histolytica* is usually associated with an amebic hepatic abscess, and the pus from empyema is generally sterile unless superinfected. Serum antibodies for IgG to *E histolytica* are considered the strongest adjunct method of diagnosing extraintestinal disease [PMID 22990049]. Aspirates from the abscess can also be tested for antigen, with improved sensitivity over microscopy; however, PCR has shown to provide the best sensitivity and specificity for detecting *E histolytica* from abscess fluid [PMID 18828976]. In hydatid disease caused by *E granulosus*, typical hooklets and scolices are readily seen in the fluid aspirated from the cyst by use of light microscopy i5.34. Centrifugation of the specimen prior to performing a wet mount from the sediment will enhance detection of these structures. Pleural effusions associated with *P westermanni* often are suspected by a combination of signs and symptoms (brown/blood streaked sputum) as well as travel history and relevant exposure. Stool and sputum microscopy for the characteristic ova are diagnostic [PMID 22990049].

Unlike pleural effusions, bacteria account for only 10% of acute pericarditis [PMID 23102482]. Gram+ organisms (primarily *S aureus* and *S pneumoniae*) make up the majority (64%) of bacterial pericarditis and Gram– organisms (primarily *H influenzae*) account for 27% [PMID 23102482]. Culture and staining are described above for pericardial specimens suspicious of bacterial etiology. *M tuberculosis* is responsible for ~4% of cases of acute pericarditis, 7% of cases of cardiac tamponade, and in earlier studies, 6% of cases of constrictive pericarditis [PMID 2046135]. However, in some nonindustrialized countries, tuberculous pericarditis is still a leading cause of pericardial effusion. The resurgence of tuberculosis in all industrial countries due to AIDS makes tuberculous pericarditis an increasingly important consideration. Culture and stains are described above. The utility of ADA in this specimen type is dubious at best, and a recent study showed no significant difference between tuberculous and nontuberculous pericarditis in a developing country with high tuberculosis rates [PMID 23945888].

Viruses account for 90% of all infectious pericarditis cases [PMID 23102482]. The viruses attributed to these cases are numerous and diverse t5.9 [PMID 23102482], and as a result, culture and direct fluorescent antibody microscopy is of limited utility on these specimens. Pericardial fluid should therefore be submitted for real time PCR for any or all viruses considered in the differential diagnosis. Coxsackieviruses and echoviruses account for the majority of cases and should be strongly considered in suspected cases of pericarditis [PMID 23102482]. Consultation with the microbiology laboratory is critical to ensure adequate specimen volume is available to test for all appropriate viral etiologies.

t5.9	Viruses attributed to infective pericarditis
Adenovirus	
Coxsackie virus A&B	
Cytomegalovirus	
Echovirus	
Epstein-Barr virus	
Hepatitis B&C	
Human herpesvirus 6	
Human immunodeficiency virus	
Influenza A	
Parvovirus B19	
Measles	
Mumps	
Varicella zoster virus	

Adapted from Htwe and Khardori [PMID 23102482]

Artifacts & pitfalls

- None of the current laboratory tests are 100% effective in separating transudates from exudates. The Light criteria misclassify ~25% of transudates as exudates, and most of these patients are on diuretics.
- Mesothelial cells, because of their variable appearance, frequently cause difficulty in the microscopic examination and may be mistaken for malignant cells.
- Artifacts are often introduced by cytocentrifugation and degenerative changes in cell morphology are often seen in longstanding effusions.
- There is no single microscopic feature that is diagnostic of malignancy.

Key points

- A thoracentesis is indicated for any undiagnosed pleural effusion. Aliquots for aerobic and anaerobic bacterial cultures are best inoculated into blood culture media at the bedside. When malignancy, mycobacterial infection or fungal infection is suspected, at least 100 mL should be submitted.
- The 4 leading causes of pleural effusions in order of incidence are congestive heart failure, malignancy, pneumonia and pulmonary embolism.
- The main usefulness in defining a pleural effusion as a transudate or an exudate is to determine which effusions need further laboratory evaluation. If the effusion is a transudate, usually no further diagnostic procedures are needed.
- The purpose of laboratory testing of serous effusions is
  - to differentiate transudates from exudates
  - to differentiate malignant from nonmalignant effusions
  - to diagnose specific causes of serous effusions, eg, infection.
- The most reliable test for differentiating between transudates and exudates is the simultaneous analysis of pleural fluid and serum for total protein and lactic dehydrogenase concentration (Light criteria).
- Microscopic examination for malignant cells may be the most important part of the examination of an undiagnosed exudative fluid. Lung cancer is the leading cause of malignant pleural effusion. The 2nd most common is breast carcinoma.
- The use of a blood gas analyzer for pleural fluid pH measurements is the preferred method for categorizing and managing parapneumonic effusions.
- Several tumor markers have been investigated as potential biomarkers to help distinguish malignant from benign effusions. To date most have poor sensitivity and specificity. Soluble mesothelin related peptides (SMRP), however, have diagnostic value in mesothelioma.

References

PMID 1115469 Galen MA, Stenberg SM, Lowrie EG et al [1975] Hemorrhagic pleural effusion in patients undergoing chronic hemodialysis. *Ann Intern Med* 82(3):359-361

PMID 10385010 Ferrer A, Osset J, Alegre J et al [1999] Prospective clinical and microbiologic study of pleural effusions. *Eur J Clin Microbiol Infect Dis* 18(4):237-41

PMID 10516908 Heffner JE [1999] Infection of the pleural space. *Clin Chest Med* Sep;20(3):607-22

PMID 11035692 Colice GL, Curtis A, Deslauriers J et al [2000] Medical and surgical treatment of parapneumonic effusions : an evidence-based guideline. *Chest* 118(4),1158-1171

PMID 11091267 Fischer A [2000] Severe combined immunodeficiencies (SCID). *Clin Exp Immunol* 122(2):143-149

PMID 1115470 Berger HW, Rammiohan G, Neff MS et al [1975] Uremic pleural effusion: A study of 14 patients on chronic dialysis. *Ann Intern Med* 82(3):362-364

PMID 11176736 Branca P, Rodriguez RM, Rogers JT et al [2001] Routine measurement of pleural fluid amylase is not indicated. *Arch Intern Med* 161(2):228-232

PMID 11403751 Romero-Candeira S, Fernandez C, Martin et al [2001] Influence of diuretics on the concentration of proteins and other components of pleural transudates in patients with heart failure. *Am J Med* 110:681-6

PMID 12075059 Light RW [2002] Clinical practice. Pleural effusion. *N Eng J Med* 346:1971

PMID 1247347 Bynum LJ, Wilson JE [1976] Characteristics of pleural effusions associated with pulmonary embolism. *Arch Intern Med* 136:159-162

PMID 12728146 Maskell NA, Butland RJA, Pleural Diseases Group, Standards of Care Committee, British Thoracic Society [2003] BTS guidelines for the investigation of a unilateral pleural effusion in adults. *Thorax* 58Suppl 2:ii8-17

PMID 12796164 Heffner JE, Heffner JN, Brown LK [2003] Multilevel and continuous pleural fluid pH likelihood ratios for evaluating malignant pleural effusions. *Chest* 123(6):1887-1894

PMID 13223169 Harvey AM [1954] Systemic lupus erythematosus: review of the literature and clinical analysis of 138 cases. *Medicine* 33:291-437

PMID 15115678 Burgess LJ [2004] Biochemical analysis of pleural, peritoneal and pericardial effusions. *Clin Chim Acta* 343(1-2),61-84

PMID 15596670 Porcel, JM, Vives M, Esquerda A et al [2004] Use of a panel of tumor markers (carcinoembryonic antigen, cancer antigen 125, carbohydrate antigen 15-3, and CK19 fragments) in pleural fluid for the differential diagnosis of benign and malignant effusions. *Chest* 126(6):1757-1763

PMID 16623208 Porcel JM, Light RW [2006] Diagnostic approach to pleural effusion in adults. *Am Fam Physician* 73(7):1211-1220

PMID 16765714 Balbir-Gurman A, Yigla M, Nahir AM et al [2006] Rheumatoid pleural effusion. *Sem Arthritis Rheum* 35(6):368-378

PMID 17121764 Reuter H, Burgess L, van Vuuren W et al [2006] Diagnosing tuberculous pericarditis. *QJM* 99(12):827-839

PMID 17283581 Porcel JM, Ordi-Ros J, Esquerda A et al [2007]. Antinuclear antibody testing in pleural fluid for the diagnosis of lupus pleuritis. *Lupus* 16(1):25-27

PMID 17356060 Creaney J, Yeoman D, Naumoff LK et al [2007] Soluble mesothelin in effusions: a useful tool for the diagnosis of malignant mesothelioma. *Thorax* 62(7):569-576

PMID 17625694 Tuon FF, Silva VID, Almeida GMD de et al [2007] The usefulness of adenosine deaminase in the diagnosis of tuberculous pericarditis. *Rev Inst Med Trop Sao Paulo* 49(3):165-170

PMID 18195577 Sahn SA [2008] The value of pleural fluid analysis. *Am J Med Sci* 335(1): 7-15. doi:10.1097/MAJ.0b013e31815d25e6

PMID 18195577 Sahn SA [2008] The value of pleural fluid analysis. *Am J Med Sci* 335(1):7-15

PMID 18344697 Arroyo M, Soberman JE [2008] Adenosine deaminase in the diagnosis of tuberculous pericardial effusion. *Am J Med Sci* 335(3):227-229

PMID 18556632 Rahman NM, Mishra EK, Davies HE et al [2008] Clinically important factors influencing the diagnostic measurement of pleural fluid pH and glucose. *Am J Respir Crit Care Med* 178(5):483-490

PMID 18828976 Pritt BS, Clark CG [2008] Amebiasis. *Mayo Clin Proc* 83(10):1154-9; quiz 1159-60

PMID 18986277 Nolte FS [2008] Molecular diagnostics for detection of bacterial and viral pathogens in community-acquired pneumonia. *Clin Infect Dis* 47Suppl3:S123-6

PMID 19181646 Maldonado F, Hawkins FJ, Daniels CE et al [2009] Pleural fluid characteristics of chylothorax. *Mayo Clin Proc* 84(2):129-133

PMID 19299498 Davies HE, Sadler RS, Bielsa S et al [2009] Clinical impact and reliability of pleural fluid mesothelin in undiagnosed pleural effusions. *Am J Respir Crit Care Med* 180(5):437-444

PMID 19363209 Porcel JM, Martínez-Alonso M, Cao G et al [2009] Biomarkers of heart failure in pleural fluid. *Chest* 136(3):671-677

PMID 19386693 Dheda K, van Zyl-Smit RN, Sechi LA et al [2009] Utility of quantitative T cell responses vs unstimulated interferon-g for the diagnosis of pleural tuberculosis. *Eur Respir J* 34:1118-26

PMID 19672657 Porcel JM [2009] Tuberculous pleural effusion. *Lung* 187(5):263-70

PMID 20392619 McGrath EE, Warriner D, Anderson PB [2010] The use of nonroutine pleural fluid analysis in the diagnosis of pleural effusion. *Resp Med* 104(8):1092-1100

PMID 2046135 Fowler NO [1991] Tuberculous pericarditis. *JAMA* 266:99-103

PMID 20473171 Krenke R, Korczyński P [2010] Use of pleural fluid levels of adenosine deaminase and interferon γ in the diagnosis of tuberculous pleuritis. *Curr Opin Pulm Med* 16(4):367-75

PMID 20529669 Hackbarth JS, Murata K, Reilly WM et al [2010] Performance of CEA and CA19-9 in identifying pleural effusions caused by specific malignancies. *Clin Biochem* 43(13-14):1051-1055

PMID 20573057 Porcel JM [2011] Pearls and myths in pleural fluid analysis. *Respirology* 16(1):44-52

PMID 20816597 Porcel JM, Esquerda A, Bielsa S [2010] Diagnostic performance of adenosine deaminase activity in pleural fluid: a single-center experience with over 2100 consecutive patients. *Eur J Intern Med* 21(5):419-423

PMID 21459855 Menzies SM, Rahman NM, Wrightson JM et al [2011] Blood culture bottle culture of pleural fluid in pleural infection. *Thorax* 66(8):658-62

PMID 22448326 Hassan T, Al-Alawi M, Chotirmall SH et al [2012] Pleural fluid analysis: standstill or a work in progress? *Pulm Med* 716235

PMID 22474483 Aljohaney A, Amjadi K, Alvarez GG [2012] A systematic review of the epidemiology, immunopathogenesis, diagnosis, and treatment of pleural TB in HIV-infected patients. *Clin Dev Immunol* 842045. Epub 2012 Mar 14.

PMID 22579767 Lu J, Grenache DG [2012] Development of a rapid, microplate-based kinetic assay for measuring adenosine deaminase activity in body fluids. *Clin Chim Acta* 413:1637-1640

PMID 22982641 Považan A, Vukelić A, Kurucin T et al [2012] The most common isolates from pleural infections. *Acta Microbiol Immunol Hung* 59(3):375-85

PMID 22990049 Lal C, Huggins JT, Sahn SA [2013] Parasitic diseases of the pleura. *Am J Med Sci* 345(5):385-9

PMID 23102482 Htwe TH, Khardori NM [2012] Cardiac emergencies: infective endocarditis, pericarditis, and myocarditis. *Med Clin North Am* 96(6):1149-69

PMID 23508114 Porcel JM [2013] Identifying transudates misclassified by Light's criteria. *Curr Opin Pulm Med* 19(4):362-367

PMID 23945888 Emadi Koochak H, Davoudi S, Salehi Omran A et al [2013] Diagnostic value of interferon-γ assay in tuberculosis pericardial effusions: study on a cohort of Iranian patients. *Acta Med Iran* 7;51(7):449-53

PMID 2751171 American Thoracic Society [1989] Guidelines for thoracentesis and needle biopsy of the pleura. *Am Rev Respir Dis* 140:257-258

PMID 3062725 Sahn SA [1988] Pleural effusions in the atypical pneumonias. *Semin Respir Infect* 3:322-334

PMID 3062727 Heffner JE [1988] Pleuropulmonary manifestations of actinomycosis and nocardiosis. *Semin Respir Infect* 3:352

PMID 3259069 Kim YK, Mohsenifar Z, Koerner SK [1988] Lymphocytic pleural effusion in postpericardiotomy syndrome. *Am Heart J* 115:1077-1079.

PMID 3341671 Sahn SA, Good JT [1988] Pleural fluid pH in malignant effusions. Diagnostic, prognostic, and therapeutic implications. *Ann Intern Med* 108(3):345-349

PMID 3358655 Hanes VE, Lucia H [1988] Acridine orange as a screen for organisms in clinical specimens and comparison with Gram's stain. *Arch Pathol Lab Med* 112:529-532

PMID 3548191 Das DK, Gupta SK, Amyagari S et al [1987] Pleural effusions in non-Hodgkin lymphoma. A cytomorphologic, cytochemical and immunologic study. *Acta Cytol* 31(2):119-124

PMID 3653300 van Keimpema AR, Slaats EH, Wagenaar JP [1987] Adenosine deaminase activity, not diagnostic for tuberculous pleurisy. *Eur J Resp Dis* 71(1):15-8

PMID 4051357 Health and Public Policy Committee, American College of Physicians [1985] Diagnostic thoracentesis and pleural biopsy in pleural effusions. Position Paper. *Ann Intern Med* 103:799-802

PMID 4131173 Bartlett JG, Thadepalli H, Gorback SL et al [1974] Bacteriology of empyema. *Lancet* 1:338-340

PMID 4630686 Berger HW, Mejia E [1973] Tuberculous pleurisy. *Chest* 63:88-92

PMID 4642731 Light RW, MacGregor MI, Luchsinger PC et al [1972] Pleural effusions: the diagnostic separation of transudates and exudates. *Ann Intern Med* 77:507-513

PMID 4872925 Kay M [1968] Pleuropulmonary complications of pancreatitis. *Thorax* 23(3):297-306

PMID 4988357 Levine H, Metzger W, Lacera O et al [1970] Diagnosis of tuberculous pleurisy by culture of pleural biopsy specimen. *Arch Intern Med* 126:269-271

PMID 5027585 Sherr HP, Light RW, Merson MH et al [1972] Origin of pleural fluid amylase in esophageal rupture. *Ann Intern Med* 76(6):985-986

PMID 5676332 Nosanchuk JS, Naylor B [1968] A unique cytologic picture in pleural fluid from patients with rheumatoid arthritis. *Am J Clin Pathol* 50:330-335

PMID 6066230 Walker WC, Wright V [1967] Rheumatoid pleuritis. *Ann Rheum Dis* 26(6):467-474.

PMID 6170424 Raju RN, Kardinal CG [1981] Pleural effusion in breast carcinoma: analysis of 122 cases. *Cancer* 48(11):2524-2527

PMID 6261936 Fentiman JS, Millis R, Sexton S [1981] Pleural effusion in breast cancer: a review of 105 cases. *Cancer* 47(8):2087-2092

PMID 6605838 Good JT, King TE, Antony VB et al [1983] Lupus pleuritis: clinical features and pleural fluid characteristics with special reference to pleural fluid antinuclear antibodies. *Chest* 84:714-718

PMID 6788249 Kumar 5, Seshadri MS, Koshi G et al [1981] Diagnosing tuberculous pleural effusion: comparative sensitivity of mycobacterial culture and histopathology. *Br Med* 283(6283):20

PMID 6933801 Yazdi HM, Hajdu SI, Melamed MR [1980] Cytopathology of pericardial effusions. *Acta Cytol* 24:401-412

PMID 6981226 Pettersson T, Klockars M, Hellström PE [1982] Chemical and immunological features of pleural effusions: comparison between rheumatoid arthritis and other diseases. *Thorax* 37(5):354-361

PMID 6992663 Young EJ, Hirsh DD, Fainstein V et al [1980] Pleural effusions due to Cryptococcus neoformans: a review of the literature and report of 2 cases with cryptococcal antigen determinations. *Am Rev Respir Dis* 121(4):743-7

PMID 7047062 Sahn SA [1982] Pleural effusion in lung cancer. Symposium on recent advances in lung cancer. *Clin Chest Med* 3(2):443-452

PMID 7316625 Varkey B, Rose HD, Kutty CP et al [1981] Empyema thoracic during a 10-year period: analysis of 72 cases and comparison to a previous study (1952-1967). *Arch Intern Med* 141:1771-1776

PMID 7424940 Light RW, Girard WM, Jenkinson SG et al [1980] Parapneumonic effusions. *Am J Med* 69:507-512

PMID 7587426 Costa M, Quiroga T, Cruz E [1995] Measurement of pleural fluid cholesterol and lactate dehydrogenase. A simple and accurate set of indicators for separating exudates from transudates. *Chest* 108(5):1260-1263

PMID 7767510 Heffner JE, Brown LK, Barbieri C et al [1995] Pleural fluid chemical analysis in parapneumonic effusions. A meta-analysis. *Am J Respir Crit Care Med* 151(6):1700-1708

PMID 8222811 Sanchez-Armengol A, Rodriguez-Panadero F [1993] Survival and talc pleurodesis in metastatic pleural carcinoma, revisited. Report of 125 cases. *Chest* 104(5):1482-1485

PMID 8325082 Joseph J, Sahn SA [1993] Connective tissue diseases and the pleura. *Chest* 104(1):262-270

PMID 8339626 Romero S, Candela A, Martín C et al [1993] Evaluation of different criteria for the separation of pleural transudates from exudates. *Chest* 104(2):399-404

PMID 8915232 Rubins JB, Rubins HB [1996] Etiology and prognostic significance of eosinophilic effusions. *Chest* 110:1271-74

PMID 9106577 Heffner JE, Brown LK, Barbieri CA [1997] Diagnostic value of tests that discriminate between exudative and transudative pleural effusions. Primary Study Investigators. *Chest* 111(4):970-980.

PMID 9149572 Meyers DG, Meyers RE, Prendergast TW [1997] The usefulness of diagnostic tests on pericardial fluid. *Chest* 111:1213-21

PMID 9713637 Gaguez I, Porcel JM, Vives M et al [1998] Comparative analysis of Light's criteria and other biochemical parameters for distinguishing transudates from exudates. *Resp Med* 92:762

PMID 9824016 Cheng DS, Rodriguez RM, Rogers J et al [1998] Comparison of pleural fluid pH values obtained using blood gas machine, pH meter, and pH indicator strip. *Chest* 114(5):1368-1372

CLSI C49-A: CLSI [2007] Analysis of Body Fluids in Clinical Chemistry; Approved Guideline. CLSI document C49-A. Wayne, PA: Clinical and Laboratory Standards Institute

Light RW [2007] *Pleural Diseases*, 5e. Lippencott Williams & Wilkins, a Wolter Kluwer Business

Punchalski J, ed [2013] *Pleural Disease. Clinics in Medicine*, vol 34, no 1

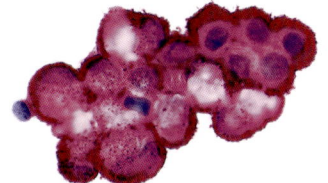

Kjeldsberg CR, Straseski JA, Couturier MR, Cohen MB

Peritoneal Fluid
Chapter 6

Anatomy & pathophysiology

The peritoneum (Greek: to stretch over) is a delicate, smooth serous membrane that covers the walls and viscera of the abdomen and pelvis. It consists of 2 layers that are contiguous with one another with the space between them forming the peritoneal cavity. This cavity is lined by a single layer of mesothelial cells. The peritoneal cavity is not a true cavity but only becomes so in the presence of disease that causes fluid to accumulate within it. The accumulation of fluid within the peritoneal cavity constitutes a peritoneal effusion that signals that the patient has ascites. The fluid is also called ascitic fluid.

Peritoneal fluid is an ultrafiltrate of plasma. The accumulation of peritoneal fluid may result from increased hydrostatic pressure of the systemic circulation (as seen in congestive heart failure [CHF]), decreased plasma oncotic pressure (as seen with hypoproteinemia), increased permeability of the capillaries in the peritoneum (as seen with peritonitis), and decreased reabsorption (as may be seen in neoplasms).

Causes of peritoneal effusions are listed in **t6.1**. In North America and Europe, alcoholic cirrhosis is the most common cause. As with pleural fluid, peritoneal fluid can be divided into transudates and exudates. However, the laboratory criteria for separating transudates from exudates are less clearly defined in peritoneal fluid. The serum ascites albumin gradient (SAAG) is commonly used as a reasonably reliable test for separating transudates from exudates [PMID 1616215]. As will be discussed in the chemical analysis sections, there are a number of other methods. However, there are to date no absolutely reliable methods for separating the 2.

Specimen collection & clinical indications

>400 mL of peritoneal fluid is usually required before an effusion can be detected by physical examination or imaging. The indications for paracentesis are ascites of unknown origin, suspected intestinal perforation, hemorrhage, or infarct. The 2 most common indications for paracentesis are to rule out bacterial peritonitis and a suspected intraabdominal malignant neoplasm.

t6.1	Causes of peritoneal effusions
Transudates	
Cirrhosis	
Congestive heart failure	
Nephrotic syndrome	
Postpartum	
Postsurgery	
Portal vein obstruction	
Exudates	
Infections	
Bacterial peritonitis (primary & secondary)	
Tuberculosis	
Fungal	
Parasitic	
Neoplastic disease	
Metastatic malignancy—carcinoma; sarcoma	
Hepatocellular carcinoma	
Mesothelioma	
Lymphoma	
Gastrointestinal disease	
Abscess—subphrenic, hepatic	
Pancreatitis	
Bile peritonitis	
Trauma	
Chylous effusion	
Trauma	
Malignancy—carcinoma, lymphoma	
Tuberculosis	

The procedure of removing fluid from the peritoneal cavity is called paracentesis and the fluid submitted to the laboratory is called paracentesis fluid, peritoneal fluid, or ascitic fluid. A minimum of 30 mL is usually needed for a complete laboratory evaluation but this amount depends on the clinical situation. For cytologic examination in a suspected malignancy at least 100 mL is desirable.

Diagnostic peritoneal lavage (DPL) consists of the insertion of a perforated peritoneal dialysis catheter into the peritoneal cavity through a small, midline, infraumbilical incision. The catheter is aspirated and if blood is not observed grossly, 1 L of a saline based solution is infused.

The fluid is immediately retrieved by gravity and analyzed. If the result is "indeterminate," the catheter is left in place and the procedure repeated in 1-2 hours.

DPL is no longer recommended as a routine technique for the evaluation of abdominal trauma, because noninvasive procedures such as computed tomography and ultrasound have limited its common use to rapid screening for significant abdominal hemorrhage and for evaluation of possible viscous injury. DPL is also sometimes used in evaluation of patients with suspected acute peritonitis or pancreatitis.

t6.2 lists criteria that may be used for diagnosing trauma by peritoneal fluid analysis. In acute situations (within 4 hours of injury) WBC counts may have little diagnostic value, as the WBC may not yet be elevated.

t6.2 Criteria for diagnosing blunt & penetrating trauma by peritoneal lavage fluid analysis

Diagnosis	Gross findings	Findings on laboratory analysis
Positive	Blood noted in aspirate or lavage return Lavage fluid retrieved via Foley catheter or chest tube Evidence of food, foreign particle, or bile	RBC count >100,000/mL (>50,000 mL in cases of penetrating trauma—stab or gunshot wounds) WBC count >500/mL Amylase level >2× that of serum amylase level
Indeterminate	Small amount of bloody fluid noted in dialysis catheter on insertion	RBC count 50,000-100,000/mL (10,000-50,000/mL in cases of penetrating trauma) WBC count 100-500/mL Amylase level slightly higher than serum amylase level
Negative	Clear, pale yellow	RBC count <50,000/mL (<1,000/mL in cases of penetrating trauma) WBC count <100/mL Amylase level lower than serum amylase level

Data adapted from Alyono D, et al [PMID 7123495]

Peritoneal wash is a specialized sampling of the abdominal cavity for women with suspected or confirmed gynecologic malignancies. Typically a large volume of saline, ~1 L, is used to wash the abdomen and pelvis. Evaluation is usually limited to cytologic examination for the detection of metastatic carcinoma, often of ovarian origin.

For cell counts a specimen should be put in an EDTA anticoagulated venipuncture tube. Specimens for culture should include blood culture bottles that have been inoculated at the bedside.

Recommended tests

The most useful laboratory tests for evaluation of peritoneal fluid are listed in t6.3.

t6.3 Laboratory tests in peritoneal effusions

Useful in most patients
Gross examination
Cytology
Stains and cultures for microorganisms
Serum ascites albumin concentration gradient (SAAG)

Useful in selected patients
Leukocyte count and differential
Enzymes: lipase, amylase, alkaline phosphatase
Cholesterol, triglycerides
Immunohistochemistry/flow cytometry
Tumor markers
RBC count (lavage in trauma patients)

Gross examination

The gross examination gives immediate information in the clinical and laboratory triage. Transudates are usually clear and pale yellow t6.4. Exudates are cloudy or turbid because of large numbers of leukocytes, elevated protein concentrations and/or microorganisms. Such fluids may be seen with peritonitis, perforated or infarcted intestine, and pancreatitis. Bile stained fluid is green and may be seen with perforation of the gallbladder or small intestine, or with a perforated duodenal ulcer. A green fluid may also be present in cholecystitis and acute pancreatitis. The presence of bile can be confirmed by a spot test for bilirubin. Grossly hemorrhagic peritoneal fluids may be seen in trauma (ruptured spleen or liver), intestinal infarction, pancreatitis, and malignant disorders. If pathologic hemorrhage must be distinguished from a traumatic tap, a visual quantitation of blood in the peritoneal fluid may be useful. Traumatic tap typically shows clearing on continued aspiration. Peritoneal lavage is a sensitive method for detecting the presence of blood. As few as 8 drops per liter of saline will cause a pink discoloration. >25 mL of blood per liter of lavage fluid gives a bright red opaque appearance.

t6.4 Peritoneal fluid gross appearance & clinical significance

Appearance	Significance
Transudates	
Clear straw colored	Cirrhosis; further analysis often not necessary
Exudates	
Cloudy, purulent	Infectious process, peritonitis
Red tinged to bloody	If not traumatic tap: trauma, malignancy, intestinal infarction, pancreatitis
Milky white	Chylous or pseudochylous effusion
Viscous, hemorrhagic or clear	Mesothelioma
Green (bile stained)	Perforation of gallbladder or small intestine, acute pancreatitis
Anchovy paste color	Rupture of amebic liver
"Chocolate sauce"	Abscess

True chylous peritoneal fluid is very rare. When present, it is creamy and has the consistency of milk. Chylous ascites is caused by leakage of lymphatic vessels resulting from trauma, malignancy, tuberculosis, and rarely cirrhosis of the liver. Malignant lymphoma and carcinoma are the 2 most common causes. Pseudochylous fluid, which may be associated with chronic effusions of any cause, has a milky, golden or green appearance because of cell debris and cholesterol crystals.

Cell counts

The total ascitic leukocyte count (WBC) may be useful in distinguishing between peritoneal transudates (eg, in uncomplicated cirrhosis) from spontaneous bacterial peritonitis (SBP). ~90% of patients with SBP have a WBC count of >250/mL, most of which are neutrophils [PMID 6724512]. However, a wide range exists for patients with chronic liver disease because of extracellular shifts in fluid associated with ascites formation and resolution. The same patient may have transudative and exudative patterns at different times [PMID 7586905].

Microscopic examination & clinical considerations

An examination of the cells present in the peritoneal fluid and a differential cell count should be performed on a stained smear made by using cytocentrifugation, or other methods. When malignancy is suspected, cell blocks may be useful in addition to smear preparation to perform "ancillary" studies such as immunohistochemistry.

The cell types encountered in peritoneal fluid are similar to those described in Chapter 5 under "Microscopic examination" and include neutrophils (polymorphonuclear leukocytes [PMNs]), eosinophils and basophils, lymphocytes, plasma cells, mononuclear phagocytes (monocytes, histiocytes, and macrophages), mesothelial cells, and malignant cells.

Exudative peritoneal effusions are characterized by a variable number of neutrophils, lymphocytes, macrophages, mesothelial cells, eosinophils, and basophils in decreasing order of frequency. Mononuclear phagocytes (monocytes, histiocytes, macrophages) are seen in variable numbers in peritoneal effusions depending on the etiology. As with mesothelial cells, these cells have a variable appearance and a number of different types of mononuclear phagocytes are seen (as described in Chapter 5) i6.1-i6.6.

Lymphocytes are present in variable numbers in peritoneal effusions and may exhibit a variety of morphologic features during transformation in response to various stimuli (as also illustrated in Chapter 5) i6.7-i6.10. A predominance of lymphocytes is seen in transudates resulting from congestive heart failure (CHF), cirrhosis, and nephrotic syndrome. A predominance of lymphocytes may also be seen in chylous effusions, tuberculous peritonitis, and cancer. Distinguishing a benign lymphocyte rich effusion from malignant lymphoma may be difficult morphologically, especially in small lymphocytic lymphomas. In such

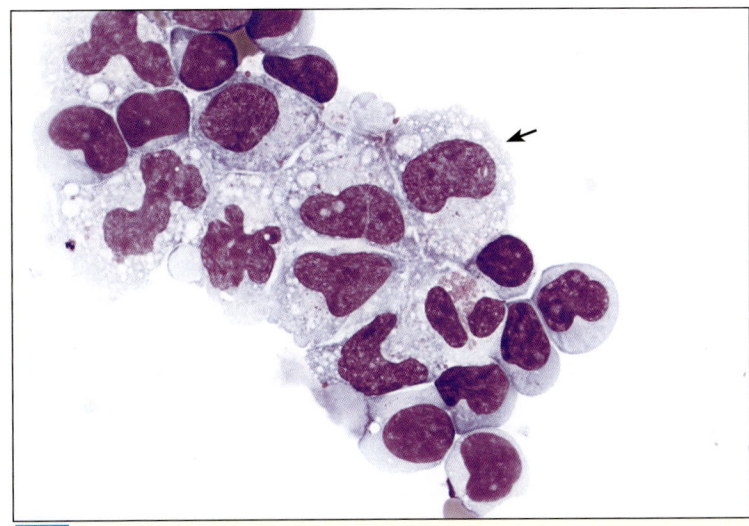

i6.1 Histiocytes (arrow) surrounded by several lymphocytes

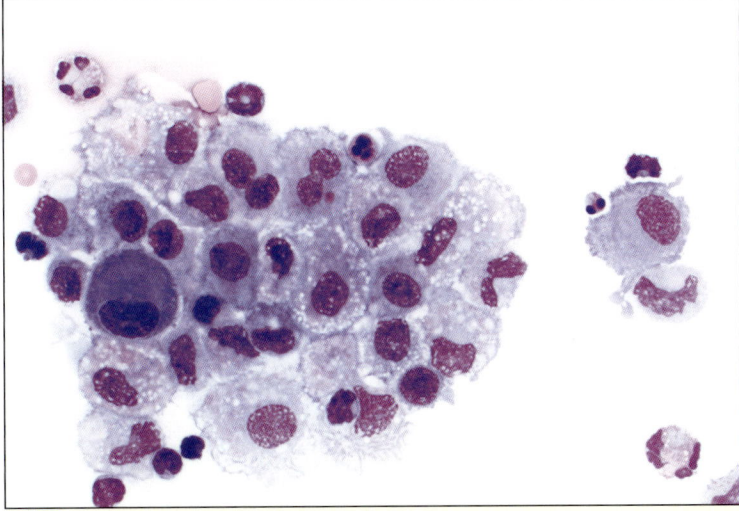

i6.2 Cluster of histiocytes & 1 mesothelial cell

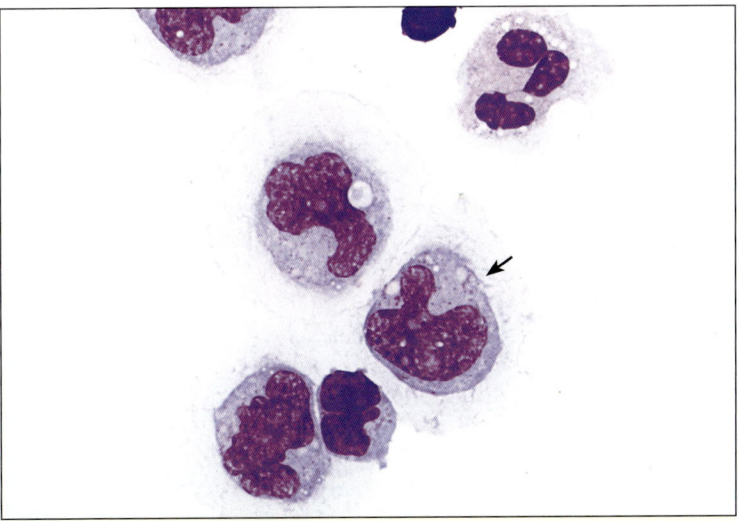

i6.3 Several histiocytes (arrow)

6: Peritoneal Fluid

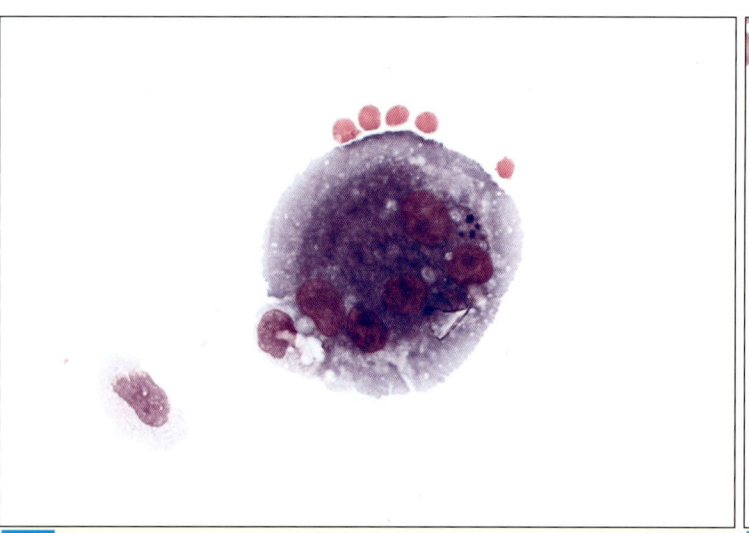

i6.4 A multinucleate histiocyte or possibly a multinucleate mesothelial cell

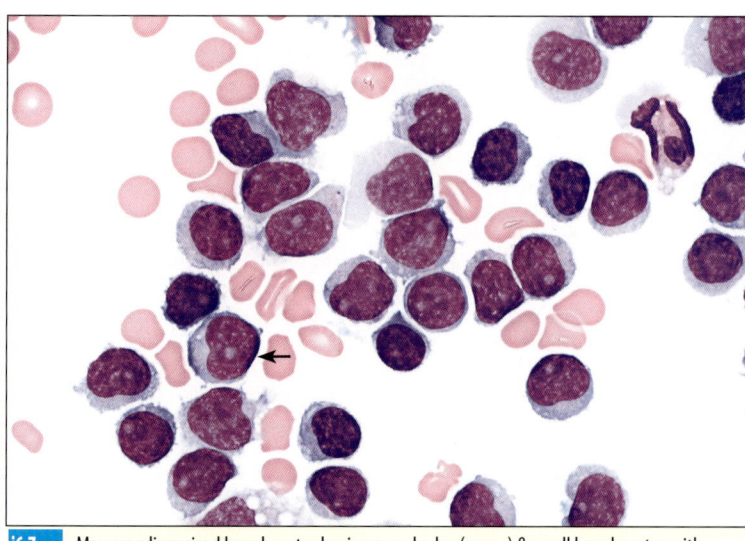

i6.7 Many medium sized lymphocytes having a nucleolus (arrow) & small lymphocytes with condensed chromatin

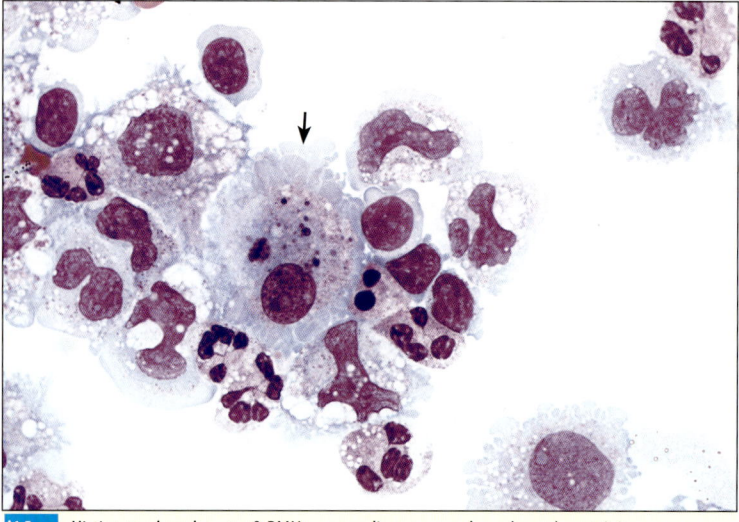

i6.5 Histiocytes, lymphocytes & PMNs surrounding a macrophage (arrow) containing phagocytosed material

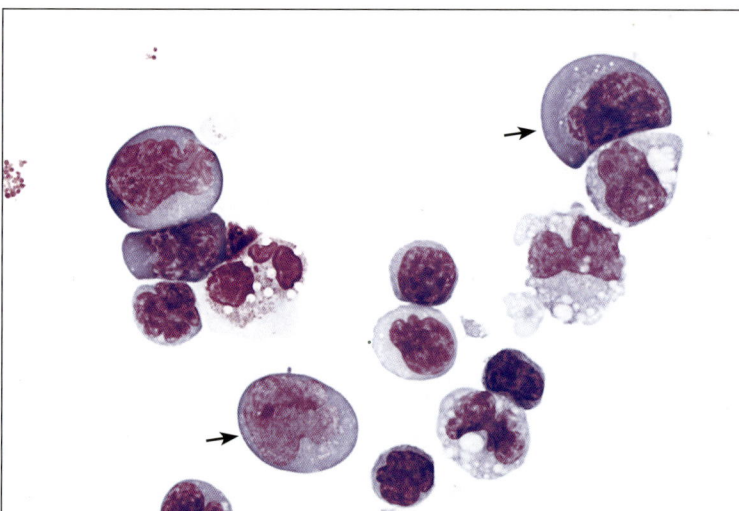

i6.8 Several transformed lymphocytes (immunocytes [arrows])

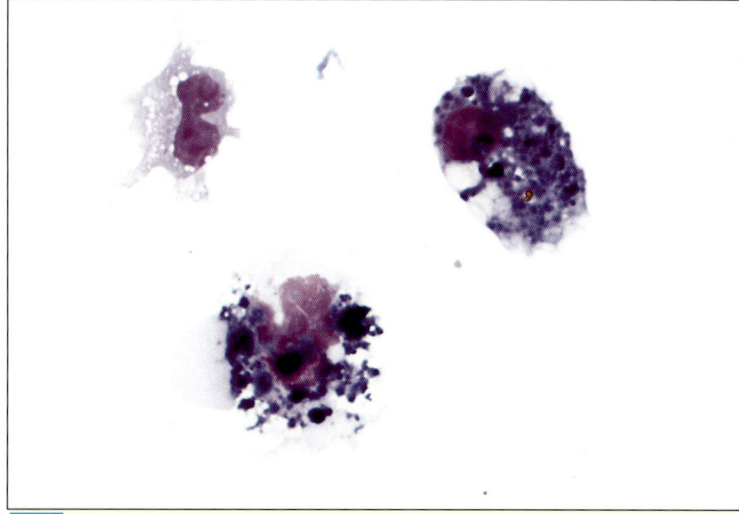

i6.6 2 macrophages filled with hemosiderin

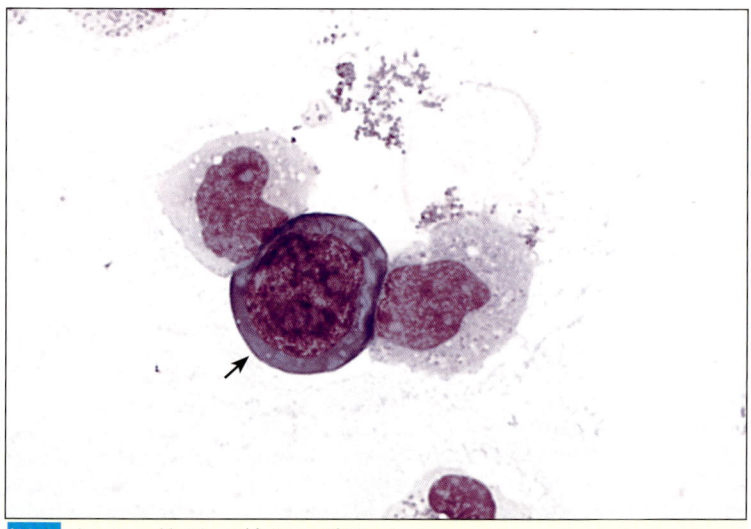

i6.9 An immunoblast (arrow) between 2 histiocytes

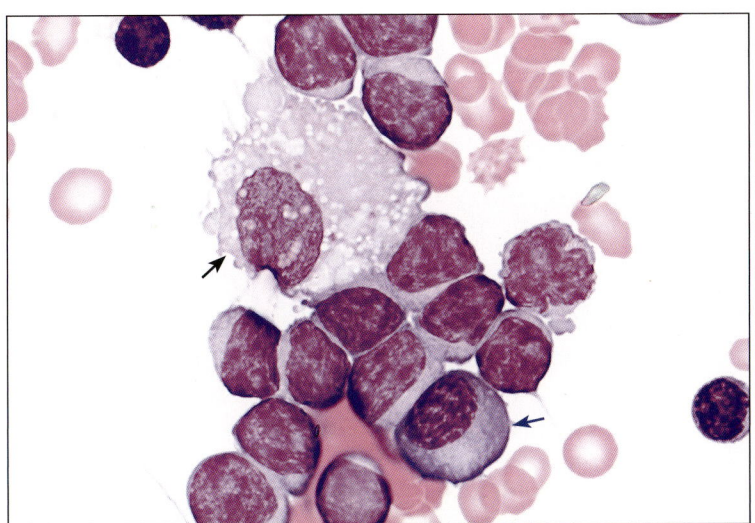

i6.10 A plasma cell (blue arrow), many lymphocytes & a histiocyte (black arrow)

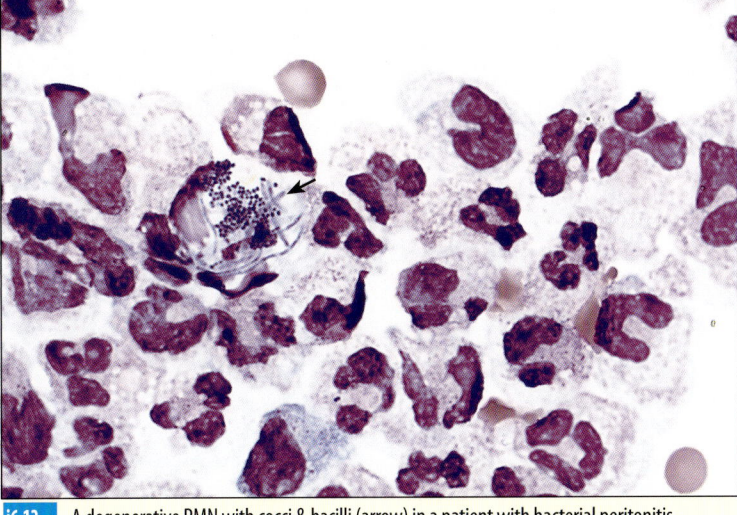

i6.12 A degenerative PMN with cocci & bacilli (arrow) in a patient with bacterial peritonitis

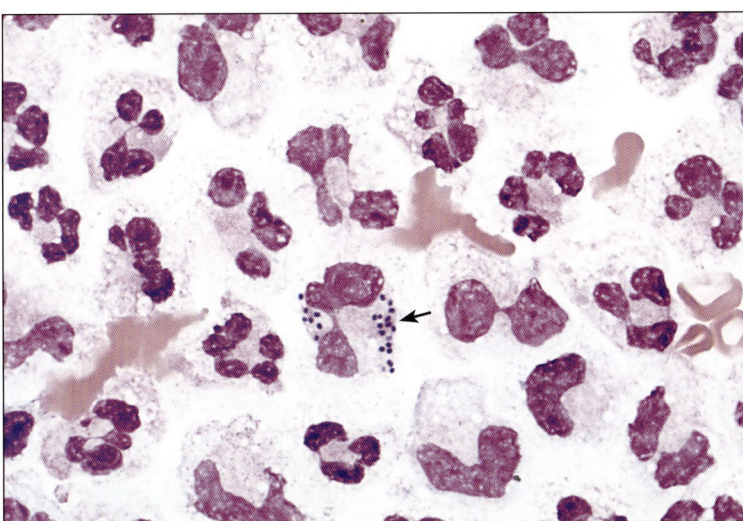

i6.11 Multiple PMNs with 1 containing intracellular bacterial cocci (arrow) in a patient with bacterial peritonitis

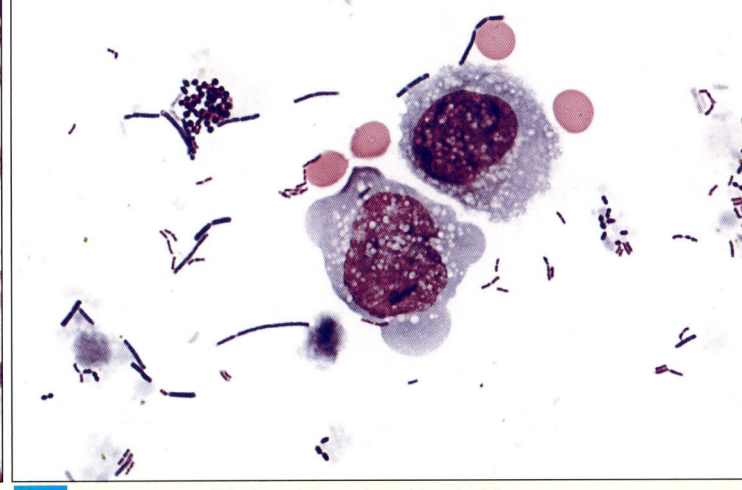

i6.13 Numerous extracellular bacteria in a patient with peritonitis

instances, immunophenotyping using either immunohistochemical techniques or flow cytometry is essential.

Neutrophils in longstanding effusions may have a decrease in the number of cytoplasmic granules and the nuclei may appear as densely stained spherical fragments sometimes mistaken for nucleated RBCs. In bacterial peritonitis, the PMNs may show degeneration in the form of vacuolization, loss of granules, and blurring of the nuclei. A PMN count of >250/mL is a reliable discriminatory test for bacterial peritonitis i6.11-i6.13. In fungal peritonitis both intracellular and extracellular organisms may be seen i6.14-i6.15.

Peritoneal fluid eosinophilia is particularly evident in patients undergoing continuous ambulatory peritoneal dialysis (CAPD) but has also been associated with congestive heart failure, vasculitis, malignant lymphoma, and ruptured hydatid cyst i6.16 [PMID 3341375]. Mast cells and basophils often accompany eosinophils and small numbers of these cells may be seen in cases of peritoneal fluid eosinophilia i6.17.

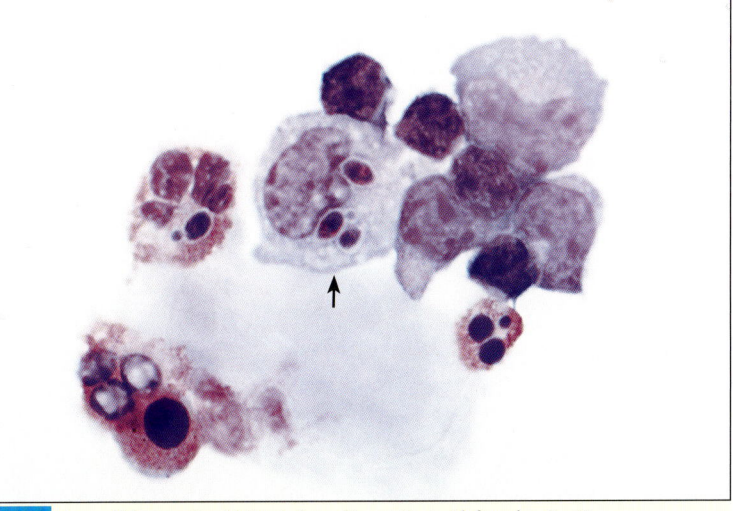

i6.14 Intracellular yeast in a histiocyte (arrow) in a patient with fungal peritonitis

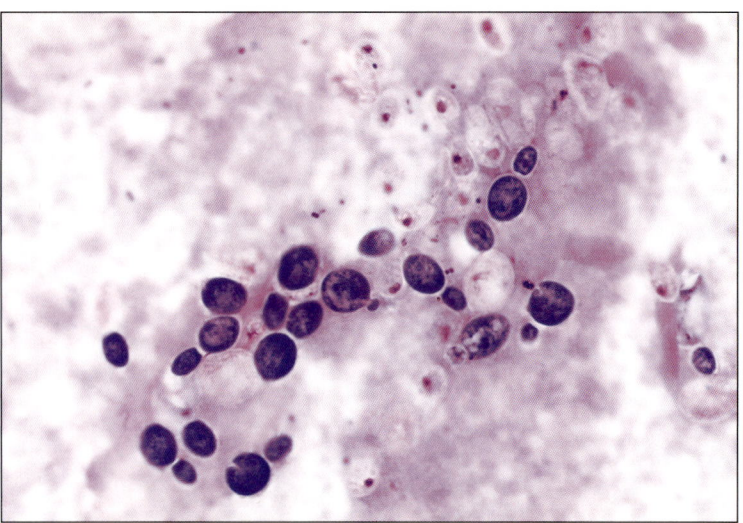
i6.15 Extracellular yeast (*Candida*) in patient with fungal peritonitis

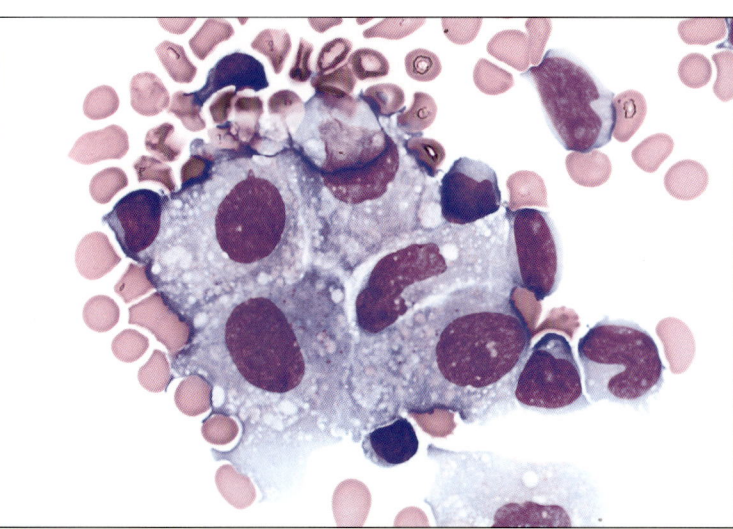
i6.18 A cluster of mesothelial cells with vacuolated cytoplasm

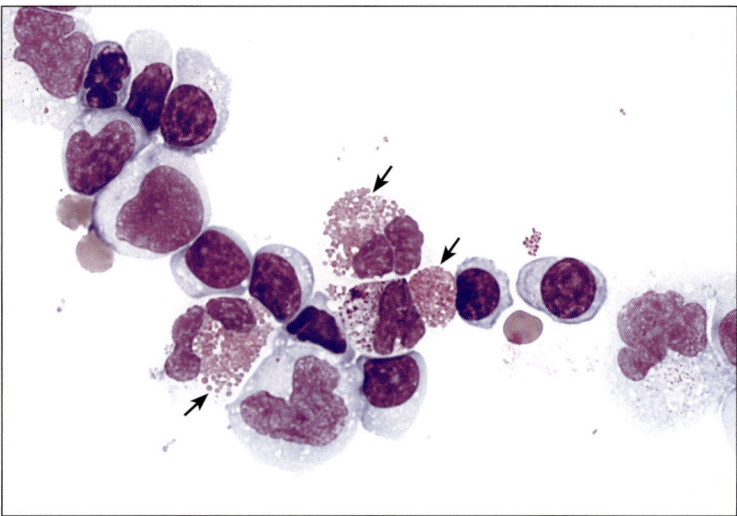
i6.16 Lymphocytes & several eosinophils (arrows)

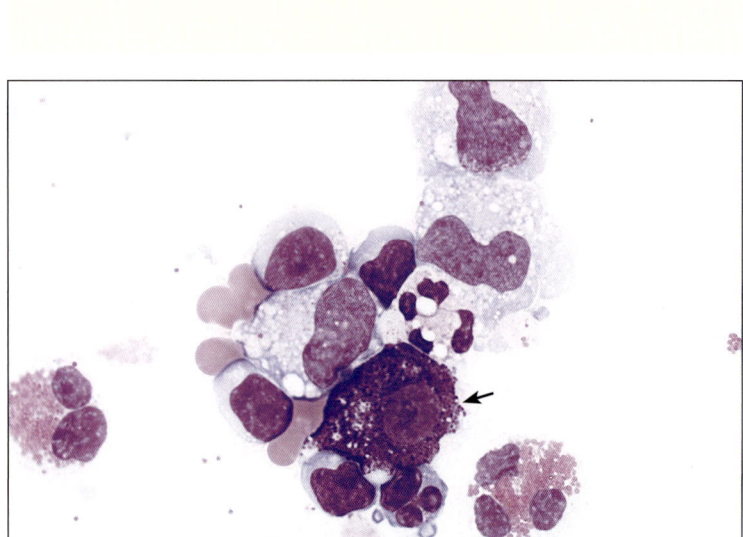
i6.17 Histiocytes, lymphocytes, 1 eosinophil & a mast cell (arrow)

LE (lupus erythematosus) cells have been reported in peritoneal fluid, as in other serous effusions.

The examiner must be familiar with the wide range of appearances of benign mesothelial cells in order not to mistake these for malignant cells (see Chapter 5) i6.18-i6.24. "Atypical" mesothelial cells, resembling malignant cells, are often seen in longstanding effusions and in ascites associated with cirrhosis of the liver.

In addition to performing a differential cell count, the smear should be examined for possible malignant cells t6.5. When a malignant condition is suspected, the specimen should always be submitted for full cytologic examination i6.25-i6.40.

t6.5	Incidence of malignant neoplasms associated with peritoneal effusion
Ovarian carcinoma	32%
Breast carcinoma	13%
Lymphoma/leukemia	7%
Gastric carcinoma	6%
Colorectal carcinoma	5%
Endometrial carcinoma	5%
Pancreatic carcinoma	4%
Adenocarcinoma of unknown origin	15%
Other	9%

Megakaryocytes, immature leukocytes, and nucleated red blood cells may rarely be seen in peritoneal fluid secondary to peritoneal myeloid metaplasia i6.41. Megakaryocytes may be mistaken for a metastatic malignancy.

Malignancies

As with pleural fluid, cancer is one of the most common causes of peritoneal effusion. Therefore, one of the most important parts of the laboratory investigation is the cytologic examination for malignant cells. These samples are often evaluated simultaneously in the clinical hematology laboratory and in the cytology laboratory. Peritoneal fluid

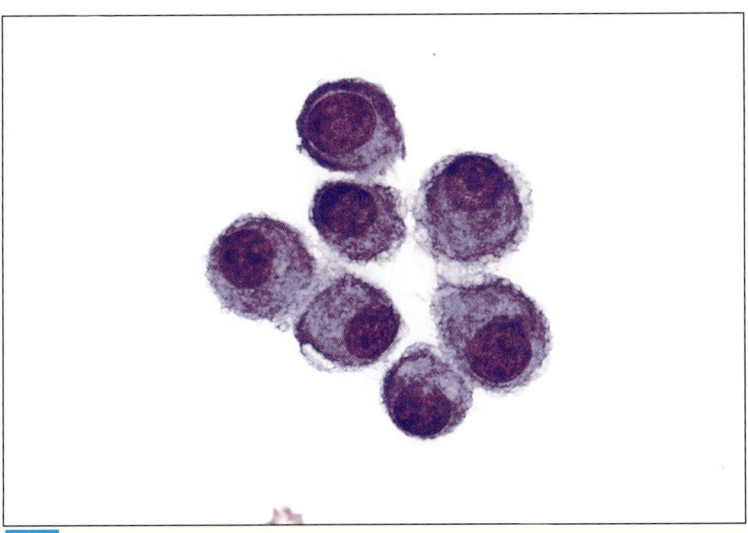

i6.19 Many small mesothelial cells

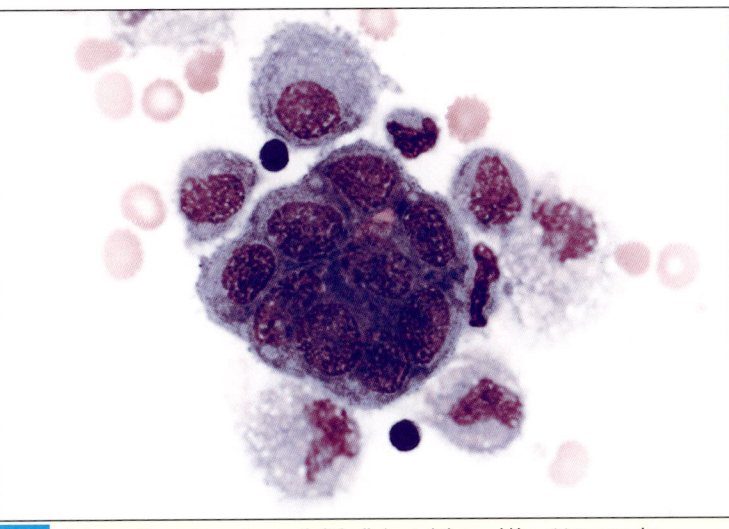

i6.22 A clump of hyperchromatic mesothelial cells (center) that could be misinterpreted as malignant cells

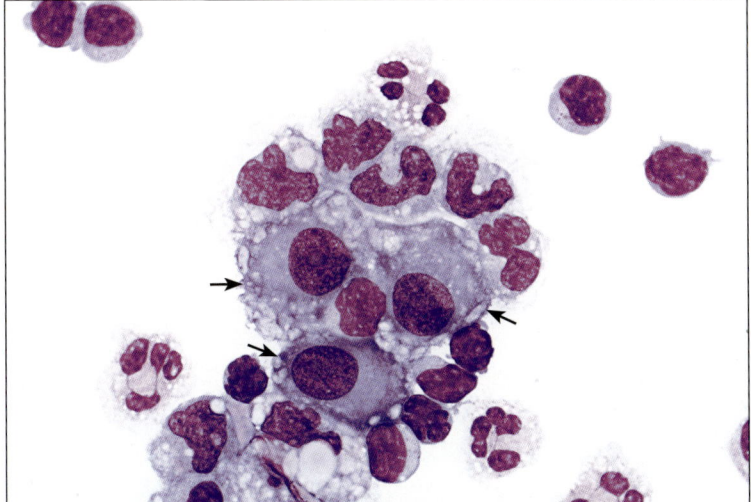

i6.20 3 mesothelial cells (arrows) surrounded by histiocytes, lymphocytes & PMNs

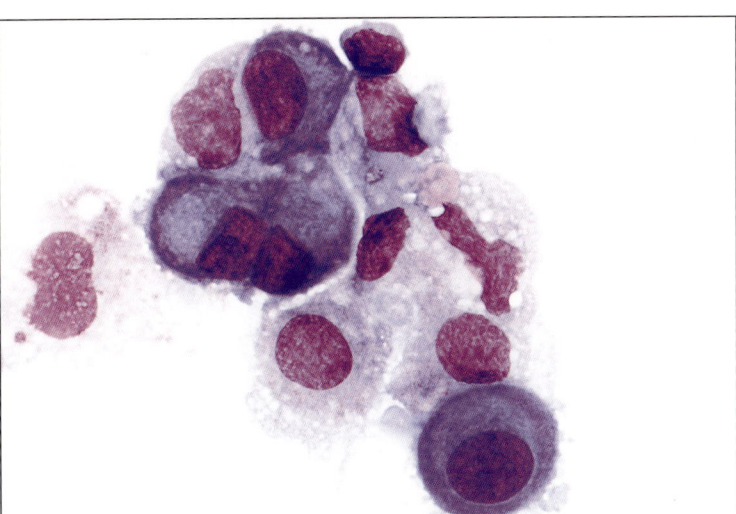

i6.23 Several mesothelial cells with deep blue cytoplasm & histiocytes

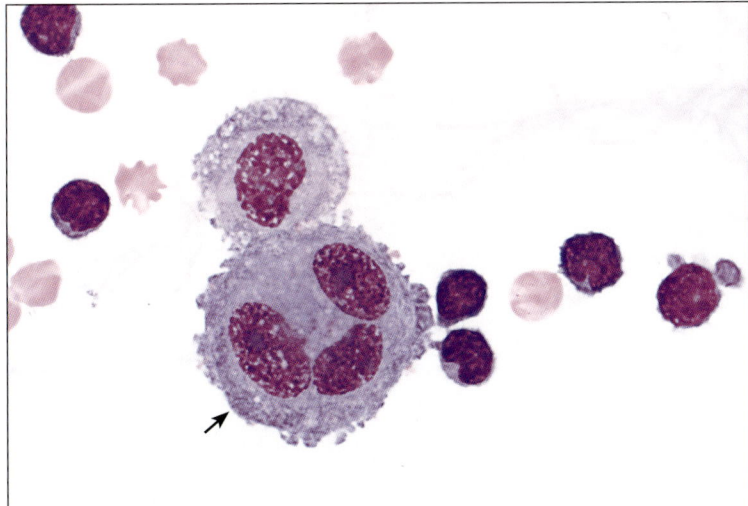

i6.21 A multinucleate mesothelial cell (arrow)

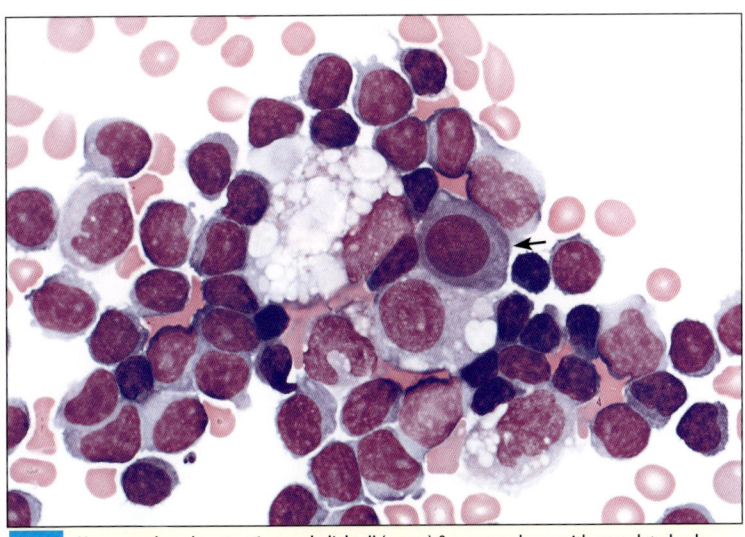

i6.24 Numerous lymphocytes, 1 mesothelial cell (arrow) & a macrophage with vacuolated pale cytoplasm

6: Peritoneal Fluid

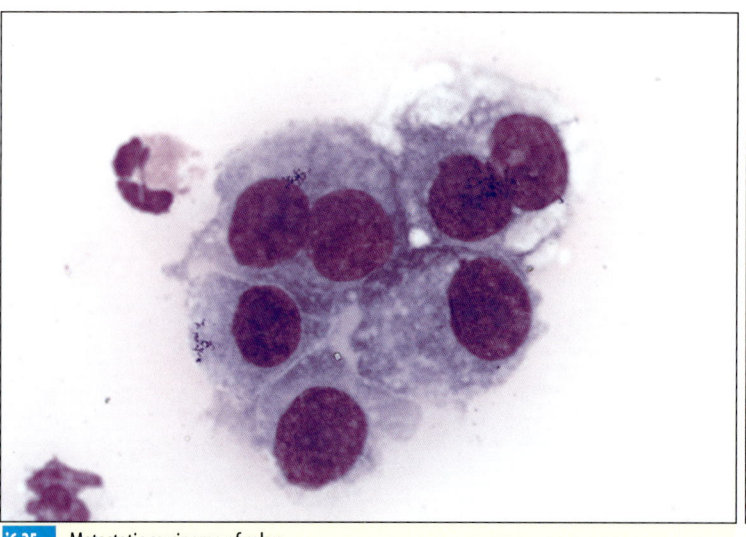

i6.25 Metastatic carcinoma of colon

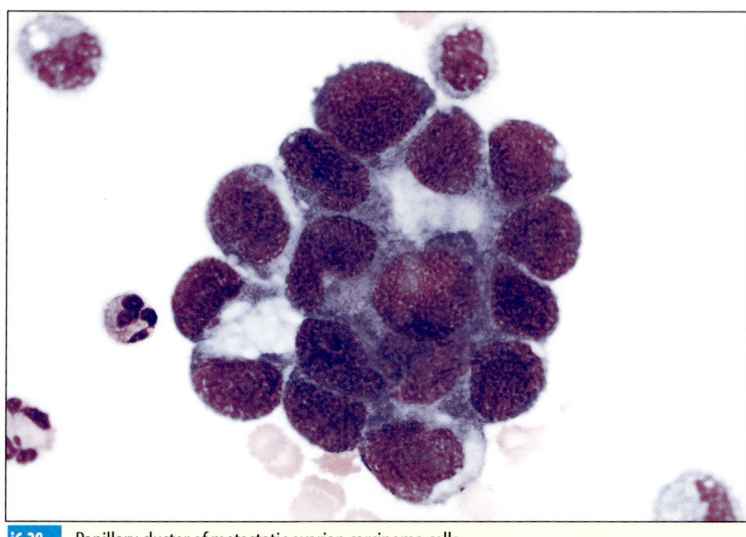

i6.28 Papillary cluster of metastatic ovarian carcinoma cells

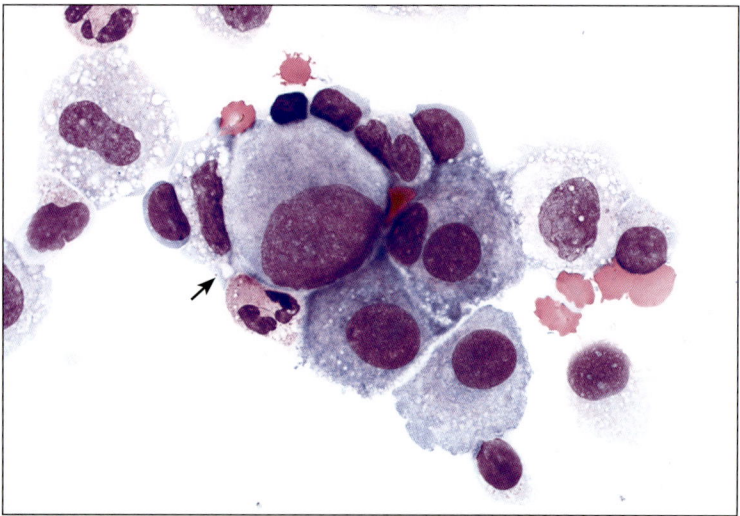

i6.26 A malignant cell (arrow) from carcinoma of stomach surrounded by mesothelial cells, lymphocytes & histiocytes

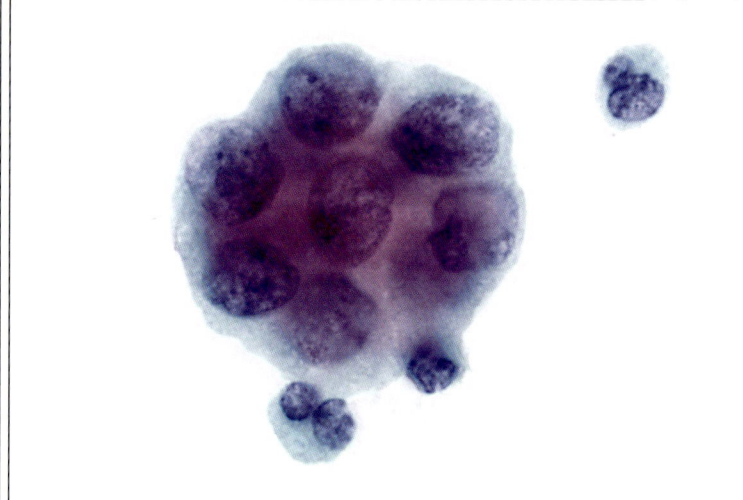

i6.29 Papillary cluster of ovarian carcinoma cells. Papanicolaou stain

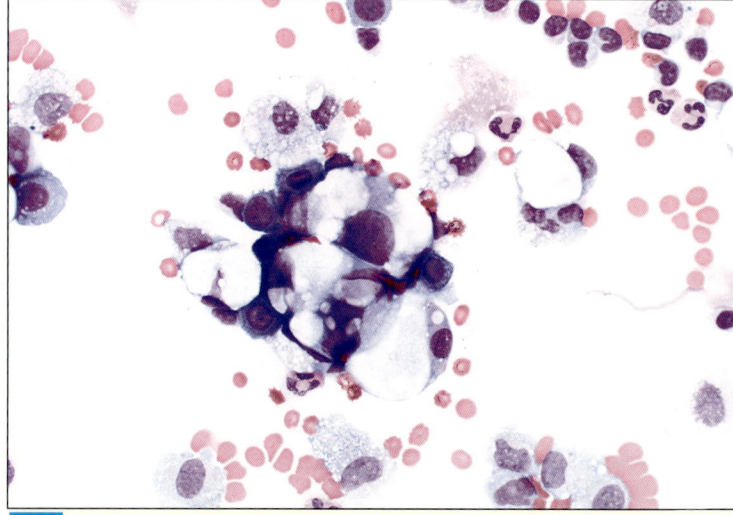

i6.27 A cluster of large malignant cells (center) with abundant pale cytoplasm from patient with adenocarcinoma of stomach

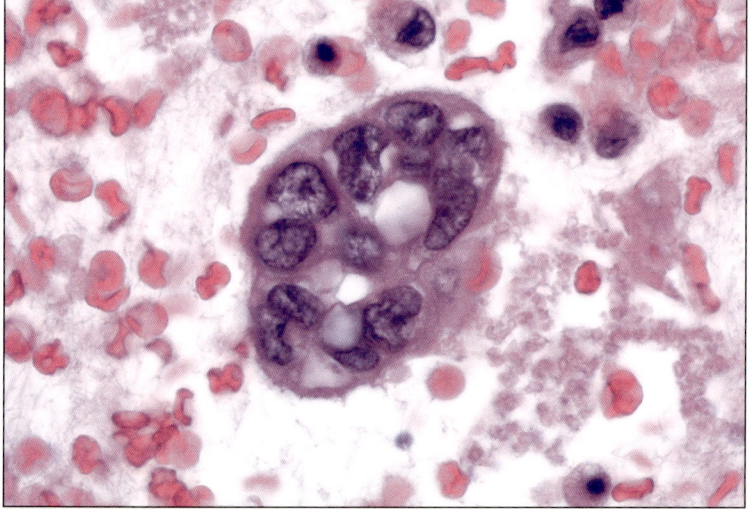

i6.30 Ovarian carcinoma. Cell block (H&E stain).

6: Peritoneal Fluid

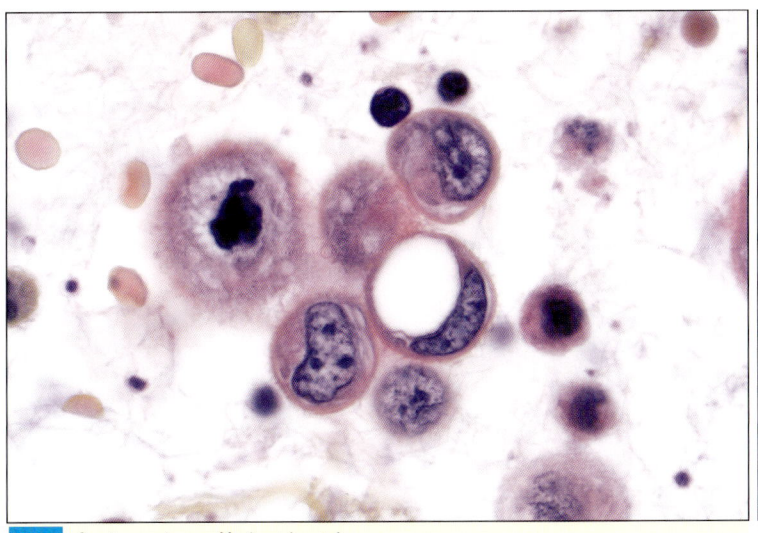

i6.31 Ovarian carcinoma. Mucicarmine stain.

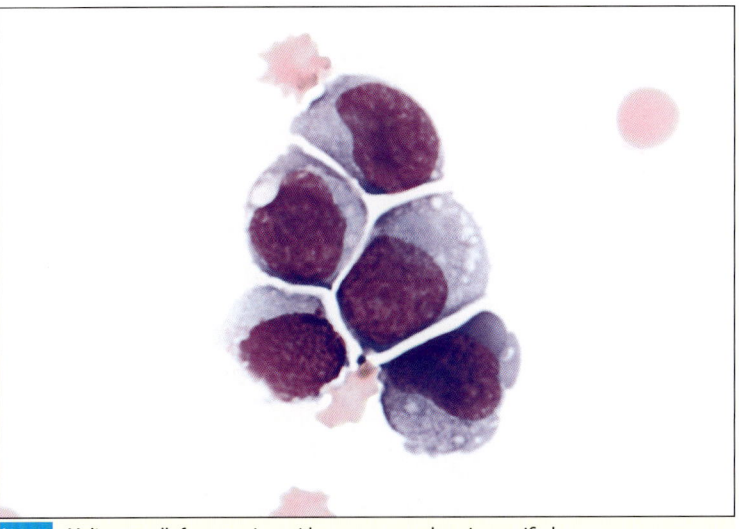

i6.34 Malignant cells from a patient with sarcoma, not otherwise specified

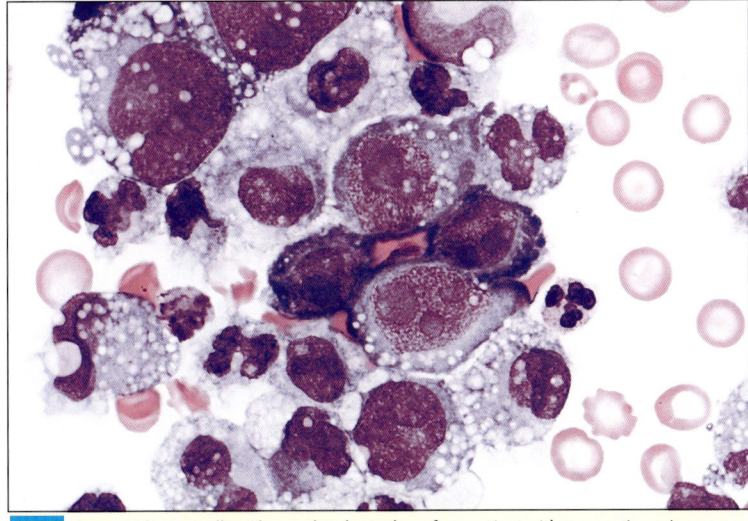

i6.32 Large malignant cells with vacuolated cytoplasm from patient with pancreatic carcinoma

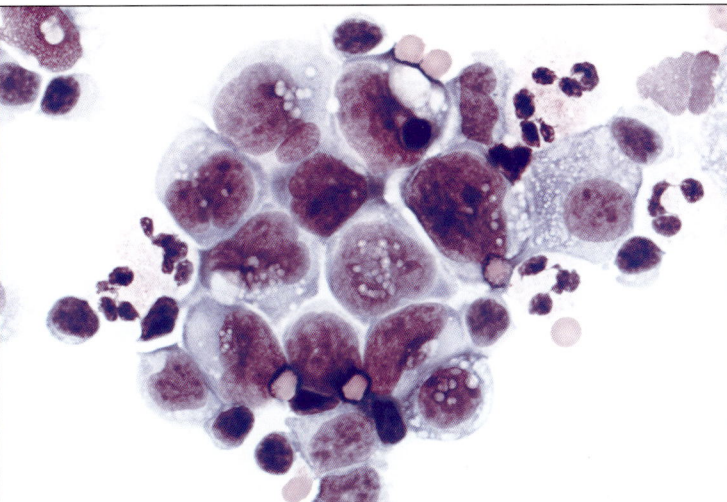

i6.35 Cluster of malignant cells from a patient with metastatic rhabdomyosarcoma

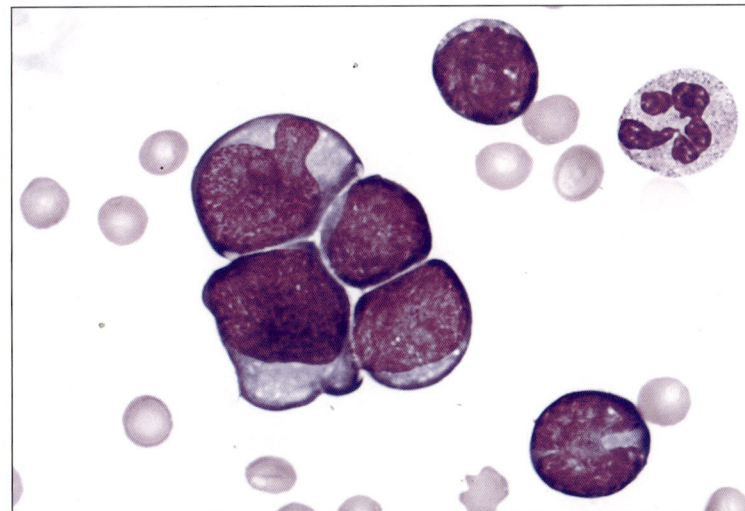

i6.33 Blastlike cells from patient with carcinoma of prostate

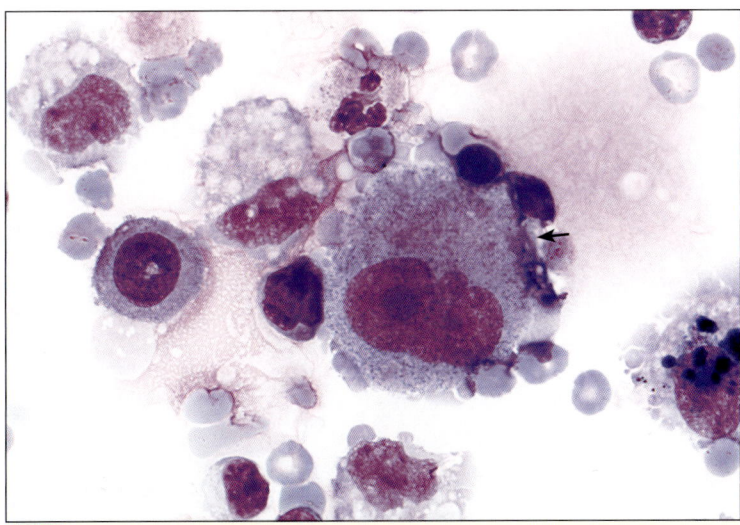

i6.36 A large binucleate malignant cell (arrow) from a patient with metastatic melanoma

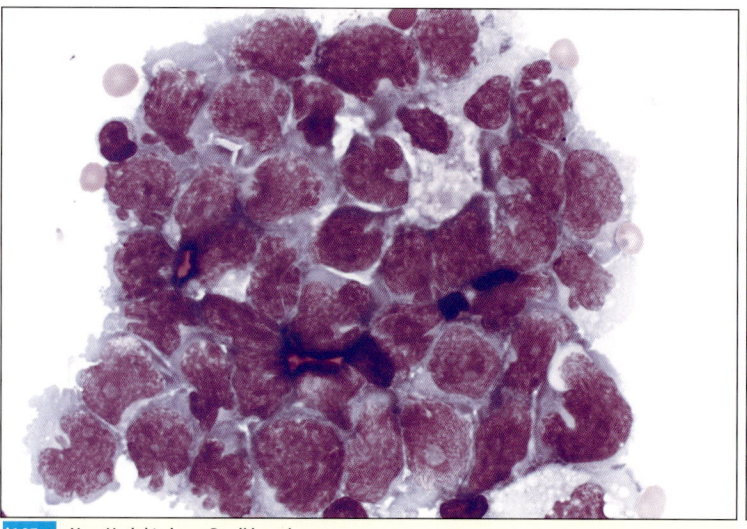

i6.37 Non-Hodgkin large B cell lymphoma

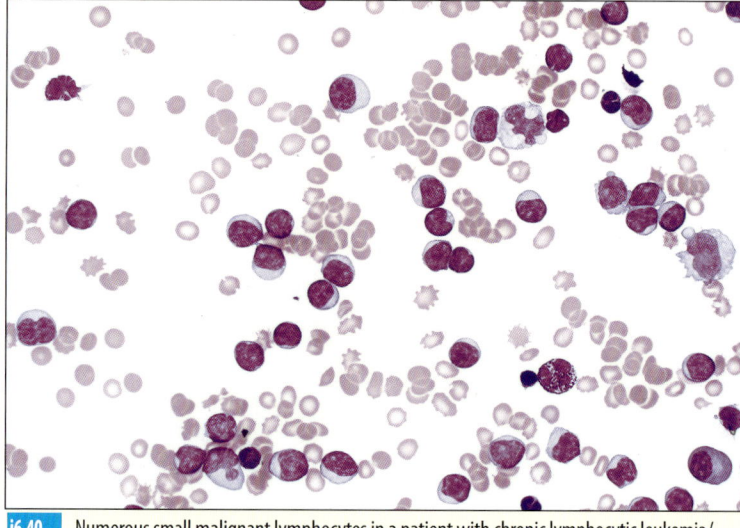

i6.40 Numerous small malignant lymphocytes in a patient with chronic lymphocytic leukemia/small lymphocytic lymphoma

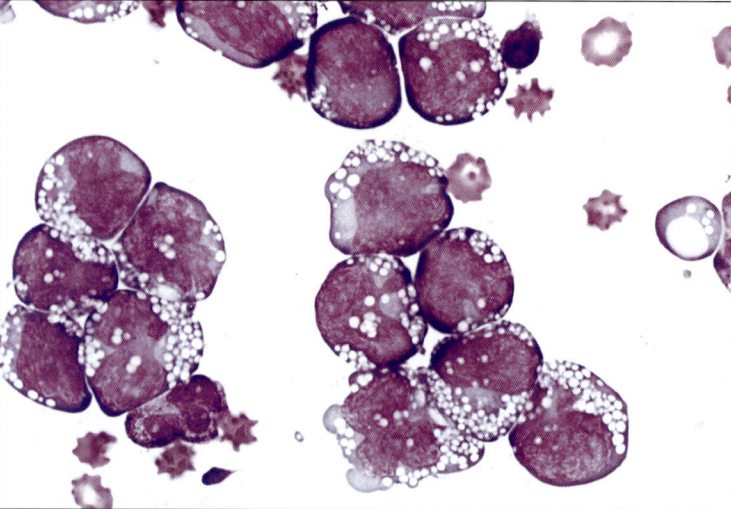

i6.38 Non-Hodgkin large B cell lymphoma cells with vacuolated cytoplasm

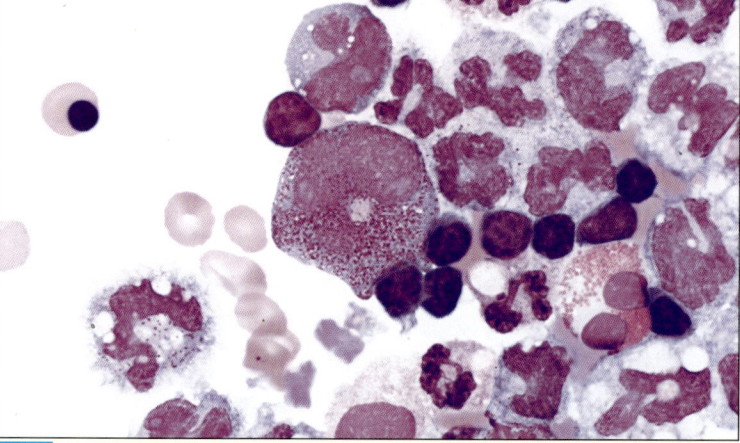

i6.41 Immature myeloid cells & nucleated red blood cells in a patient with a myeloproliferative neoplasm

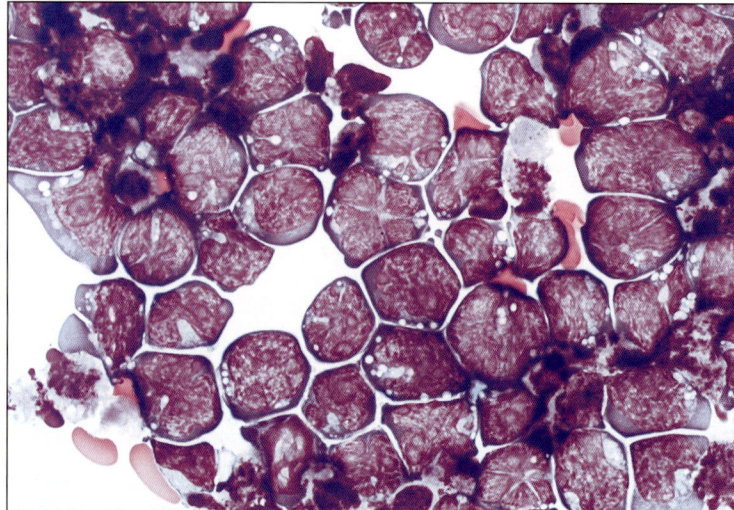

i6.39 Burkitt lymphoma from a child with intestinal obstruction

cytology has good sensitivity for detecting peritoneal carcinomatosis. Malignant neoplasms produce peritoneal effusions through a variety of mechanisms and all effusions do not contain malignant cells. The cytologic examination is only expected to be positive in patients who have tumor cells lining the peritoneum with shedding of cells into the peritoneal fluid. Malignant ascites is almost always associated with a poor prognosis.

The most common malignant neoplasms associated with peritoneal effusion, in decreasing order of frequency, are ovarian carcinoma, breast carcinoma, malignant lymphoma/leukemia, and adenocarcinomas of the stomach, colon, and rectum **t6.5** [PMID 3469856].

Malignant peritoneal effusions are usually exudates. The leukocyte count is variable and usually shows a predominance of lymphocytes but a variable number of neutrophils may also be present. Often many mesothelial cells are seen. Again, it is essential that the examiner be familiar with the variable appearance of mesothelial cells since they frequently may resemble malignant cells.

No single microscopic feature allows one to distinguish malignancy from a reactive benign process with certainty, but malignant cells frequently have a large cell size, a higher N:C ratio, nuclear hyperchromasia with irregularities of the chromatin pattern, large nucleoli, and increased mitotic activity i6.25-i6.40. However, many exceptions to this exist. For a more detailed discussion of different types of malignant cells, the reader is referred to Chapter 5. Immunohistochemistry is frequently helpful in difficult cases in determining the type/origin of the malignancy. Flow cytometry immunophenotyping is used in evaluating leukemias and lymphomas.

Of the malignant lymphomas associated with peritoneal effusions, the most common are non-Hodgkin lymphomas i6.37-i6.40. In children, the lymphomas usually involve the small intestine and may be associated with acute intestinal obstruction due to intussusception. When this is associated with a peritoneal effusion, a cytologic examination may be diagnostic. >80% of the non-Hodgkin lymphomas involving the peritoneal cavity are of the B cell phenotype.

Peritoneal washings are used to document early signs of intraabdominal spread in ovarian and other gynecologic carcinomas and sometimes in carcinoma of the gastrointestinal tract. Some of the difficulties involved in the interpretation of peritoneal washings are the frequent presence of sheets of mesothelial cells (coelomic epithelium), Müllerian inclusions, ciliated columnar epithelial cells from the Fallopian tube, and endometrial cells (endometriosis). Since these cellular elements are usually not present in paracentesis fluid, they may cause problems in the cytologic examination and be mistaken for malignant cells [PMID 3348055].

Immunohistochemical studies may be confusing unless carefully interpreted in conjunction with morphologic finding and the clinical history.

A number of other laboratory parameters may be useful in the differentiation between malignancy related ascites and nonmalignant ascites. These are discussed further in the chemical analysis and tumor marker sections.

Chemical analysis

Most chemical measurements of ascites are performed in order to distinguish between transudative and exudative processes. The SAAG is the recommended firstline test for this purpose [PMID 20595402]. The utility of all other chemical testing is more limited and should be restricted to specific clinical inquiries that align with patient symptoms t6.6. Measurement of most of the analytes discussed within this chapter may be performed similarly to serum measurements. Caution should be taken to first confirm the analyte can be detected in ascitic fluid and that lower concentrations can be detected by the serum assay.

t6.6	Miscellaneous peritoneal fluid analysis
Analyte	Associated clinical disorder(s)
Albumin	Transudate vs exudate
Bilirubin	Gall bladder rupture
Cholesterol	Malignant ascites
Lactate	Bacterial peritonitis
Alkaline phosphatase	Bowel perforation
Adenosine deaminase	Tuberculosis
Amylase isoenzymes	Pancreatitis, ovarian and Fallopian tube carcinoma
Lipase	Pancreatic ascites*

*Inflammation, pseudocyst, traumatic injury, malignancy

Protein & albumin

The measurement of total protein in peritoneal fluid has generally been limited to classification of the fluid as either a transudate or exudate. Classically, fluids containing <30 g/L (3.0 g/dL) of total protein have been defined as transudates, while those having ≥30 g/L have been classified as exudates. However, this classification is an oversimplification and there are many exceptions. As a result, the measurement of total protein is only of limited value in the assessment of peritoneal fluid.

Measurement of albumin to calculate the SAAG provides considerably more useful and reliable information and is the recommended test for separating transudates from exudates [PMID 20595402]. Gradients >1.1 g/dL are indicative of transudates caused by high hydrostatic pressure often due to cirrhosis [PMID 9308124]. Gradients below this cutoff are usually associated with malignancy. Additionally, tuberculosis and most cases of bacterial peritonitis, pancreatic ascites, chronic renal failure and intraabdominal neoplasms are usually associated with fluids having protein concentrations >30 g/L (3.0 g/dL). Conversely, in spontaneous bacterial peritonitis the protein concentration reportedly averages 18 g/L (1.8 g/dL) [PMID 4938274]. Serum and ascites specimens should be obtained and measured simultaneously in order to properly calculate the gradient.

Bilirubin, urea nitrogen & creatinine

Choleperitoneum, the presence of bile in the peritoneal cavity, is a rare but critically important disorder to identify. Bilirubin provides the best and most direct marker for the presence of bile in the peritoneal space [PMID 3680904]. In studying the total bilirubin content in the ascitic fluid and serum of patients with various causes of ascites, Runyon [PMID 3680904] established the "normal range" of ascitic fluid bilirubin and the ascitic fluid/serum bilirubin ratio (mean ± SD) as 0.7 ± 0.8 mg/dL and 0.38 ± 0.44, respectively. Ascitic fluid bilirubin >6.0 mg/dL and an ascitic fluid/serum bilirubin ratio >1.0 is characteristic of choleperitoneum due to a ruptured gall bladder. While the SAAG provides the best overall accuracy for identifying transudates vs exudates, ascitic fluid/serum bilirubin ratios >0.6 have been statistically associated with exudative processes [PMID 9517648].

Of note, bile is comprised of conjugated bilirubin. Therefore, both direct and total bilirubin assays routinely used to measure serum concentrations are acceptable for use in ascites fluid.

Similar to determining inappropriate bile leakage into the peritoneum by utilizing bile measurements, urea nitrogen and creatinine measurements may help identify inappropriate sample acquisition or rupture of the urinary bladder. Significantly increased concentrations of urea nitrogen and creatinine in the peritoneal fluid compared with normal serum values indicate sample aspiration from the urinary bladder. Elevated concentrations of these analytes in the fluid with a high serum urea nitrogen value and normal serum creatinine concentrations suggest rupture of the urinary bladder. Leakage or rupture may be attributed to surgery or other trauma.

Amylase & lipase

Under normal conditions, peritoneal fluid amylase values are comparable to plasma concentrations. An amylase determination may be useful for determining pancreas related causes of ascites [PMID 14206200]. Elevations of ascitic fluid amylase concentrations 3× above the reference serum value reportedly occur in up to 90% of patients with acute or traumatic pancreatitis or pancreatic pseudocyst [PMID 2437177]. Conversely, ~10% of patients with pancreatic disease have normal serum and ascitic fluid amylase concentrations. Striking differences between the ascitic fluid and serum amylase concentrations have generally been considered a highly reliable indicator of pancreatic disease. Nevertheless, increased ascitic fluid amylase activity is not limited to pancreatic disorders and increased fluid amylase concentrations have been reported in 77% of 26 cases with gastroduodenal perforation [PMID 13498647], small bowel strangulation with or without perforation [PMID 14206200] and acute mesenteric venous thrombosis [PMID 13563173]. Due to this finding and the low prevalence of pancreatic ascites, amylase measurements are not recommended for routine fluid analysis.

Determination of the serum amylase activity on admission has been advocated by some as an aid in the diagnosis of traumatic injury to the pancreas; others have argued that serum amylase levels lack adequate sensitivity and specificity in the evaluation of pancreatic injury. Salivary amylase isoenzyme determination may be useful in the identification of nonpancreatic sources of amylase elevations. The measurement of ascitic fluid lipase activity has been considered complementary to—and perhaps more reliable than—amylase determination in the diagnosis of pancreatic ascites [PMID 1200007]. Differences in clearance rates may result in lipase concentrations being elevated longer than amylase with less fluctuation.

Cholesterol & triglycerides

Cholesterol concentrations have been reported to be significantly higher in malignant ascitic fluids than nonmalignant or cirrhotic fluids. A cholesterol cutoff of 48 mg/dL has been reported to have 96.5% sensitivity and 96.6% specificity, with overall diagnostic accuracy for diagnosing malignant ascites of 96.6% [PMID 8294324]. Other studies have reported a cholesterol cutoff of 46 mg/dL was associated with 97% [PMID 2837370] and 87.5% [PMID 3247589] diagnostic accuracy for malignancy. Jungst et al [PMID 3957233] also noted that the best discrimination between malignant and cirrhotic ascites was attributed to cutoff values of 48 mg/dL for cholesterol, 0.6 mmol/L for phospholipids, and 65 mg/dL for triglycerides. These values resulted in a diagnostic efficiency of 92.3% for cholesterol, 79.4% for phospholipids and 72.8% for triglycerides. They and others have concluded that the measurement of ascitic fluid cholesterol is an excellent, cost effective general method to discriminate ascites due to cirrhosis from that caused by malignant disease [PMID 7548806]. However, Runyon warned of the lack of specificity of markers such as cholesterol and fibronectin in ascitic fluid, possibly leading to exhaustive searches for nonexistent tumors [PMID 8289030].

Extravasation of milky chyle (lymph) into the peritoneal cavity due to trauma or obstruction of the lymphatic system results in chylous ascites (chyloperitoneum). Chyle is composed of triglyceride rich chylomicrons. The diagnosis of chylous ascites is commonly made by noting a milky or creamy appearance of the fluid. Lipid determinations may be useful for determining chylous from pseudochylous effusions. Cholesterol concentrations are elevated in pseudochylous effusions, while triglyceride concentrations are often higher in chylous effusions. Large numbers of leukocytes and/or necrotic debris can add to the suggestion of a chylous effusion. It has been suggested that the most reliable way to be certain that an ascitic fluid is truly chylous is to demonstrate the presence of chylomicrons by lipoprotein electrophoresis [PMID 841541]. Nevertheless, the occurrence of chylous ascites is rare. The major disorders associated with chylous ascites are metastatic carcinoma, lymphoma, congenital anomalies of lymphatic vessels, and postsurgical trauma.

Lactate dehydrogenase (LDH)

LDH concentrations are often elevated in malignant abdominal effusions when compared with simultaneously determined serum values. Benign effusions usually have LDH levels comparable to or less than those in the serum. For example, Boyer et al [PMID 666469] noted that none of the ascitic fluids from their patients with liver disease had levels >350 sigma units (SU). On the other hand, 8 of 14 patients (57%) with malignant effusions had LDH activities >500 SU. Ascitic fluid LDH to serum LDH ratios >0.6 increased the diagnostic sensitivity to 80%.

Lee et al reported the utility of ascitic fluid/serum LDH ratios in the early diagnosis of spontaneous bacterial peritonitis [PMID 3666966]. A cutoff value of 0.4 resulted in a diagnostic accuracy of ~74%, essentially the same as a WBC count cutoff of >300/μL or total neutrophil count of >240/μL. They found that the use of multiple tests had a better positive predictive value than a single test. Similarly, Castaldo et al reported that the combination of ascitic fluid LDH and cholesterol values discriminated between malignant ascites and cirrhotic ascites and/or hepatocellular carcinoma in 100% of cases [PMID 8131285].

pH

The pH of ascitic fluid has been proposed as a means to detect spontaneous bacterial peritonitis. pH values from the sterile ascites of cirrhotic patients may be used to approximate expected values in noninfected individuals and range from 7.35-7.59 [PMID 2029997]. Infection is suggested when ascitic fluid pH of <7.31 is observed in cirrhotic alcoholics in the absence of systemic acidosis [PMID 6807793]. Other studies have also supported the measurement of ascitic fluid pH as a useful aid in differentiating spontaneous bacterial peritonitis from noninfectious hepatic ascites. An arterial ascitic fluid pH gradient >0.10 was supportive of spontaneous bacterial peritonitis [PMID 3967867, PMID 3967868, PMID 3956943, PMID 3956944]. These studies also recommended that total leukocyte counts >1,000/µL and total neutrophil counts >500/µL supported the diagnosis. Esophogeal ruptures may also cause acidic pH values. Furthermore, Attali et al [PMID 3956944] noted that cirrhotic patients with an ascitic fluid pH <7.15 had a poor prognosis.

However, due to the lack of sensitivity and specificity of this measurement, it is reported that ascitic pH does not contribute to clinical decision making in the case of peritoneal infection. While ascitic pH does correlate well with neutrophil counts, the pH measurement was 0% sensitive in detecting the presence of bacteria when neutrophils were not present [PMID 2029997].

Lactate

Similar to pH, lactate measurements in ascitic fluid have been proposed to aid in identification of spontaneous bacterial peritonitis or other infectious processes, particularly in the cirrhotic patient [PMID 7307856]. The authors noted a significantly higher lactate concentration in patients with bacterial peritonitis (mean 77 mg/dL) compared to those with uninfected ascites (mean 14 mg/dL). Lactate measurement was at least as sensitive as WBC counts for diagnosing peritonitis. Stassen et al report 90% sensitivity and specificity when a lactate concentration of 40 mg/dL is used as a cutoff [PMID 3956943].

Glucose

The measurement of glucose in peritoneal fluid has generally been considered clinically useful only in selected cases, particularly in bacterial peritonitis and in differentiating infectious and malignant ascites from other causes. An ascitic fluid/serum glucose ratio of <1.0 has been reported in 70%-80% of patients with spontaneous bacterial peritonitis [PMID 3666966]. Ascitic fluid glucose concentrations are reportedly 50 mg/dL or less in 30%-60% of tuberculosis peritonitis cases [PMID 4793122, PMID 998592] and in ~50% of cases with abdominal carcinomatosis [PMID 4793122].

Runyon and Hoefs analyzed the ascitic fluid of 22 patients prior to the onset of spontaneous bacterial peritonitis, during infection and/or following treatment [PMID 3979958]. They found that although the ascitic fluid/serum glucose ratio did decrease significantly with infection, neither ascitic fluid total protein nor absolute ascitic fluid glucose concentrations changed during the infection or after treatment.

It is evident from these and other studies that, in general, the measurement of ascitic fluid glucose has relatively low sensitivity and specificity. As such, it is usually not helpful in elucidating the etiology of a peritoneal effusion.

Alkaline phosphatase

Alkaline phosphatase activity is high in the intestinal tract; therefore measurement in peritoneal fluid may be helpful for evaluating certain abdominal disorders. Alkaline phosphatase concentrations in peritoneal fluid may be significantly elevated over serum reference values in patients with simple or ischemic obstruction, strangulation, intestinal perforation or traumatic hemoperitoneum [PMID 5044540, PMID 1246661]. Importantly, serum alkaline phosphatase concentrations are usually normal in these patients.

Measurement of alkaline phosphatase in peritoneal fluid has reported utility in the differentiation between primary bacterial peritonitis and bacterial peritonitis caused by perforation of the bowel. The latter condition will present with higher concentrations of alkaline phosphatase (>240 U/L) in the peritoneal fluid than the former, with 92% sensitivity and 88% specificity [PMID 11281549].

Measurement of alkaline phosphatase in peritoneal lavage fluid is a sensitive marker for small intestinal injury in the immediate posttraumatic period [PMID 3964997]. The activity of other enzymes, notably LDH, aldolase, aspartate aminotransferase and creatine kinase is also elevated; however, these measurements are much less specific than alkaline phosphatase for diagnosis [PMID 5044540, PMID 1246661]. In isolated traumatic liver injuries, both serum and peritoneal fluid may show pronounced elevations of aspartate aminotransferase, alanine aminotransferase and LDH.

Electrolytes

Evaluation of electrolyte concentrations in peritoneal fluid does not offer diagnostic information beyond that provided by plasma concentrations. Measurement of potassium, chloride, sodium, calcium, bicarbonate and magnesium are therefore not recommended in this fluid type.

Markers of malignancy

The differential diagnosis of ascites remains a problem in clinical practice. Although ascites is most often the result of chronic liver disease or malignant neoplasms, the complete separation of these 2 causes has not been possible to date. Conventional cytology, the classic diagnostic tool for detecting malignant cells in pleural and peritoneal effusions, has varying sensitivity and specificity and is often not capable of detecting all cases of malignancy. Some reports indicate cytology alone is capable of detecting tumor cells in only 30%-40% of cases [PMID 2454957, PMID 646247]. Biochemical markers of malignancy may therefore be useful measurements in certain clinical scenarios, despite low sensitivity and specificity. It should be noted that these biochemical determinations, also referred to as tumor markers, have particular utility in monitoring response to therapy and tumor recurrence and are not used as general screening tools. A myriad of markers have been reported for use in ascitic fluid including carcinoembryonic antigen (CEA), CA125, CA19-9, fibronectin and AFP to name a few.

Early studies have shown that CEA measurements in ascitic fluid have considerable diagnostic value. Cutoffs from 3 ng/mL to 10 ng/mL have been reported [PMID 2454957, PMID 646247, PMID 11684715, PMID 23454392] with values greater than these cutoffs associated with malignant effusions. A 5 ng/mL cutoff for CEA reportedly provided the highest sensitivity and specificity (51% and 97%, respectively) [PMID 11684715].

CA125 may also prove useful in ascitic fluid determinations. Although CA125 concentrations may be elevated in numerous nonmalignant situations, very high values are often associated with ovarian malignancy. Hunter et al found that patients with ovarian cancer had CA125 concentrations >200 U/mL with 95% sensitivity and 99% specificity [PMID 2404835]. Only 2 of 165 patients with benign gynecologic disorders had peritoneal fluid CA125 concentrations above this cutoff. However, other reports indicate contradictory findings and question the utility of CA125 in ascitic samples.

Many studies investigate the utility of measuring several tumor markers and/or proteins at once, with or without additional cytologic examination. Pinto et al used cutoffs of 6.3 ng/mL for CEA and 3,652 U/mL for CA125 to identify malignant effusions due to carcinomas of the lung, breast, gastrointestinal tract and ovarian mucinous carcinoma in pleural and peritoneal fluid [PMID 1616424]. They reported sensitivities between 75% and 100% and overall specificity of 98%. These authors concluded that the adjunctive measurement of CEA and CA125 in pleural and peritoneal effusions enhances the sensitivity of cytologic diagnosis. In addition, these measurements may be helpful in predicting the primary tumor site in patients who present with effusions secondary to carcinoma of an unknown primary origin.

In a study of 9 separate measurements, Gerbes et al found that cholesterol and fibronectin measurements were the most sensitive for determining malignant from nonmalignant ascites [PMID 1913524]. Each had a negative predictive value of 92%, which was increased to 100% when CEA and cytology were added after the initial screening tests. They proposed ascitic fluid samples with >45 mg/dL of cholesterol should be further tested for CEA and cytology for optimum diagnostic power. Another study found the combined measurement of 5 different proteins in ascitic fluid (total protein, LDH, TNF-α, C4 and haptoglobin) correctly classified 89% of cases in a multivariate analysis study [PMID 10749324]. Similarly, Alexandrakis et al reported that the ascites:serum ratios of albumin and IL-1α allowed for 100% correct classification of malignant ascites [PMID 11288954].

However, another investigation has concluded that measuring tumor markers in ascitic fluid offers no advantage over serum analysis when malignant ascites is suspected [PMID 19215676]. Among other markers, they included CEA, CA125, CA19-9 and AFP in their studies comparing ascites and serum measurements from adults with malignant and benign disease. These markers were highly correlated between the sample types, indicating adequacy of serum measurement.

Microbiologic examination

Infection of the peritoneal cavity may occur spontaneously in patients with chronic ascites, such as in those with cirrhosis. It may also occur as a result of leakage or rupture of the gastrointestinal tract, during chronic continuous peritoneal dialysis, or as a complication of a surgical procedure. In cases of rupture or leakage from hollow organs or following surgery, infection is often evident as a localized abscess or generalized peritonitis. Cultures typically grow mixed aerobic and anaerobic flora [PMID 4028657]. Early diagnosis of bacterial peritonitis is often difficult due to insensitive and nonspecific testing mechanisms.

Spontaneous bacterial peritonitis (SBP) is relatively common in patients with hepatic cirrhosis, and since its first description in 1963, the mortality rate has dropped dramatically from upwards of 90% to ~30%, largely due to prompt diagnosis and appropriate antimicrobial therapy [PMID 16680233]. In fact, 1 study showed overall mortality in patients admitted with SBP of 27.8%, but only 2.2% were directly attributable to the infection [PMID 2019378]. Despite this mortality decrease, SBP still remains the most common bacterial infection in patients with advanced cirrhosis (more common than pneumonia and urinary tract infections) [PMID 15920324].

The ascitic fluid in SBP is cloudy, and the polymorphonuclear (PMN) lymphocyte count must exceed 250 cells/mL and a single (typically hematogenously seeded) microorganism should be recovered in culture t6.7 [PMID 4028657, ISBN-10:1416061894, ISBN-10:0192629220]. *Escherichia coli* and *Klebsiella pneumoniae* account for the majority of SBP, while *Streptococcus* species (especially *S pneumoniae* and viridans group *Streptococci*) are the second most frequently isolated [PMID 19266595]. Various Gram– and Gram+ organisms have been described and account for ~25% of SBP [PMID 19266595]. Despite the fact that the bowel is comprised of mostly anaerobes, SBP is rarely attributed to anaerobes. The protein content in ascitic fluid specimens from patients with SBP is unusually low (<2.0 g/dL) in most cases, often <1.0 g/dL [PMID 3770358].

t6.7 Test patterns for ascitic fluid infections*

	PMNs (cells/mL)	Bacterial culture results
Spontaneous bacterial peritonitis	≥250	Monomicrobial
Secondary bacterial peritonitis	≥250	Polymicrobial
Culture negative granulocytic ascites	≥250	Culture negative
Polymicrobial ascites	<250	Polymicrobial
Monomicrobial nongranulocytic ascites	<250	Monomicrobial

*Adapted from Sheer et al [PMID 15920324]

Specimens for culture and stain should be submitted to the microbiology laboratory promptly in sterile collection tubes at room temperature and if possible, blood culture liquid broth bottles should be inoculated at bedside to maximize the yield of causative organisms. Conventional culture on solid media may be performed; however the utility of blood culture bottles has been shown in a prospective study to improve organism recovery in culture from 43% (solid media) to 93% (blood bottles) [PMID 3049220]. The recommended volume of inoculum is 10 mL, which not only improves recovery by 50%, but also shortens the turnaround time to culture positivity [PMID 3049220]. Gram stains may only be positive in <25% of cases of SBP (cytocentrifugation cannot typically be performed due to turbidity); however the Gram stain is important to establish whether an ascitic fluid represents a monomicrobial infection (eg, SBP or monomicrobial nongranulocytic ascites), indicative of a polymicrobial infection (eg, secondary bacterial peritonitis, polymicrobial ascites), and also whether yeast (eg, *Candida*) is present (a factor that would dramatically alter empiric antimicrobial therapy). The spectrum of ascitic fluid infections are characterized in t6.7.

To satisfy the criteria for secondary bacterial peritonitis (versus spontaneous) 2 of the following characteristics must be established for the ascitic fluid: glucose concentration <50 mg/dL, total protein content >1 g/dL, or LD greater than the upper limit of normal for the assay being performed [PMID 2293571]. Using these criteria, bowel perforation can be predicted with 100% sensitivity, though the specificity is only 45% [PMID 2293571]. The leukocyte and neutrophil counts are generally not useful in distinguishing between spontaneous and secondary bacterial peritonitis because they typically overlap for each condition. However, 1 pattern that may further characterize the 2 presentations is that neutrophil counts decrease exponentially after antimicrobial therapy in cases of SBP, whereas neutrophil counts remain relatively constant or increase in subsequent testing in secondary bacterial peritonitis [PMID 3729637].

Peritonitis is a common problem in patients with chronic renal disease undergoing continuous ambulatory peritoneal dialysis (CAPD). The offending organisms may include bacteria, mycobacteria, or fungi. The spectrum of bacteria is quite broad and includes Gram+ (~70%), Gram– (~28%), and anaerobes (2%) [Troidle 2006]. Many of these bacteria are of environmental origin in addition to normal human gut and skin flora. Recent reports have also described animal derived *Pasturella* peritonitis in patients with CAPD [PMID 15109592]. A common risk appears to be pet cats and/or dogs biting/scratching dialysis tubing and introducing *Pasteurella* species [PMID 15109592].

In addition to *Mycobacterium tuberculosis*, *M avium/intercellulare* and the rapid growing mycobacteria (Runyon group IV) are considered environmental mycobacteria associated with CAPD peritonitis [PMID 8452953, PMID 8110951]. *Candida* species are the most common cause of fungal peritonitis, and this is true in CAPD as well [PMID 21976010]. *Aspergillus* and zygomycetes have also been reported as causative agents of peritonitis in CAPD; however their incidence is considered rare in comparison to *Candida* [PMID 12742319].

In up to 20% of cases, no organisms will be identified by culture [PMID 7999819]. There are several reasons that this may occur: the organism load may be below the sensitivity of the culture method, cultures were not appropriately performed or were exclusively selective (eg, no fungal or mycobacterial growth media incorporated), or a noninfectious inflammatory response was present (eg, no organisms were involved despite a cloudy dialysate [PMID 11208038]). As an additional aid in the diagnosis of bacterial peritonitis, acridine orange stain can provide better visualization of bacteria than Gram stain for evaluating cases of peritonitis in CAPD (particularly in a very cloudy specimen), though this method requires a fluorescent microscope with appropriate filters in the microbiology laboratory [PMID 3729637].

Tuberculous peritonitis (TBP) is a common cause of ascites in developing countries; however with increasing rates of pulmonary tuberculosis in developed countries, it is not surprising that the incidence of extrapulmonary tuberculosis have also increased. This is true particularly for TBP in CAPD patients [PMID 10913399]. The diagnosis of TBP is often difficult to make and is frequently overlooked, since the classic features of prolonged fever (59%), weight loss (61%), exudative ascites (73%), and a positive skin test result (53%) may not always be present or may not be clinically recognized [PMID 16197489]. TBP often presents as culture negative peritonitis or culture positive peritonitis for which standard antimicrobials are not effective and for which there is no suspicion of tuberculosis [PMID 19270209].

In cases of TBP, the peritoneal fluid total protein level exceeds 2.5 g/dL. However, the SAAG value is thought to be of more diagnostic value than the total protein level and is typically very low (<11 g/L) in 100% of cases of TBP [ISBN-10: 0721648363]. The specificity of SAAG is however quite low [PMID 16197489]. SAAG is calculated by measuring the serum and ascitic albumin at the same time and subtracting the ascitic value from the serum value. When either elevated total protein or low SAAG is demonstrated, and the cause of the effusion is unknown, acid-fast stains and cultures for acid-fast bacilli should be initiated. It should be noted however, that acid-fast stains may be positive in only 3% of TBP cases [PMID 16197489]. Fluid cultures are positive in up to 83% of cases, particularly when 1 L of peritoneal fluid is concentrated and inoculated in a mycobacterial blood culture bottle; however standard mycobacterial cultures are only positive in 35% of cases [PMID 16197489].

Adenosine deaminase is also a valuable diagnostic tool in TBP, with a metaanalysis revealing excellent sensitivity and specificity (exceeding 90%) in over 16 well designed studies using a cutoff of >30 U/L [PMID 16197489, PMID 24049517]. A peritoneal biopsy may also be of diagnostic assistance, but may not be appropriate in all patients depending on clinical stability and overall presentation. Despite its value in smear positive pulmonary tuberculosis, molecular methods have not been studied in depth for TBP.

Special studies

Most of the studies that are discussed here are related to malignancy. Those relevant to, for example, microbiologic studies, eg, PCR, are discussed in the corresponding section. As noted above, there are a number of serum tumor markers that can be assayed in peritoneal fluid. They are generally of limited clinical utility since they do not significantly add to what can be obtained from serum measurements of the same antigen, eg, CEA or CA125. In contrast, there is great utility for flow cytometric analysis in lymphocyte rich fluids for the detection of monoclonal populations that herald a non-Hodgkin lymphoma diagnosis. Similarly, immunohistochemistry, typically performed on cell blocks is useful for the identification of malignancies, the large majority of which are carcinomas and then, more specifically, adenocarcinomas. The key distinction is generally focused on separating "reactive/atypical" mesothelial cells from a metastatic adenocarcinoma, and much less frequently is focused on distinguishing between malignant mesothelioma and a metastatic adenocarcinoma. For these it is recommended that a panel of antibodies be used in order to reliably make a definitive diagnosis. For further reading the reader is referred to Chapter 2, which is focused on methods and special techniques, or to specialized books and articles.

Artifacts & pitfalls

- Careful correlation with clinical history is essential in the interpretation of all laboratory analyses.
- The examiner must be familiar with the many morphologic changes/artifacts seen in both benign and malignant cells in serous fluid specimens.

Key points

- The 2 most common indications for paracentesis are to rule out bacterial peritonitis and to rule out a suspected malignant neoplasm.
- The most useful tests in most patients are gross examination, cytology, stains and culture for microorganism and SAAG.
- The examiner of the microscopic examination of the peritoneal fluid specimen must be familiar with the wide range in appearance of benign mesothelial cells in order not to mistake them for malignant cells.
- The most common malignant neoplasms associated with a peritoneal effusion are, in decreasing order of frequency, ovarian carcinoma, breast carcinoma, malignant lymphoma/leukemia, and adenocarcinomas of the stomach, colon and rectum.
- The examiner must be aware that many morphologic changes/artifacts are commonly seen in both benign and malignant cells from serous fluids. In addition to the morphologic changes caused by the cells sitting in the fluid for variable periods of time, there are often changes brought about by the cytocentrifugation procedure.
- Immunohistochemistry, best done in cell blocks, using a panel of antibodies, are often very helpful in determining the type of malignancy. Flow cytometry is essential in evaluating hematologic malignancies.
- Most chemical measurements are performed in order to distinguish between transudative and exudative processes. The SAAG test is the firstline test. The utility of the other chemical tests is more limited and should be restricted to specific clinical situations.

- Spontaneous bacterial peritonitis (SBP) remains the most common bacterial infection in patients with advanced cirrhosis.
- Specimens for culture and stain should be submitted to the microbiology laboratory promptly, and if possible culture liquid broth bottles should be inoculated at bedside to maximize the yield of causative organisms. The utility of blood culture bottles will improve organism recovery in culture.
- To satisfy criteria for secondary bacterial peritonitis (vs spontaneous), 2 of the following characteristics must be established: glucose concentration <50 mg/dL, total protein content >1 g/dL, or LD greater than upper limit for the assay being performed. Using these criteria, bowel perforation can be predicted with 100% sensitivity, though specificity is only 45%.
- Tuberculous peritonitis is a common cause of ascites in developing countries. It is also seen in CAPD patients, and is often overlooked.

References

PMID 2019378 Runyon BA, McHutchison JG, Antillon MR et al [1991] Short-course vs long-course antibiotic treatment of spontaneous bacterial peritonitis. *Gastroenterology* 100:1737-1742.

PMID 2293571 Akriviadis EA, Runyon BA [1990] Utility of an algorithm in differentiating spontaneous from secondary bacterial peritonitis. *Gastroenterology* 98:127-133.

PMID 3049220 Runyon BA, Canawati HN, Akriviadis EA [1988] Optimization of ascitic fluid culture technique. *Gastroenterology* 95:1351-1355.

PMID: :3469856 Sears D, Hajdu SI [1987] The cytologic diagnosis of malignant neoplasms in pleural and peritoneal effusions. *Acta Cytol* 31:85-97.

PMID 10749324 Alexandrakis MG, Moschandrea JA, Koulocheri SA et al [2000] Discrimination between malignant and nonmalignant ascites using serum and ascitic fluid proteins in a multivariate analysis model. *Dig Dis Sci* 45(3):500-8.

PMID 10913399 Talwani R, Horvath JA [2000] Tuberculous peritonitis in patients undergoing continuous ambulatory peritoneal dialysis: case report and review. *Clin Infect Dis* 31(1):70-5.

PMID 11208038 Rocklin M, Teitelbaum I [2001] Noninfectious causes of cloudy peritoneal dialysate. *Semin Dial* 14(1):37-40.

PMID 11281549 Wu SS, Lin OS, Chen YY et al [2001] Ascitic fluid carcinoembryonic antigen and alkaline phosphatase levels for the differentiation of primary from secondary bacterial peritonitis with intestinal perforation. *J Hepatol* 34(2):215-21.

PMID 11288954 Alexandrakis MG, Moschandrea J, Kyriakou DS et al [2001] Use of a variety of biological parameters in distinguishing cirrhotic from malignant ascites. *Int J Biol Markers* 16(1):45-9.

PMID 11684715 Gulyás M, Kaposi AD, Elek G et al [2001] Value of carcinoembryonic antigen (CEA) and cholesterol assays of ascitic fluid in cases of inconclusive cytology. *J Clin Pathol* 54(11):831-5.

PMID 1200007 Sileo AV, Chawla SK, LoPresti PA [1975] Pancreatic ascites: diagnostic importance of ascitic lipase. *Am J Dig Dis* 20(12):1110-4.

PMID 1246661 Delany HM, Moss CM, Carnevale N [1976] The use of enzyme analysis of peritoneal blood in the clinical assessment of abdominal organ injury. *Surg Gynecol Obstet* 142(2):167-7.

PMID 12742319 Nannini EC, Paphitou NI, Ostrosky-Zeichner L [2003] Peritonitis due to *Aspergillus* and zygomycetes in patients undergoing peritoneal dialysis: report of 2 cases and review of the literature. *Diagn Microbiol Infect Dis* 46(1):49-54.

PMID: 13498647] Amerson JR, Howard JM, Vowles KD [1958] The amylase concentration in serum and peritoneal fluid following acute perforation of gastroduodenal ulcers. *Ann Surg* 147(2):245-50.

PMID 13563173 Gray EB Jr, Amadore E [1958] Acute mesenteric venous thrombosis simulating acute pancreatitis; the value of peritoneal fluid analysis. *JAMA* 167(14):1734-6.

PMID 14206200 Mansberger AR Jr [1964] The diagnostic value of abdominal paracentesis with special reference to peritoneal fluid ammonial levels. *Am J Gastroenterol* 42:150-64.

PMID 15109592 Cooke FJ, Kodjo A, Clutterbuck EJ et al [2004] A case of *Pasteurella multocida* peritoneal dialysis-associated peritonitis and review of the literature. *Int J Infect Dis* 8(3):171-4.

PMID 15920324 Sheer TA, Runyon BA [2005] Spontaneous bacterial peritonitis. *Dig Dis* 23(1):39-46.

PMID 1616215 Runyon BA, Montano AA, Evangelos A, et al. The SAAG is superior to the exudate–transudate concept in the differential diagnosis of ascites. *Ann Intern Med* 1992;117:215.

PMID 1616424 Pinto MM, Bernstein LH, Rudolph RA et al [1992] Diagnostic efficiency of carcinoembryonic antigen and CA125 in the cytologic evaluation of effusions. *Arch Pathol Lab Med* 116(6):626-31.

PMID 16197489 Sanai FM, Bzeizi KI [2005] Systematic review: tuberculous peritonitis—presenting features, diagnostic strategies and treatment. *Aliment Pharmacol Ther* 22(8):685-700.

PMID 16680233 Caruntu FA, Benea L [2006] Spontaneous bacterial peritonitis: pathogenesis, diagnosis, treatment. *J Gastrointestin Liver Dis* 15(1):51-6.

PMID 1913524 Gerbes AL, Jüngst D, Xie YN et al [1991] Ascitic fluid analysis for the differentiation of malignancy-related and nonmalignant ascites. Proposal of a diagnostic sequence. *Cancer* 68(8):1808-14.

PMID 19215676 Tuzun Y, Celik Y, Bayan K et al [2009] Correlation of tumour markers in ascitic fluid and serum: are measurements of ascitic tumour markers a futile attempt? *J Int Med Res* 37(1):79-86.

PMID 19266595 Koulaouzidis A, Bhat S, Saeed AA [2009] Spontaneous bacterial peritonitis. *World J Gastroenterol* 15(9):1042-9.

PMID 19270209 Akpolat T [2009] Tuberculous peritonitis. *Perit Dial Int* 29Suppl2:S166-9.

PMID 2029997 Runyon BA, Antillon MR [1991] Ascitic fluid pH and lactate: insensitive and nonspecific tests in detecting ascitic fluid infection. *Hepatology* 13(5):929-35.

PMID 20595402 Tarn AC, Lapworth R [2010] Biochemical analysis of ascitic (peritoneal) fluid: what should we measure? *Ann Clin Biochem* 47(Pt 5):397-407.

PMID 21976010 Carneiro HA, Mavrakis A, Mylonakis E [2011] *Candida* peritonitis: an update on the latest research and treatments. *World J Surg* 35(12):2650-9.

PMID 23454392 Kaleta EJ, Tolan NV, Ness KA et al [2013] CEA, AFP and CA19-9 analysis in peritoneal fluid to differentiate causes of ascites formation. *Clin Biochem* 46(9):814-8. doi: 10.1016/j.clinbiochem.2013.02.010. Epub 2013 Feb 27.

PMID 2404835 Hunter VJ, Weinberg JB, Haney AF et al [1990] CA125 in peritoneal fluid and serum from patients with benign gynecologic conditions and ovarian cancer. *Gynecol Oncol* 36(2):161-5.

PMID 24049517 Shen YC, Wang T, Chen L et al [2013] Diagnostic accuracy of adenosine deaminase for tuberculous peritonitis: a meta-analysis. *Arch Med Sci* 9(4):601-7.

PMID 2437177 Runyon BA [1987] Amylase levels in ascitic fluid. *J Clin Gastroenterol* 9(2):172-4.

PMID 2454957 Mezger J, Permanetter W, Gerbes AL et al [1988] Tumour associated antigens in diagnosis of serous effusions. *J Clin Pathol* 41(6):633-43.

PMID 2837370 Prieto M, Gómez-Lechón MJ, Hoyos M et al [1988] Diagnosis of malignant ascites. Comparison of ascitic fibronectin, cholesterol, and serum ascites albumin difference. *Dig Dis Sci* 33(7):833-8.

PMID 3247589 Mortensen PB, Kristensen SD, Bloch A et al [1988] Diagnostic value of ascitic fluid cholesterol levels in the prediction of malignancy. *Scand J Gastroenterol* 23(9):1085-8.

PMID 3341375 Chan MK, Chow L, Lam SS, et al [1988] Peritoneal eosinophilia in patients on continuous ambulatory peritoneal dialysis: a prospective study. *Am J Kidney Dis* 11:180-183.

PMID 3348055 Zuna RE, Mitchell ML [1988] Cytologic findings in peritoneal washings associated with benign gynecologic disease. *Acta Cytol* 32:139-147.

PMID 3666966 Lee HH, Carlson RW, Bull DM [1987] Early diagnosis of spontaneous bacterial peritonitis: values of ascitic fluid variables. *Infection* 15(4):232-6.

PMID 3680904 Runyon BA [1987] Ascitic fluid bilirubin concentration as a key to choleperitoneum. *J Clin Gastroenterol* 9(5):543-5.

PMID 3729637 Runyon BA, Hoefs JC [1986] Spontaneous vs secondary bacterial peritonitis. *Arch Intern Med* 146:1563-1565.

PMID 3770358 Runyon BA [1986] Low-protein-concentration ascitic fluid is predisposed to spontaneous bacterial peritonitis. *Gastroenterology* 91:1343-1346.

PMID 3956943 Stassen WN, McCullough AJ, Bacon BR et al [1986] Immediate diagnostic criteria for bacterial infection of ascitic fluid. Evaluation of ascitic fluid polymorphonuclear leukocyte count, pH, and lactate concentration, alone and in combination. *Gastroenterology* 90(5 Pt 1):1247-54.

PMID 3956944 Attali P, Turner K, Pelletier G et al [1986] pH of ascitic fluid: diagnostic and prognostic value in cirrhotic and noncirrhotic patients. *Gastroenterology* 90(5 Pt 1):1255-60.

PMID 3957233 Jüngst D, Gerbes AL, Martin R et al [1986] Value of ascitic lipids in the differentiation between cirrhotic and malignant ascites. *Hepatology* 6(2):239-43.

PMID 3964997 Marx JA, Bar-Or D, Moore EE et al [1985] Utility of lavage alkaline phosphatase in detection of isolated small intestinal injury. *Ann Emerg Med* 14(1):10-4.

PMID 3967867 Yang CY, Liaw YF, Chu CM et al [1985] White count, pH and lactate in ascites in the diagnosis of spontaneous bacterial peritonitis. *Hepatology* 5(1):85-90.

PMID 3967868 Garcia-Tsao G, Conn HO, Lerner E [1985] The diagnosis of bacterial peritonitis: comparison of pH, lactate concentration and leukocyte count. *Hepatology* 5(1):91-6.

PMID 3979958 Runyon BA, Hoefs JC [1985] Ascitic fluid chemical analysis before, during and after spontaneous bacterial peritonitis. *Hepatology* 5(2):257-9.

PMID 4028657 Reimer LG [1985] Approach to the analysis of body fluids for the detection of infection. *Clin Lab Med* 5:209-222

PMID 4938274 Conn HO, Fessel JM [1971] Spontaneous bacterial peritonitis in cirrhosis: variations on a theme. *Med (Baltimore)* 50(3):161-97.

PMID 5044540 Rush BF Jr, Host WR, Fewel J et al [1972] Intestinal ischemia and some organic substances in serum and abdominal fluid. *Arch Surg* 105(2):151-7.

PMID 646247 Loewenstein MS, Rittgers RA, Feinerman AE [1978] Carcinoembryonic antigen assay of ascites and detection of malignancy. *Ann Intern Med* 88(5):635-8.

PMID 666469 Boyer TD, Kahn AM, Reynolds TB [1978] Diagnostic value of ascitic fluid lactic dehydrogenase, protein, and WBC levels. *Arch Intern Med* 138(7):1103-5.

PMID 6724512 Runyon BA, Hoefs JC [1984] Ascitic fluid analysis in the differentiation of spontaneous bacterial peritonitis from gastrointestinal tract perforation into ascitic fluid. *Hepatology* 4:447-450.

PMID 6741988 Rector WG Jr, Reynolds TB [1984] Superiority of the serum ascites albumin difference over the ascites total protein concentration in separation of "transudative" and "exudative" ascites. *Am J Med* 77(1):83-5.

PMID 6807793 Gitlin N, Stauffer JL, Silvestri RC [1982] The pH of ascitic fluid in the diagnosis of spontaneous bacterial peritonitis in alcoholic cirrhosis. *Hepatology* 2(4):408-11.

PMID 6862152 Paré P, Talbot J, Hoefs JC [1983] Serum ascites albumin concentration gradient: a physiologic approach to the differential diagnosis of ascites. *Gastroenterology* 85(2):240-4.

PMID 7123495 Alyono D, Morrow CE, Perry JF [1982] Reappraisal of diagnostic peritoneal lavage criteria for operation in penetrating and blunt trauma. *Surgery* 92:751-757.

PMID 7286905 Hoefs JC [1981] Increase in ascites white blood cell and protein concentrations during diuresis in patients with chronic liver disease. *Hepatology* 1:249-254.

PMID 7307856 Brook I, Altman RS, Loebman WW et al [1981] Measurement of lactate in ascitic fluid: an aid in the diagnosis of peritonitis with particular relevance to spontaneous bacterial peritonitis of the cirrhotic. *Dig Dis Sci* 26(12):1089-94.

PMID 7548806 Gupta R, Misra SP, Dwivedi M et al [1995] Diagnosing ascites: value of ascitic fluid total protein, albumin, cholesterol, their ratios, serum ascites albumin and cholesterol gradient. *J Gastroenterol Hepatol* 10(3):295-9.

PMID 7999819 Lye WC, Wong PL, Leong SO et al [1994] Isolation of organisms in CAPD peritonitis: a comparison of 2 techniques. *Adv Perit Dial* 10:166-8.

PMID 8110951 Perlino CA [1993] *Mycobacterium avium* complex: an unusual cause of peritonitis in patients undergoing continuous ambulatory peritoneal dialysis. *Clin Infect Dis* 17(6):1083-4.

PMID 8131285 Castaldo G, Oriani G, Cimino L et al [1994] Total discrimination of peritoneal malignant ascites from cirrhosis- and hepatocarcinoma-associated ascites by assays of ascitic cholesterol and lactate dehydrogenase. *Clin Chem* 40(3):478-83.

PMID 8289030 Runyon BA [1994] Malignancy-related ascites and ascitic fluid "humoral tests of malignancy." *J Clin Gastroenterol* 18(2):94-8.

PMID 8294324 Garg R, Sood A, Arora S et al [1993] Ascitic fluid cholesterol in differential diagnosis of ascites. *J Assoc Physicians India* 41(10):644-6.

PMID 841541 Seriff NS, Cohen ML, Samuel P et al [1977] Chylothorax: diagnosis by lipoprotein electrophoresis of serum and pleural fluid. *Thorax* 32(1):98-100.

PMID 8452953 Hakim A, Hisam N, Reuman PD [1993] Environmental mycobacterial peritonitis complicating peritoneal dialysis: 3 cases and review. *Clin Infect Dis* 16(3):426-31.

PMID 9308124 McHutchison JG [1997] Differential diagnosis of ascites. *Semin Liver Dis* 17(3):191-202.

PMID 9517648 Elis A, Meisel S, Tishler T et al [1998] Ascitic fluid to serum bilirubin concentration ratio for the classification of transudates or exudates. *Am J Gastroenterol* 93(3):401-3.

PMID 998592 Brown JD, Dac An N [1976] Tuberculous peritonitis. Low ascitic fluid glucose concentration as a diagnostic aid. *Am J Gastroenterol* 66(3):277-82.

ISBN 0192629220 Moore K [2003] Spontaneous bacterial peritonitis (SBP). In: Warrel DA et al. *Oxford Textbook of Medicine*, 4th ed. Oxford University, pp739-741.

ISBN 0721648363 Boyer TD [2003] Diagnosis and management of cirrhotic ascites. In: Zakim, D, Boyer, TD, ed. *Hepatology: A Textbook of Liver Disease*, 4th ed. Philadelphia: WB Saunders, pp631-58.

ISBN 1416061894 Runyon B [2006] Ascites and spontaneous bacterial peritonitis. In: Feldman M, Friedman LS, Sleisenger MH, ed. *Sleisenger and Fordran's Gastrointestinal and Liver Disease*, 8th ed. Philadelphia: Saunders, pp1935-1964.

Troidle L, Finkelstein F [2006] Treatment outcome of CPD-associated peritonitis. *Annals of Clinical Microbiology and Antimicrobials* 5(6). http://www.ann-clinmicrob.com/content/5/1/6.

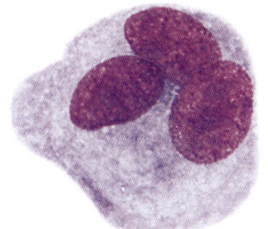

Couturier MR, Straseski JA, Kjeldsberg CR

Synovial Fluid
Chapter 7

Anatomy & pathophysiology

Synovial fluid is an ultrafiltrate of plasma that is passed through fenestrations of the subsynovial capillary endothelium into the synovial cavity. There it is combined with hyaluronic acid, a glycosaminoglycan of high molecular weight secreted by the synovial lining cells [ISBN 978-1-4377-1738-9 Goldring]. Diarthrodial joints are lined at their margins by synovial membrane (synovium), with synovial cells lining the joint space f7.1. The synovial cells are arranged in a layer 1-3 cells thick, embedded in a ground substance without a basement membrane i7.1. In addition to having the capacity for protein synthesis, the synovial cells phagocytose debris presented at the fluid-cell interface. The functions of the synovial fluid are to lubricate the joint space and to transport nutrients to the articular cartilage. The protein and immunoglobulin concentrations of the synovial fluid are ~1/4 those of plasma, while electrolytes, glucose, and uric acid concentrations are similar to those of the blood.

Immunologic, mechanical, chemical, or bacteriologic damage may alter the permeability of the membranes and capillaries to produce varying degrees of inflammatory response i7.2. Various disorders produce changes in the chemical constituents of the joint fluid and in the type of cell population present.

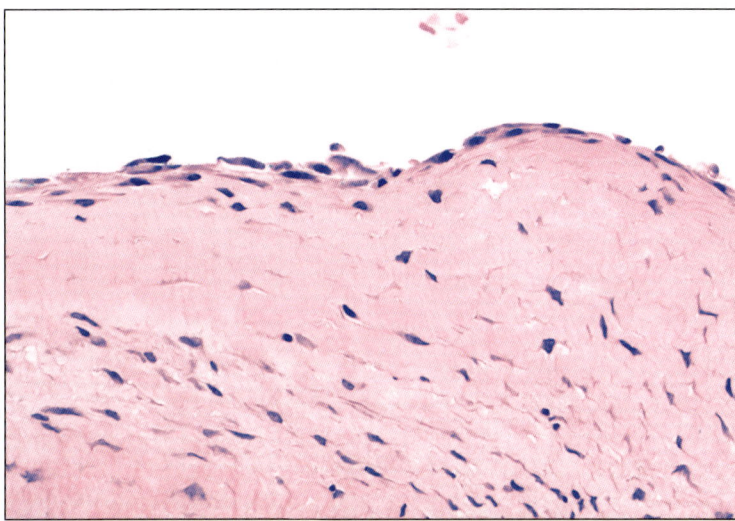

i7.1 Histologic section showing synovial membrane with a single layer of flat, synovial lining cells (synoviocytes)

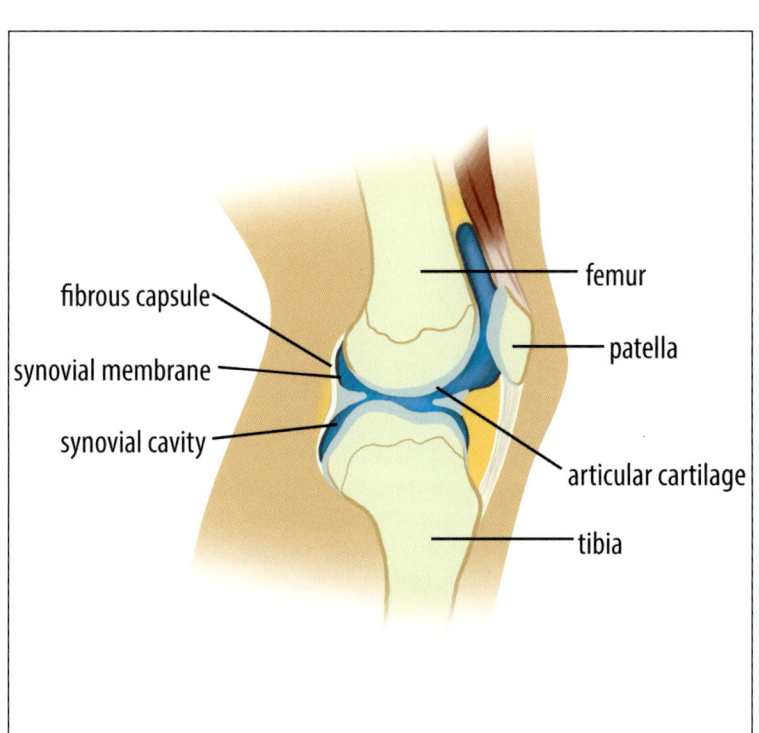

f7.1 Schematic drawing showing anatomic relationship of parts in a diarthrodial joint.

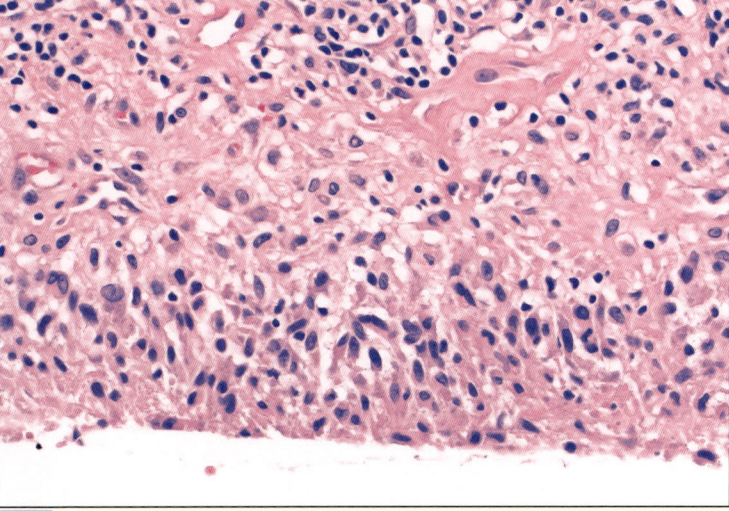

i7.2 Histologic section of synovial membrane in a patient with rheumatoid arthritis. There is hyperplasia of the synovial lining cells, with underlying inflammatory infiltrate.

Normal adult reference values for the components of synovial fluid are presented in t7.1.

t7.1 Adult reference values for synovial fluid

	Conventional units	SI units
Leukocyte	<150/µL	<0.15×10⁹/L
Differential white blood cell (WBC) count		
Polymorphonuclear leukocytes (PMNs)	<25%	<0.25
Lymphocytes	<75%	<0.75
Monocytes	<70%	<0.70
Glucose level (blood-synovial fluid difference)	<10 mg/dL	<0.55 mmol/L
Hyaluronate	0.30-0.41 g/dL	3.0-4.1 g/L
Lactate	<25 mg/dL	<2.8 mmol/L
Protein	1-3 g/dL	10-30 g/L
Uric acid		
Males	<8.0 mg/dL	<476 µmol/L
Females	<6.0 mg/dL	<357 µmol/L

Through clinical and laboratory examination of the synovial fluid, joint disorders can be divided into 5 categories t7.2. Such a classification is useful as long as one realizes that considerable overlap may occur in synovial fluid findings among different groups and that, on occasion, >1 diagnosis may be present. The 5 major disease categories are as follows

- group I, noninflammatory
- group II, inflammatory
- group III, infectious
- group IV, crystal associated
- group V, hemorrhagic

Impaired function of synovial fluid with age or disease may play a role in the development of degenerative joint disease such as osteoarthritis. Inflammatory joint fluids contain various lytic enzymes that produce depolymerization of hyaluronic acid, which greatly impairs the lubricating ability of the fluid.

t7.2 Classification of arthritides

Group I (noninflammatory)
Osteoarthritis
Traumatic arthritis
Osteochondritis dissecans
Osteochondromatosis
Neuropathic osteoarthropathy
Pigmented villonodular synovitis
Early rheumatoic arthritis
Paget disease
Acromegaly
Ochronosis
Hyperparathyroidism

Group II (inflammatory)
Rheumatoid arthritis
Lupus erythematosus
Reiter syndrome
Rheumatic fever
Ankylosing spondylitis
Regional enteritis
Ulcerative colitis
Psoriatic arthritis
Fat droplet synovitis
Sarcoidosis
Scleroderma
Polymyalgia rheumatica
Erythema multiforme

Group III (infectious)
Bacterial
Mycobacterial
Fungal
Spirochetal

Group IV (crystal induced)
Gout
Calcium pyrophosphate dihydrate (CPPD) crystal deposition disease
Apatite associated arthropathy

Group V (hemorrhagic)
Traumatic arthritis
Hemophiliac arthropathy
Anticoagulation
Pigmented villonodular synovitis
Neuropathic osteoarthropathy
Synovial hemangioma
Hemangioma

Specimen collection, requirements & stability

The collection of joint fluid through needle aspiration (arthrocentesis) requires expertise and should be performed with extreme care. The sterility of the technique is of utmost importance to avoid unintentional introduction of contaminants into the joint. Arthrocentesis should in fact be limited to patients with an undiagnosed effusion or a significant clinical change in an already established effusion. Collection of synovial fluid must be performed with a sterile disposable needle in order to avoid contamination of the joint as well as contamination of the collection with birefringent particulates and resident skin flora (including coagulase negative *Staphylococcus* species and *Propionibacterium acnes*).

Oxalate, lithium heparin, and powdered EDTA should be avoided in the syringe due to their propensity to form crystalline artifacts. As well, both heparin and EDTA have antimicrobial properties and should not be used to collect specimens intended for microbiologic cultures. The total volume of collected fluid is variable and depends on the joint involved and the nature of the effusion.

3 specific lines of interrogation should be initiated for comprehensive evaluation of synovial fluid, and (given sufficient specimen volume) should be divided as follows: 5 mL collected in a plain tube used for chemical analysis, 5 mL in an anticoagulated tube containing EDTA or heparin for microscopic analysis, and >5 mL divided into an anaerobic transport tube and blood culture bottle for microbiologic analysis. Any additional specimen should be submitted in a clean sterile tube for additional microbiologic analysis such as fungal or acid-fast bacterial cultures (see Chapter 2).

For microbiologic specimens, all collection tubes should be maintained at room temperature and expedited to the laboratory for culture setup within 24 hours. Results from synovial fluid specimens that are received >24 hours from the time of collection should contain a comment explaining the possibility of a false negative culture due to suboptimal specimen handling.

The specimen tube for chemical analysis is allowed to clot at room temperature (normal fluid does not clot). The specimen is then centrifuged to remove all the cells. The cells in synovial fluid may alter the chemical composition of the fluid; therefore, centrifugation should not be delayed. This is particularly important when complement levels are to be determined. The supernatant can be used for assays of rheumatoid factor, antinuclear antibody, complement, or other biochemical procedures. For complement determinations, the tests must be performed within 2-3 hours after collection of the specimen since complement is heat labile. If the specimen cannot be examined immediately, the fluid should be frozen and stored at –70°C until examined.

It is recommended that the synovial fluid be microscopically examined within an hour after arthrocentesis, as storage for 5-6 hours can reduce the visible cells count from "inflammatory" to "noninflammatory" in this time period [PMID 2930602]. Such delays in examination may therefore lead to a misdiagnosis. The decrease in WBC count over time is also paralleled by a decrease in the percentages of polymorphonuclear neutrophils (PMNs). In contrast, fluids with a predominance of mononuclear cells typically have a slower decrease in cell counts over time [PMID 2930602]. Viscid synovial fluid interferes with accurate cell counts, and therefore digestion with hyaluronidase prior to the analysis should be employed (see Chapter 2).

The effects of specimen storage on crystals can also lead to misleading results. MSU crystals do not decrease in numbers significantly over the first 3 days of storage but they do decrease over a period of weeks (an effect slowed by refrigeration) [PMID 2930602]. CPPD crystals decrease significantly after 2-3 days in storage, and refrigeration does not protect CPPD crystals from dissolution [PMID 2930602]. Apatite crystal containing clumps appear to be resistant to dissolution over a period of several weeks [PMID 2930602].

If arthrocentesis results in a dry tap, a few drops of fluid may still be in the needle that can be used for the most essential portions of the examination, namely Gram stain, bacteriologic culture, and microscopic examination for leukocytes and crystals. Therefore, communication with the laboratory should be initiated to ensure appropriate submission can be achieved. Many laboratories will not accept syringes with the needle attached, so this communication is paramount to ensure appropriate processing.

It has been reported that lipid inclusions may develop in synovial fluid specimens incubated for 48 hours [PMID 188502]. These inclusions and membrane lipids, thought to be released from disintegrated cells, give rise to positively birefringent Maltese crosses [PMID 188502]. Hematinlike crystals may be seen in stored bloody synovial fluid specimens due to degradation of hemoglobin.

If a delay in the examination of the specimen is unavoidable, or if the specimen is being sent for consultation, it should be refrigerated (excluding microbiologic submissions). Synovial fluid should be handled in a sterile manner since infectious agents could generate oxalate and become a source of crystal formation [PMID 2930602].

Laboratory studies

The laboratory analyses performed on synovial fluid are listed in t7.3. The special studies listed are only performed in specific circumstances and are usually not of diagnostic value.

t7.3	Laboratory examination of synovial fluid
Routine studies	
Gross examination for color & clarity	
Leukocyte count and differential count	
Gram stain & microbiologic culture	
Crystal examination with polarizing microscope & compensator	
Special studies	
Glucose	
Protein	
Lactate	
Uric acid	
Enzymes	
Lipids	
Immunologic studies	

Gross examination

The analysis of synovial fluid starts with the recording of volume and the gross appearance of the removed fluid. Effusions of all arthritides produce variable amounts of synovial fluid. For example, an aspirated volume of >4 mL from the knee is considered abnormal. Furthermore, joint effusions may sometimes be difficult to aspirate because of thick fibrin, rice bodies, and other debris. It is also possible that the fluid may be loculated and thus not easily obtained. However, there is little correlation between the volume of fluid obtained and the type or severity of the joint disease. A specific diagnosis is rarely made from gross examination alone, but it may help categorize the joint fluid into 1 of the 5 groups described in t7.4 [ISBN 978-1-4377-0974-5 El-Gabalawy].

Normal joint fluid is colorless, like water, or light yellow. It is thought that diapedesis of red blood cells, which accompanies most inflammatory situations, and breakdown of hemoglobin to bilirubin are responsible for the light yellow color of most fluids aspirated from patients with group I disease. The effusion is cloudy or turbid when print cannot be read easily through the fluid i7.3. Usually the cloudier the fluid is, the more cells that are present. Turbidity, which usually indicates leukocytosis, increases with the degree of inflammation.

With inflammatory conditions, fibrinogen and other coagulation factors are present, and clot formation often occurs. The presence of clear, light yellow, viscous fluid usually indicates a noninflammatory disease from group I. Fluid from group II patients (those with inflammatory diseases) is frequently cloudy, appears turbid and yellow, and clots while standing. Fluid from patients in group III (infectious disease) is often grossly purulent.

The color varies in different types of bacterial infections, depending on the chromogen of the invading bacteria. *Staphylococcus aureus* organisms may produce a golden pigmented color, and *Serratia marcescens* may produce a red hue [ISBN 978-0-8121-1123-1]. Cartilage debris and the presence of crystals may also produce a cloudy or turbid fluid. Fluid from a joint with crystal associated synovitis may appear purulent or opaque white and occasionally green in color. The presence of so called rice bodies, products of degenerating proliferative synovial lining cells or of microinfarction of the synovium, may cause the fluid to resemble pus on gross examination [PMID 7352946]. Rice bodies have been demonstrated to be present in 72% of patients with rheumatoid arthritis using a specially designed wide bore needle for aspirate before and after saline lavage. Using a regular fine gauge needle, however, the incidence of rice bodies is much smaller, presumably because the bodies block the lumen of the needle. Cloudy, fatty fluid usually indicates the presence of cholesterol crystals, often seen in chronic arthritides. Droplets of free floating fat, however, frequently occur in association with trauma with or without infarction. In such patients, bone marrow particles have also been described.

Hemorrhagic fluid is homogeneously bloody. Streaks of blood are seen in a traumatic aspirate. Centrifugation of the fluid may be necessary to differentiate between a traumatic tap and hemarthrosis. Xanthochromia of the supernatant usually indicates that blood has been present in the synovial fluid for some time. Xanthochromia may, however, be difficult to interpret because of the normal light yellow appearance of the synovial fluid. A dark red or bloody supernatant in the presence of grossly observed blood suggests hemarthrosis rather than a traumatic tap. A hematocrit obtained on a true bloody effusion may determine whether it is blood or whether it is blood mixed with joint fluid. A true bloody effusion, in contrast to that caused by a traumatic tap, often does not clot.

Ochronotic fluid may have dark speckled particles ("ground pepper" sign) [PMID 4459470]. Metal or plastic fragments from prosthetic arthroplasty may be associated with black or gray discoloration of the synovial fluid [PMID 5823923]. In pigmented villonodular synovitis the fluid may be grossly bloody or have an orange-brown color. Cholesterol containing fluid may be dark yellow in color. Cholesterol rich synovial effusions may be seen in rheumatoid arthritis. At first sight, the fluid grossly may have the appearance of pus. The fluid, however, has a more uniform consistency. In bright light, it has a shimmering, gold-pink appearance, and cholesterol crystals may be seen. Urate or apatite laden fluid can be white or yellow and sometimes pasty in appearance i7.3.

In general, noninflammatory fluid is more viscous than inflammatory fluid. However, tests for synovial fluid viscosity and the mucin clot test are not described as they are not reliable or useful in the classification of synovial effusions.

t7.4 Synovial fluid findings by disease category

Finding	Normal	Group I (noninflammatory)	Group II (inflammatory)	Group III (infectious)	Group IV (crystal induced)	Group V (hemorrhagic)
Appearance	Clear to straw colored	Yellow, transparent	Yellow, cloudy, turbid, or bloody	Yellow, purulent	Cloudy, turbid, or white-opaque	Red-brown or xanthochromic
WBCs	0-150/µL (0-0.15×10^9/L)	<3,000/µL (0-3×10^9/L)	3,000-75,000/µL (3-75×10^9/L)	50,000-200,000/µL (50-200×10^9/L)	500-200,000/µL (0.5-200×10^9/L)	50-10,000/µL (0.05-10×10^9/L)
Polymorphonuclear leukocytes	<25%	<30%	>50%	>90%	<90%	<50%
Crystals present	–	–	–	–	+	–
RBCs present	–	–	–	+	–	+
Blood glucose to synovial fluid glucose ratio (mg/dL)*	0-10 mg/dL (0-0.56 mmol/L)	0-10 mg/dL (0-0.56 mmol/L)	0-40 mg/dL (0-2.22 mmol/L)	20-100 mg/dL (1.11-5.55 mmol/L)	0-80 mg/dL (0-4.44 mmol/L)	0-20 mg/dL (0-1.11 mmol/L)
Culture	–	–	–	Often +	–	–

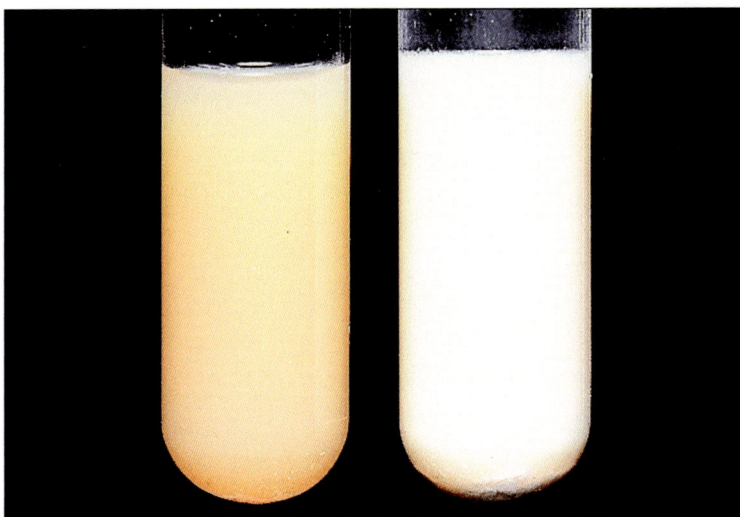

i7.3 The tube to the left shows turbid synovial fluid containing inflammatory cells and increased protein. The tube to the right shows the pink-white color that may be present in urate-laden fluid (gout).

Cell counts

The leukocyte count is an important test for classification of an effusion as septic, inflammatory, or noninflammatory t7.4. Together with the volume of the synovial fluid, the leukocyte count may be used as a rough measure of the intensity of inflammation in sequential samples. However, considerable overlap may occur in all ranges, and a high leukocyte count in synovial fluid is not diagnostic by itself. For example, in the early phase of bacterial infection, the leukocyte count may be normal. In addition, fluid samples from cases of gout or rheumatoid arthritis may demonstrate leukocyte counts in the range usually associated with septic arthritis. There have also been occasional reports of acute gout and acute pseudogout without synovial fluid leukocytosis, which suggests an alternate inflammatory mechanism.

The leukocyte count is usually performed in a standard hemocytometer (see Chapter 2). Unless the leukocyte count is very high (>50,000/µL) a total count can be performed with undiluted fluid. Physiologic saline should be used as a diluent instead of one containing acetic acid, as the latter will precipitate hyaluronic acid, produce cell clumping, and result in a spuriously low WBC count. The fluid must be properly agitated before being added to the counting chamber. The addition of hyaluronidase with toluidine blue is useful in viscid specimens and is always used with automated cell counters (see Chapter 2). Cells sediment in vivo, and when the patient has been in the supine position for an extended period, the joint contents should be mixed by barbotage before arthrocentesis [McCarty ISBN 978-0-8121-1123-1].

Automated cell counters like Iris iQ200 (Iris Diagnostics, Chatsworth, California, USA; initially designed for urine samples), Beckman-Coulter LH750 (Beckman-Coulter, Brea, CA, USA), Advia 120 (Bayer, Barcelona, Spain), and Sysmex XE-5000 (Kobe, Japan) are now being used successfully with a variety of body fluids [PMID 14649464, PMID 19228639, PMID 20236183, PMID 21836038, PMID 23647736, Williams 2011]. For automated cell counters like Iris iQ200, all synovial fluid specimens must be pretreated with hyaluronidase to reduce viscosity and prevent the formation of blue coagulate when lysing reagent is added. If clots are found in the specimen, a manual count should be done.

Normal synovial fluid contains usually only up to 50 WBC/µL, and polymorphonuclear cells are rarely seen. Most authors, however, consider 150-200/µL to be the upper limit of normal. Group I (noninflammatory) disorders are usually associated with a leukocyte count of 200-3,000/µL; group II (inflammatory) disorders are usually associated with a leukocyte count of 3,000-75,000/µL; group III (infectious) disorders usually have a leukocyte count of 50,000-200,000/µL; and group IV (crystal associated) disorders have a leukocyte count that may vary from 500-200,000/µL t7.4.

Again, considerable overlap may occur in the leukocyte counts, and these values are not specific for any one group. In one study, 70% of patients with culture proven infectious arthritis had synovial fluid leukocyte counts >50,000/µL, while 12.5% of patients with gout, 10% of those with pseudogout, and 4% of those with rheumatoid arthritis also had leukocyte counts in this range [PMID 474588]. In 1/4 of the fluid specimens containing monosodium urate crystals and 1/3 of those with calcium pyrophosphate crystals, the leukocyte counts were <2,555/µL [PMID 474588]. This study emphasizes the need for a careful search for crystals in fluid specimens with high, as well as low, leukocyte counts. Furthermore, septic arthritis can coexist with other types of arthritis, such as gout, pseudogout, systemic lupus erythematosus, and rheumatoid arthritis. Very high leukocyte counts (>100,000/µL with the majority being PMNs) are most commonly seen in septic arthritis, but they are also sometimes seen in psoriatic arthritis and Reiter syndrome. Reiter syndrome is often associated with genitourinary *Chlamydia trachomatis* infection; importantly the organism is not found in the synovial fluid, so testing is not indicated from this source.

Microscopic examination & clinical considerations

As described under "Specimen collection," the differential count and cytologic examination should preferably be done within 1 hour of the arthrocentesis. Wright stained cytospin preparations should be made. If the specimen is viscous, treatment with hyaluronidase is helpful (Chapter 2). If cytospin instruments are not available, smears of centrifuged specimens can be used. The smears should be made as thin as possible, since the purple-blue staining of the mucopolysaccharides and mucoproteins in synovial fluid may make the cytologic examination difficult. Synovial fluids that are allowed to clot will often trap cells in the clot-like structure, and smears produced from such specimens characteristically reveal cells with poor staining properties.

The types of cells that may be seen on microscopic examination of abnormal synovial fluid include neutrophils, lymphocytes, plasma cells, monocytes, eosinophils, mononuclear phagocytes (monocytes, macrophages, and histiocytes), synovial lining cells, and lupus erythematosus cells. Neutrophils and lymphocytes generally show a morphologic structure identical to that of the corresponding cells of the blood. Neutrophils may contain vacuoles, fat droplets, bacteria, or crystals. It is common for the nuclei to

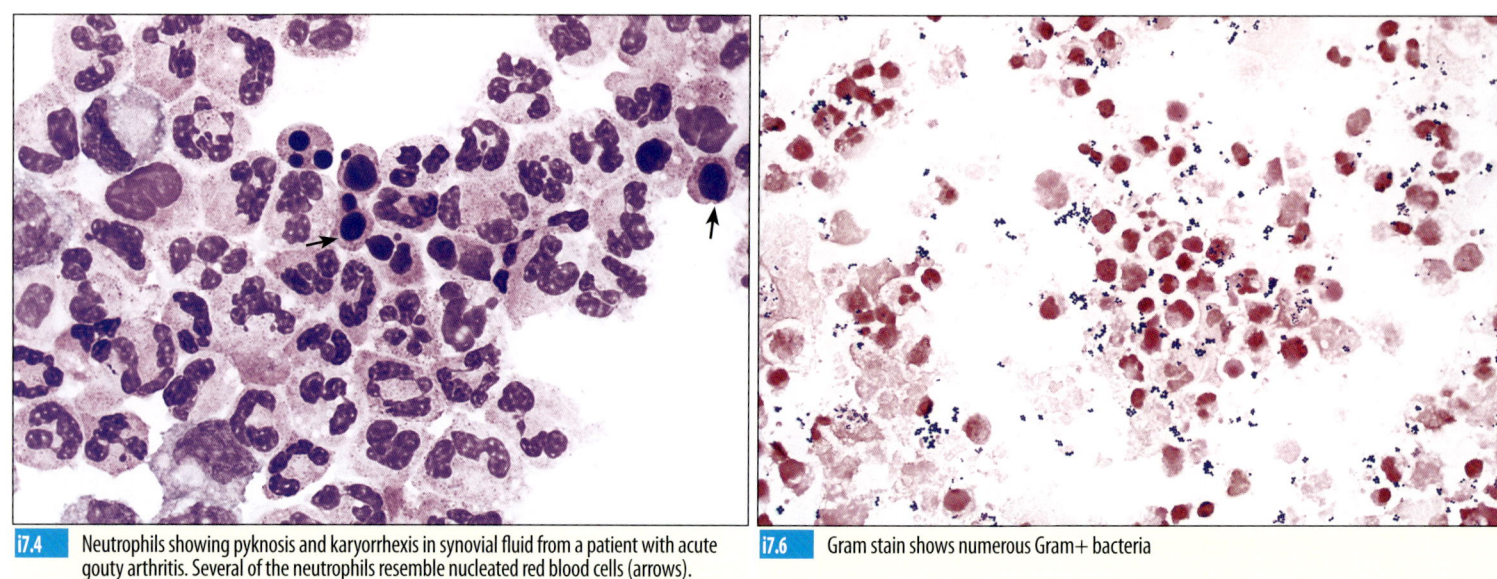

| i7.4 | Neutrophils showing pyknosis and karyorrhexis in synovial fluid from a patient with acute gouty arthritis. Several of the neutrophils resemble nucleated red blood cells (arrows). |
| i7.6 | Gram stain shows numerous Gram+ bacteria |

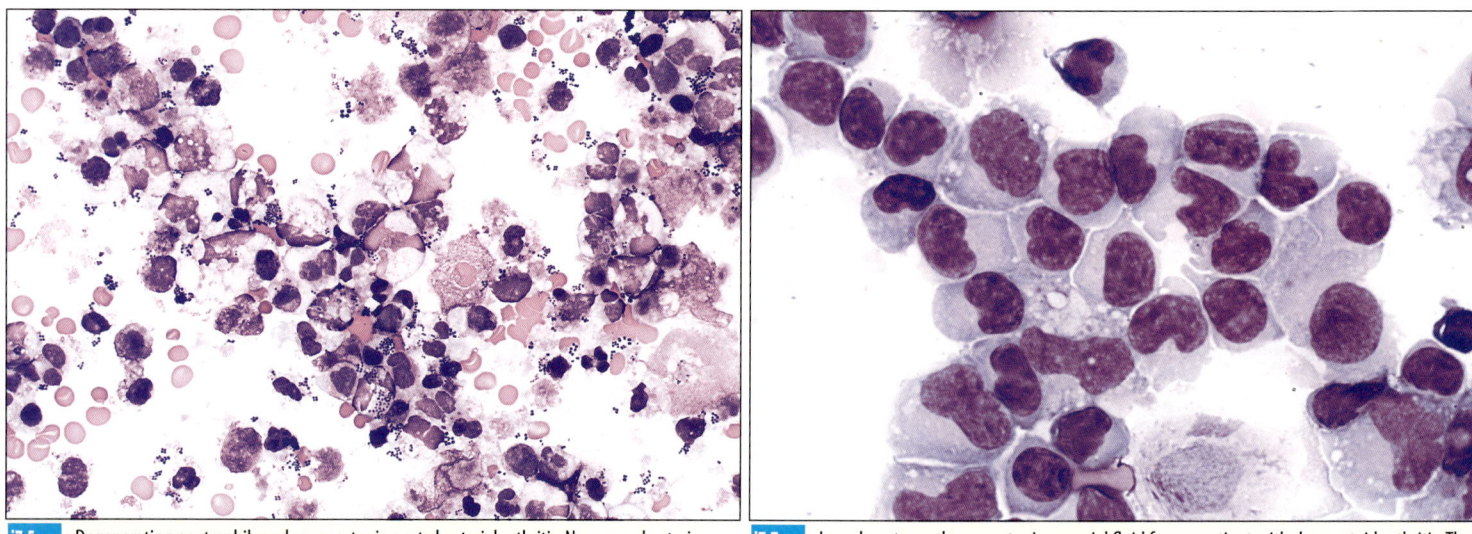

| i7.5 | Degenerating neutrophils and monocytes in acute bacterial arthritis. Numerous bacteria are also present. |
| i7.7 | Lymphocytes and monocytes in synovial fluid from a patient with rheumatoid arthritis. The irregular nuclear contours of the lymphocytes are probably artifactual. |

show pyknosis and karyorrhexis i7.4. These degenerating nuclear fragments should not be mistaken for organisms. Mucin may also cause artifacts and complicate the interpretation of a Gram stain. A high percentage of neutrophils (>80%) is highly suggestive of septic arthritis, regardless of the magnitude of the total leukocyte count. When the percentage of neutrophils is markedly elevated, a Gram stain should always be performed i7.5, i7.6. The absence of bacteria on the Gram stain, however, does not exclude the possibility of a septic joint. A predominance of neutrophils is also often seen in crystal induced arthritis (urate gout and pseudogout) and in various inflammatory conditions.

Lymphocytes, including transformed lymphocytes (immunocytes & immunoblasts), are the predominant cell type in early stages of rheumatoid arthritis, but later neutrophils may predominate [PMID 171408]. A predominance of lymphocytes is often seen in patients with rheumatoid arthritis, but also in chronic infections, nonspecific arthritis, systemic lupus erythematosus, and other collagen disorders i7.7.

A predominance of monocytes may be seen in arthritis associated with serum sickness and certain viral infections (hepatitis & rubella) and occasionally with crystal associated arthritis i7.8 [PMID 420721, PMID 6847731]. Chronic monocytosis has been found in patients with lupus erythematosus [PMID 6847731].

Synovial lining cells have morphologic features similar to those of mesothelial cells in pleural and peritoneal fluids i7.9, i7.10. Synovial lining cells may be difficult to differentiate from monocytes and histiocytes. The presence of synovial lining cells does not appear to have any specific diagnostic significance.

Synovial fluid eosinophilia, defined as >2% of WBCs, has been reported in association with rheumatoid arthritis, rheumatic fever, metastatic carcinoma to the synovium, Guinea worm infestation of the joints, Lyme disease, reactive arthritis associated with *Strongyloides* infection, following radiation therapy, chronic urticaria, and angioedema t7.5, i7.11 [PMID 3056421, PMID 3357226, PMID 7092970, PMID 7417355].

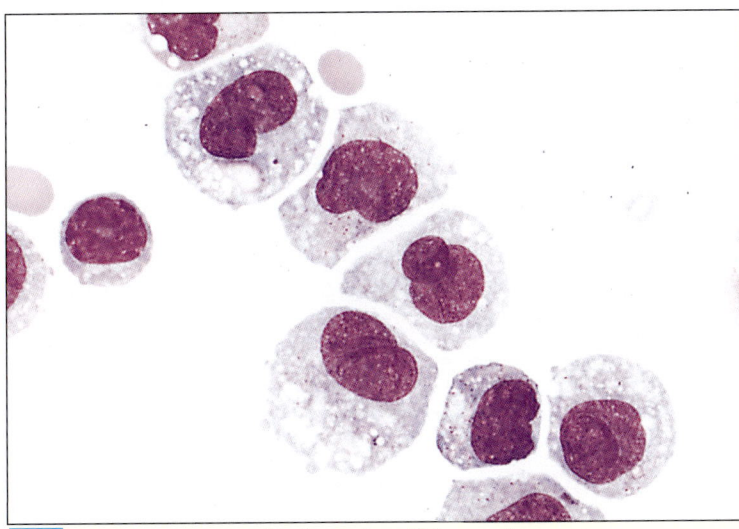

i7.8 Monocytes seen in synovial fluid in a patient with lupus erythematosus

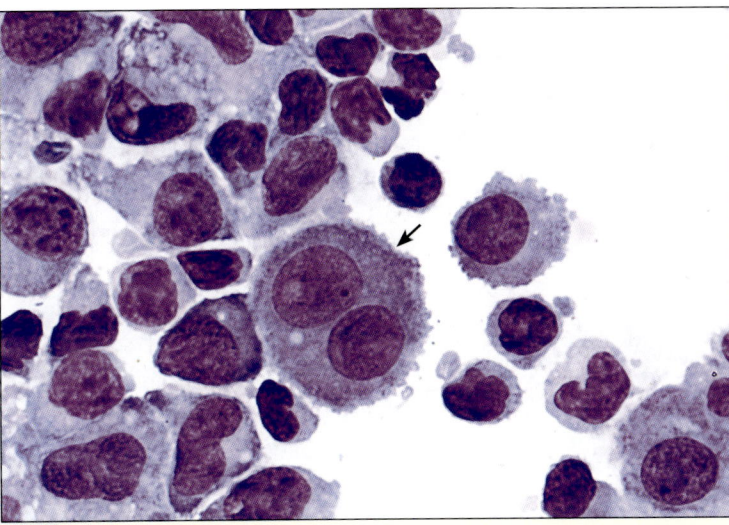

i7.10 Binucleate synovial lining cell (arrow)

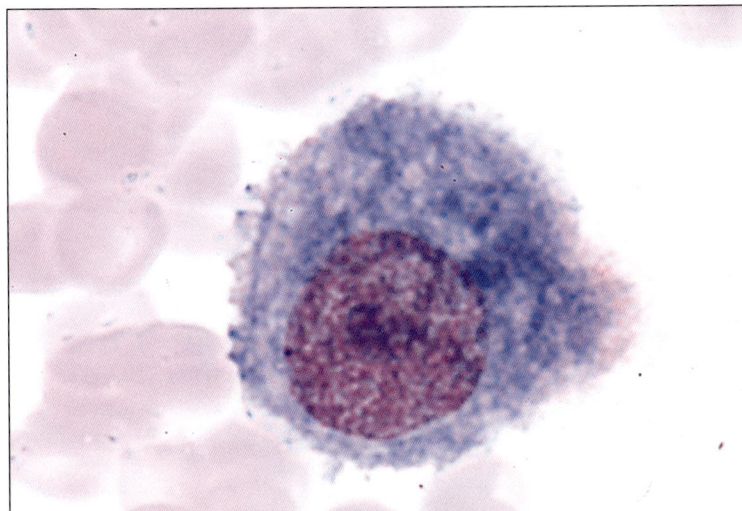

i7.9 Synovial lining cells (arrows) resembling mesothelial cells

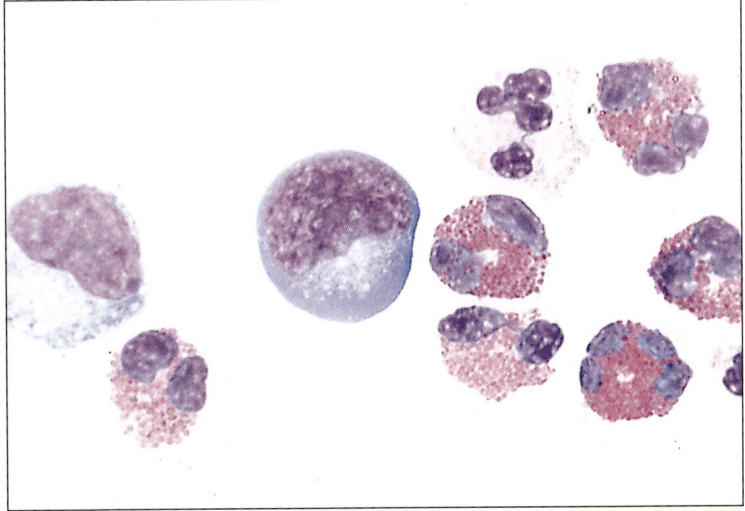

i7.11 Eosinophils & transformed lymphocyte in the synovial fluid from a patient with Lyme disease

t7.5 Causes of synovial fluid eosinophilia

Rheumatic disease
Parasitic arthritides
Lyme disease
Hypereosinophilic syndrome
Allergic disease with arthritis
Metastatic disease to synovium
Therapeutic radiation
Arthrography
Idiopathic

A small number of mast cells may be observed in the synovial fluid from patients with a variety of arthritides, including rheumatoid arthritis, systemic lupus erythematosus, osteoarthritis, Crohn disease, and that associated with trauma [PMID 2427093, PMID 4004360].

A variety of lipid bodies have been described in synovial fluids. Extracellular lipid globules have been reported in traumatic arthritis, aseptic necrosis, and rheumatoid arthritis with ordinary and polarized light microscopy [PMID 623698]. A few large extracellular fat droplets are frequently seen in joint effusions and are thought to originate from surrounding tissues by the needle during the arthrocentesis. Large amounts of extracellular lipid may be seen in synovial fluid following trauma to the adjacent bone and/or supporting structures [PMID 679544]. Occasionally, lipid droplets have been seen both extracellularly and intracellularly in patients with traumatic arthritis and aseptic necrosis, which occasionally may be accompanied by marked synovial fluid leukocytosis [PMID 5559440, PMID 6244798]. These lipid droplets may sometimes only be visible under polarized light microscopy as Maltese crosses. Spuriously elevated leukocyte counts have been associated with the presence of fat globules due to fractures. A factitious high WBC count may be present because the automated electronic counter may record fat globules as leukocyte [PMID 7458972].

So called Reiter cells are vacuolated macrophages containing either neutrophilic or basophilic globular material or both i7.12 [PMID 6023534]. Such cells, however, are not specific indicators for Reiter disease and have been found in many types of inflammatory joint fluids. Dark purple inclusions in mononuclear phagocytes may also be clumps of apatite crystals [PMID 199097].

LE cells occur in ~10% of effusions from patients with systemic lupus erythematosus (SLE) i7.13 [PMID 4931742]. In some patients, LE cells may initially be present in synovial fluid and not in the peripheral blood [PMID 4193825]. LE cells may also be seen in synovial fluid samples from patients with rheumatoid arthritis.

Cartilage cells (chondrocytes) are occasionally seen in the synovial fluid of patients with osteoarthritis, but isolated cartilage cells may also appear in a number of arthritides, including traumatic arthritis and pseudogout. Cartilage cells have a central, small, round, pyknotic nucleus surrounded by a clear zone and a distinct burgundy cytoplasm i7.14.

In septic arthritis associated with pyogenic bacteria, white blood cell counts usually exceed 50,000/µL, and the majority of the cells are polymorphonuclear leukocytes. This type of leukocyte count may, however, also be seen in infections due to mycobacteria, fungi, viruses, and helminths. In addition, conditions such crystal associated arthritis and rheumatoid arthritis may be associated with similar high white blood cell counts. Intra-articular injections of gold salts and corticosteroids may also produce elevation of synovial fluid white blood cell count. White blood cell counts <50,000/µL do not exclude infection, particularly in immunocompromised patients.

In bacterial arthritis due to pyogenic organisms, the polymorphonuclear leukocytes usually account for >85% of the white blood cells. In mycobacterial infection, neutrophils predominate initially and lymphocytes and monocytes predominate later. In fungal arthritis, the findings are variable. In viral arthritis, lymphocytes usually predominate, but initially neutrophils may predominate.

Many organisms are usually present in synovial fluid of patients with bacterial infection i7.15, i7.16; however, they may not always be detected with a routine Gram stain. This is especially true with Gram– bacteria, which may be difficult to see against the background of many leukocytes, mucin, and debris. Mycobacteria may be identified with acid-fast stains or fluorescent stains. Fungi may be identified with PAS and Gomori methenamine silver (GMS) stains; however the identification of the causative organism is reliably made when the organism is isolated in culture. Recent advances in molecular diagnostics may provide a more rapid diagnosis and supplement the classic microbiologic techniques in selected cases (see "Microbiologic examination").

Joint infection complicating rheumatoid arthritis is common (most often the knee), but the diagnosis is often delayed [PMID 2650687]. In such patients, the synovial fluid leukocyte count ranges from 30,000/µL to >400,000/µL and the Gram stain is often positive (since the predominant organism is *Staphylococcus aureus*). Septic arthritis may also

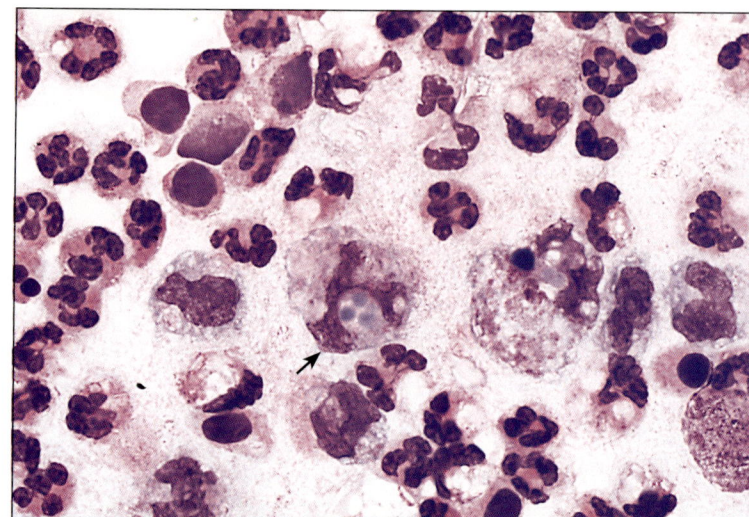

i7.12 So called Reiter cell in synovial fluid. Blue intracytoplasmic inclusions in macrophages represent phagocytosed nuclear material (arrow). This finding is not a specific indicator for Reiter disease and is seen in a variety of conditions. Similar intracytoplasmic inclusions may also be seen in serous effusions.

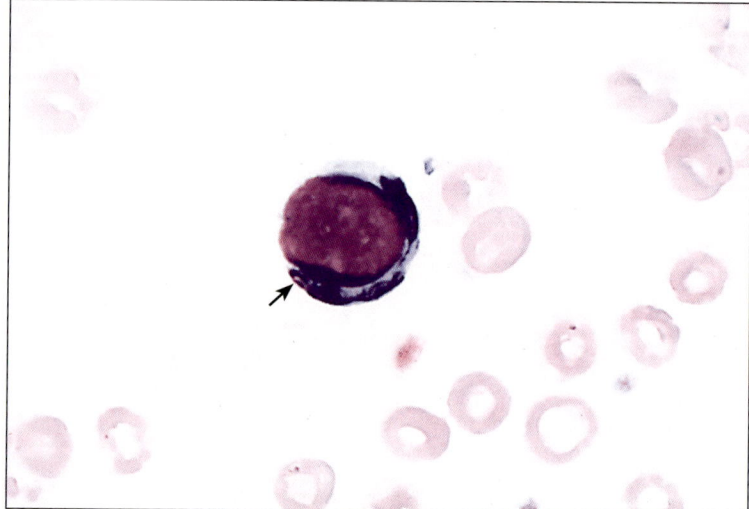

i7.13 Lupus erythematosus cell (arrow) in synovial fluid from patient with lupus erythematosus

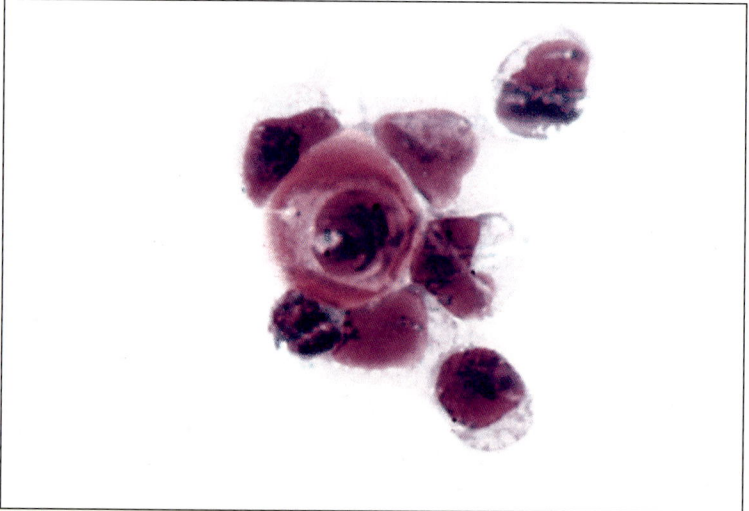

i7.14 A chondrocyte (cartilage cell) in synovial fluid from a patient with osteoarthritis. Note the characteristic clear zone surrounding the nucleus and distinct burgundy cytoplasm.

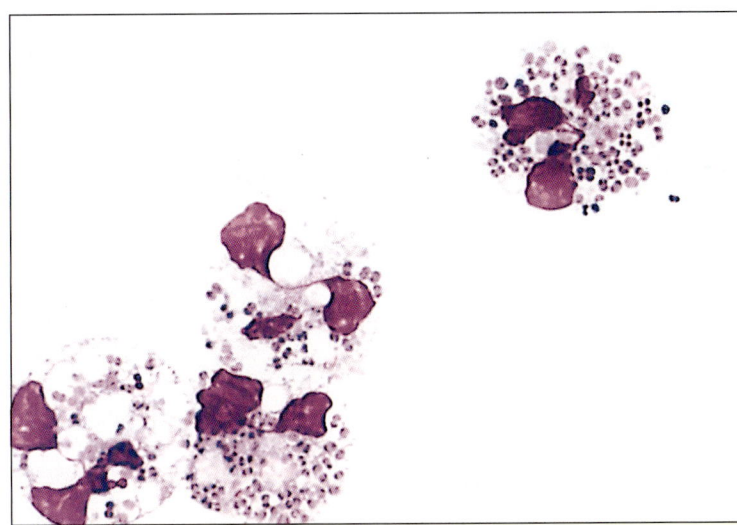

i7.15 Many intracellular bacteria are seen in neutrophils in synovial fluid from patient with gonorrhea

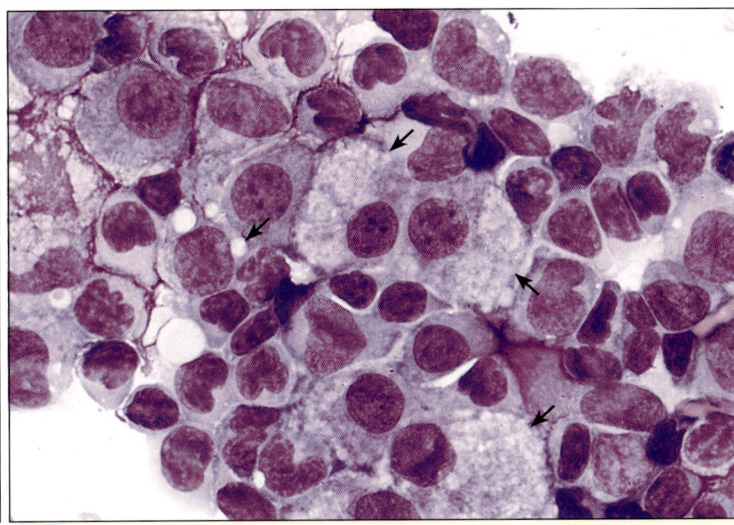

i7.17 Degenerative (vacuolated) synovial lining cells (arrows) in a patient with traumatic arthritis

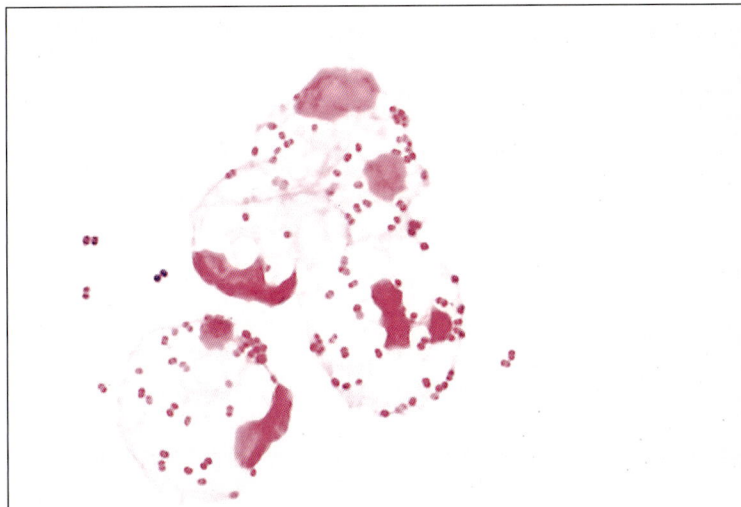

i7.16 Gram stain of synovial fluid showing *Neisseria gonorrhoeae*

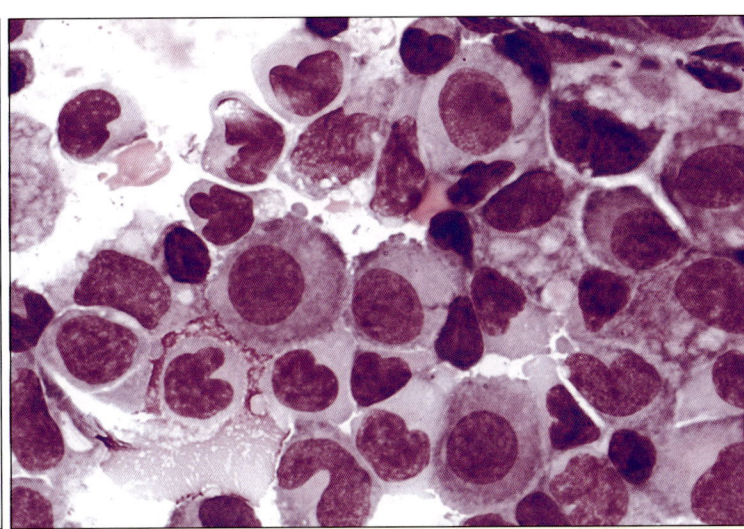

i7.18 Multiple synovial lining cells in a patient with osteoarthritis

occur in patients with systemic lupus erythematosus and in patients with crystal associated arthritides. Whenever septic arthritis is a possibility, culture of synovial fluid and a Gram stain should be performed immediately to arrive at the correct diagnosis and to determine the appropriate therapy.

In traumatic arthritis hemosiderin containing histiocytes and foreign body giant cells may be seen. In addition, a variable number of synovial cells frequently occur in sheets and show variable degrees of degeneration i7.17. Cartilage cells may be numerous. Lipid droplets may be seen in leukocytes or lying free in the fluid and, when present with hemorrhagic fluid, are associated with trauma. The lipid droplets may cause an inflammatory reaction. The presence of fat cells together with bone marrow spicules indicate that a fracture has occurred. In patients with longstanding internal derangement (eg, torn meniscus) fragments of fibrocartilage may be seen [PMID 1998384].

In osteoarthritis, frequently many cartilage cells are present that sometimes are multinucleated. Synovial cells, often in sheets, are frequently seen i7.18.

In pigmented villonodular synovitis, papillary aggregates of synovial cells are characteristic, and hemosiderin inclusions may be seen within synovial cells and histiocytic cells. A Prussian blue stain can identify iron in the cells. Many multinucleated foreign body giant cells may also be seen.

Amyloid arthropathy sometimes occurs in patients with amyloidosis. Amorphous material, which shows typical apple green birefringence with Congo red stain under polarized light, may be seen [PMID 3580010]. Localized amyloid deposits may, on occasion, be related to age or trauma.

In ochronosis, which refers to the accumulation of melaninlike pigment in connective tissues of patients with alkaptonuria, synovial fluid speckled with dark particles resembling ground pepper may be seen [ISBN 978-0-8121-1332-7]. Microscopic examination of this fluid reveals fragments of pigmented cartilage [PMID 4459470].

In Whipple disease, inclusions in synovial fluid macrophages may be seen with a periodic acid Schiff stain (PAS).

Malignant cells are rarely seen in synovial fluid and usually represent metastatic disease [PMID 7354476].

Crystal examination, identification & clinical considerations

The identification of crystals in the synovial fluid is one of the few pathognomonic tests in the study of arthritides t7.6. The exact mechanism of crystal deposition is not completely understood, but crystals develop as a result of crystallization of an elevated plasma level that becomes highly concentrated in the joint (urate gout). Formation of crystals may also be associated with hyperparathyroidism, hypomagnesemia, hemochromatosis, severe hypothyroidism, and hypercalcemia (pseudogout, calcium pyrophosphate deposition). Because of these metabolic associations, recommended laboratory screening studies include serum calcium, phosphorus, magnesium, and tests for thyroid function and diabetes mellitus in patients with pseudogout (calcium pyrophosphate deposition disorder).

t7.6 Crystals & associated clinical disorders

Crystal	Clinical disorder
Monosodium urate monohydrate	Urate gout
Calcium pyrophosphate dihydrate (CPPD)	CPPD deposition disease; pseudogout; pyrophosphate gout; chondrocalcinosis
Basic calcium phosphates: hydroxyapatite, octacalcium phosphate, tricalcium phosphate (Whitlockite); dicalcium phosphate (Brushite)	Apatite gout
Calcium oxalate monohydrate (Whewellite); calcium oxalate dihydrate (Weddelite)	Oxalate gout (renal dialysis patients)
Cholesterol esters	Cholesterol gout (chronic effusions, rheumatoid arthritis)

Pseudogout is often associated with various types of degenerative arthritis [ISBN 978-1-4377-1738-9 Terkeltaub]. There is abnormal formation of calcium pyrophosphate crystals in the cartilage, which is later followed by release of crystals into the synovial fluid. Hydroxyapatite and other members of the basic calcium phosphate (BCP) family of crystals are much less often associated with crystal deposition disease. Calcium oxalate crystals may be seen in patients on long term renal dialysis.

Gouty arthritis is a disorder that can be treated successfully, but may require lifelong therapy [ISBN 978-1-4377-1738-9 Burns, Keenan]. Therefore, it is essential that the laboratory examining synovial fluid apply appropriate techniques, and that the examiner have experience in identification of the crystals. It is also important that the specimen be appropriately collected, as described previously (Chapter 2). Ideally, the specimen should be examined for crystals within an hour, but crystal dissolution may be less of a problem than previously thought. Calcium pyrophosphate dihydrate (CPPD) crystals are fairly stable for several weeks and can be maintained for longer periods by freezing.

The types of crystals that may be seen in synovial fluid include monosodium urate monohydrate, calcium pyrophosphate dehydrate, apatite and other calcium phosphates, calcium oxalate monohydrate/dihydrate, cholesterol, and lipids t7.6 [ISBN 978-0-8121-1123-1, ISBN 978-0-8121-1332-7]. Other crystalline structures that may be seen include Charcot-Leyden crystals, cryoglobulin crystals, amyloid fragments, aluminum phosphate crystals, metal fragments from prostheses, fragments of cartilage, and collagen fibrils t7.7.

t7.7 Artifacts that may be seen with polarized microscopic examination

Glass fragments
Dust particles
Fibrils from lens paper
Lipids from degenerated cells
Nail polish used to seal cover slip
Starch from gloves
Drying artifact
Collagen fibrils
Corticosteroids
Cartilage fragments
Metal fragments from prosthesis
Threads
Scratches in glass slide

MSU crystals are the most important crystals to identify since their presence is usually diagnostic of gout. The MSU crystals have a characteristic needlelike appearance and may be intracellular, extracellular, or both i7.19-i7.22. Intracellular MSU crystals are considered specific for the diagnosis of gout; extracellular crystals provide less specific information. A detailed description of examination for crystals is present in Chapter 2. MSU crystals are seen in ~90% of patients during acute attacks of gout. Between acute attacks, they may be seen in ~75% of patients. Crystals may also be found in asymptomatic joints many weeks after an acute attack. In a small number of patients, even during acute attacks, monosodium urate monohydrate crystals may not be found. The reasons for this are many and include aspiration from the wrong site, failure to mix the fluid prior to the examination, loculation within the joint, crystal dissolution, inadequate equipment, examiner inexperience, and insufficient search for crystals. Therefore, a repeat of the examinations for crystals may be required occasionally for a definitive diagnosis. When serum uric acid levels return to normal the MSU crystals slowly dissolve.

Following recurrent attacks of acute gouty arthritis, chalky deposits of urates known as "tophi" develop in articular and periarticular joint tissues (joint capsule, cartilage, and bone). The urates become surrounded by chronic inflammatory cells, foreign body giant cells, and fibrosis i7.23, i7.24. Destruction of the capsular tissue and bone eventually may lead to deforming chronic arthritis if the patient is not treated.

MSU crystals may also occasionally be seen in synovial fluids as a result of inflammation. MSU and CPPD crystals may be seen in patients with septic arthritis. Thus, it is important to consider the possibility of septic arthritis in patients with very high synovial fluid white blood cell counts or in patients who do not respond to treatment with colchicine or nonsteroidal anti-inflammatory agents [PMID 199097, PMID 3051151].

In the majority of patients with acute gouty arthritis, the white blood cell count is 20,000-30,000/µL with ~90% polymorphonuclear leukocytes i7.25. Occasionally, levels as high

7: Synovial Fluid

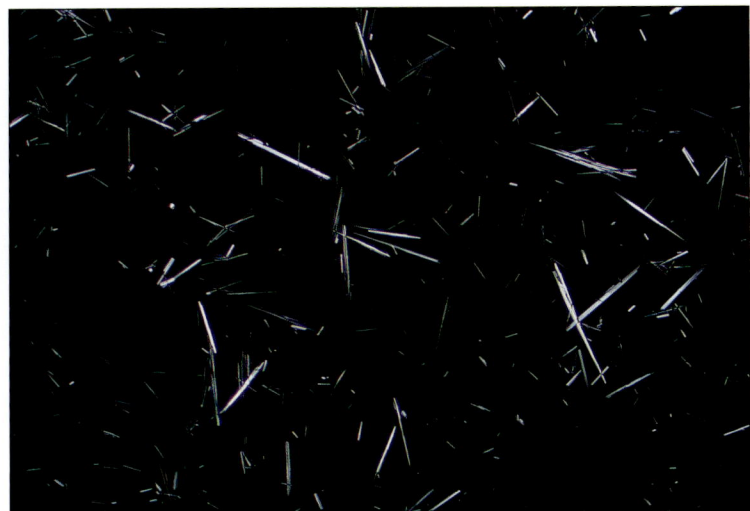

i7.19 Extracellular needle shaped MSU crystals. Polarized light.

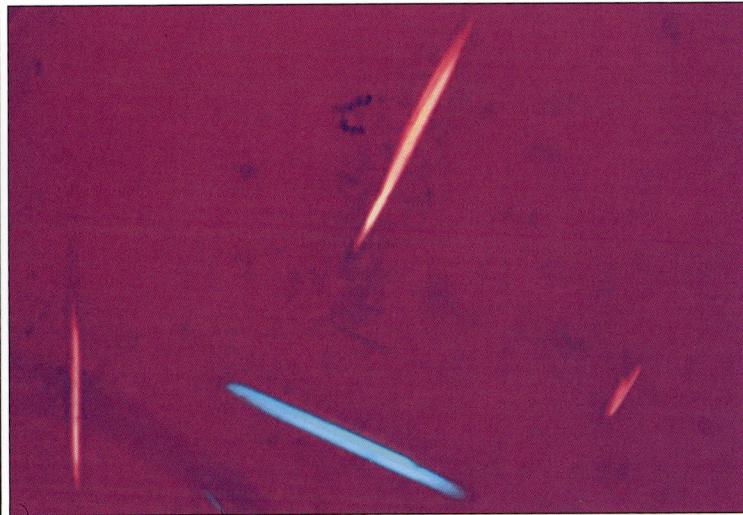

i7.22 Several monosodium urate MSU crystals seen under polarized light and a red compensator. Color of crystals (blue or yellow) depends on orientation of crystals in relation to axis of compensator (see Chapter 2).

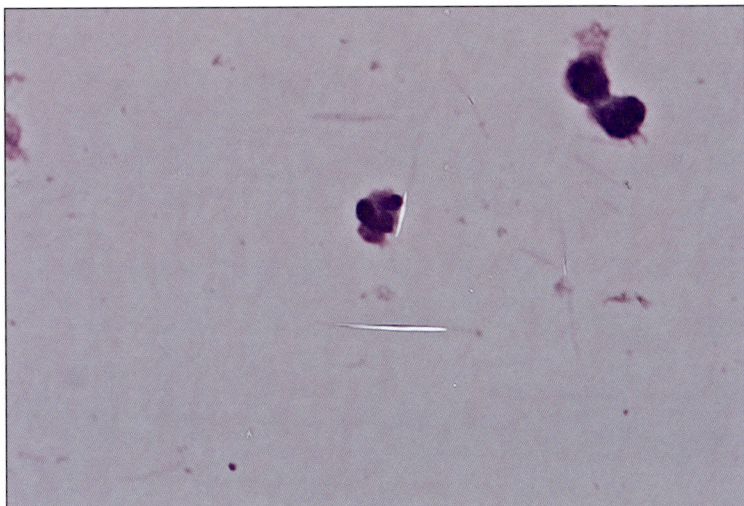

i7.20 1 extracellular and 1 intracellular MSU crystal. Polarized light.

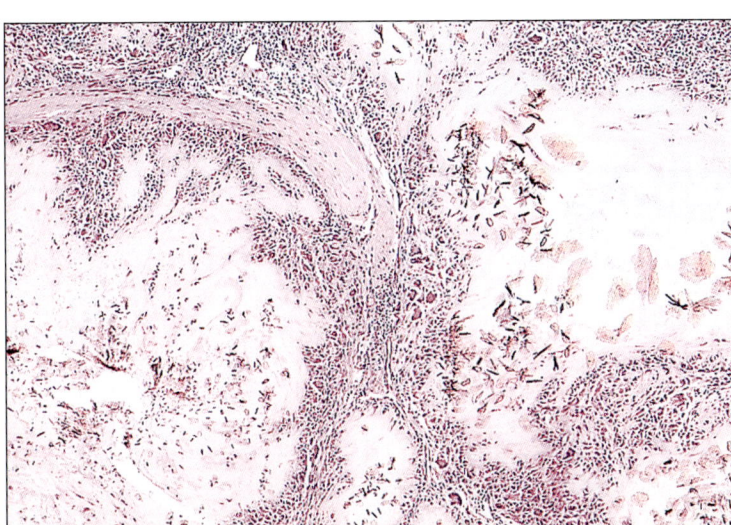

i7.23 Histologic section of synovium from patient with gout showing tophus containing clusters of monosodium urate crystals and chronic inflammatory cells and giant cells (H&E stain)

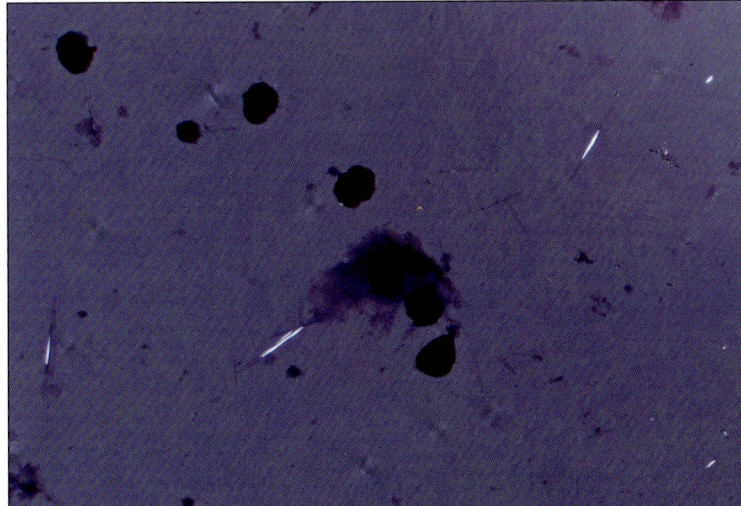

i7.21 Extracellular MSU crystals. Polarized light & red compensator.

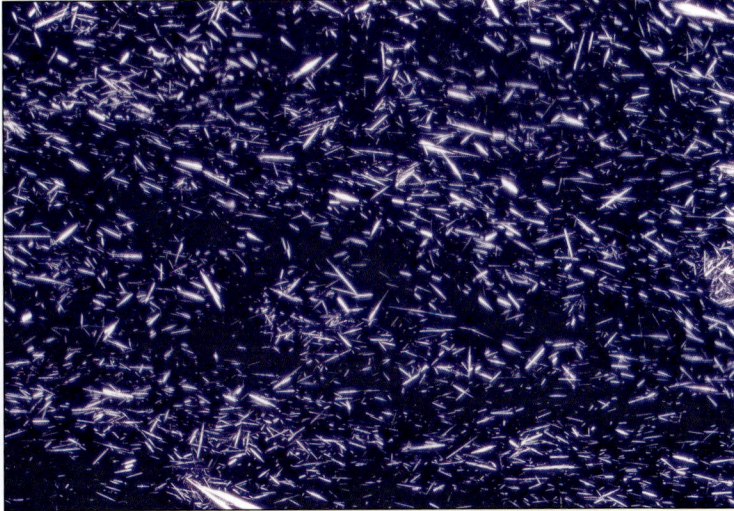

i7.24 Numerous MSU crystals from a tophus. Polarized light.

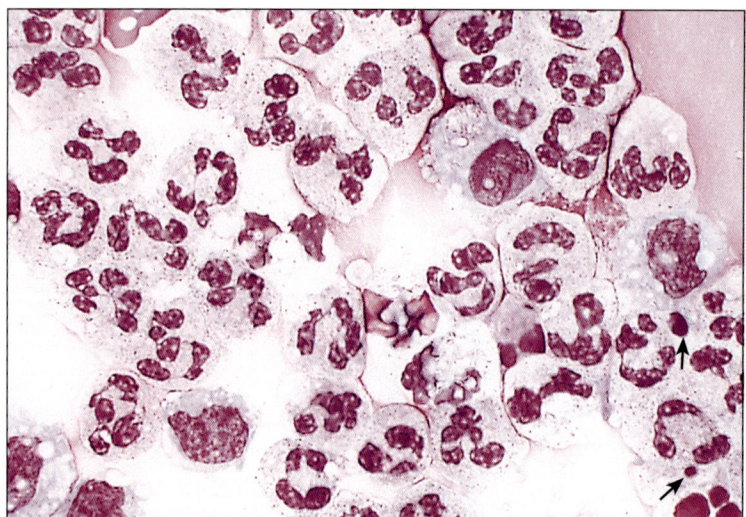

i7.25 Numerous PMNs in synovial fluid from patient with acute gouty arthritis. The karyorrhectic PMN nuclei must not be mistaken for organisms (arrows).

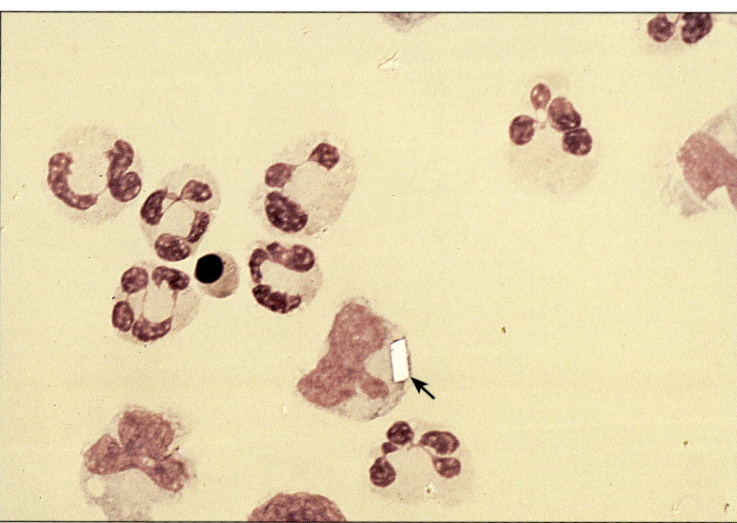

i7.26 A CPPD crystal (arrow). Wright stain, polarized light.

as 200,000/µL or as low as 2,000/µL may occur. Low leukocyte levels usually indicate that the attack is subsiding.

The presence of CPPD crystals is characteristic of a group of disorders collectively called "calcium pyrophosphate deposition disease" (CPDD) [ISBN 978-1-4377-1738-9 Terkeltaub]. Other terms that are used include "pseudogout," "pyrophosphate gout," and "chondrocalcinosis."

CPPD crystals are more difficult to identify than MSU crystals as they are only weakly birefringent with polarized light. Since the majority of CPPD crystals are weakly or not birefringent in ordinary light, microscopy sometimes is better in seeing the crystals. However, polarized microscopy is required for definitive crystal definition. Polarized light on Wright-Giemsa stained cytospin preparations works better than wet preparations. CPPD crystals have a rodlike, platelike, or rhomboid appearance i7.26, i7.27 [ISBN 978-0-8121-1123-1, ISBN 978-0-8121-1332-7]. They may also appear as needles and be mistaken for MSU crystals i7.28. Reliable differentiation from MSU crystals requires a red compensator.

The clinical features of calcium pyrophosphate deposition disease are extremely variable and may mimic many different types of disorders [ISBN 978-1-4377-1738-9 Terkeltaub]. ~1/2 of these patients have a clinical picture similar to that of osteoarthritis, with progressive degeneration of many joints, particularly the knees, wrists, metacarpophalangeal joints, hips, shoulders, elbows, and ankles (in order of frequency). Other patients may initially be seen with clinical features resembling gout—hence the term pseudogout. These patients experience acute or semiacute attacks of arthritis, often involving 1 joint at a time. Septic arthritis must always be ruled out in these cases. A small number

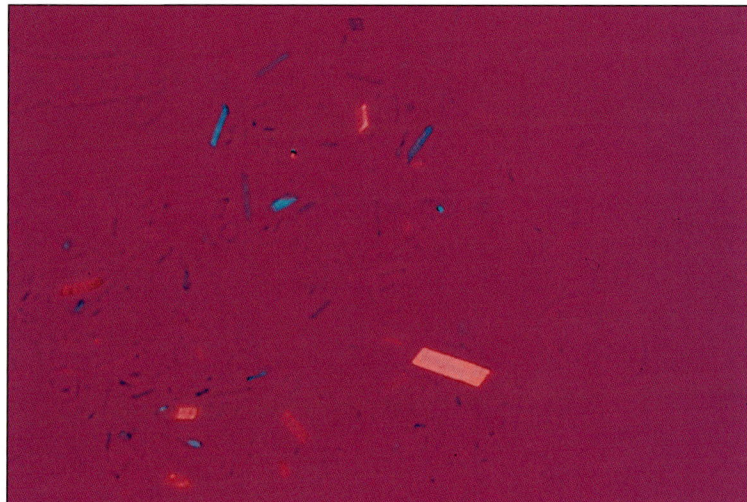

i7.27 Several calcium pyrophosphate crystals as seen with polarized light and red compensator (see Chapter 2)

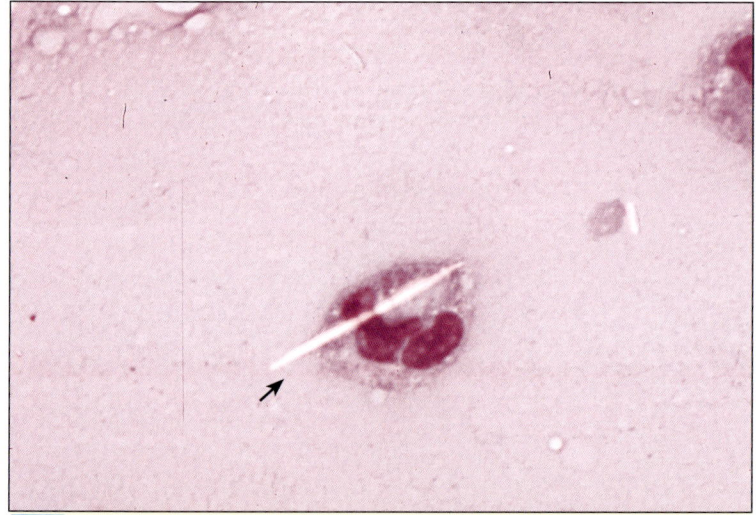

i7.28 This intracellular needle shaped crystal (arrow) could be either a CPPD or an MSU crystal; differentiation can only be achieved with a red compensator (see **f2.6**)

of patients, comprising yet another group, display clinical features resembling rheumatoid arthritis.

The synovial leukocyte count in CPPD deposition disease is usually <50,000/µL, but may occasionally be as high as that seen in septic arthritis.

The histologic changes in CPDD are similar to those seen in MSU arthritis. After a time, crystalline deposits occur in articular tissue, surrounded by chronic inflammatory cells, giant cells, and fibrosis i7.29, i7.30.

Basic calcium phosphate (BCP) crystals include crystals composed of hexagonal carbonate substituted hydroxyapatite occurring together with octacalcium phosphate or occasionally with tricalcium phosphate [ISBN 978-1-4377-1738-9 Terkeltaub]. These crystals are usually too small and too weakly birefringent to be identified by conventional polarized light microscopy. The crystals can be identified by a scanning electron microscope and with the use of X ray energy dispersive (EDAX) analysis coupled with a scanning electron microscope. Alizarin red dye may also be used, but it lacks specificity. Occasionally, BCP crystals may be identified as shiny nonbirefringent irregular cytoplasmic inclusions by light microscopy. Purple cytoplasmic inclusions may be seen on Wright stained smears to suggest the diagnosis.

Several major syndromes have been associated with hydroxyapatite (HA) crystals [PMID 199097]. In acute calcific periarthritis, in which there is periarticular inflammation and transient calcification in the vicinity of the joint, HA crystals are seen in calcific deposits. In a second syndrome, acute calcific arthritis associated with calcification in and/or around the joint, HA crystals are found in synovial fluid and calcific deposits. Finally, HA crystals may be seen in synovial fluid samples from patients with subacute chronic arthritis resembling osteoarthritis. The terms "apatite associated arthropathy," "apatite gout," and "basic calcium phosphate deposition diseases" have been suggested to describe these heterogeneous disorders. In a large study using polarized light microscopy, after instilling alizarin red dye under the coverslip, crystals of hydroxyapatite were found in osteoarthritis (76%) and rheumatoid arthritis (13%) [PMID 1998384].

It is difficult to identify BCP crystals in synovial fluid with certainty in a typical clinical laboratory. Fortunately, their identification does not, at this time, appear to be important for a diagnosis, for a prognosis, or as a guide to treatment in arthritic diseases.

A combination of urate and pyrophosphate crystals in the same synovial fluid is occasionally seen. An increased incidence chondrocalcinosis has been described in patients with hyperuricemia [PMID 7114915]. Hydroxyapatite deposition has been described in patients with gout. In patients with osteoarthritis, the mixture of hydroxyapatite and CPPD

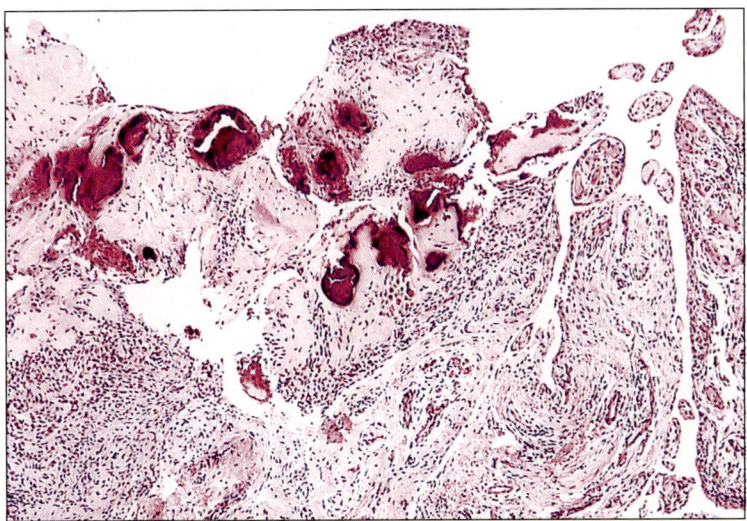

i7.29 Histologic section of synovium from patient with calcium pyrophosphate dehydrate crystal disposition disease. Dark purple areas represent calcium. Surrounding tissue shows chronic inflammation & fibrosis (H&E stain).

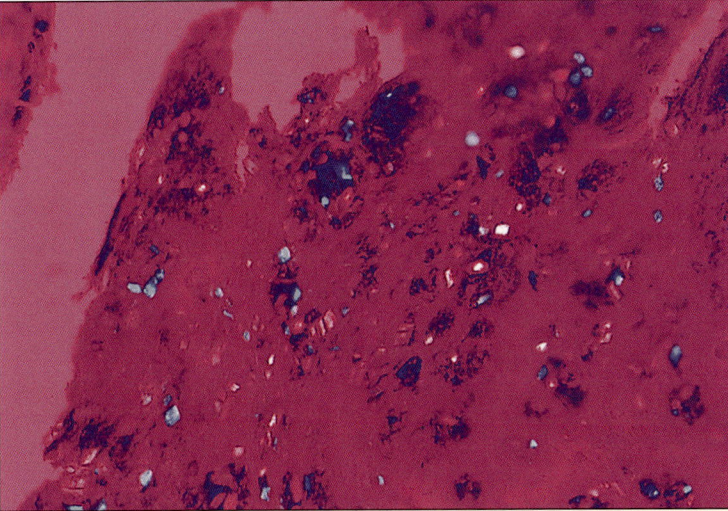

i7.30 Many CPPD crystals seen with polarized light & red compensator in same tissue illustrated in i7.29

crystals in the same joint is as common as the presence of either crystal on its own. In one study, 60% of the synovial fluids from osteoarthritis patients contained CPPD crystals, hydroxyapatite crystals, or both. In a recent retrospective study of 100 synovial fluid samples from patients with osteoarthritis, CPPD crystals were seen in 22% [PMID 20971716]. Furthermore, the prevalence of CPPD crystals in synovial fluid from patients with gout was 7.7%.

Cholesterol crystals in synovial fluid are a rare observation, and most of the patients who have been described have had rheumatoid arthritis of long duration [PMID 3690136,

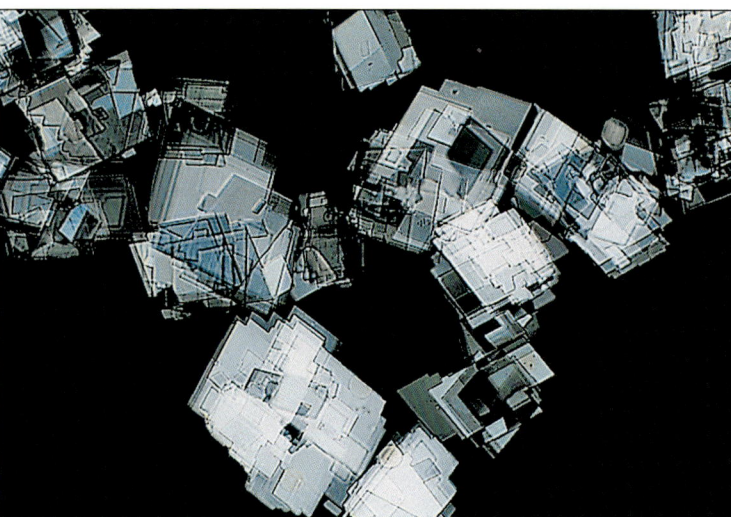

i7.31 Numerous platelike cholesterol crystals in synovial fluid seen with polarized light

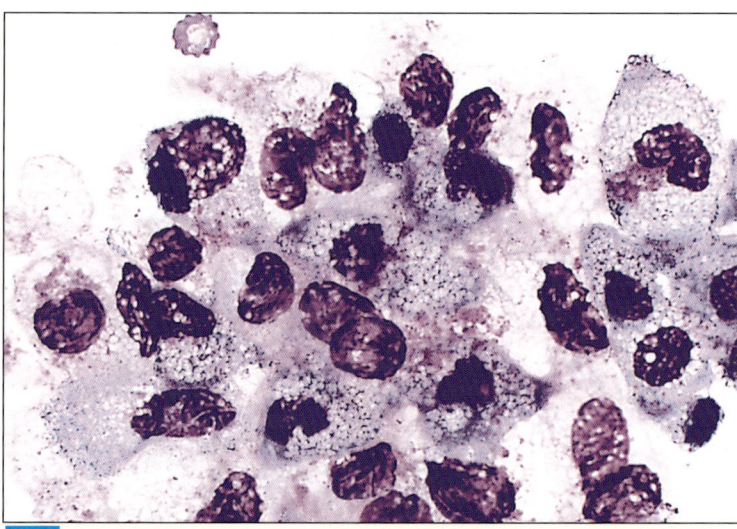

i7.33 Many lipophages (lipid laden macrophages) in synovial fluid (which also contained cholesterol crystals) in a patient with longstanding rheumatoid arthritis

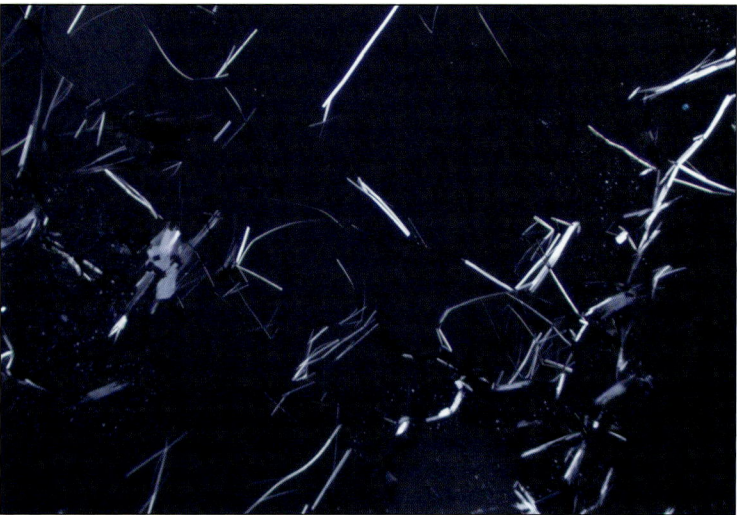

i7.32 Cholesterol crystals resembling MSU or CPPD crystals. Polarlized light.

[PMID 449407]. Cholesterol crystals usually have the appearance of rectangular, notched plates i7.31 [ISBN 978-0-8121-1332-7]. They may be easier to see with regular light microscopy than polarized light. A variety of cholesterol crystal forms may be seen, and some simulate MSU and CPPD crystals i7.32 (see Chapter 2). Cholesterol crystals have also been described in patients with longstanding osteoarthritis and in ankylosing spondylitis [PMID 7230158]. Synovial fluid effusions containing cholesterol crystals appear to be particularly prevalent in the shoulder joint [PMID 3690136]. The mechanism of cholesterol crystal formation is thought to involve cholesterol from cell membranes of degenerating cells associated with impaired drainage of the joint. In addition to cholesterol crystals, many lipophages may be found during the microscopic examination i7.33.

Calcium oxalate crystals may be deposited in primary oxalosis, a rare inborn error of metabolism, in a number of tissues, including joints. More common is calcium oxalate associated arthropathy in patients with chronic renal failure undergoing maintenance hemodialysis [PMID 7092004]. This condition has been particularly striking in patients who have had longstanding renal failure and who are taking large doses of ascorbic acid [PMID 3778544]. Calcium oxalate associated arthropathy has also been described in a patient treated with peritoneal dialysis who did not receive large doses of ascorbic acid [PMID 3404640]. Calcium oxalate dihydrate has a characteristic double pyramid appearance, as seen more frequently in the urine [ISBN 978-0-8121-1332-7]. The monohydrate form of calcium oxalate is nondescript, and the classic pyramid type may sometimes be difficult to find.

It is important in the interpretation of synovial fluid to know whether intra-articular injection of corticosteroids has occurred. Corticosteroid ester crystals may be present extracellularly or intracellularly, being phagocytosed by leukocytes and/or synovial lining cells [PMID 4320615]. Triamcinolone hexacetonide crystals are negatively birefringent, but most of the other steroid crystals utilized are positively birefringent [PMID 3051151]. Although they resemble MSU or CPPD crystals, corticosteroid esters usually have irregular outlines and ragged edges i7.34 [PMID 4320615, ISBN 978-0-8121-1332-7]. The presence of corticosteroid ester crystals particularly may occur when diagnostic aspiration and injection of a joint are done at the same time, and this may be seen in synovial fluid >1 month following injection.

As mentioned previously, liquid lipid crystals, or spherules, with a Maltese cross appearance by polarized light, may be associated with acute arthritis, usually involving trauma, but they have also been described in atraumatic acute arthritis [PMID 2542545].

Charcot-Leyden crystals have been described in eosinophilic synovitis and are canoe shaped particles composed of crystallized lysolecithinase from eosinophils [PMID 3753540, ISBN 978-0-8121-1332-7]. Cryoglobulins have been reported to crystallize in synovial fluid [PMID 6767403]. Aluminum phosphate crystals have been described in patients with chronic renal failure who are taking large amounts of aluminum containing gels. Metal fragments have been described in fluids removed from patients who had metal prosthetic parts [PMID 5823923].

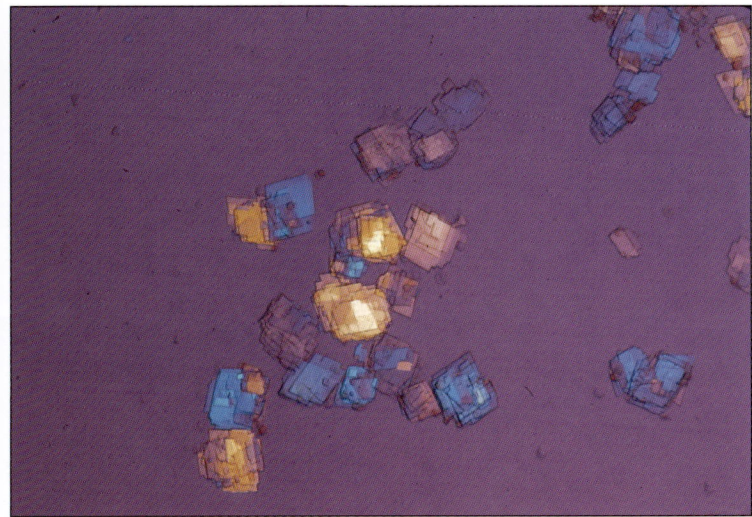

i7.34 Steroid crystals. Polarized light with red compensator.

Chemical & immunologic analysis

Overall, chemical analysis of synovial fluid has little clinical utility and may provide misleading information [PMID 12006320, PMID 16677989, PMID 17405973, PMID 2198352]. Shmerling et al [PMID 2198352] published one of the few studies investigating the clinical sensitivity and specificity of synovial fluid testing. Glucose, protein, and lactate dehydrogenase had low sensitivity and specificity for detecting inflammatory joint disease or septic arthritis and could not differentiate between the disease states. WBC counts and percentage of PMNs contributed independent diagnostic information, but lactate dehydrogenase did not. To date, cell count, culture and crystal identification remain the most informative analyses in synovial fluid [PMID 12006320].

However, select analyses may provide supportive (rather than diagnostic) information in certain cases, particularly in differentiating arthritides. Similar to other fluids, interpretation of biochemical analyte concentrations in synovial fluid are most useful when compared to concurrently collected serum or plasma values. For most analytes, biochemical and immunological analysis of synovial fluid is performed similarly to serum measurements.

Glucose

Glucose is one of the more commonly measured analytes in synovial fluid; however, abnormal concentrations are not indicative of any specific disease process. Measurement may provide clues to leukocyte or bacterial infiltration, pointing the clinician toward a possible disease process. Equilibrium of glucose between plasma and synovial fluid must be reached before measurement, with collections ideally obtained 6-8 hours postprandial. Unless synovial fluid glucose is analyzed within 1 hour of collection, artifactual lowering due to the glycolytic action of leukocytes may take place. Therefore, samples for glucose analysis should be collected in tubes containing sodium fluoride if prompt analysis is not possible [PMID 579389]. Glucose measurement in synovial fluid mimics serum measurement, employing glucose oxidase or hexokinase reactions on routine chemistry analyzers.

At equilibrium, the synovial fluid glucose concentration is normally equal to or slightly lower than (within 10 mg/dL) the serum glucose concentration. In general, glucose concentrations are much lower in the synovial fluid of patients with joint inflammation or infection. Patients with noninflammatory joint disorders (eg, degenerative joint disease, neuropathic osteoarthropathy, pigmented villonodular synovitis, trauma) have synovial fluid glucose concentrations <25 mg/dL below the simultaneously measured serum t7.6. Patients with inflammatory joint diseases (eg, rheumatoid arthritis, rheumatic fever, SLE, and Reiter syndrome) have concentrations that are >25 mg/dL lower than the serum concentrations. In cases of septic arthritis, the synovial fluid glucose concentration is often >40 mg/dL lower than the serum concentration t7.4 [Rippey]. This may help support diagnosis in the event that an initial Gram stain or culture is negative. However, it has been reported that synovial fluid glucose concentrations are decreased in only ~50% of patients with septic arthritis [PMID 3883171]. There is considerable overlap of concentrations in noninflammatory and inflammatory joint disorders and septic arthritis, thus limiting the clinical utility of this measurement.

Protein

Normal synovial fluid is generally considered to be a plasma ultrafiltrate. The filter, however, is not perfect. It permits passage not only of normal electrolytes and other small solutes but also a significant number of plasma proteins. These proteins enter the joint cavity after leaving the synovial capillaries. It is generally assumed that this occurs via passive diffusion rather than active transport. Molecular charge, size and shape may all also affect the rate of protein trans-synovial exchange. Alteration in the vascular or synovial membrane permeability may result from local inflammation.

Total protein concentrations within the synovial fluid space may be determined using traditional biuret or pyrogallol red reagents, with spectrophotometric detection of a colored end product. Mean synovial fluid protein concentrations from various studies have ranged from 1.3-2.8 g/dL with a mean of 1.49 g/dL from all studies (1.88 g/dL in cadavers and 1.38 g/dL in living volunteers). The major differences in these studies may be due to the use of varying methods of protein analysis. In addition, essentially all studies measured the protein concentration in synovial fluid from knee joints. However, abundant animal data indicate that significant differences in concentration between locations are the rule, not the exception [PMID 2672342].

Protein concentrations >3.0 g/dL usually indicate an inflammatory, infectious or hemorrhagic exudate and are observed in RA, gout, septic arthritis, SLE, the inflammatory arthropathies accompanying Crohn disease, Reiter syndrome, ankylosing spondylitis, psoriasis, and ulcerative colitis. Most of these proteins are derived from plasma due to increased vascular permeability. Local immunoglobulin synthesis also occurs.

As inflammation progresses and permeability becomes affected, larger proteins will increasingly be found within the synovial space. Fibronectin is a high molecular weight glycoprotein found in body fluids, the connective tissue matrix and basement membranes. Early studies have reported significantly higher fibronectin concentrations in the synovial fluid of patients with RA, as compared with plasma concentrations [PMID 7056032]. Fibronectin concentrations in these patients did not correlate with other measures of inflammation, such as erythrocyte sedimentation rate or synovial fluid cell counts, indicating local production of fibronectin by the synovium. β_2 microglobulin and C-reactive protein are smaller molecular weight proteins that have also been identified in the synovial fluid of patients with RA [PMID 2512862, PMID 6158572].

An early report indicated that total protein measurements in synovial fluid are unable to discriminate between inflammatory arthropathies [Hasselbacher 1986]. This and other findings point to the limited utility of this measurement and do not recommend it as part of routine testing of synovial fluid.

Uric acid

As mentioned, the preferred laboratory diagnosis of gout is made by MSU crystal identification in synovial fluid. As a result, quantitation of synovial fluid uric acid is seldom recommended. However, polarized microscopy and adequate technical expertise may not be available in all laboratories. Reports detailing this lack of expertise include a quality assurance survey of 6 teaching hospitals in Australia that revealed false positive crystal identification (11% of samples) and missed MSU crystals (21% of samples), with 2 laboratories reporting 50% or fewer correct results [PMID 1759919, PMID 3606682]. Thus, uric acid analysis of synovial fluid may be more commonly requested than is recommended in order to supplement microscopy studies. It may be particularly useful in cases where symptoms are indicative of a gout diagnosis but crystals are not identified.

Most automated chemistry analyzers utilize the uricase reaction for measurement of uric acid. Uric acid concentrations in synovial fluid typically correlate with serum concentrations [PMID 7226556]. As a result, many believe that joint effusions in gout also have urate concentrations essentially identical to that of serum [ISBN 978-0-3161-5004-0]. However, others have reported that the measurement of synovial fluid uric acid is a better single diagnostic factor than its measurement in serum [PMID 5855250, PMID 8809438]. As such, a synovial fluid uric acid concentration significantly higher than the upper reference range for serum may be diagnostic of gout [PMID 51606, PMID 5855250]. Of course, in untreated gout, both synovial fluid and serum uric acid levels are usually elevated.

Enzymes

Many enzymes have been studied in synovial fluid, including lactate dehydrogenase (LD), aspartate aminotransferase (AST), acid and alkaline phosphatase, muramidase (lysozyme), N-acetyl-D-glucosaminidase, 5'-nucleotidase, γ–glutamyltransferase, adenosine deaminase and cytidine deaminase. Of these, LD is the most common enzyme measured in synovial fluid. It can be measured using routine enzymatic methods on automated chemistry analyzers.

While sensitive to bacterial infection, elevated LD concentrations are not specific and may lead to false positive determinations of septic arthritis [PMID 2198352, PMID 6497466]. Elevated LD concentrations may also be found in the synovial fluid of patients with noninfectious inflammatory processes such as RA and gout. LD presence in the fluid of these patients is presumably due to the high concentration of LD found in the infiltrating neutrophils [PMID 14212943, PMID 1593572]. In contrast, the LD activity is normal in synovial fluid from patients with (noninflammatory) osteoarthritis. Its concentration appears to be related to the severity of inflammation in patients with RA, with concentrations between 400 and 700 U/L indicating moderate inflammation and concentrations >750 U/L corresponding to high levels of inflammation [PMID 1593572]. However, as mentioned, the Shmerling et al study [PMID 2198352] indicated that LD provided no independent diagnostic information when detecting inflammatory joint disease or septic arthritis.

Overall, while numerous enzymes have been investigated for measurement in synovial fluid, definitive association of enzyme concentrations and disease severity or prognostic ability has yet to be elucidated.

Lactate

Numerous publications have established that synovial fluid lactic acid concentrations are increased in patients with monoarticular septic arthritis when compared with nonseptic monoarticular arthritis [PMID 1794370, PMID 7473474, PMID 7747151]. The reasons for increased synovial fluid lactate levels in infected joints are uncertain. Although small amounts of lactate are undoubtedly produced by the neutrophils and bacteria that are present, the major contributor is probably the synovial tissue. It has been suggested that the increased metabolic demand within the inflamed synovium leads to relative hypoxia, resulting in the synovial tissue conversion from aerobic to anaerobic glycolysis, in which lactic acid is the end product [PMID 7313579, PMID 7472474].

The predominant measurement is by automated chemistry analyzers monitoring the conversion of lactate to pyruvate, but blood gas analyzers may be used to obtain more rapid results. Gas liquid chromatography methods for lactic acid have also been described [PMID 697948, PMID 7076866, PMID 7115453, PMID 7472474], and measurements of both L-lactic acid and its optical isomer D-lactic acid have been explored [PMID 7472474]. Although lactic acid reference intervals for synovial fluid have not been specifically established, it can be reasonably assumed that they are similar to those found in blood and cerebrospinal fluid (9-29 mg/dL; 0.98-3.7 mmol/L) of normal individuals [PMID 7273404, PMID 7313579].

Rapid lactate determinations can be readily obtained in most laboratories; thus this measurement appears to be useful for the quick diagnosis of septic arthritis [PMID 7076866]. This may be particularly helpful in cases in which bacterial stains are negative or in which antimicrobial treatment may have preceded diagnostic techniques [PMID 7076866]. Moreover, the use of large amounts of local anesthetic may inhibit the growth of many microorganisms [PMID 4393033] and prevent a conclusive diagnosis. In this situation, the estimation of synovial fluid lactic acid becomes a valuable diagnostic tool. However, it should be noted that a normal lactate concentration does not definitively rule out infection.

There are 4 primary limitations that one should take into consideration in interpreting synovial fluid lactate concentrations. First, normal or intermediate values may neither confirm nor exclude infection. Second, concentrations may be low or normal in gonococcal arthritis [PMID 6886455]. Third, although elevated lactate concentrations are indicative of septic arthritis, they may also be elevated in nonseptic arthritis, particularly RA [PMID 6886455]. Fourth, the test gives no clue to the specific nature of the infecting organism, and the physician will have to treat the patient empirically until the culture results are known.

Lipids

As with other body soft tissues, lipids constitute a significant part of the areas in and around joints. This is especially true of the synovium, intra-articular fat pad, and bone marrow, which are composed of 70%-90% lipids by dry weight [PMID 3547659]. Although various lipids are normally present in synovial fluid, their concentrations are much lower (average 40%) than those found in plasma [PMID 14223919, PMID 7548857]. The concentrations are reportedly significantly higher in inflammatory and crystal induced arthritis (eg, RA, SLE and gout), as compared to noninflammatory (osteoarthritis) effusions [PMID 14223919, PMID 22037510]. Enzymatic measurements of cholesterol and triglycerides can be performed with automated chemistry analyzers.

Synovial fluid lipid effusions may loosely be categorized into 3 groups: (1) cholesterol rich effusions, (2) lipid droplets within joint fluid, and (3) chylous synovial effusions [PMID 3547659].

Cholesterol rich effusions not only have high cholesterol concentrations, but usually contain microscopically identifiable cholesterol crystals and are associated with chronic RA. These fluids, however, are relatively rare and constitute only 0.1-0.3% of all fluids examined [PMID 3547659]. Nevertheless, a few reports have noted them in other inflammatory joint disorders [PMID 449407, PMID 951619]. Synovial fluid cholesterol concentrations in these fluids range from that normally present in serum to as high as 2,600 mg/dL, whereas triglyceride levels range from normal to 2-3× that normally seen in serum [PMID 3547659].

Neutrophils within the synovial fluid may contain lipid droplets, which can be visualized with Sudan or oil red O stains. They are associated with many forms of arthritis, but are nonspecific. Large lipid droplets are often associated with trauma [PMID 3547659]. When present in combination with gross blood, intra-articular fracture or serious cartilage or ligamentous injury may be suspected.

Chylous synovial effusions are extremely rare. Although they may appear purulent, leukocyte counts are usually only mildly elevated. Chylous effusions have been reported in association with RA, SLE, filariasis, pancreatitis and trauma [PMID 3547659].

Cholesterol concentrations may offer assistance in cases of inconclusive microscopic crystal analysis, as cholesterol crystals may resemble MSU or other crystal types. However, there is no definitive documentation that supports routine lipid measurement in synovial fluid.

pH

Synovial fluid from an inflamed joint may have a lower (acidic) pH than noninflamed fluid. Glucose utilization by WBC leads to lactic acid production, thus increasing hydrogen ion concentrations. However, there is little clinical utility in the measurement of pH in synovial fluid. Proper (anaerobic) specimen handling is difficult to ensure and comparable clinical information can be more easily gleaned from other measurements already mentioned.

Immunologic analysis

Rheumatoid factor (RF) is one type of autoantibody produced by patients with RA. It reacts with the Fc region of IgG and has been associated with IgA, IgG and (most often) IgM globulins. RF is present in the synovial fluid of ~60% of RA patients, usually in slightly lower titers than those found in the serum [PMID 4341270]. Occasionally, patients with seronegative test results will have positive results for RF in synovial fluid [PMID 14057620, PMID 5316357]. Since a wide variety of other chronic inflammatory processes are characterized by persistent antigenic stimuli, false positive results are common [PMID 4118982, PMID 5316357, PMID 5548446]. In general, however, assays for RF have not been helpful for disease diagnosis or prognosis [ISBN 978-0-8121-1123-1].

~70% of patients with SLE and ~20% of patients with RA will have antinuclear antibodies (ANAs) in the synovial fluid [PMID 4341270]. However, ANA measurement in synovial fluid is not specific enough to be used diagnostically [PMID 4118982].

Complement components are a group of nonspecific serum factors that interact in a cascading sequence during immunologic reactions. The end result of their activation is increased blood vessel permeability, recruitment of neutrophils from the circulation and eventual phagocytosis of antigen-antibody complexes found within the joint space. Complement proteins normally enter the joint space in proportion to their size and total serum protein concentration. Therefore, interpretation of complement levels depends not only on the total serum complement but also on the total protein concentration. Patients with RA and SLE often have a preponderance of antigen-antibody complexes present in the synovial fluid, thus complement activity can be a useful measure in these individuals.

Historically, total hemolytic complement (CH50) was used to measure the functional activity of all complement components. The CH50 value represents the ability of the fluid to lyse 50% of a standard suspension of sheep erythrocytes coated with rabbit antibody. Today individual complement components, most commonly C2, C3 and C4, can be measured by automated nephelometric, turbidimetric or immunoturbidimetric methods. In general, normal synovial fluid complement concentrations are ~10% of the total serum complement concentration [PMID 729254]. Additionally, t7.8 relates complement and protein values in normal synovial fluid.

t7.8 Correlation of protein & complement levels in normal synovial fluid

Total Protein (mg/mL)	Complement (CH50 U/mL)
20	8-38
30	11-42
40	15-46
50	19-50

As inflammation occurs and joint permeability is enhanced, protein, including complement, enters the articular cavity. For most inflammatory fluids, complement concentrations are ~40%-70% of serum activity [PMID 729254]. However, in RA and SLE complement is consumed locally and the synovial fluid complement level will be therefore be decreased. Synovial fluid complement concentrations in these patients may be 30% of the serum complement concentration [PMID 4330119]. RA and SLE may be distinguished from each other if serum complement is included in the analysis; serum complement may be decreased in SLE but increased in RA. Decreased synovial fluid complement concentrations may also be observed in septic and crystal induced arthritis. Normal or slightly elevated total complement concentrations may be present in the synovial fluid of patients with traumatic or degenerative joint disease, Reiter syndrome, psoriatic arthritis, ankylosing spondylitis, seronegative juvenile RA and seronegative RA t7.9 [PMID 4330119, PMID 7470168].

t7.9 Complement levels in patients with joint disease

Disease	Serum levels	Synovial fluid levels
Seropositive rheumatoid arthritis	Normal or ↑	Normal or ↓
Seronegative rheumatoid arthritis	Normal or ↑	Normal
Seronegative juvenile rheumatoid arthritis	Normal or ↑	Normal
Systemic lupus erythematosus	Normal or ↓	↓
Reiter syndrome	Normal or ↑	Normal or ↑
Ankylosing spondylitis	Normal or ↑	Normal
Psoriatic arthritis	Normal or ↑	Normal
Septic arthritis	Normal or ↑	Normal or ↓
Crystal induced arthritis	Normal or ↑	Normal or ↓

Newer biomarkers

A multitude of reports highlight newer biomarkers of joint disease that may be found in synovial fluid. Substances as varied as lubricin, fibronectin, bradykinin, fractalkine, leptin, glucosamine, cytokines (eg, TNF-α, IL-8, IL-6, IL-1β), matrix metalloproteinases and autoantibodies to glucose-6-phospate isomerase have been proposed for diagnostic and prognostic uses for a variety of disorders. Their utility has yet to be confirmed. Drug concentrations have been measured in synovial fluid and may be helpful [PMID 6360465]; however interpretation is difficult due to lack of clinical data. Additionally, the use of synovial fluid in postmortem analysis has been proposed. Comparisons with vitreous humor show that a subset of chemical analytes has similar stabilities and concentrations in both fluids [PMID 11343852]. This may be useful in cases where vitreous humor is unavailable, compromised or depleted by other testing.

Microbiologic examination

Septic arthritis is the most rapidly destructive disease of joints. As such, all suspected cases should be considered as medical emergencies since permanent joint damage is a common complication. These infections are usually hematogenously acquired since the synovium is extremely vascular, which promotes access to the joint space. Although viruses, *Mycobacterium* species, and fungi may all be causative agents, aerobic bacteria are clearly the most common infectious organisms. Certain bacteria, such as *Neisseria gonorrhoeae* i7.15, i7.16 and *Staphylococcus aureus*, are particularly likely to infect a joint during a bacteremic episode. Bacteremia is less common in septic arthritis attributed to Gram– bacilli, with blood cultures only positive in ~50% of cases, whereas the synovial fluid is culture positive in 90% of cases [PMID 12364368]. Less commonly, bacterial entry may be facilitated by a deep penetrating wound, intra-articular steroid injection, arthroscopy, prosthetic joint surgery, contiguous rupture of osteomyelitis into the joint, or neighboring soft tissue sepsis. [PMID 22100289]. Furthermore, arthritis, recent or past joint trauma, and surgery (particularly prosthetic joint implantation) are all important risk factors in developing synovial infections.

Septic arthritis can be conceptually grouped into 3 major causations: gonococcal i7.35, nongonococcal, and other (including Lyme disease, *Mycobacterium* species, and fungi). The majority (>80%) of septic arthritis cases are nongonococcal, and an invaluable predictor of the offending agent is patient age [PMID 22100289, PMID 9449882]. *Staphylococcus aureus* i7.36 is the most common organism identified in all age groups (~44%), regardless of specific risk factors [PMID 12539074]. *S aureus* and *Streptococcus agalactiae* account for the majority of septic arthritis in children <2 months of age, while *Kingella kingae*, *Streptococcus pyogenes*, and *S aureus* account for the majority of infections in children 2 months to 5 years of age [PMID 22100289]. *Haemophilus influenzae* once accounted for 30% of septic arthritis cases in patients younger than 2 years of age, but in recent decades its incidence has rapidly declined likely due to widespread vaccination against *H influenzae* serogroup b [PMID 10573336, PMID 22100289]. In the case of *K kingae*, which is extremely fastidious, direct inoculation of the specimen into a blood culture bottle is paramount for culture based recovery of this organism [PMID 15172344]. This awareness and improved culture practice likely accounts for *K kingae* being considered an emerging cause of pediatric septic arthritis, thought to account for up to 50% of septic arthritis cases in children <24 months [PMID 12364368, PMID 21321033, PMID 9725094].

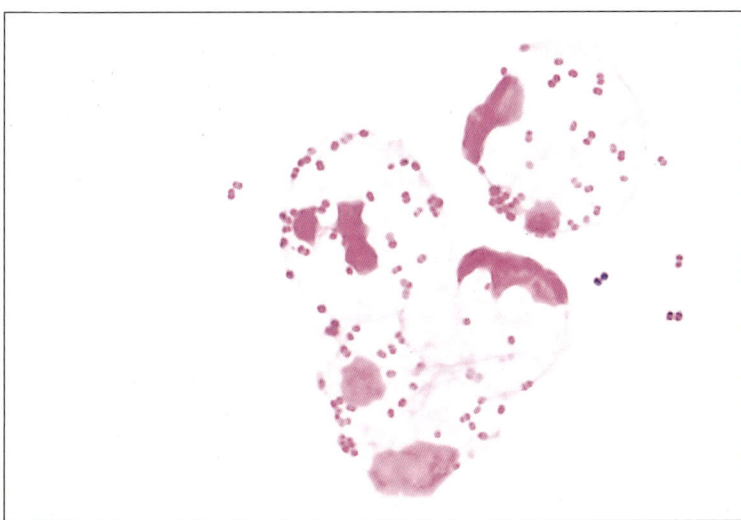

i7.35 Gram stain of synovial fluid showing *Neisseria gonorrhoeae*

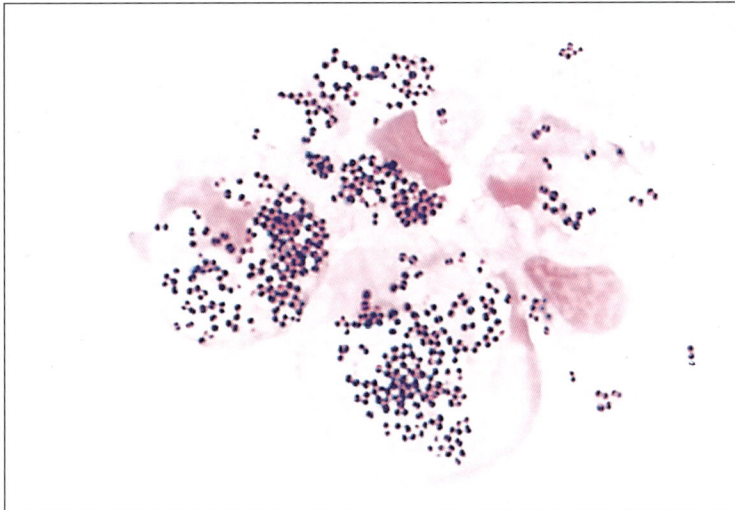

i7.36 Gram stain of synovial fluid showing *S aureus*

Collectively, children <2 years of age account for ~1/3 of all septic arthritis cases. In children aged 2-15 years, *S aureus*, *S pyogenes*, and *S pneumoniae* account for ~85% of cases, with *S aureus* responsible for nearly 1/2 of those. In patients aged 16-50 years, *N gonorrhoeae* once accounted for up to 75% of cases in the United States (through the 1970s); however public health initiatives lead to substantial reductions in those rates, though increasing fluoroquinolone resistance may lead to a resurgence in these infections in the future [PMID 10923855]. *S aureus* is now the most frequently recovered cause of septic arthritis in patients >2 years old, accounting for ~40% of cases. [PMID 21916390]. Septic arthritis with methicillin resistant *S aureus* (MRSA) is a major concern for treatment outcome, and estimates (based on case reports) suggest that 5%-25% of *S aureus* septic arthritis is due to MRSA [PMID 21916390].

In addition to age specific predictors, patient specific risk factors can also account for variability in expected pathogens in synovial fluids. Intravenous drug users are at particular risk for infections with opportunistic pathogens and unusual environmental Gram− bacilli in addition to MRSA [PMID 22100289]. Adults with RA are particularly prone to develop joint infections (~10-fold the normal population); the majority caused by *S aureus* [PMID 8849354]. Septic arthritis with a variety of Gram− bacilli is also found in patients with a wide array of immune disorders (both inherited and drug induced). In particular, patients with complement deficiencies are at increased risk for gonococcal and meningococcal (*Neisseria menigitidis*) septic arthritis [PMID 21916390]. Though gonococcal arthritis has declined dramatically, women remain at highest risk of infections due to asymptomatic infections that disseminate during pregnancy and shortly after menses. Men who have sex with men are also at increased risk of gonococcal arthritis due to the recent rise of infections specifically in this population, often in concert with HIV infections. Patients with HIV infections are additionally at risk for *S aureus* (most frequent), *Mycobacterium* species, and fungal infections of the joint [PMID 9133965]. The final risk factor of particular concern in recent years is patients undergoing prosthetic joint surgeries. This group has been shown to be at particular risk for hospital acquired MRSA in addition to significant infection with typically avirulent skin flora such as *Propionibacterium acnes* and coagulase negative *Staphylococcus* species [PMID 22100289].

The outcome of treatment depends on multiple interrelated factors, each being important in the eventual outcome. These factors can include

- duration of symptoms
- host defense mechanisms
- prior joint disease
- type of bacteria present (and resistance factors)
- specific joint infected
- history of prosthetic joint placement

Generally speaking, when septic arthritis is diagnosed and treated early, the clinical outcome is universally favorable. Generally considered, drug resistant organisms tend to be more difficult to treat, and prosthetic joint infections typically involve complex biofilms that are difficult to eradicate with antimicrobial therapy alone. Importantly the majority of patients with gonococcal arthritis completely recover, whereas ~50% of staphylococcal arthritis have serious residual joint disease and patients with polyarticular, septic, nongonococcal arthritis have mortality rates of 30%-40% [PMID 22100289].

The routine examination of synovial fluid should include a cytocentrifuged Gram stain if the fluid is turbid (but not opaque), as well as routine aerobic and anaerobic bacterial cultures. Failure to culture various microorganisms often depends on their stringent growth requirements. Applying a blood culture procedure to culture synovial fluid is the most important step to improve recovery of fastidious organisms attributed to these infections (see Chapter 2). An additional problem that may complicate the isolation of microorganisms from septic joint fluid is the antimicrobial activity of tubes containing EDTA and to a lesser extent heparin and sodium polyanethol sulfonate (SPS). Tubes containing these substances should be avoided. If tuberculosis, fungi, or anaerobic bacteria are suspected, special handling and culture media are needed as described in Chapter 2. Synovial fluid smears are positive for acid-fast bacilli in ~20% of proven cases, while cultures are usually positive in ~80% of proven cases. In the case of tuberculosis, a closed synovial biopsy specimen taken for histologic examination may provide the most rapid diagnosis. Whenever a joint effusion is noted, careful consideration of the possible causes should precede aspiration to assure proper specimen collection and testing is ordered. A consultation at this stage with a clinical microbiologist may prove helpful, by saving considerable time and possibly leading to a diagnosis that otherwise might be missed. In early or mild bacterial infections, for example, the gross fluid examination alone may suggest a nonseptic origin. Furthermore, prominent fluid leukocytosis is present not only in septic arthritis, but in inflammatory and crystal induced arthritis as well t7.4. Moreover, infectious arthritis can readily complicate the inflammatory and crystal induced arthritides. Hence, failure to adequately culture the specimen may result in a missed or delayed diagnosis, a prolonged clinical course, and possible permanent injury to the joint in the case of nongonococcal disease.

Despite its recent decline, *N gonorrhoeae* remains an important causative agent of septic arthritis; it is imperative that the proper media be inoculated immediately after fluid aspiration. *Neisseria gonorrhoeae* is best recovered on prewarmed modified Thayer Martin media and should be inoculated at bedside and immediately transferred to a CO_2 containing incubator (5%-10%). This is not always practical, leading to consistent difficulties in recovering viable *N gonorrhoeae* in culture. In fact, *N gonorrhoeae* is recovered in <50% of infected joints in patients with disseminated gonococcal infections. In culture negative cases, a positive Gram stain of Gram– diplococci from a synovial fluid is still consistent with presumptive gonococcal septic arthritis.

Routine microbiologic studies frequently require 2 or more days before culture results are available. Molecular testing holds great promise for the investigation of culture negative "septic" arthritis; however the wide array of potential pathogens poses as a barrier to conventional PCR assays. An alternative method is PCR amplification of conserved housekeeping genes directly from a synovial fluid (eg, 16S rRNA for bacteria, 18S rRNA for fungi) and subsequent sequencing of the gene product (see Chapter 2). This method is has been conventionally applied to biopsy specimens and formalin fixed, paraffin embedded tissues, but can theoretically be applied to all normally sterile body fluids. One limitation is that this technique is prone to exogenous and laboratory derived bacterial DNA, so results should be interpreted with care in the context of the clinical presentation.

Lyme arthritis

Lyme disease was first described in Old Lyme, Connecticut, in 1976 [PMID 836338], although historical records indicate a similar clinical syndrome existed in Europe in at least 1921 (likely before then) [Afzelius 1921]. Once thought to be a local disease of New England, the causative spirochete *Borrelia burgdorferi* is actually found throughout the United States and Canada, wherever the host ticks *Ixodes scapularis* or *I pacificus* are found. The majority of endemic Lyme disease cases are reported from states in the northeastern United States, the northern Midwest states, and eastern Canada [PMID 22962880]. Between the years of 1992 and 2006, the incidence of Lyme disease increased from ~9,900 cases per year to nearly 20,000 cases per year [PMID 22962880].

Diagnosing Lyme disease is challenging and has become controversial in recent years. While the medical community largely follows specific criteria for defining Lyme disease, several patient advocacy groups contest that the recommended testing and treatment algorithms drafted by the Infectious Disease Society of America (IDSA) and the Centers for Disease Control and Prevention are inadequate [PMID 17029130, PMID 7623762]. The currently accepted diagnostic algorithm for Lyme disease includes a 2 step serological testing algorithm, which involves a screen with a total serum antibody ELISA or IFA, and subsequent confirmatory testing with IgM and/or IgG Western blot(s) from the same serum sample [PMID 7623762]. IgM Western blots can remain positive for several years, and are not recommended for patients with signs and symptoms that have persisted for >30 days [PMID 7623762]. Specific criteria for the blot interpretation are followed in order to provide standardized case definitions based on these test results. Lyme Western blots can be difficult to interpret (open to subjectivity), which further drives the controversy underlying this disease. The same testing algorithm can be applied to CSF specimens to aid in the diagnosis of neuroborreliosis, and demonstration of intrathecal production of Lyme antibodies is preferred by the IDSA over other methods [PMID 17029130]. Like other spirochetal infections (eg, syphilis), molecular tests have proven to be of limited utility in diagnosis (defined by specific clinical circumstances of suspected neuroborreliosis and early Lyme arthritis) [PMID 17266710]. The spirochete is difficult to capture in a given clinical specimen, rendering molecular tests insensitive largely due to sampling error. The sensitivity in synovial fluid particularly is significantly lower in patients who received therapy for Lyme disease, and studies suggest that synovial tissue provides better sensitivity than the fluid [PMID 11257206 PMID 18452806, PMID 8639170].

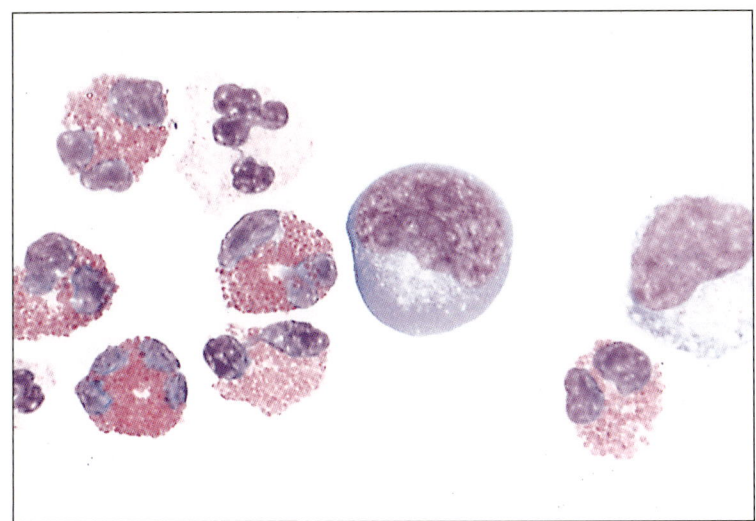

i7.37 Synovial eosinophilia in a case of Lyme disease

Many patients with Lyme disease present with a characteristic skin rash known as erythema migrans, or more commonly the "bull's eye rash." As the acute infection progresses, transient oligoarticular symptoms of arthralgia or myalgia may develop. In some cases, joint swelling may be clinically documented. Lyme arthritis is typically a symptom of late stage disease and may develop in upwards of 60% of untreated patients [PMID 20425509]. Importantly, many patients successfully treated for Lyme disease may still develop symptoms of late Lyme infection, including arthritis [PMID 18452806, PMID 20425509]. Many of these arthritis cases are considered to be largely autoimmune mediated, with no evidence of active Lyme disease [PMID 18452806]. The large joints (hips & knees) are most commonly afflicted by Lyme arthritis. Analysis of the synovial fluid will reveal a typical inflammatory profile, and may include eosinophilia t7.7, i7.37. Serological testing from the synovial fluid is not recommended. Culture and PCR from the synovial fluid both lack sensitivity (see above); though a positive result would be considered diagnostic. Importantly, these methods should not replace serological testing, but may be performed as adjunct diagnostic measures in specific clinical situations [PMID 11257206, PMID 17266710].

Artifacts & pitfalls

- Specimen storage and incubation can lead to spurious results for crystal detection. MSU crystals decrease in numbers significantly when stored for >3 days (an effect slowed by refrigeration). CPPD crystals however decrease significantly after 2-3 days in storage (regardless of refrigeration) [PMID 2930602]. Falsely negative results can be obtained if improper storage conditions are maintained or specimen processing is delayed.

- Artifacts that resemble MSU crystals and CPPD crystals may be found in the synovial fluid, including collagen fibrils, cartilage fragments, metallic fragments after prosthetic arthroplasty, and microcrystalline corticosteroid esters t7.7 [ISBN 978-0-8121-1332-7]. These can lead to falsely positive reports of crystals from synovial fluid.

- Polarized light examination is also subject to generating microscopic artifacts. Examples from synovial fluid include a fluid drying out effect, glass fragments, fibrils from lens paper, dust, starch from gloves, and nail polish (if used to seal coverslips) t7.7 [ISBN 978-0-8121-1332-7]. Calcium oxalate powder, EDTA, and lithium heparin can form birefringent crystals that may be phagocytosed by neutrophils. These crystalline artifacts usually have indistinct, amorphous form or nonparallel, jagged edges.

- Anticoagulants such as EDTA, and to a lesser extent heparin and SPS, can lead to spurious results of microbiologic studies. Each has antimicrobial properties that can result in falsely negative cultures, which in the setting of a negative Gram stain, could lead to a missed diagnosis of septic arthritis.

- Time and temperature stability of microbiologic specimens is also crucial for avoiding falsely negative cultures. Collection tubes should be maintained at room temperature and expedited to the laboratory for culture setup within 24 hours. Due to the invasive nature of synovial fluid collection, cultures should still be performed past 24 hours; however the results must carry a strongly worded disclaimer explaining the possibility of a false negative culture due to suboptimal specimen handling. Conversely, false positive culture results can be achieved if sterile technique is not maintained during collection of the synovial fluid. Complicating the result interpretations for contaminated cultures is the fact that contaminating skin flora are possible pathogens in septic joints (eg, coagulase negative *Staphylococcus* and *Propionibacterium acnes*) [PMID 22100289].

- The association of genitourinary *Chlamydia trachomatis* infection with Reiter syndrome can lead to unnecessary microbiologic interrogation of synovial fluid. The organism is not found in the synovial fluid and testing will invariably be negative, which can lead to misinterpretation of clinical causation.

Key points

- Microscopic crystal examination/identification and microbiologic testing are the most important lines of interrogation for synovial fluid

- Chemical analysis is not clinically useful in most cases

References

PMID 10573336 Howard AW, Viskontas D, Sabbagh C [1999] Reduction in osteomyelitis and septic arthritis related to *Haemophilus influenzae* type B vaccination. *J Pediatr Orthop* 19(6):705-9.

PMID 10923855 Centers for Disease Control and Prevention (CDC) [2000] Gonorrhea—United States, 1998. *MMWR Morb Mortal Wkly Rep* 49(24):538-42

PMID 11257206 Dumler JS [2001] Molecular diagnosis of Lyme disease: review and meta-analysis. *Mol Diagn* 6(1):1-11

PMID 11343852 Madea B, Kreuser C, Banaschak S [2001] Postmortem biochemical examination of synovial fluid—a preliminary study. *Forensic Sci Int* 118(1):29-35

PMID 12006320 Swan A, Amer H, Dieppe P [2002] The value of synovial fluid assays in the diagnosis of joint disease: a literature survey. *Ann Rheum Dis* 61(6):493-8

PMID 12364368 Shirtliff ME, Mader JT [2002] Acute septic arthritis. *Clin Microbiol Rev* 15(4):527-44

PMID 12539074 Ross JJ, Saltzman CL, Carling P et al [2003] Pneumococcal septic arthritis: review of 190 cases. *Clin Infect Dis* 36(3):319-27

PMID 14057620 Rodnan GP, Eisenbeis CH Jr, Creighton AS [1963] The occurrence of rheumatoid factor in synovial fluid. *Am J Med* 35:182-8

PMID 14212943 Cohen AS [1964] Lactic dehydrogenase (LDH) and transaminase (GOT) activity of synovial fluid and serum in rheumatic disease states, with a note on synovial fluid LDH isozymes. *Arthritis Rheum* 7:490-501

PMID 14223919 Small DM, Cohen AS, Schmid K. [1964] Lipoproteins of synovial fluid as studied by analytical ultracentrifugation. *J Clin Invest* 43:2070-9

PMID 14649464 Aulesa C, Mainar I, Prieta M, et al [2003] Use of the Advia 120 hematology analyzer in the differential cytologic analysis of biological fluids (cerebrospinal, peritoneal, pleural, pericardial, synovial, and others). *Lab Hematol* 9(4):214-24

PMID 15172344 Yagupsky P [2004] *Kingella kingae*: from medical rarity to an emerging paediatric pathogen. *Lancet Infect Dis* 4(6):358-67

PMID 1593572 Pejovic M, Stankovic A, Mitrovic DR [1992] Lactate dehydrogenase activity and its isoenzymes in serum and synovial fluid of patients with rheumatoid arthritis and osteoarthritis. *J Rheumatol* 19(4):529-33

PMID 16677989 Brannan SR, Jerrard DA [2006] Synovial fluid analysis. *J Emerg Med* 30(3):331-9

PMID 17029130 Wormser GP, Dattwyler RJ, Shapiro ED et al [2006] The clinical assessment, treatment, and prevention of Lyme disease, human granulocytic anaplasmosis, and babesiosis: clinical practice guidelines by the Infectious Diseases Society of America. *Clin Infect Dis* 43(9):1089-134

PMID 171408 Gatter RA, Richmond JD [1975] Predominance of synovial fluid lymphocytes in early rheumatoid arthritis. *J Rheumatol* 2(3):340-5

PMID 17266710 Wilske B, Fingerle V, Schulte-Spechtel U [2007] Microbiological and serological diagnosis of Lyme borreliosis. *FEMS Immunol Med Microbiol* 49(1):13-21

PMID 17405973 Margaretten ME, Kohlwes J, Moore D et al [2007] Does this adult patient have septic arthritis? *JAMA* 297(13):1478-88

PMID 1759919 McGill NW, York HF [1991] Reproducibility of synovial fluid examination for crystals. *Aust N Z J Med* 21(5):710-3

PMID 1794370 Marcos MA, Vila J, Gratacos J et al [1991] Determination of D-lactate concentration for rapid diagnosis of bacterial infections of body fluids. *Eur J Clin Microbiol Infect Dis* 10(11):966-9

PMID 18452806 Marques A [2008] Chronic Lyme disease: a review. *Infect Dis Clin North Am* 22(2):341-60, vii-viii

PMID 188502 Lutas EM, Zucker-Franklin D [1977] Formation of lipid inclusions in normal leukocytes. *Blood* 49(2):309-20

PMID 19228639 Walker TJ, Nelson LD, Dunphy BW, et al [2009] Comparative evaluation of the Iris iQ200 body fluid module with manual hemacytometer count. *Am J Clin Pathol* 131(3):333-8

PMID 199097 Schumacher HR, Smolyo AP, Tse RL et al [1977] Arthritis associated with apatite crystals. *Ann Intern Med* 87(4):411-6

PMID 1998384 Freemont AJ, Denton J, Chuck A, et al [1991] Diagnostic value of synovial fluid microscopy: a reassessment and rationalization. *Ann Rheum Dis* 50(2):101-7

PMID 20236183 Paris A, Nhan T, Cornet E, et al [2010] Performance evaluation of the body fluid mode on the platform Sysmex XE-5000 series automated hematology analyzer. *Int J Lab Hematol* 32(5):539-47

PMID 20971716 Robier C, Neubauer M, Quehenberger F, et al [2011] Coincidence of calcium pyrophosphate and monosodium urate crystals in the synovial fluid of patients with gout determined by the cytocentrifugation technique. *Ann Rheum Dis* 70(6):1163-4

PMID 21321033 Yagupsky P, Porsch E, St Geme JW 3rd [2011] *Kingella kingae*: an emerging pathogen in young children. *Pediatrics* 127(3):557-65

PMID 21836038 Goubard A, Marzouk M, Canoui-Poitrine F, et al [2011] Performance of the Iris iQ(R)200 Elite analyzer in the cell counting of serous effusion fluids and cerebrospinal drainage fluids. *J Clin Path* 64(12):1123-7

PMID 21916390 Horowitz DL, Katzap E, Horowitz S et al [2011] Approach to septic arthritis. *Am Fam Physician* 84(6):653-60

PMID 2198352 Shmerling RH, Delbanco TL, Tosteson AN et al [1990] Synovial fluid tests. What should be ordered? *JAMA* 264(8):1009-14

PMID 22037510 Oliviero F, Lo Nigro A, Bernardi D et al [2012] A comparative study of serum and synovial fluid lipoprotein levels in patients with various arthritides. *Clin Chim Acta* 413(1-2):303-7

PMID 22100289 García-Arias M, Balsa A, Mola EM [2011] Septic arthritis. *Best Pract Res Clin Rheumatol* 25(3):407-21

PMID 22962880 Wright WF, Riedel DJ, Talwani R et al [2012] Diagnosis and management of Lyme disease. *Am Fam Physician* 85(11):1086-93

PMID 23647736 Danise P, Maconi M, Rovetti A, et al [2013] Cell counting of body fluids: comparison between 3 automated hematology analyzers and the manual microscope method. *Int J Lab Hematol* 35(6):608-13

PMID 2427093 Malone DG, Irani AM, Schwartz LB, et al [1986] Mast cell numbers and histamine levels in synovial fluids from patients with diverse arthritides. *Arthritis Rheum* 29(8):956-63

PMID 2512862 Walters MT, Stevenson FK, Goswami R et al [1989] Comparison of serum and synovial fluid concentrations of β_2-microglobulin and C reactive protein in relation to clinical disease activity and synovial inflammation in rheumatoid arthritis. *Ann Rheum Dis* 48(11):905-11

PMID 2542545 Gardner GC, Terkeltaub RA [1989] Acute monoarthritis associated with intracellular positively birefringent maltese cross appearing spherules. *J Rheumatol* 16(3):394-6

PMID 2650687 Goldenberg DL [1989] Infectious arthritis complicating rheumatoid arthritis and other chronic rheumatic disorders. *Arthritis Rheum* 32(4):496-502

PMID 2672342 Weinberger A, Simkin PA [1989] Plasma proteins in synovial fluids of normal human joints. *Semin Arthritis Rheum* 19(1):66-76

PMID 2930602 Kerolus G, Clayburne G, Schumacher HR [1989] Is it mandatory to examine synovial fluids promptly after arthrocentesis? *Arthritis Rheum* 32(3):271-8

PMID 3051151 McCarty DJ [1988] Crystal identification in human synovial fluids. Methods and interpretation. *Rheum Dis Clin North Am* 14(2):253-67

PMID 3056421 Kay J, Eichenfield AH, Athreya BH, et al [1988] Synovial fluid eosinophilia in Lyme disease. *Arthritis Rheum* 31(11):1384-9

PMID 3404640 Rosenthal A, Ryan LM, McCarty DJ [1988] Arthritis associated with calcium oxalate crystals in an anephric patient treated with peritoneal dialysis. *JAMA* 260(9):1280-2

PMID 3547659 Wise CM, White RE, Agudelo CA [1987] Synovial fluid lipid abnormalities in various disease states: review and classification. *Semin Arthritis Rheum* 16(3):222-30

PMID 3580010 Lakhanpal S, Li CY, Gertz MA, et al [1987] Synovial fluid analysis for diagnosis of amyloid arthropathy. *Arthritis Rheum* 30(4):419-23

PMID 3606682 Hasselbacher P [1987] Variation in synovial fluid analysis by hospital laboratories. *Arthritis Rheum* 30(6):637-42

PMID 3690136 Riordan JW, Dieppe PA [1987] Cholesterol crystals in shoulder synovial fluid. *Br J Rheumatol* 26(6):430-2

PMID 3735282 Bauer PA, Teneubaum J, Fam AG, et al [1986] Coexistent septic and crystal arthritis: report of 4 cases and literature review. *J Rheumatol* 13(3):604-7

PMID 3753540 Brown JP, Plaszczynsk MR, Menard HA, et al [1986] Eosinophilic synovitis: clinical observations on a newly recognized subset of patients with dermatographism. *Arthritis Rheum* 29(9):1147-51

PMID 3778544 Reginato AJ, Seoane JLF, Alvarez CB, et al [1986] Arthropathy and cutaneous cabinosis in hemodialysis oxalosis. *Arthritis Rheum* 29(11):1387-96

PMID 3883171 Goldenberg DL, Reed JI [1985] Bacterial arthritis. *N Engl J Med* 312(12):764-71

PMID 4004360 Freemont AJ, Denton J [1985] Disease distribution of synovial fluid mast cells and cytophagocytic mononuclear cells in inflammatory arthritis. *Ann Rheum Dis* 44(5):312-5

PMID 4118982 Seward CW, Osterland CK [1973] The pattern of anti-immunoglobulin activities in serum, pleural, and synovial fluids. *J Lab Clin Med* 81(2):230-40

PMID 4193825 Hunder GC, Pierre RV [1970] In vivo LE cell formation in synovial fluid. *Arthritis Rheum* 13(4):448-54

PMID 420721 Brawer AE, Cathcart ES [1979] Acute monocytic arthritis. *Arthritis Rheum* 22(3):294-300

PMID 4320615 Kahn CB, Hollander JL, Schumacher HR [1970] Corticosteroid crystals in synovial fluid. *JAMA* 211(5):807-9

PMID 4330119 Cracchiolo A [1971] Joint fluid analysis. *Am Fam Physician* 4(5):87-94

PMID 4341270 Cracchiolo A, Barnett EV [1972] The role of immunological tests in routine synovial fluid analysis. *J Bone Joint Surg Am* 54(4):828-40

PMID 4393033 Schmidt RM, Rosenkranz HS [1970] Antimicrobial activity of local anesthetics lidocaine and procaine. *J Infect Dis* 121(6):597-607

PMID 4459470 Hunter T, Gordon DA, Ogryzlo MA [1974] The ground pepper sign of synovial fluid: a new diagnostic feature of ochronosis. *J Rheumatol* 1(1):45-53

PMID 449407 Ettlinger RE, Hunder GG [1979] Synovial effusions containing cholesterol crystals report of 12 patients and review. *Mayo Clin Proc* 54(6):366-74

PMID 474588 Krey PR, Bailen DA [1979] Synovial fluid leukocytosis: a study of extremes. *Am J Med* 67(3):436-42

PMID 4931742 Labowitz R, Schumacher HR Jr [1971] The articular manifestations of systemic lupus erythematosus. *Ann Intern Med* 74(6):911-21

PMID 51606 Teloh HA [1975] Clinical pathology of synovial fluid. *Ann Clin Lab* 5(4):282-7

PMID 5316357 Panush RS, Bianco NE, Schur PH [1971] Serum and synovial fluid IgG, IgA and IgM antigammaglobulins in rheumatoid arthritis. *Arthritis Rheum* 14(6):737-47

PMID 5548446 Huskisson EC, Hart FD, Lacey BW [1971] Synovial fluid Waaler-Rose and latex tests. *Ann Rheum Dis* 30(1):67-72

PMID 5559440 Lawrence C, Seife B [1971] Bone marrow in joint fluid: a clue to fracture. *Ann Intern Med* 74(5):740-2

PMID 579389 Owen DS [1978] Synovial fluid glucose. *JAMA* 239(3):193

PMID 5823923 Kitridou RC, Schumacher HR Jr, Sbarbaro JL et al [1969] Recurrent hemarthrosis after prosthetic knee arthroplasty: identification of metal particles in the synovial fluid. *Arthritis Rheum* 12(5):520-8

PMID 5855250 Reeves B [1965] Significance of joint fluid uric acid levels in gout. *Ann Rheum Dis* 24(6):569-71

PMID 6023534 Pekin TJ, Malinin TI, Zvaifler NJ [1967] Unusual synovial fluid findings in Reiter syndrome. *Ann Intern Med* 66(4):677-84

PMID 6066820 Hasselbacher P [1987] Variation in synovial fluid analysis by hospital laboratories. *Arthritis Rheum* 30(6):637-42

PMID 6158572 Todesco S, Punzi L, Montanaro D et al [1980] β_2-microglobulin in synovial fluid of rheumatoid arthritis. *J Rheumatol* 7(4):555-8

PMID 623698 Graham J, Golman JA [1978] Fat droplets and synovial fluid leukocytosis in traumatic arthritis. *Arthritis Rheum* 21(1):76-80

PMID 6244798 Weinstein J [1980] Synovial fluid leukocytosis associated with intracellular lipid inclusions. *Arch Intern Med* 140(4):560-1

PMID 6360465 Wallis WJ, Simkin PA [1983] Antirheumatic drug concentrations in human synovial fluid and synovial tissue. Observations on extravascular pharmacokinetics. *Clin Pharmacokinet* 8(6):496-522

PMID 6497466 Gobelet C, Gerster JC [1984] Synovial fluid lactate levels in septic and nonseptic arthritides. *Ann Rheum Dis* 43(5):742-5

PMID 6712368 Eisenberg JM, Schumacher HR, Davidson PK et al [1984] Usefulness of synovial fluid analysis in evaluation of joint effusions. *Arch Intern Med* 144(4):715-9

PMID 6767403 Langlands DR, Dawkins RL, Matz LR et al [1980] Arthritis associated with crystallizing cryoprecipitable LIg paraprotein. *Am J Med* 68(3):461-5

PMID 679544 Gregg JR, Nixon JE, DiStefano V [1978] Neutral fat globules in traumatized knees. *Clin Orthop Relat Res* (132):219-24

PMID 6847731 George D [1983] Chronic monocytic arthritis. *Arthritis Rheum* 26(5):674-7

PMID 6886455 Curtis GD, Newman RJ, Slack MP [1983] Synovial fluid lactate and the diagnosis of septic arthritis. *J Infect* 6(3):239-46

PMID 697948 Brook I, Reza MJ, Bricknell KS et al [1978] Synovial fluid lactic acid. A diagnostic aid in septic arthritis. *Arthritis Rheum* 21(7):774-9

PMID 7056032 Scott DL, Farr M, Crockson AP et al [1982] Synovial fluid and plasma fibronectin levels in rheumatoid arthritis. *Clin Sci (Lond)* 62(1):71-6

PMID 7076866 Riordan T, Doyle D, Tabaqchali S [1982] Synovial fluid lactic acid measurement in the diagnosis and management of septic arthritis. *J Clin Pathol* 35(4):390-4

PMID 7092004 Hoffman GS, Schumacher HR, Paul H et al [1982] Calcium oxalate microcrystalline-associated arthritis in end-stage renal disease. *Ann Intern Med* 97(1):36-42

PMID 7092970 Klofkorn RW, Lehman TJA [1982] Eosinophilic synovial effusions complicating chronic urticaria and angioedema. *Arthritis Rheum* 25(6):708-9

PMID 7114915 Hollingworth P, Williams PL, Scott JT [1982] Frequency of chondrocalcinosis of the knee in asymptomatic hyperuricaemia and rheumatoid arthritis: a controlled study. *Ann Rheum Dis* 41(4):344-6

PMID 7115453 Borenstein DG, Gibbs CA, Jacobs RP [1982] Gas-liquid chromatographic analysis of synovial fluid. Succinic acid and lactic acid as markers for septic arthritis. *Arthritis Rheum* 25(8):947-53

PMID 7226556 Weinberger A, Wysenbeck A, Agam G et al [1981] Synovial fluid urate concentration in normouricemic and hyperuricemic subjects without joint diseases. *Clin Chim Acta* 111(2-3):279-80

PMID 7230158 Fam AG, Pritzker KPH et al [1981] Cholesterol crystals in osteoarthritis joint effusions. *J Rheumatol* 8(2):273-80

PMID 7273404 Knight JA, Dudek SM, Haymond RE [1981] Early (chemical) diagnosis of bacterial meningitis—cerebrospinal fluid glucose, lactate, and lactate dehydrogenase compared. *Clin Chem* 27(8):1431-4

PMID 729254 Wolf AW, Benson DR, Shoji H et al [1978] Current concepts in synovial fluid analysis. *Clin Orthop Relat Res* (134):261-5

PMID 7313579 Paulsen O, Berghard G [1981] Synovial fluid lactate determinations as a diagnostic aid in cases of monoarticular arthritis. *Scand J Infect Dis* 13(3):239-40

PMID 7352946 Cheung HS, Ryan LM, Kozin F, et al [1980] Synovial origins of rice bodies in joint fluid. *Arthritis Rheum* 23(1):72-6

PMID 7354476 Fam AG, Kolin A, Lewis AJ [1980] Metastatic carcinomatous arthritis and carcinoma of the lung. A report of 2 cases diagnosed by synovial fluid cytology. *J Rheumatol* 7(1):98-104

PMID 7417355 Podell TE, Ault M, Sullam P, et al [1980] Synovial fluid eosinophilia. *Arthritis Rheum* 23(9):1060-1

PMID 7458972 Vincent J, Korn JH, Podewell C et al [1980] Synovial fluid pseudoleukocytosis. *Arthritis Rheum* 23(12):1399-400

PMID 7470168 Swann DA, Hendren RB, Radin EL et al [1981] The lubricating activity of synovial fluid glycoproteins. *Arthritis Rheum* 24(1):22-30

PMID 7473474 Gratacós J, Vila J, Moyá F et al [1995] D-lactic acid in synovial fluid. A rapid diagnostic test for bacterial synovitis. *J Rheumatol* 22(8):1504-8

PMID 7548857 Prete PE, Gurakar-Osborne A, Kashyap ML [1995] Synovial fluid lipids and apolipoproteins: a contemporary perspective. *Biorheology* 32(1):1-16

PMID 7623762 Centers for Disease Control and Prevention (CDC) [1995] Recommendations for test performance and interpretation from the Second National Conference on Serologic Diagnosis of Lyme Disease. *MMWR Morb Mortal Wkly Rep* 44(31):590-1

PMID 7747151 Kortekangas P, Peltola O, Toivanen A et al [1995] Synovial fluid L-lactic acid in acute arthritis of the adult knee joint. *Scand J Rheumatol* 24(2):98-101

PMID 8639170 Jaulhac B, Chary-Valckenaere I, Sibilia J et al [1996] Detection of *Borrelia burgdorferi* by DNA amplification in synovial tissue samples from patients with Lyme arthritis. *Arthritis Rheum* 39(5):736-45

PMID 8809438 Beutler AM, Keenan GF, Soloway S et al [1996] Soluble urate in sera and synovial fluids from patients with different joint disorders. *Clin Exp Rheumatol* 14(3):249-54

PMID 8849354 Kaandorp CJ, Van Schaardenburg D, Krijnen P et al [1995] Risk factors for septic arthritis in patients with joint disease. A prospective study. *Arthritis Rheum* 38(12):1819-25

PMID 9133965 Saraux A, Taelman H, Blanche P et al [1998] HIV infection as a risk factor for septic arthritis. *Br J Rheumatol* 36(3):333-7

PMID 9449882 Goldenberg DL [1998] Septic arthritis. *Lancet* 351(9097):197-202

PMID 951619 Meyers OL, Watermeyer GS [1976] Cholesterol-rich synovial effusions. *S Afr Med J* 50(25):973-5

PMID 9725094 Ike RW [1988] Bacterial arthritis. *Curr Opin Rheumatol* 10(4):330-4

ISBN 978-0-3161-5004-0 Cohen AS, Brandt KD, Krey PR. Synovial fluid. In: Cohen AS, ed. *Laboratory Diagnostic Procedures in the Rheumatic Diseases*. Little Brown & Co

ISBN 978-0-8121-1123-1 McCarty DJ [1989] Synovial fluid. In: McCarty DJ, ed. *Arthritis and Allied Conditions: A Textbook of Rheumatology*, 11e. Lea & Febiger, p69-90.

ISBN 978-0-8121-1332-7 Schumacher HR, Regineto AJ. *Atlas of Synovial Fluid and Crystal Identification*. Philadelphia, Pa Leá & Febiger; 1991.

ISBN 978-1-4377-0974-5 Karcher DS, McPherson RA. Cerebrospinal, synovial, serous body fluids and alternative specimens. In: McPherson RA, Pincus MR eds. *Henry's Clinical Diagnosis and Management by Laboratory Methods*, Philadelphia, Pa Elsevier, Saunders; 2011:480-506.

ISBN 978-1-4377-1738-9 Burns CM, Wortman RL [2010] Clinical features and treatment of Gout In: Firestein GS, Budd RC, Gabriel SE et al, ed. *Kelley's Textbook of Rheumatology*, 9e. Elsevier, Saunders, p1554-1575

ISBN 978-1-4377-1738-9 El-Gabalawy HS [2010] Synovial fluid analysis, synovial biopsy, and synovial pathology. In: Firestein GS, Budd RC, Gabriel SE et al, ed. *Kelley's Textbook of Rheumatology*, 9e. Elsevier, Saunders, p753-769

ISBN 978-1-4377-1738-9 Goldring RS, Goldring MB [2010] Biology of the normal joint. In: Firestein GS, Budd RC, Gabriel SE et al, ed. *Kelley's Textbook of Rheumatology*, 9e. Elsevier, Saunders, p1-19

ISBN 978-1-4377-1738-9 Keenan RT, Nowatzky J, Pillinger MH [2010] Etiology and pathogenesis of hyperuricemia and gout. In: Firestein GS, Budd RC, Gabriel SE et al, ed. *Kelley's Textbook of Rheumatology*, 9e. Elsevier, Saunders, p1533-1553

ISBN 978-1-4377-1738-9 Terkeltaub R [2010] Calcium crystal disease: calcium pyrophosphate dehydrate and basic calcium phosphate. In: Firestein GS, Budd RC, Gabriel SE et al, ed. *Kelley's Textbook of Rheumatology*, 9e. Elsevier, Saunders, p1576-1596.

ISBN 978-1-4377-1738-9 Wise CM [2010] Arthrocentesis and injection of joints and soft tissue. In: Firestein GS, Budd RC, Gabriel SE et al, ed. *Kelley's Textbook of Rheumatology*, 9e. Elsevier, Saunders, p770-788

Afzelius A [1921] Erythema chronicum migrans. *Acta Derm Venereol* 2:120-125

Hasselbacher P [1986] Protein measurement in synovial fluid: a test without value. *Arthritis Rheum* 1896;29:S63

Rippey JH [1979] Synovial fluid analysis. *Lab Med* 10:140-145

Williams JE, Walters J, Kabb K [2011] Gaining efficiency in the laboratory—automated body fluid cell counts: evaluation of the body fluid application on the Sysmex XE-500 Hematology Analyser. *Lab Med* 42:395-401

Carrell DT, Emery BR, Farley JD, Shamsi MB

Seminal Fluid
Chapter 8

Accurate diagnosis of male infertility requires not only an accurate description of the number of motile sperm, but also includes assays that span the spectrum of sperm function. Under in vivo conditions, abundant numbers of sperm must be able to traverse through the female tract to reach the oocyte, and while doing so must undergo sperm capacitation, a series of chemical reactions that facilitate the acrosome reaction. The acrosome reaction biochemically and morphologically prepares the sperm to penetrate the zona pellucida and fuse with the oocyte's oolemma to deliver intact and functional paternal DNA that can help initiate and maintain embryonic development. Defects in any of the stages of sperm production, sperm delivery, sperm function, or genetic competence, may culminate in male infertility [PMID 24194470].

Semen analysis has been, and still is, the primary method for the initial evaluation of male infertility. The information from a semen analysis, along with the patient's history, helps to develop a differential diagnosis which is then used in conjunction with other sperm tests to not only diagnose etiologies, but also direct future care, including the possible use of assisted reproductive technologies (ART) such as in vitro fertilization (IVF) and intracytoplasmic sperm injection (ICSI). For example, either a decreased sperm count or a diminished sperm function test may be indicators of the need for IVF with ICSI rather than a clinical plan of artificial insemination (AI).

Although fertile men as a group have higher mean sperm quality for parameters of the semen analysis compared to infertile men, there is significant overlap and the semen analysis is of poor predictive power [PMID 11794171]. Therefore, it is not surprising that a significant percentage of infertile men have been reported to have normal semen analysis results [PMID 9696208]. This highlights that extreme care must be taken to not "overinterpret" semen analysis results. Nevertheless, semen analysis is the starting point for evaluation and can provide valuable information in assessing the potential benefit of other sperm function tests and the potential effectiveness of specific therapies. This chapter describes the utility and standard procedures of the basic semen analysis, and also describes other valuable assays of sperm functional ability and chromatin status that should be available in the analysis of male infertility.

Normal human reproductive physiology

The duration of spermatogenesis is 60-72 days [PMID 16406920]. Therefore, semen analysis results may represent the cumulative effects of influential biological, physical and environmental exposures occurring for at least 2 months prior to semen collection. The production of sperm involves delicate endocrine regulation by the hypothalamus (gonadotropin releasing hormone [GnRH]), the anterior pituitary gland (follicle stimulating hormone [FSH] and luteinizing hormone [LH]) and the testes (testosterone & inhibin), as well as paracrine and autocrine factors within the testes. Sertoli cells are the key support cells, are intimately involved in the regulation of spermatogenesis, provide the blood testes barrier through tight junctions, and are involved in support of the germ cells and delivery of spermatozoa into the tubular lumen. The spermatozoa released into the lumen of the seminiferous tubules are transported to the epididymis where the sperm undergo maturation and acquire increased motility and capacity to fertilize f8.1 [PMID 7484449].

After ejaculation, the movement of the sperm in the female reproductive tract depends on the ability of the sperm to penetrate the cervical mucus barrier, then traverse

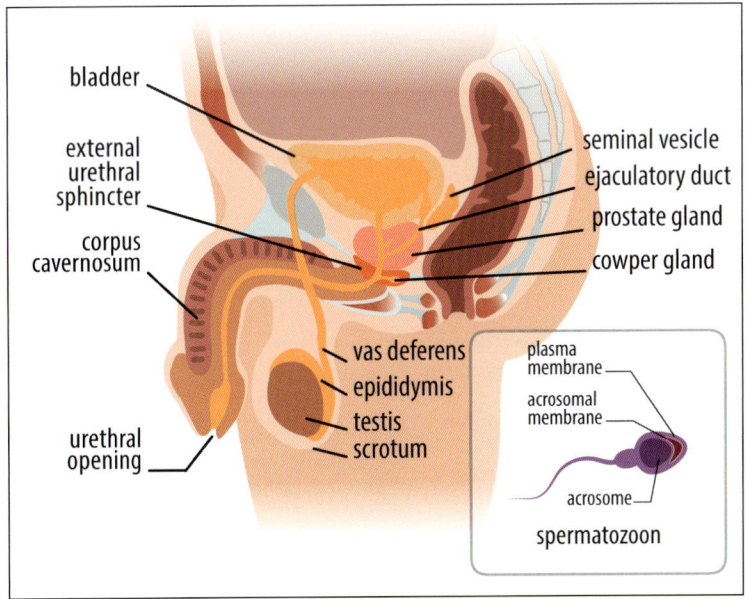

f8.1 The anatomic relationships of the male genital tract components

the uterus and Fallopian tubes where a percentage of competent sperm undergo capacitation, a series of chemical reactions that result in an influx of calcium ions, efflux of hydrogen ions, and increased fluidity of the sperm plasma and acrosome membranes that ultimately lead to the acrosome reaction. The acrosome reaction is a process that sperm undergo in which the sperm acrosome membranes and plasma membranes fuse, resulting in the release of proteolytic enzymes enabling the sperm to penetrate through the zona pellucida, and morphologically and biochemically prepare the sperm for fusion to the oocyte plasma membrane [PMID 15817522]. Postpenetration sperm functions include decondensation of the chromatin, formation of a functional pronucleus, formation of centrioles from the sperm centrosome, and chromatin remodeling, including epigenetic changes [PMID 16467269]. Recent data clearly indicate a role for epigenetic contributions of the sperm to embryogenesis, and it is likely that future sperm testing will include the evaluation of epigenetic integrity of the sperm [PMID 22289286, PMID 23955672].

Semen analysis

The conventional semen analysis is the first diagnostic step in the assessment of male infertility. It not only evaluates basic sperm parameters, but also evaluates the seminal plasma and nonsperm cells, providing information on the functional status of the seminiferous tubules, the epididymis, and the accessory glands. This chapter will largely reflect the procedures and normal values espoused by the guidelines of World Health Organization (WHO), especially for the basic semen analysis. The latest edition, *WHO Laboratory Manual for the Examination and Processing of Human Semen*, 5th edition (WHO 5), published in 2010, provided significant changes to standard procedures, and appears to have improved accuracy and predictive power. Additionally, the WHO 5 guidelines provide new reference ranges and values for the semen quality parameters of the analysis t8.1. Specific studies and methodologies for the semen analysis are described below and summarized in t8.2.

t8.2 Semen analysis studies & methodologies

Assay	Tissue	Objective	Benefits	Limitations
Gross examination of semen	Semen	Evaluation of the seminal component of the ejaculate for color and consistency	Diagnosis of abnormalities of the ejaculatory ducts and accessory glands, and possible presence of red blood cells	Low probability of diagnosing disorders based on gross examination only
Microscopic examination of semen	Semen	To evaluate semen for presence or absence of sperm, amorphous cells, bacteria, sperm clumping, and sperm agglutination	Diagnosis of pyospermia, and bacteriospermia; absence of sperm is suggestive of azoospermia	Followup for diagnosis is required for prostatic infection and the seminal fluid must be concentrated and reexamined for sperm to diagnose azoospermia
Sperm count	Semen	To evaluate the concentration of sperm per volume of semen and total sperm count	Diagnosis of azoospermia or oligozoospermia. Sometimes suggestive of Y chromosome microdeletion, cystic fibrosis-related gene mutations, Klinefelter syndrome, and other causes of reduced sperm counts.	Needs replicate counts to be accurate; performed by specially trained, high complexity certified technicians. Thorough laboratory quality control is required. Azoospermia and severe oligozoospermia need to be followed up with additional diagnostic procedures to be well defined.
Sperm motility	Semen	To evaluate the percentage of sperm that are moving and their characteristic pattern	Diagnosis of asthenozoospermia, helpful in the diagnosis of antisperm antibodies and other sperm motility defects	Needs replicate counts to be accurate; performed by specially trained, high complexity certified technicians. Thorough laboratory quality control is required. Abnormal factors need to be followed with additional testing for patient diagnosis.
Sperm morphology	Semen	To evaluate the shape of the sperm	Diagnosis of teratozoospermia, globozoospermia, microcephaly, macrocephaly; helpful in diagnosis of sperm function in fertilization (capacitation and acrosome reaction). Severe teratozoospermia is associated with sperm aneuploidy. Tapered sperm suggestive of a possible varicocele.	Needs replicate counts to be accurate; performed by specially trained, high complexity certified technicians. Thorough laboratory quality control is required. Abnormal factors need to be followed with additional testing for patient diagnosis. Including ultrastructural analysis by transmission electron microscopy, sperm penetration assay, and sperm aneuploidy testing.
Sperm viability	Semen	To evaluate the percent of viable sperm in the ejaculate	Diagnosis of necrospermia and helpful in the diagnosis of antisperm antibodies	The sperm hypoosmotic swelling test has the potential for overestimation due to the presence of morphologic tail abnormalities
Leukocytes and immature germ cells	Semen	To evaluate and classify round cells in the semen	Diagnosis of pyospermia, potential identification of immature germ cells in the semen. Pyospermia may be suggestive of an infection or increased sperm DNA damage.	Not all round cell types are readily identifiable by staining and evaluation in the routine diagnostic laboratory
Postvasectomy semen analysis	Semen	To evaluate the ejaculate for the concentration of sperm (sterilization) following a vasectomy procedure	Easily adapted to most clinical laboratories; rapid test for determination of a successful procedure.	Analysis should be performed within one hour of collection following standard collection procedures as described for a full semen analysis
Antisperm antibody testing	Isolated sperm, semen, blood, cervical mucus	To evaluate bodily fluids for the presence of sperm binding antibodies that can contribute to infertility	Helpful in the determination of the cause of asthenospermia and necrospermia	Time consuming testing protocols, which require strict controls. Must be performed by specially trained, high complexity certified technicians. Thorough laboratory quality control is required.

t8.1 Comparison of reference ranges for semen parameter according to different WHO guidelines

	1980	1987	1992	1999	2010
Semen Volume (mL)	–	>2.0	>2.0	>2.0	>1.5
pH	–	7.2-7.8	7.2-7.8	7.2	>7.2
Sperm concentration (×10^6/mL)	>20	>20	>20	>20	>15
Total sperm number (×10^6)	–	>40	>40	>40	>39
Progressive motility (%)	>60	>50	>50	>50	>32
Normal morphology (%)	>80	>50	>30	–	>4
Vitality (% alive)	–	>50	>75	>50	>58
White blood cells	<5.0	<1.0	<1.0	<1.0	<1.0
Antibody coated sperm (%)	–	<10	<20	<50	<50

Preanalytic considerations

Human semen and sperm exhibit marked heterogeneity within an ejaculate, as well as substantial variation between ejaculates of the same male, therefore a minimum of 2 samples should typically be examined [PMID 9886521]. Samples should be collected after a period of abstinence of >48 hours, but <7 days. Semen samples should be collected either by masturbation or ejaculation into a specialized, nonlatex, spermicidal free collection condom. Any collection container should be evaluated for sperm toxicity for each manufactured lot using a sperm survival assay [PMID 16021863]. Patients should be counseled regarding precautions to be taken during semen collection to avoid spillage of the sample and the important need to notify the technician of such events. If the sample is collected away from the diagnostic laboratory, the specimen container should be kept at body temperature during transport and the sample should be analyzed within 1 hour of collection.

t8.2 Semen analysis studies & methodologies (continued)

Assay	Tissue	Objective	Benefits	Limitations
Sperm penetration assay	Motile sperm, isolated from the ejaculate	To evaluate the sperm fertilizing potential (sperm oolema binding and nuclear decondensation)	Helpful in the determination of infertility treatment and the diagnosis of idiopathic malefactor infertility	Strict adherence to protocols and tightly run controls are required for validity
Acrosome reaction assays	Capacitated sperm	To evaluate the ability of sperm to acrosome react in the presence of a stimulus	Helpful in the determination of infertility treatment and the diagnosis of idiopathic malefactor infertility	The assay is time consuming and requires tightly run controls; questionable predictive ability in some reports
Hemizona assay	Capacitated sperm	To evaluate the ability of sperm to bind to the zona	Helpful in the determination of infertility treatment and the diagnosis of idiopathic malefactor infertility	The assay is time consuming and requires tightly run controls; requires collection of human zona from an IVF clinic
Assessment of reactive oxygen species (ROS)	Semen, washed sperm	To evaluate the level of ROS present in semen and produced by washed sperm	Helpful in determining the amount of oxidative stress on sperm	ROS compounds are highly reactive and short lived with a high degree of variability between measurements and time points. The assay must be done at the site of collection due to the unstable nature of the ROS.
Acridine orange (DNA damage)	Sperm	To evaluate the amount of DNA damage in sperm	Rapid test with a simple protocol; may be helpful in the diagnosis of idiopathic male factor infertility and poor outcomes in IVF failure	Poor repeatability due to heterogeneous staining, rapid photobleaching and qualitative judgment of double stained cells
Sperm chromatin structure assay (SCSA; DNA damage)	Sperm	To evaluate the amount of DNA damage in sperm	Highly reproducible with low inter- and intralab variations; helpful in the diagnosis of idiopathic malefactor infertility and poor outcomes in IVF failure	A flow cytometer and specialized software are required for analysis
TUNEL assay (DNA damage)	Sperm	To evaluate the amount of DNA damage in sperm	Can be done with bright field microscopy, easily performed on low sperm numbers with reliable data. Sensitive to both double and single strand breaks. Helpful in the diagnosis of idiopathic malefactor infertility and poor outcomes in IVF failure.	More laborious than other assays for DNA damage
Sperm chromatin dispersion (SCD; DNA damage)	Sperm	To evaluate the amount of DNA damage in sperm	Simple technique that does not require any special instrumentation; helpful in the diagnosis of idiopathic malefactor infertility and poor outcomes in IVF failure	In comparison to other DNA damage testing, there are fewer published reports validating predictive ability
Comet assay (DNA damage)	Sperm	To evaluate the amount of DNA damage in sperm	Can detect only double strand breaks or both depending on the type of assay setup. The assay is widely used and generally well accepted with good data on where to set reporting cutoff values. Helpful in the diagnosis of idiopathic malefactor infertility and poor outcomes in IVF failure.	Testing requires long assay time and tech hours for evaluation. If the software is not used there is more qualitative assessment of the tail properties.
Sperm aneuploidy (FISH)	Sperm	To evaluate the percent of sperm with chromosome aneuploidies	Helpful in the diagnosis of recurrent pregnancy loss, failed IVF cycles, or high blastocyst aneuploidy	The assay requires specialized equipment and a large investment of technician time. Only a subset of chromosomes can be analyzed on a single sperm

Gross examination of semen

Freshly ejaculated semen appears as a coagulum that spontaneously liquefies at room temperature within 15-60 minutes. A 30 minute liquefaction period should precede the semen analysis. If the sample remains viscous after 30 minutes it should be left to liquefy and checked for full liquefaction every 10 minutes, up to a total liquefaction time of 1 hour. Once the initial liquefaction period has lapsed, semen viscosity is analyzed by allowing it to drop by gravity from a wide bore pipette. Normal semen falls in drops, whereas hyperviscous semen forms threads >2 cm long. Infection, defects in prostatic proteolytic enzymes, or absence of the seminal vesicle or prostatic components may lead to abnormalities in the liquefaction and viscosity.

Semen is normally gray opalescent in color and a change in semen color may be indicative of pathology. Reddish to pink semen is indicative of hematospermia, yellow semen is a potential symptom of jaundice, and dense white and turbid semen may indicate inflammation in the urethra or associated glands. Any variation from the normal color should be noted, and reported in the semen analysis report.

The pH of semen reflects the balance between the pH values of the different accessory gland secretions, mainly the alkaline seminal vesicular secretion and the acidic prostatic secretion. Normal semen has a slightly alkaline pH >7.2. The pH should be measured soon after liquefaction as loss of CO_2 may influence the pH of the sample. The acceptable method for measurement of semen pH is using paper pH strips (range of pH 6.0-10). Spread a drop of semen onto the paper, wait for the semen to fully impregnate the paper and compare to the calibration strip provided with the paper. Alternatively, a calibrated pH meter placed in contact with the semen sample may be used. Low pH values are indicative of semen composed mainly of prostatic secretions resulting from aplasia of vasa deferens and seminal vesicles or blockage of ejaculatory ducts due to inflammation. Prostate infections may also reduce the seminal pH.

The volume of the ejaculate is contributed mainly by the seminal vesicles and prostate gland, with a small amount from the bulbourethral glands and epididymides. Precise measurement of volume is essential, because it allows the total number of spermatozoa and nonsperm cells in the ejaculate to be calculated and may indicate pathologies of the ejaculatory duct or accessory glands. Obstructions of the vas deferens or ejaculatory dysfunctions, such as retrograde ejaculation, are the most probable cause of low semen volumes. Measurement of semen volume by decanting the semen into a graduated cylinder or by pipetting has been shown to introduce a significant amount of error [PMID 7816062, PMID 15223853, PMID 16957135, PMID 19871256]. Therefore, the suggested method is to use a preweighed vessel for collection and then reweighing the container after collection. The density of semen is reported to be ~1 g/mL, with a range of 1.043-1.102 [PMID 7816062, PMID 15223853, PMID 16957135, PMID 19871256].

Microscopic examination of semen

An initial microscopic investigation of semen must be performed to look for contamination, the presence of epithelial cells, urethral or prostatic bacteria, and round cells (immature germ cells or leukocytes). Additionally, the microscopic overview includes an analysis of sperm aggregation/agglutination and determination of the dilution required for accurate assessment of sperm number. Aggregation refers to adherence of immotile sperm to each other or of motile sperm with mucus strands, nonsperm cells or debris, while agglutination refers to motile spermatozoa sticking to each other in consistent patterns, such as head to head, tail to tail, or in a mixed way i8.1a. Severe agglutination may affect the assessment of sperm number and motility. Agglutination is categorized as grade 1 (isolated; <10 sperm per agglutinate), grade 2 (moderate; 10-50 sperm per agglutinate), grade 3 (large; agglutinates of >50), grade 4 (gross; all sperm agglutinated and agglutinates interconnected). Further, the site of attachment, head to head, tail to tail, tailtip to tailtip, mixed, or tangled, should also be documented during the analysis. The presence of agglutination, across several samples from the same individual, is suggestive of the presence of antisperm antibodies and in such cases the semen and serum from the male should be evaluated for antisperm antibodies, as discussed below.

Sperm count

The number of sperm in the ejaculate is reported as both sperm concentration (millions of sperm per mL of semen) and as total sperm count (semen volume multiplied by the sperm concentration). The sperm concentration is a function of both testicular and accessary gland function, whereas the total sperm count provides information on testicular function alone. Commercially available Neubauer hemocytometer counting chamber slides are generally preferred for determining sperm concentration, but many labs have found the Makler counting chamber preferable for evaluation of the sperm concentration and an addendum has been made for their use in the most current WHO manual. Sperm counts with the Makler chamber are easily performed. A free falling drop of ~10 μL of semen is placed onto the lower disk of the chamber and coverslipped using the provided crystal cover. Care should be taken that the semen is filling the area of the counting chamber without any bubbles and the semen is not overlapping onto the crystal pedestals. At least, 200 sperm should be counted in duplicate, using 2 different counting chambers i8.1b. The variance between the 2 values should be monitored to ensure the sampling error is within limits provided in WHO guidelines.

Samples where no sperm are observed should be further evaluated by centrifuging at least 1.0 mL of the well mixed semen sample at 3,000 g for 15 minutes, followed by microscopic examination of the pellet for the presence of sperm <2 separate preparations of 10 μL aliquots <22 × 22 coverslips. Fructose should be measured in samples without sperm to determine the integrity of vas deferens and seminal vesicles. Azoospermia, the lack of sperm in the ejaculate, may be due to obstructions of the ejaculatory tract or due to absence of

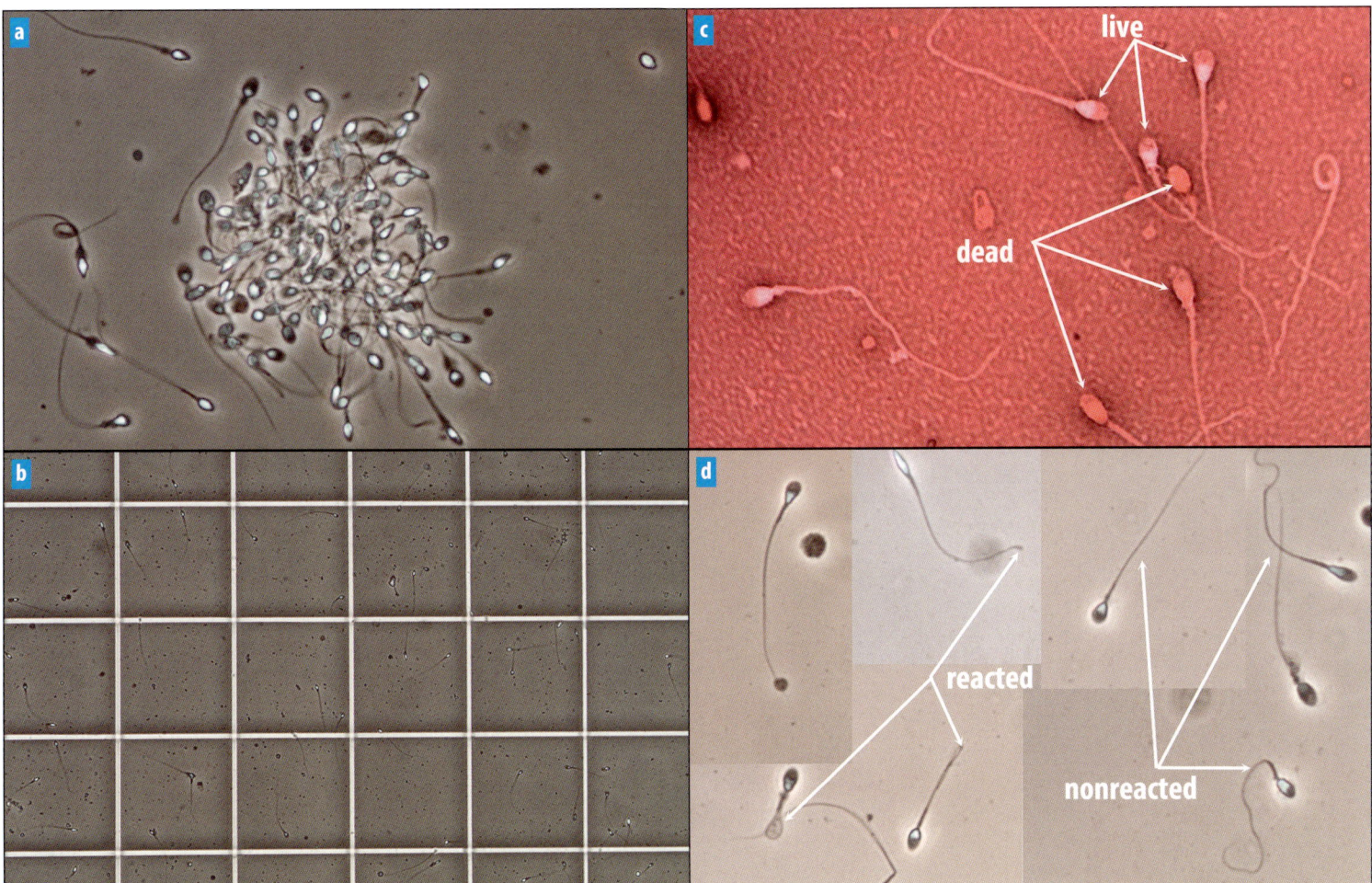

i8.1 Photomicrographs of 4 semen analysis components
  a sperm agglutination observed during the initial microscopic evaluation of the semen
  b a Makler chamber being used for the determination of sperm concentration
  c viability staining using the eosin nigrosin viability stain. Sperm heads stained pink are an indication of nonviability
  d characteristic changes that take place on a sperm tail in reaction to being placed in a hypoosmotic solution, an alternative assay for evaluation of membrane integrity

spermatogenesis (nonobstructive azoospermia). The identification of obstructive or nonobstructive azoospermia is based on the results of the patient history, physical exam, semen analysis, and endocrine profile. For men with nonobstructive azoospermia or impaired sperm production, a karyotype and Yq microdeletion analysis is recommended [PMID 17554051]. Genetic conditions such as Y chromosome microdeletions, cystic fibrosis related gene polymorphisms, Klinefelter syndrome, structural chromosome anomalies, or gene polymorphisms are the most common causes of azoospermia and oligozoospermia, but other exogenous factors, such as scrotal heat, iatrogenic factors, infection (systemic) or gonad toxins or endogenous factors such as varicocele, endocrinopathy, febrile or systemic illness, or cryptorchidism can also be factors.

Sperm motility

Sperm motility should be assessed as soon as possible after liquefaction, since it is affected by dehydration and changes in pH or temperature. The latest WHO guidelines recommend a simplified analysis of sperm motility that distinguishes spermatozoa with progressive or nonprogressive motility from those that are nonmotile. Progressively motile sperm are those that are in active motion, either linearly or in a large circular pattern, regardless of speed. Nonprogressive motility is defined as all other patterns of motility with an absence of progression, eg, swimming in small circles or immobilized motility (a flagella beat without sperm progression). Low sperm motility may be an indication of sperm ultrastructural defects, particularly defects in the microtubule arrangement of the sperm axoneme or the presence of antisperm antibodies [PMID 21586547, PMID 19297071]. Typically, the majority of nonmotile sperm are not viable, but in cases of ultrastructural defects or antisperm antibodies, a significant proportion of the nonmotile sperm may be viable. Additionally, defects in energy generation due to mutations in the sperm mitochondrial genome has been implicated in patients with poor sperm motility [PMID 22381250].

Grading sperm motility can be done using a Makler Counting Chamber or on a plain glass slide with the use of a microscope grid reticle. In either case, the semen should be examined under phase contrast microscopy at 200× magnification. The slide should be prewarmed to 37°C and assessment of motility should be done immediately after fluid drifting on the slide has stopped. A warmed microscope stage is useful, but in any case the evaluation should be done quickly to avoid effects from drying under

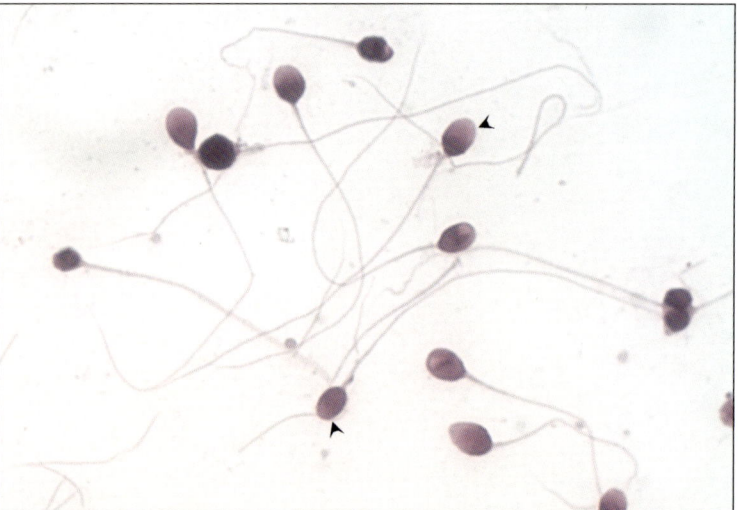

i8.2 Sperm stained with the hematoxylin and eosin for morphology analysis. The arrows indicate morphologically normal sperm.

the coverslip. Drying is more pronounced near the edges; therefore, counting in those areas should be avoided.

The actual grading of the 3 classes is most accurately done by grading motile sperm first within a defined area, separately tallying the cells as progressive and nonprogressive, then counting nonmotile sperm in a second tally. As the evaluator becomes more proficient, tallying all 3 categories at once is possible. 2 well mixed drops should be observed and counting 200 sperm per drop is suggested. The average of the 2 evaluations are reported after they are validated for statistical variation from sampling error. Only whole sperm (excluding microcephalic or pinheaded sperm) should be counted in the evaluation. While raw semen will typically contain some cellular debris, microcephalic sperm, sperm fragments, and round cells of varying origins (including epithelial cells), the observer should always note the presence of any predominant abnormality or observation in the semen analysis report as a comment.

Sperm morphology

Human sperm morphology is heterogeneous, and some amorphous sperm are capable of fertilization; however, a reduced percentage of morphologically normal sperm is sometimes associated with defects that may decrease fertilization ability or affect patient health, such as a varicocele. Therefore, evaluation of sperm morphology may add valuable insights to the clinical prognosis [PMID 8844314]. However, the direct relationship of sperm morphology and fertilizing ability remains controversial [PMID 15482758]. The most commonly used technique, "strict criteria" analysis, identifies a normal sperm as having a single ellipse shaped head with specific measurements and proportions i8.2 [PMID 2394790]. Morphologic defects in the sperm are categorized as defects of the head, the neck or midpiece, and of the tail. Defects of the sperm head are categorized as large, small, tapered, pyriform, round, amorphous, vacuolated and double head i8.3. Common defects of the neck and mid piece include bent neck and cytoplasmic droplets, while tail defects include short, double, broken, or bent tails i8.4.

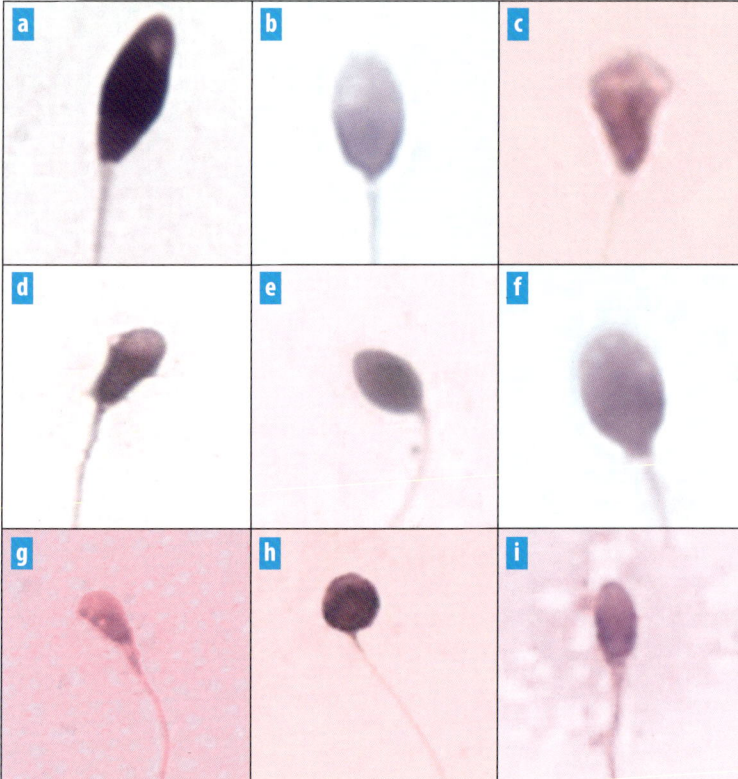

i8.3 Examples of abnormal sperm head morphology. Abnormal morphologies include:
a tapered
b amorphous with irregular membrane
c amorphous abnormal head shape
d pyriform
e no acrosome
f increased acrosomal vacuoles (enlarged for better viewing of vacuoles)
g postacrosomal vacuole
h round
i tapered

Studies have reported that subtle morphologic defects are not a reliable predictor in chromosomal aberrations [PMID 15205404] or genetic constituents [PMID 11704105]. However, more dramatic defects, such as globozoospermia, macrocephaly, and microcephaly, are associated with an elevated risk of sperm aneuploidy. The absence of an acrosome is also associated with globozoospermia; therefore, an acrosome reaction test is suggested [PMID 22571172, PMID 17127284]. Increased residual cytoplasmic droplet size is associated with increased free radical production, which may cause nuclear and mitochondrial DNA damage. Free radicals from the cytoplasmic droplet have been implicated in induction of lipid peroxidation, which affects lipoprotein architecture of sperm membranes and further deterioration of the sperm morphology, as well as possibly inducing DNA strand breaks [PMID 23543240, PMID 23159014].

Current WHO methodology suggests that 2 semen smears should be made and evaluated with 200 sperm being tallied per slide and an average reported, after evaluation for sampling error. Semen smears should be made on precleaned, plain glass microscope slides by pulling a drop of well mixed semen across the surface of the slide with a second slide held against the top surface at ~45°. This method leaves a thin layer of semen on the surface while the majority of the seminal fluid is removed so as to minimize background and interference during the morphology

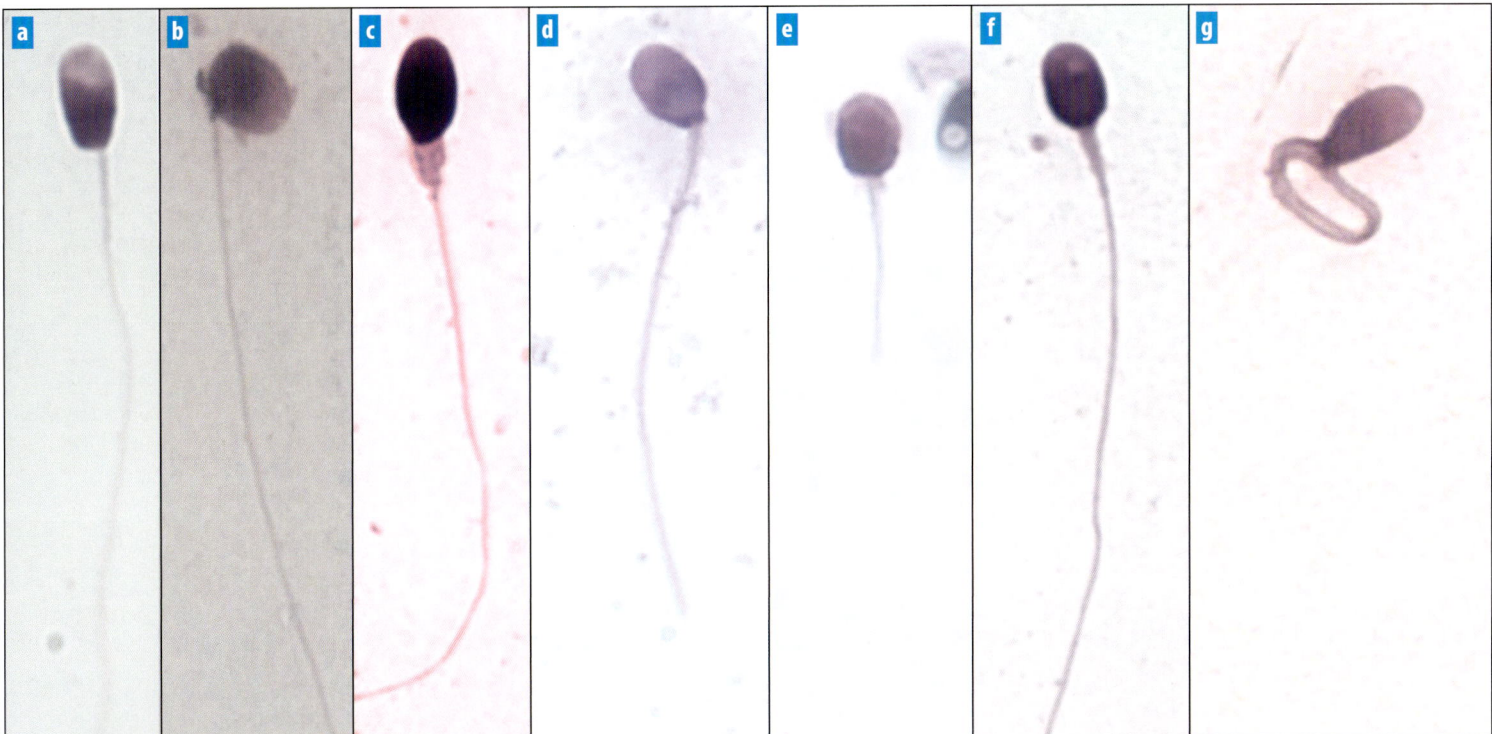

i8.4 Abnormal sperm midpiece & tail morphology. Abnormal morphologies include
a asymmetrical tail insertion
b bent neck
c excess residual cytoplasm
d, e short tail
f thick insertion
g coiled tail

interpretation. The type of staining system used can result in a large variation in the results and their interpretation; therefore, strict laboratory quality control practices should be employed. Acceptable fixation and staining protocols include the Papanicolaou stain, the Shorr stain, or the Diff-Quik stain. While there are many head, neck/midpiece, and tail defects observed in human sperm, the reporting system currently in place simply categorizes sperm as normal or abnormal. A specimen that has a preponderance of any type of abnormality should be noted, as those data may be clinically relevant.

Sperm viability

Sperm viability testing is useful to determine if nonmotile sperm are alive or dead, and is commonly used as an adjunct test for a sample with a low motility score to differentiate necrospermia from immotile, but viable sperm [ISBN: 1416031553]. A high viability with low motility indicates structural morphologic defects, such as primary ciliary dyskinesia or other defects in the sperm axoneme, which may be further evaluated with electron microscopy. For intracytoplasmic sperm injection (ICSI), often the sperm are retrieved from testis. The use of viability testing for these sperm retrieved from testis helps to determine which sperm are alive and can be used for ICSI.

Investigating the intactness of the sperm membrane by using either dye exclusion assays or the hypoosmotic swelling test can assess the percentage of viable sperm. The dye exclusion method is based on the principle that damaged plasma membranes allow entry of membrane nonpermeable stains. The hypoosmotic swelling test is based on the premise that only live sperm with intact membranes will swell in hypotonic solutions. This swelling becomes evident in the sperm tail and can be observed by phase contrast microscopy. Since, the use of stains kills the sperm, the hypoosmotic test, where the sperm are viable, is used for selection of sperm for ICSI. Viability testing is recommended for samples with ≤40% progressively motile spermatozoa [PMID 1519572]. Viability tests also provide a cross-check on the motility evaluation, since the percentage of dead cells should not exceed (within sampling error) the percentage of immotile spermatozoa. The percentage of viable cells normally exceeds that of motile cells.

The most common and well accepted dye exclusion test is eosin nigrosin staining. The procedure requires the use of a standardized eosin nigrosin solution mixed with an equal volume of well mixed raw semen. This suspension is then dropped onto 2 separate plain glass slides and a thin smear is made and allowed to air dry. Each slide is assessed for live, unstained sperm, vs the population of dead, pink stained sperm using 1,000× magnification under an oil immersion lens i8.1c. 200 sperm are tallied on each slide and the average percent of live cells per slide is compared. If the 2 replicates are within an acceptable range of sampling error, the average of the 2% ages of live, unstained, cells is recorded.

In the hypoosmotic swelling test, semen or sperm are placed in a hypoosmotic solution (15 mOsm/L or less). A live sperm will maintain an osmotic gradient and absorb fluid, resulting in plasma membrane swelling i8.1d. Dead sperm, whose plasma membranes are no longer intact, do not swell in hypotonic media. There are contradictory reports about the clinical significance and prognostic value for this test, since a high level of false positive results have been indicated [PMID 6694140, PMID 2745673]. The hypoosmotic test has a unique advantage over other viability tests that the sperm are still viable and therefore the assay can be used for selecting sperm for ICSI.

Leukocytes & immature germ cells

Semen often contains round cells including polymorphonuclear leukocytes and spermatocytes (immature germ cells). Both of these appear similar under phase contrast microscopy. Peroxidase positive granulocytes are the most common form of leukocytes present in semen and can be easily differentiated from other round cells in the population using peroxidase stain. More discrete differentiation can be performed based on differences in staining coloration and on nuclear size and shape with the aid of fixed and stained pathology slides [PMID 10972527]. In these more robust pathological techniques, polymorphonuclear leukocytes appear to be more bluish in color, as compared to immature germ cells, which stain more pinkish in color when using the Papanicolaou stain [PMID 10972527]. The nuclear diameter can also be used to determine the cell type and staging of germ cells.

Detection of increased leukocyte concentration in semen is suggestive of infection or inflammation. The threshold value for pyospermia, also termed leukocytospermia (increased peroxidase positive cells in the semen), has been set at 1.0 M/mL. Therefore, staining for peroxidase positive sperm in the semen is suggested as a routine component of the semen analysis. A simple protocol is to mix a 1:10 solution of semen to peroxidase stain in a tube, lightly vortex the sample, and incubate for 20-30 minutes. Load the sample onto a counting chamber and assess for the number of positive cells. Bear in mind that the sample has been diluted 1:10, this will change the calculation for the counting chamber you are using. When possible 200 cells should be counted over the area, in duplicate, to reduce the sampling error

It should be noted that studies have reported leukocytes and immature germ cells as a potential source of reactive oxygen species (ROS) in the semen [PMID 23898825, PMID 21076433]. The ROS generated from these round cells in their pathological concentration may induce damage to cellular biomolecules such as DNA, RNA, protein and lipids of the sperm [PMID 23543240, PMID 19293438, PMID 22749934].

Postvasectomy semen analysis

Guidelines of the American Urological Association (AUA) indicate that men undergoing a vasectomy should be evaluated 8-16 weeks after the procedure with a postvasectomy semen analysis (PVSA) to verify sterility. According to the AUA guidelines, the patient should be counseled and followed further if the sample has motile sperm present, or if >100,000 nonmotile sperm are present in the ejaculate [PMID 23098786]. These guidelines emphasize the need for analysis of a "fresh" sample so that motility can be evaluated [PMID 23098786, PMID 23917167].

Standard PVSA protocols include the same collection and handling protocols described above. The analysis should include a determination of the volume and the appearance and characteristics of the seminal fluid. Furthermore, a quantitative motility and count should be performed. Generally, sperm morphology is not performed, but any gross observations noted during the count and motility analysis should be noted.

Antisperm antibody testing

Antisperm antibodies may be present in the semen and serum of an infertile male, and are also produced in some females. In the male, antisperm antibodies are produced due to a breach in the blood testis barrier subsequent to surgery, cryptorchidism, infection or other trauma [PMID 15374685]. When the blood testis barrier is compromised, antisperm antibodies are produced that recognize specific regions of the sperm cell and may result in cell death and/or agglutination. Antisperm antibodies in semen almost exclusively belong to IgA and IgG class of immunoglobulins, since the IgM antibodies cannot normally cross the blood testis barrier due to their high molecular weight.

Antisperm antibodies are usually suspected when semen analysis indicates elevated sperm agglutination or asthenozoopermia, especially when sperm are observed to have a shaking motility, or following abnormal postcoital test results from a physician's office. The sperm antibodies may negatively affect the fertility in several ways. The antisperm antibodies may reduce the number of sperm reaching ova by agglutinating, immobilizing or opsonizing the sperm. When the antibodies are located on the tail they can immobilize the sperm or cause agglutination, and when present on sperm head they may directly affect fertilization capacity [PMID 23428233]. The antisperm antibodies may interfere with capacitation, cumulus penetration, acrosome reaction, zona binding and penetration, or sperm oocyte membrane interactions [PMID 15374685].

Current methods of detection of antisperm antibodies can be categorized as "direct" tests for the presence of antisperm antibody on sperm, or as "indirect" tests for antisperm antibodies in sperm free fluids, such as seminal plasma, serum and solubilized cervical mucus. The major limitation of the presently used assays for antisperm antibodies is their inability to quantify the antibody density on the sperm surface and to define antigenic specificities of these antibodies

Immunobead assay

The immunobead test is done on washed sperm, as compared to the neat semen used in mixed agglutination assay. Since sperm washing removes the possible masking components of seminal plasma, the immunobead test is more informative for antibodies on the sperm. In the immunobead test, washed sperm are mixed with beads that have been covalently coated with rabbit antihuman immunoglobulins against IgG or IgA. The binding of beads to motile spermatozoa indicates the presence of IgG or IgA antibodies on the surface of the spermatozoa i8.5. Both the mixed agglutination assay and the immune bead test depend on the presence of motile sperm, which is not always possible. In such cases, the indirect immunobead test may be performed.

In the indirect immunobead test, the sperm free fluid, such as seminal plasma, serum and cervical mucus, is diluted and heat inactivated. Subsequently, the sample is incubated with antibody free, control, washed sperm. If antisperm antibodies are present in the test fluid they will bind to the donor spermatozoa, which are assessed using the direct immunobead test protocol described above. For the accuracy of results, it is important that sufficient time is allowed for sperm antibody interaction as it may take up to 10 minutes for the agglutination to become visible.

Mixed agglutination assay

The mixed agglutination assay is performed on unwashed semen, and antihuman IgG or IgA are added to a suspension of semen and latex beads coated with human IgG or IgA antibody. The formation of mixed agglutinates between latex beads and motile spermatozoa indicates the presence of IgG or IgA antibodies on the spermatozoa. Sperm function has been reported to be impaired in cases where ≥50% of the motile spermatozoa have antibody bound to them [PMID 1519572]. Assessment of nonprogressive sperm that are close to the beads may lead to overestimation of antisperm antibodies. Particle binding restricted to the tailtip is not associated with impaired fertility and can also be present in fertile men [PMID 15374685].

ELISA assay for antisperm antibodies

In the ELISA assay, antibodies to isotype specific immunoglobulins are covalently linked to an enzyme and added to a sample (fixed sperm, sperm extracts, cervical mucus extracts, or sera). The formation of the antibody enzyme immunoglobulin complexes is detected by adding a specific enzyme substrate that results in a color change and can be quantified spectrophotometrically. This technique has the advantage of being specific and quantitative, but the site of antibody binding is not discernible.

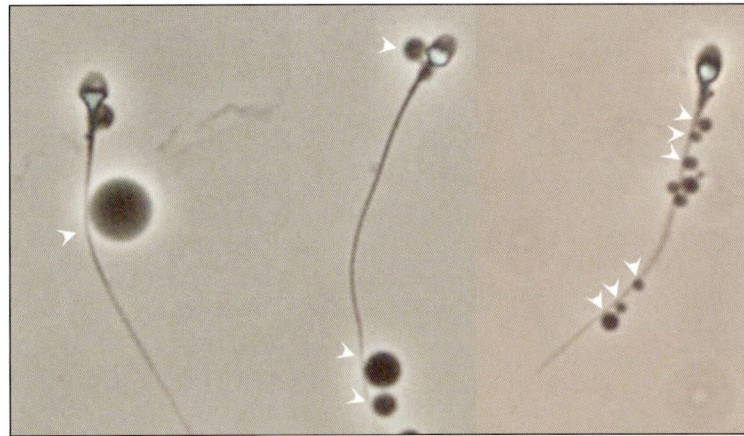

i8.5 Phase contrast micrograph of immunobead staining to various regions of the sperm cell as a result of antisperm antibodies; arrows indicate various regions of immunobead binding on sperm

Assays of sperm functional ability

As described above, fertilization requires various sperm functional capabilities, including capacitation, the acrosome reaction, zona penetration, sperm oocyte membrane fusion and penetration of the oolemma. The following assays are of use in evaluating these sperm functional abilities.

Sperm penetration assay

The sperm penetration assay (SPA) was developed by Yanagimachi et al as a test system to evaluate sperm fertilizing ability using zona free hamster oocytes as a surrogate for human oocytes. Specifically, the SPA evaluates the ability of sperm to undergo capacitation, fuse with the oocyte membrane, and decondense once oocyte penetration has occurred. Essentially, the sperm penetration assay is a bioassay similar to IVF, but using hamster ova from which zonae have been enzymatically removed. The assay is scored by calculating the percentage of ova that are penetrated or by the average number of sperm penetrations per ovum (polyspermy is present due to removal of the zona) i8.6. A modification of this assay, which is far less commonly employed, implements direct injection of the human sperm into the hamster oocytes to identify male factor patients who may fail to fertilize human oocytes after IVF/ICSI due to a defect in sperm head decondensation [PMID 10685549].

Early studies of the SPA were plagued by variations in the protocol that can dramatically alter results, and by poor quality control procedures. However, several studies have demonstrated the usefulness of the assay when strict protocols and validation studies are employed. The studies have reported a positive correlation for sperm penetration assay and IVF fertilization rates and also for pregnancy outcome in couples with idiopathic infertility [PMID 11730736, PMID 1521652, PMID 3110205, PMID 1992700], suggesting it to be an efficient diagnostic test for assessment of sperm quality. Additionally, the assay may be used to determine the necessity of ICSI for patients undergoing IVF.

The disadvantages of the SPA are primarily cost, the technical nature of the assay, and the need for intralaboratory control systems, since national proficiency testing is

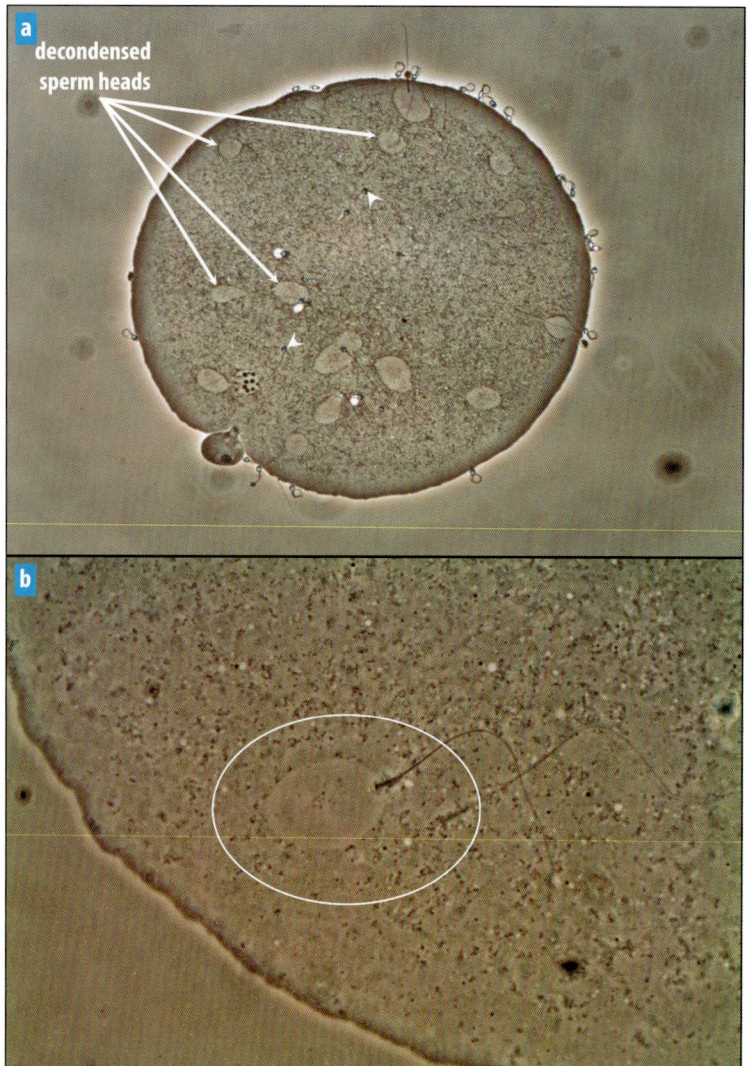

i8.6 The sperm penetration assay (SPA). Phase contrast photomicrograph of a zona free hamster egg following incubation with human sperm.
  a a hamster egg with several decondensed sperm nuclei that indicate penetration of the sperm into the oocyte (as indicated by the arrows) as compared to sperm bound to the surface of the oocyte (arrowheads).
  b a close up view of a decondensed (penetrated) sperm head (circled)

not available for this assay. However, the assay does provide valuable clinical information, such as distinguishing patients that should undergo ICSI rather than "standard" IVF.

Acrosome reaction assays

The sperm acrosome covers up to 2/3 of the sperm head and consists of enzymes, including acrosin, hyaluronidase and neuraminidase, that help to digest the zona pellucida. The absence or dysfunction of the acrosome may impair the acrosome reaction, leading to fertilization failure. Several methods can be used for assessment of acrosome status. These methods include light microscopy and fluorescence microscopy using fluorescently labeled lectins and monoclonal antibodies that bind to either the outer membrane or acrosome contents.

The acrosome reaction assay is clinically more informative if 3 parameters are measured: the percentage of sperm with a morphologically normal acrosome (>1/2 head is brightly and uniformly fluorescing following labeling), the percentage of sperm undergoing a spontaneous acrosome reaction during in vitro incubation (fluorescent band at the equatorial segment of the sperm and no fluorescence at in the remainder of the acrosome region), and the percentage of sperm undergoing an acrosome reaction after stimulated with a chemical inducer of the acrosome reaction, such as calcium ionophore A23187, progesterone, and the human zona pellucida [PMID 2050585, PMID 12524067, PMID 8299795]. The percent difference between stimulated and spontaneous acrosome reaction is termed the acrosome response to ionophore challenge score (ARIC score) **i8.7**. The normal difference is 15% acrosome reacted, values <10% acrosome reacted are considered abnormal and those between 10%-15% suggest that sperm function may be abnormal [PMID 1519572].

Studies have shown a significant correlation between normal sperm acrosome morphology and sperm zona pellucida binding [PMID 3135205, PMID 8774300] and normal sperm morphology and inducibility of acrosome reaction [PMID 9430436]. Acrosome reaction assays are most commonly performed for patients with round headed sperm (globozoospermia), who in some cases have a total absence of acrosome, and for patients with prior IVF failure. Patients with poor acrosome reaction are advised to undergo ICSI in conjunction with IVF therapy.

Hemizona assay

The hemizona assay is a bioassay in which human oocyte zona pellucidae are isolated from discarded human IVF oocytes, then microdissected into 2 equal halves. Each half is exposed to the same concentration of patient or control sperm. The sperm bound to zona in each half is observed and calculated and the hemizona ratio is calculated by dividing the number of patient sperm bound by the number of fertile control sperm bound to each respective half of the zona. A hemizona ratio <30%-40% is generally considered as an abnormal result [PMID 16682031].

The sperm/zona binding assay is a variation of the hemizona assay, however, in this assay the sperm from patient and fertile control are labeled with different fluorochromes (eg, fluorescein, rhodamine) so that creation of a hemizona is not required. Instead, the zona intact oocytes are incubated with equal numbers of differently fluorochrome labeled sperm. The number of spermatozoa from the patient and fertile control samples bound to the same intact zona are counted and reported as a ratio.

These tests are recommended in cases of low or failed in vitro fertilization, idiopathic infertility and teratozoospermia [PMID 14747159]. The binding of few or no spermatozoa to the zona pellucida usually indicates a sperm function defect and results from both zona binding tests have been shown to be correlated with fertilization rates in vitro [PMID 12524067]. Patients who are undergoing ART but have had abnormal sperm binding test results should consider ICSI therapy. The hemizona assay has been reported to be a predictor for pregnancy in couples with male factor infertility,

Assessment of reactive oxygen species (ROS)

In recent years, oxidative stress and DNA damage assessment have become important tools in the evaluation of male infertility. Reactive oxygen species (ROS) in the form of superoxide anions, hydrogen peroxide, and the hydroxyl free radical, are formed as a byproduct of oxygen metabolism. In the genital tract, a low level of ROS is necessary for normal function of human spermatozoa, including capacitation, acrosome reaction and sperm oocyte fusion [PMID 21086725, PMID 22777732, PMID 11013428]. Though it has been well demonstrated that human spermatozoa generate ROS during normal cellular respiration, excess production can adversely affect sperm function [PMID 16412557]. High levels of ROS have been detected in the semen of 25% of infertile men [PMID 8359932, PMID 1735495].

In semen, the potential sources for ROS are contaminating leukocytes, the retention of cytoplasmic residue within the sperm midpiece, and environmental factors. The activation of leukocytes in response to inflammation and infection induces ROS production in the seminal fluid. The presence of cytoplasmic droplets as residual cytoplasm in the sperm midpiece is positively correlated with ROS generation. Exogenous factors, such as drugs, smoking, environmental or occupational exposure to xenobiotics, radiation, and temperature may increase ROS production. Factors such as obesity or systemic and urogenital infections may also lead to elevated ROS levels. Lastly, sperm handling in the laboratory may also lead to elevated ROS levels, since procedures such as centrifugation have been shown to induce high levels of ROS [PMID 18026972].

Mitochondrial ROS have been correlated with loss of sperm motility as a consequence of lipid peroxidation [PMID 16412557, PMID 17644956, PMID 18492763] culminating in the loss of sperm function [PMID 18492763, PMID 9780307, PMID 2822642]. Elevated ROS levels have been found to affect the quality of the sperm and negatively correlated with progressive motility and normal morphology [PMID 22749934, PMID 18026972, PMID 22349386, PMID 21762187, PMID 22097888, PMID 20839089]. A direct positive correlation of ROS and sperm DNA damage has been proved in many studies using various techniques for sperm DNA damage assessment [PMID 19837155, PMID 21686150, PMID 17169183, PMID 17505572, PMID 20117780]. Elevated ROS levels may also cause nuclear and mitochondrial mutations including deletion and nucleotide substitutions [PMID 12149402, PMID 18810634]. High ROS levels negatively affect fertilization and pregnancy rates [PMID 1992700, PMID 18026972, PMID 17169183, PMID 11554990]. In one study, high levels of oxidative stress were associated with <25% fertilization rates and failure to achieve a pregnancy [PMID 14511216]. Further, studies have shown that high ROS levels are associated with poor embryogenesis after IVF/ICSI [PMID 18026972, PMID 11554990].

The quantification of ROS is done using chemiluminescence techniques. Luminol is the preferred probe because of its ability to detect intra- and extracellular ROS as compared to lucigenin, which only detects intracellular free radicals [PMID 16313680, PMID 11451353, PMID 8973665, PMID 1338331]. ROS can also be measured by using cellular probes coupled with flow cytometry. The detection of ROS is done for both the neat

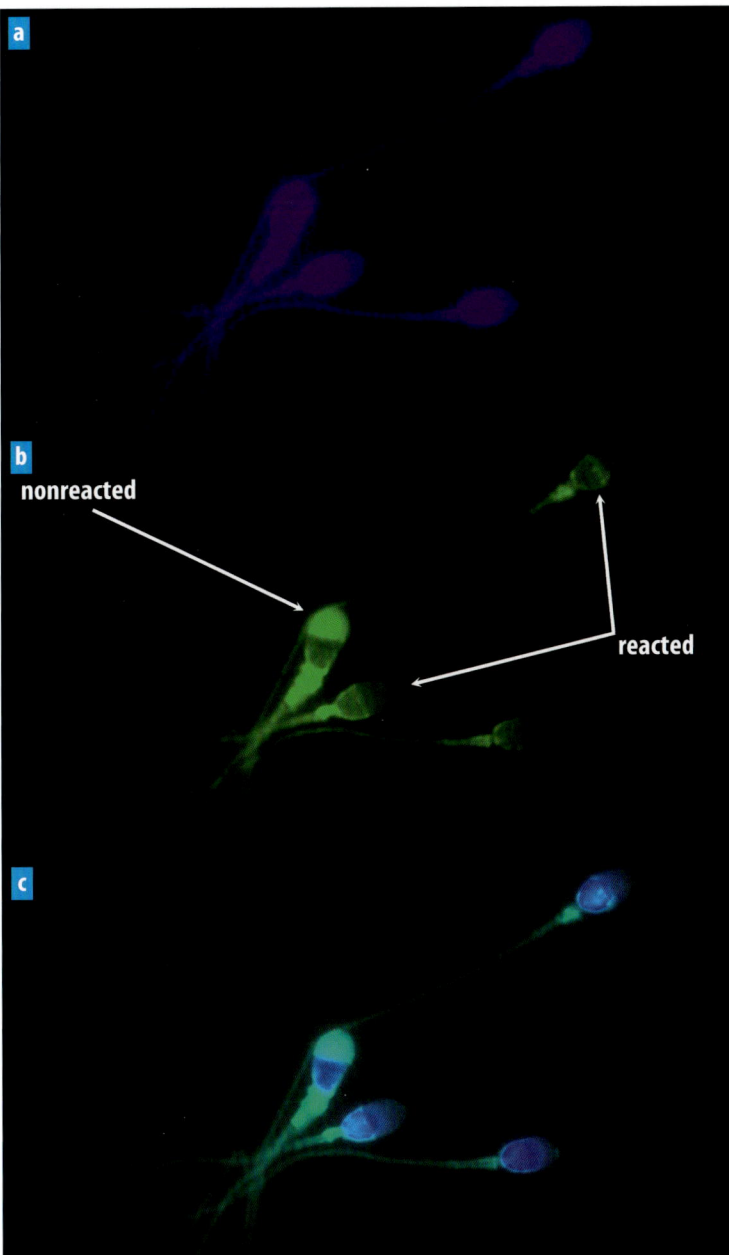

i8.7 The acrosome reaction assay. The 3 panel fluorescent micrographs indicate acrosome reacted & nonreacted sperm.
  a blue channel DAPI-stained sperm chromatin.
  b pea lectin staining with a conjugated FITC probe, which stains to the acrosome membrane of nonreacted sperm and the equatorial acrosome band of reacted sperm
  c overlay of blue green fluorescence. Reacted & nonreacted sperm are labeled & evidenced by the fluorescent band seen in the equatorial region of the sperm head.

though in the same study it was not found useful for couples with idiopathic infertility [PMID 16682031]. This assay is of limited use to most laboratories due to the unavailability of human zonae from IVF laboratories.

semen and the washed sperm. The level of neat semen ROS reflects the original oxidative status of the semen, which sperm experience in their normal milieu. The measurement of ROS levels in the washed sperm involves removal of seminal plasma by centrifugation, which is similar to the steps involved in ART processing. Hence, removal of seminal plasma results in deficiency of seminal antioxidants, whereas centrifugation has been reported to induce production of ROS [PMID 18154591]. High ROS levels in sperm post washing may be one of the reasons for ART failure, pronuclear block and slow embryo cleavage rates [PMID 16790111].

Though a valuable diagnostic assay for semen quality, ROS measurement has many inherent weaknesses. First, ROS are highly reactive and short lived and therefore must be quantified within 1 hour of semen collection. Therefore, samples cannot be stored or sent to a distant reference laboratory for ROS determination. Also it appears that ROS levels are quite variable in an individual due to physiologic or transient changes in spermatogenesis [PMID 20117777]. Finally, the protocol for ROS determination varies from laboratory to laboratory and the interpretation of ROS levels are affected by the sensitivity and type of luminometer used.

Sperm DNA damage assays

Some infertile men have normal standard sperm characteristics, but harbor DNA damage (decreased levels of DNA integrity) that can affect sperm function [PMID 19840147, PMID 18645682, PMID 16921163]. DNA integrity is defined as the absence of both single strand (ss) or double strand (ds) breaks of the DNA and absence of nucleotide modifications in the DNA [PMID 19427508]. The etiology of sperm DNA damage is multifactorial and may occur throughout spermatogenesis; therefore, DNA damage may be present in testicular sperm, epididymal sperm, or ejaculated sperm. Sperm DNA fragmentation may result from aberrant chromatin packaging during spermatogenesis [PMID 11943135, PMID 12713425, PMID 22872478, PMID 23809503], defective apoptosis [PMID 20802502], ROS production [PMID 20839089, PMID 18325925, PMID 20973394], decreased seminal antioxidants [PMID 22079708, PMID 21685925], and/or defective mitochondrial activity [PMID 19837155, PMID 15126291, PMID 20021411]. In addition, sperm DNA damage may also be induced in vitro during the ART procedures due to production of ROS [PMID 19293438]. Environmental factors, such as drugs, pollution, cigarette smoking, fever, xenobiotics, high testicular temperature, varicocele, and advanced age, have also been associated with increased sperm DNA damage [PMID 19812089, PMID 18460944, PMID 19090244, PMID 16400086, PMID 15980006, PMID 16355926].

A variety of different tests have been developed and are in routine use for the assessment of DNA damage in sperm. These assays vary in the type of damage measured and may vary in their predictive ability.

Acridine orange test

This test is based on the differential interaction of acridine orange with dsDNA and ssDNA. The dye intercalates with nonfragmented double stranded DNA, whereas with single stranded DNA or RNA the dye is bound by electrostatic interactions. When bound to dsDNA it has an excitation maximum at 502 nm and an emission maximum at 525 nm (green). When it associates with RNA or single stranded DNA, produced by ssDNA breaks, the excitation maximum shifts to 460 nm and the emission maximum shifts to 650 nm (red). The sperm with high DNA integrity emit green fluorescence while sperm with high DNA damage emit red fluorescence and the degree of damage is expressed as the percentage of sperm with red fluorescence. The advantage of this technique is that it is rapid, simple and inexpensive requiring just a fluorescence microscope. However, heterogeneous staining, rapid photobleaching, and indistinct staining are drawbacks associated with this technique.

Sperm chromatin structure assay

The sperm chromatin structure assay (SCSA) is the flow cytometry version of the acridine orange test, with other minor variations also included. The SCSA quantifies the metachromatic shift of acridine orange fluorescence from green (native DNA) to red (denatured or relaxed DNA) by using a flow cytometer as compared to visual counting of red and green cells as in the acridine orange test. The technique is highly reproducible with lower inter and intra laboratory variations. The DNA damage quantified by SCSA can be presented as the DNA fragmentation index (DFI), which is the ratio of red fluorescence to the total (sum of red and green) fluorescence. Another advantage of SCSA is that it simultaneously determines the percentage of sperm with high DNA stainability (% HDS), which is related to retained nuclear histones consistent with immature or abnormal sperm. High HDS values are predictive of pregnancy failure [PMID 22992911]. The disadvantage with the SCSA is the need for a flow cytometer and assay specific software.

Terminal deoxynucleotidyl transferase mediated dUTP nick end labeling (TUNEL) assay

The TUNEL assay quantifies the incorporation of biotinylated dUTP at double strand breaks in DNA using a reaction catalyzed by template independent terminal deoxynucleotidyl transferase. The assay scores cells with florescent or colorimetric labeled DNA i8.8. TUNEL can be applied in both bright field and fluorescence microscopy, and also using flow cytometry. The TUNEL assay is generally preferred in cases of oligozoospermia or for sperm retrieved from the epididymis or testis since the assay can be performed easily with low sperm numbers. The TUNEL assay is sensitive for both single and double stranded breaks. Some studies have shown a good correlation with the SCSA and comet assays [PMID 23843251].

Sperm chromatin dispersion (SCD)

In the sperm chromatin dispersion test, agarose embedded sperm are treated with a denaturing solution to remove the nuclear proteins and generate ssDNA from excising DNA nicks. The sperm are then subjected to lysis and the sperm with intact DNA produce a characteristic halo, while sperm with fragmented DNA exhibit a very small halo, or no halo

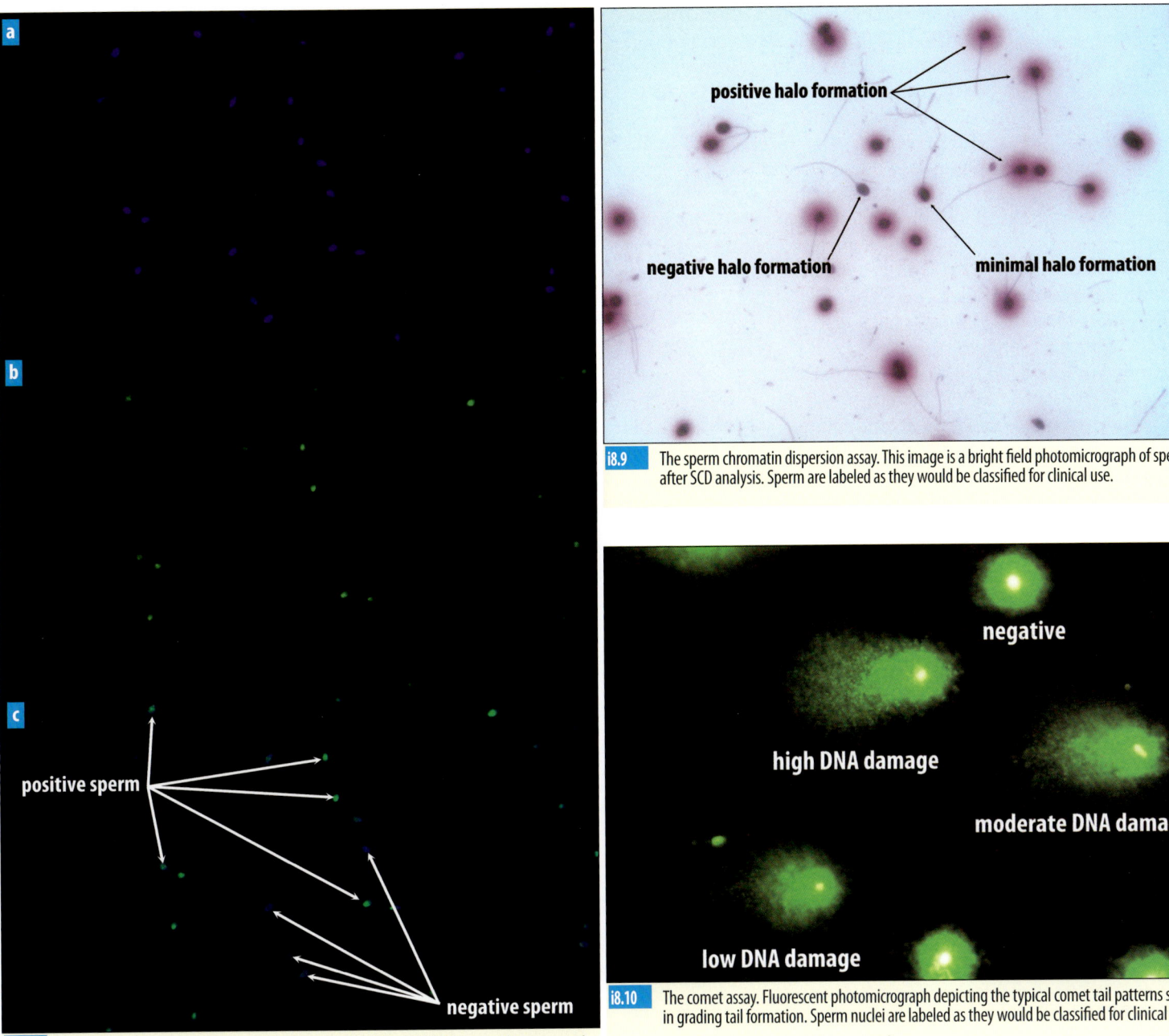

i8.8 The TUNEL assay. The 3 panel fluorescent micrographs indicate TUNEL reacted & nonreacted sperm.
a Blue channel DAPI-stained sperm nuclei
b TUNEL staining with a conjugated FITC probe that stains when there are strand breaks
c Overlay of blue green fluorescence; positive and negative sperm are labeled

i8.9 The sperm chromatin dispersion assay. This image is a bright field photomicrograph of sperm after SCD analysis. Sperm are labeled as they would be classified for clinical use.

i8.10 The comet assay. Fluorescent photomicrograph depicting the typical comet tail patterns seen in grading tail formation. Sperm nuclei are labeled as they would be classified for clinical use.

at all. The sperm chromatin dispersion test is based on the ability of intact DNA deprived of chromatin proteins to loop around the sperm nuclear matrix [PMID 11927317, PMID 10026119, PMID 12514084]. DNA breaks produce ssDNA, after treatment with denaturing agents (eg, heat, acid, or alkali) [PMID 2902165]. With the increase in DNA breaks, more ssDNA is generated and the denaturing solution transforms the regions with extensive DNA breaks into ssDNA motifs [PMID 8467513, PMID 8391465]. Halos can be observed either by bright field microscopy, if the staining is done by eosin and azure B solution i8.9, or by fluorescence microscopy if fluorochromes are used. The technique is simple and does not require complex instrumentation.

The comet assay

The comet assay is performed by sandwiching sperm between agarose layers and then lysing the cells, which results in a reduction of the sulfhydryl groups of the nuclear protamines. The lysed sperm cells are electrophoresed and the movement of fragmented DNA from damaged sperm chromatin appears similar to the tail of a comet. The staining intensity and length of the comet tail represents the amount of migrated DNA, indicating different degrees of DNA fragmentation i8.10. Dyes such as propidium iodide, SYBR-Green and YOYO-1 iodide are used for staining. The analysis for comet assay can be done both by visual scoring and by dedicated software. In subjective visual scoring, the comets are categorized on the basis of the diameter of the halo or length of the tail. Using software to analyze the comet assay provides a more detailed and objective analysis and presents the data in many formats, including length of tail (length of tail measured from periphery of comet head core), % tail DNA (percentage of DNA in the tail compared), olive tail moment (OTM; integral function of DNA in tail and pixel fluorescence of tail and head).

Depending upon the pH conditions, the comet assay has 2 distinct variants: the alkaline comet assay and the neutral comet assay. The alkaline comet assay measures both the single and the double stranded breaks and the alkali labile sites as compared to the neutral comet assay, which measures only double strand breaks. The disadvantage of alkaline comet assay is that it cannot differentiate between single or double strand breaks and overestimates true DNA strand breakage in spermatozoa because of artificial damage induced at alkali labile sites within the DNA strand [PMID 2806399]. Conversely, some suggest that alkali labile sites are predisposed to single strand breaks under high pH, their quantification along with native single and double strand breaks is more valuable for the overall assessment of sperm DNA damage [PMID 17644956]. Double strand breaks are difficult to repair by the oocyte DNA repair mechanism, making their evaluation more critical than single stranded breaks which can be repaired and hence have lower pathogenicity. The other advantage of alkaline comet assay is that it can detect damage equivalent to as few as 50 single strand breaks per cell. The major limitation of this assay is that it is labor intensive, has observer subjectivity, and requires experience to evaluate the comets, especially if software is not used in the analysis.

Sperm aneuploidy testing by fluorescent in situ hybridization (FISH)

Sperm chromosome aneuploidies (aberrant number of chromosomes) arise from errors during meiotic segregation with some errors being more common in metaphase 1, and other errors more common in metaphase 2 [PMID 11283700]. The abnormal segregation of chromosomes during meiosis may be the result of a myriad of defects, including chaotically abnormal spermatogenesis, defective checkpoint mechanisms, and interchromosomal effects resulting from translocations and other karyotype abnormalities of the patient. Sperm aneuploidy contributes to abnormal embryogenesis, usually resulting in miscarriage; however, some aneuploidies obviously increase risk of karyotype abnormalities in the offspring.

While gamete aneuploidy is clearly much more prevalent in oocytes, recent studies have clearly shown that testing is relevant in select male infertility patients [PMID 17881765]. Specifically, sperm FISH is indicated in men with severe oligozoospermia, severe teratozoospermia, unexplained recurrent pregnancy loss, and male carriers of Robertsonian translocations or other karyotype structural abnormalities [PMID 17881765].

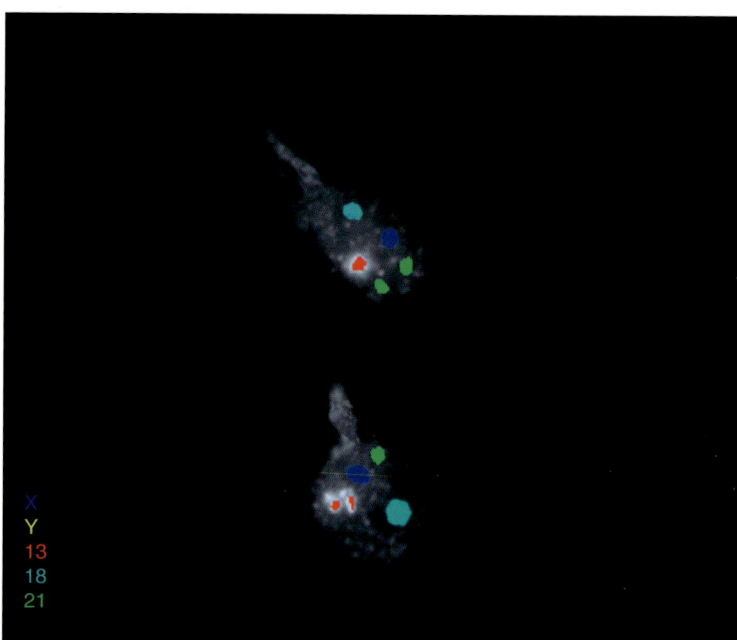

i8.11 Fluorescent micrograph of sperm hybridized with FISH probes for chromosomes X, Y, 21, 18, 13. 2 aneuploid sperm are depicted, diploid 21 (top) and diploid 13 (bottom). The color key for each chromosome is located in the bottom left corner.

The protocol for performing sperm FISH is detailed elsewhere, but is described here in brief [PMID 22992912]. Sperm nuclei are in interphase and are tightly compacted with nuclear protamine proteins; therefore, a sperm chromatin decondensation step is necessary to allow FISH probes access to the DNA. The sperm nuclei are typically decondensed using a treatment of dithiothreitol (DTT) to chemically reduce the nuclear disulfide bonding or high heat denaturation. Typically, a cocktail of 2-5 chromosomal probes are cohybridized to the sperm nuclei at once i8.11. This multicolor approach allows for more efficient counting and an internal hybridization efficiency control. The most commonly assayed chromosomes are X, Y, 13, 18, 16, 21, 22. Analysis of these chromosomes is thought be representative of the total sperm complement. Additionally, studies have shown that chromosomes 1, 15, 17, 21, and 22 are the most predictive of recurrent miscarriage [PMID 17881765, PMID 19424064]. The aneuploidy rates for counting 1,000 sperm per chromosome, using very stringent counting protocols, are in the range of 0.3%-0.5% aneuploidy per chromosome and a clinical reference range of <3.00% for X, Y, 13, 18, 21 has been widely used in the ART setting [PMID 17881765, PMID 19424064, Tempest 2010].

Artifacts & pitfalls

Semen analysis and sperm function testing results can be altered by improper collection and handling. Generally, semen/sperm must be evaluated within one hour of collection and maintained at body temperature. Some assays, such as ROS testing, may require stricter guidelines. Specimen containers must be evaluated and verified as nontoxic to sperm. Variations from these guidelines can significantly alter the results of the analysis.

Most assays are manually performed and technician training, validation, and proficiency testing are critical. Proficiency testing services for some sperm testing assays are available through national agencies; however, some assays require the establishment of careful intralaboratory proficiency testing since established proficiency testing may not be available.

Human sperm are heterogeneous within a given ejaculate. Therefore, proper mixing and sampling is critical in any assay. Additionally, generally 2 samples should be evaluated.

Some infertile men will have relatively normal semen analysis results, and conversely, some fertile men may have severely abnormal semen analysis results. Therefore, results must be viewed in conjunction with sperm function assay results and the patients' clinical history.

Recent data are demonstrating that semen quality may be variable over time due to environmental and lifestyle changes, as well as normal aging and health changes. Therefore, care must be taken to consider retesting prior to clinical decisions if the results are not within 6-12 months.

National proficiency testing services are not available for most sperm function tests and laboratories must develop accurate and adequate validation and proficiency testing of their technicians. Additionally, due to the highly technical nature of the assays technicians require advanced specialized training. Therefore, many assays are only available at a few reference laboratories.

Key points

- Semen analysis is the "starting point" for evaluation of male infertility. In many cases, additional testing evaluating sperm function, antisperm antibodies, DNA fragmentation, or sperm aneuploidy can provide valuable clinical information.

- Normal semen analysis is not a predictor of normal fertility, and abnormal semen analysis results are common in fertile men. Therefore, results must be carefully assessed in light of the clinical history of the patient.

- Postvasectomy semen analysis should be performed only on fresh semen samples and include a quantitative motility and count, as well as evaluation of the semen volume and characteristics.

- Sperm function testing is a valuable procedure when clinical history or semen analysis results indicate a possible sperm fertilization defect. The most commonly performed functional assay is the sperm penetration assay. All sperm function assay require strict quality control and validation within a laboratory.

- Sperm DNA fragmentation assays are a rapidly growing area of sperm testing. Each of the assays has inherent advantages and disadvantages. These assays may be most helpful in predicting success with ART procedures or evaluating poor ART outcomes.

References

PMID 10026119 Ward WS, Kimura Y, Yanagimachi R [1999] An intact sperm nuclear matrix may be necessary for the mouse paternal genome to participate in embryonic development. *Biol Reprod* 60(3):702-6

PMID 10685549 Gvakharia MO, Lipshultz LI, Lamb DJ [2000] Human sperm microinjection into hamster oocytes: a new tool for training and evaluation of the technical proficiency of intracytoplasmic sperm injection. *Fertil Steril* 73(2):395-401

PMID 10972527 Johanisson E, Campana A, Luthi R et al [2000] Evaluation of 'round cells' in semen analysis: a comparative study. *Hum Reprod Update* 6(4):404-12

PMID 11013428 Harrouk W, Khatabaksh S, Robaire B et al [2000] Paternal exposure to cyclophosphamide dysregulates the gene activation program in rat preimplantation embryos. *Mol Reprod Dev* 57(3):214-23

PMID 11283700 Hassold T, Hunt P [2001] To err (meiotically) is human: the genesis of human aneuploidy. *Nat Rev Genet* 2(4):280-91

PMID 11451353 Kobayashi H, Gil-Guzman E, Mahran AM et al [2001] Quality control of reactive oxygen species measurement by luminol-dependent chemiluminescence assay. *J Androl* 22(4):568-74

PMID 11554990 Hammadeh ME, Al-Hasani S, Gauss C et al [2001] Predictive value of chromatin decondensation in vitro on fertilization rate after intracytoplasmic sperm injection (ICSI). *Int J Androl* 24(5):311-6

PMID 11704105 Ryu HM, Lin WW, Lamb DJ et al [2001] Increased chromosome X, Y, and 18 nondisjunction in sperm from infertile patients that were identified as normal by strict morphology: implication for intracytoplasmic sperm injection. *Fertil Steril* 76(5):879-83

PMID 11730736 Freeman MR, Archibong AE, Mrotek JJ et al [2001] Male partner screening before in vitro fertilization: preselecting patients who require intracytoplasmic sperm injection with the sperm penetration assay. *Fertil Steril* 76(6):1113-8

PMID 11794171 Guzick DS., Overstreet JW, Factor-Litvak P et al [2001] Sperm morphology, motility, and concentration in fertile and infertile men. *N Engl J Med* 345(19):1388-93

PMID 11927317 Ankem MK, Mayer E, Ward WS et al [2002] Novel assay for determining DNA organization in human spermatozoa: implications for male factor infertility. *Urology* 59(4):575-8

PMID 11943135 Boissonneault G [2002] Chromatin remodeling during spermiogenesis: a possible role for the transition proteins in DNA strand break repair. *FEBS Lett* 514(2-3):111-4

PMID 12149402 Spiropoulos J, Turnbull DM, Chinnery PF [2002] Can mitochondrial DNA mutations cause sperm dysfunction? *Mol Hum Reprod* 8(8):719-21

PMID 12514084 Fernandez JL, Muriel L, Rivero MT et al [2003] The sperm chromatin dispersion test: a simple method for the determination of sperm DNA fragmentation. *J Androl* 24(1):59-66

PMID 12524067 Liu DY, Baker HW [2003] Disordered zona pellucida-induced acrosome reaction and failure of in vitro fertilization in patients with unexplained infertility. *Fertil Steril* 79(1):74-80

PMID 12713425 McLay DW, Clarke HJ [2003] Remodelling the paternal chromatin at fertilization in mammals. *Reproduction* 125(5):625-33

PMID 1338331 Aitken RJ, Buckingham DW, West KM [1992] Reactive oxygen species and human spermatozoa: analysis of the cellular mechanisms involved in luminol- and lucigenin-dependent chemiluminescence. *J Cell Physiol* 151(3):466-77

PMID 14511216 Zorn B, Vidmar G, Meden-Vrtovec H [2003] Seminal reactive oxygen species as predictors of fertilization, embryo quality and pregnancy rates after conventional in vitro fertilization and intracytoplasmic sperm injection. *Int J Androl* 26(5):279-85

PMID 14747159 Liu DY, Baker HW [2004] High frequency of defective sperm-zona pellucida interaction in oligozoospermic infertile men. *Hum Reprod* 19(2):228-33

PMID 15126291 Liu CY, Lee CF, Hong CH et al [2004] Mitochondrial DNA mutation and depletion increase the susceptibility of human cells to apoptosis. *Ann N Y Acad Sci* 1011:133-45

PMID 1519572 This PMID links to this article: http://www.ncbi.nlm.nih.gov/pubmed/?term=1519572 ????? World Health Organization [2010] WHO laboratory manual for the examination and processing of human semen. World Health Organization, 5e

PMID 15205404 Celik-Ozenci C, Jakab A, Kovacs T et al [2004] Sperm selection for ICSI: shape properties do not predict the absence or presence of numerical chromosomal aberrations. *Hum Reprod* 19(9):2052-9

PMID 1521652 Soffer Y, Golan A, Herman A et al [1992] Prediction of in vitro fertilization outcome by sperm penetration assay with TEST-yolk buffer preincubation. *Fertil Steril* 58(3):556-62

PMID 15223853 Brazil C, Swan SH, Drobnis EZ et al [2004] Standardized methods for semen evaluation in a multicenter research study. *J Androl* 25(4):635-44

PMID 15374685 Chiu WW, Chamley LW [2004] Clinical associations and mechanisms of action of antisperm antibodies. *Fertil Steril* 82(3):529-35

PMID 15482758 McKenzie LJ, Kovanci E, Amato P et al [2004] Pregnancy outcome of in vitro fertilization/intracytoplasmic sperm injection with profound teratospermia. *Fertil Steril* 82(4):847-9

PMID 15817522 De Jonge C [2005] Biological basis for human capacitation. *Hum Reprod Update* 11(3):205-14

PMID 15980006 Rubes J, Selevan SG, Evenson DP et al [2005] Episodic air pollution is associated with increased DNA fragmentation in human sperm without other changes in semen quality. *Hum Reprod* 20(10):2776-83

PMID 16021863 Iemmolo M, Simmons L, Matson P [2005] The rapid detection of cytotoxicity using a modified human sperm survival assay. *J Assist Reprod Genet* 22(4):177-80

PMID 16313680 Baker MA, Aitken RJ [2005] Reactive oxygen species in spermatozoa: methods for monitoring and significance for the origins of genetic disease and infertility. *Reprod Biol Endocrinol* 3:67

PMID 16355926 Weber RF, Döhle GR, Romijn JC [2005] Clinical laboratory evaluation of male subfertility. *Adv Clin Chem* 40:317-64

PMID 16400086 Enciso M, Muriel L, Fernandez JL et al [2006] Infertile men with varicocele show a high relative proportion of sperm cells with intense nuclear damage level, evidenced by the sperm chromatin dispersion test. *J Androl* 27(1):106-11

PMID 16406920 Misell LM, Holochwost D, Boban D et al [2006] A stable isotope-mass spectrometric method for measuring human spermatogenesis kinetics in vivo. *J Urol* 175(1):242-6; discussion 246

PMID 16412557 Aitken RJ, Baker MA [2006] Oxidative stress, sperm survival and fertility control. *Mol Cell Endocrinol* 250(1-2):66-9

PMID 16467269 Yanagimachi R [2005] Male gamete contributions to the embryo. *Ann N Y Acad Sci* 1061:203-7

PMID 16682031 Arslan M, Morshedi M, Arslan EO et al [2006] Predictive value of the hemizona assay for pregnancy outcome in patients undergoing controlled ovarian hyperstimulation with intrauterine insemination. *Fertil Steril* 85(6):1697-707

PMID 16790111 Agarwal A, Prabakaran S, Allamaneni SS [2006] Relationship between oxidative stress, varicocele and infertility: a meta-analysis. *Reprod Biomed Online* 12(5):630-3

PMID 16921163 Bungum M, Humaidan P, Axmon A et al [2007] Sperm DNA integrity assessment in prediction of assisted reproduction technology outcome. *Hum Reprod* 22(1):174-9

PMID 16957135 Cooper TG, Brazil C, Swan SH et al [2007] Ejaculate volume is seriously underestimated when semen is pipetted or decanted into cylinders from the collection vessel. *J Androl* 28(1):1-4

PMID 17127284 Francavilla S, Cordeschi G, Pelliccione F et al [2007] Isolated teratozoospermia: a cause of male sterility in the era of ICSI? *Front Biosci* 12:69-88

PMID 17169183 Hammadeh ME, Radwan M, Al-Hasani S et al [2006] Comparison of reactive oxygen species concentration in seminal plasma and semen parameters in partners of pregnant and nonpregnant patients after IVF/ICSI. *Reprod Biomed Online* 13(5):696-706

PMID 1735495 Iwasaki A, Gagnon C [1992] Formation of reactive oxygen species in spermatozoa of infertile patients. *Fertil Steril* 57(2):409-16

PMID 17505572 Smith R, Kaune H, Parodi D et al [2007] [Extent of sperm DNA damage in spermatozoa from men examined for infertility. Relationship with oxidative stress. *Rev Med Chil* 135(3):279-86

PMID 17554051 Bhasin S [2007] Approach to the infertile male. *J Clin Endocrinol Metab* 92(6):1995-2004

PMID 17644956 Aitken RJ, De Iuliis GN [2007] Value of DNA integrity assays for fertility evaluation. *Soc Reprod Fertil Suppl* 65:81-92

PMID 17881765 Carrell DT [2008] The clinical implementation of sperm chromosome aneuploidy testing: pitfalls and promises. *J Androl* 29(2):124-33

PMID 18026972 Hammadeh ME, Al Hasani S, Rosenbaum P et al [2008] Reactive oxygen species, total antioxidant concentration of seminal plasma and their effect on sperm parameters and outcome of IVF/ICSI patients. *Arch Gynecol Obstet* 277(6):515-26

PMID 18154591 Agarwal A, Makker K, Sharma R [2008] Clinical relevance of oxidative stress in male factor infertility: an update. *Am J Reprod Immunol* 59(1):2-11

PMID 18325925 Lewis SE, Agbaje IM [2008] Using the alkaline comet assay in prognostic tests for male infertility and assisted reproductive technology outcomes. *Mutagenesis* 23(3):163-70

PMID 18460944 Soares SR, Melo MA [2008] Cigarette smoking and reproductive function. *Curr Opin Obstet Gynecol* 20(3):281-91

PMID 18492763 Koppers AJ, De Iuliis GN, Finnie JM et al [2008] Significance of mitochondrial reactive oxygen species in the generation of oxidative stress in spermatozoa. *J Clin Endocrinol Metab* 93(8):3199-207

PMID 18645682 Erenpreiss J, Elzanaty S, Giwercman A [2008] Sperm DNA damage in men from infertile couples. *Asian J Androl* 10(5):786-90

PMID 18810634 Sharma N, Singh M, Acharya N et al [2008] Implication of the cystic fibrosis transmembrane conductance regulator gene in infertile family members of Indian CF patients. *Biochem Genet* 46(11-12):847-56

PMID 19090244 Colagar AH, Jorsaraee GA, Marzony ET [2007] Cigarette smoking and the risk of male infertility. *Pak J Biol Sci* 10(21):3870-4

PMID 19293438 Venkatesh S, Deecaraman M, Kumar R et al [2009] Role of reactive oxygen species in the pathogenesis of mitochondrial DNA (mtDNA) mutations in male infertility. *Indian J Med Res* 129(2):127-37

PMID 19297071 El-Taieb MA, Herwig R, Nada EA et al [2009] Oxidative stress and epididymal sperm transport, motility and morphologic defects. *Eur J Obstet Gynecol Reprod Biol* 144(Suppl1):S199-203

PMID 19424064 Tempest HG, Martin RH [2009] Cytogenetic risks in chromosomally normal infertile men. *Curr Opin Obstet Gynecol* 21(3):223-7

PMID 19427508 Shamsi MB, Venkatesh S, Tanwar M et al [2009] DNA integrity and semen quality in men with low seminal antioxidant levels. *Mutat Res* 665(1-2):29-36

PMID 19812089 Delbes G, Hales BF, Robaire B [2010] Toxicants and human sperm chromatin integrity. *Mol Hum Reprod* 16(1):14-22

PMID 19837155 Koppers AJ, Garg ML, Aitken RJ [2010] Stimulation of mitochondrial reactive oxygen species production by unesterified, unsaturated fatty acids in defective human spermatozoa. *Free Radic Biol Med* 48(1):112-9

PMID 19840147 Giwercman A, Lindstedt L, Larsson M et al [2010] Sperm chromatin structure assay as an independent predictor of fertility in vivo: a case-control study. *Int J Androl* 33(1):e221-7

PMID 19871256 Huggins C, Neal W [1942] Coagulation and liquefaction of semen: proteolytic enzymes and citrate in prostatic fluid. *J Exp Med* 76(6):527-41

PMID 1992700 Aitken RJ, Irvine DS, Wu FC [1991] Prospective analysis of sperm-oocyte fusion and reactive oxygen species generation as criteria for the diagnosis of infertility. *Am J Obstet Gynecol* 164(2):542-51

PMID 20021411 Amaral S, Ramalho-Santos J [2009] Aging, mitochondria and male reproductive function. *Curr Aging Sci* 2(3):165-73

PMID 20117777 Desai NR, Mahfouz R, Sharma R et al [2010] Reactive oxygen species levels are independent of sperm concentration, motility, and abstinence in a normal, healthy, proven fertile male: a longitudinal study. *Fertil Steril* 94(4):1541-3

PMID 20117780 Mahfouz R, Sharma R, Thiyagarajan A et al [2010] Semen characteristics and sperm DNA fragmentation in infertile men with low and high levels of seminal reactive oxygen species. *Fertil Steril* 94(6):2141-6

PMID 2050585 Cummins JM, Pember SM, Jequier AM et al [1991] A test of the human sperm acrosome reaction following ionophore challenge. Relationship to fertility and other seminal parameters. *J Androl* 12(2):98-103

PMID 20802502 Aitken RJ, Koppers AJ [2011] Apoptosis and DNA damage in human spermatozoa. *Asian J Androl* 13(1):36-42

PMID 20839089 Aitken RJ, Baker MA, De Iuliis GN et al [2010] New insights into sperm physiology and pathology. *Handb Exp Pharmacol* 198:99-115

PMID 20973394 Saalu LC [2010] The incriminating role of reactive oxygen species in idiopathic male infertility: an evidence based evaluation. *Pak J Biol Sci* 13(9):413-22

PMID 21076433 Henkel RR [2011] Leukocytes and oxidative stress: dilemma for sperm function and male fertility. *Asian J Androl* 13(1):43-52

PMID 21086725 Dada R, Kumar R, Shamsi MB et al [2008] Genetic screening in couples experiencing recurrent assisted procreation failure. *Indian J Biochem Biophys* 45(2):116-20

PMID 21586547 Inaba K [2011] Sperm flagella: comparative and phylogenetic perspectives of protein components. *Mol Hum Reprod* 17(8):524-38

PMID 21685925 Lombardo F, Sansone A, Romanelli F et al [2011] The role of antioxidant therapy in the treatment of male infertility: an overview. *Asian J Androl* 13(5):690-7

PMID 21686150 Cemeli E, Anderson D [2011] Mechanistic investigation of ROS-induced DNA damage by oestrogenic compounds in lymphocytes and sperm using the comet assay. *Int J Mol Sci* 12(5): 2783-96

PMID 21762187 Dada R, Mahfouz RZ, Kumar R et al [2011] A comprehensive work up for an asthenozoospermic male with repeated intracytoplasmic sperm injection (ICSI) failure. *Andrologia* 43(5):368-72

PMID 22079708 Tvrda E, Knazicka Z, Bardos L et al [2011] Impact of oxidative stress on male fertility - a review. *Acta Vet Hung* 59(4):465-84

PMID 22097888 Shi TY, Chen G, Huang X et al [2012] Effects of reactive oxygen species from activated leukocytes on human sperm motility, viability and morphology. *Andrologia* 44(Suppl 1):696-703.

PMID 22289286 Carrell DT [2012] Epigenetics of the male gamete. *Fertil Steril* 97(2):267-74

PMID 22349386 Wang X, Liu N [2012] [Sperm DNA oxidative damage in patients with idiopathic asthenozoospermia. *Zhong Nan Da Xue Xue Bao Yi Xue Ban* 37(1):100-5

PMID 22381250 Ferramosca A, Provenzano SP, Coppola L et al [2012] Mitochondrial respiratory efficiency is positively correlated with human sperm motility. *Urology* 79(4):809-14

PMID 22571172 Perrin A, Coat C, Nguyen MH et al [2013] Molecular cytogenetic and genetic aspects of globozoospermia: a review. *Andrologia* 45(1):1-9

PMID 22749934 Lavranos G, Balla M, Tzortzopoulou A et al [2012] Investigating ROS sources in male infertility: a common end for numerous pathways. *Reprod Toxicol* 34(3):298-307

PMID 22777732 Shamsi MB, Kumar R, Malhotra N et al [2012] Chromosomal aberrations, Yq microdeletion, and sperm DNA fragmentation in infertile men opting for assisted reproduction. *Mol Reprod Dev* 79(9):637-50

PMID 22872478 Chu DS, Shakes DC [2013] Spermatogenesis. *Adv Exp Med Biol* 757:171-203

PMID 22992911 Evenson DP [2013] Sperm chromatin structure assay (SCSA(R)). *Methods Mol Biol* 927:147-64

PMID 22992912 Emery BR [2013] Sperm aneuploidy testing using fluorescence in situ hybridization. *Methods Mol Biol* 927:167-73

PMID 23098786 Sharlip ID, Belker AM, Honig S et al [2012] Vasectomy: AUA guideline. *J Urol* 188(6Suppl):2482-91

PMID 23159014 Rengan AK, Agarwal A, van der Linde M et al [2012] An investigation of excess residual cytoplasm in human spermatozoa and its distinction from the cytoplasmic droplet. *Reprod Biol Endocrinol* 10:92

PMID 23428233 Restrepo B, Cardona-Maya W [2013] Antisperm antibodies and fertility association. *Actas Urol Esp* 37(9):571-8

PMID 23543240 Chen SJ, Allam JP, Duan YG et al [2013] Influence of reactive oxygen species on human sperm functions and fertilizing capacity including therapeutical approaches. *Arch Gynecol Obstet* 288(1):191-9

PMID 23809503 Jenkins TG, Aston KI, Cairns BR et al [2013] Paternal aging and associated intraindividual alterations of global sperm 5-methylcytosine and 5-hydroxymethylcytosine levels. *Fertil Steril* 100(4):945-51

PMID 23843251 Ribas-Maynou J, Garcia-Peiro A, Fernandez-Encinas A et al [2013] Comprehensive analysis of sperm DNA fragmentation by 5 different assays: TUNEL assay, SCSA, SCD test and alkaline and neutral Comet assay. *Andrology* 1(5):715-22

PMID 23898825 Mupfiga C, Fisher D, Kruger T et al [2013] The relationship between seminal leukocytes, oxidative status in the ejaculate, and apoptotic markers in human spermatozoa. *Syst Biol Reprod Med* 59(6):304-11

PMID 23917167 Coward RM, Badhiwala NG, Kovac JR et al [2014] Impact of the 2012 American Urological Association vasectomy guidelines on post-vasectomy outcomes. *J Urol* 191(1):169-74

PMID 2394790 Menkveld R, Stander FS, Kotze TJ et al [1990] The evaluation of morphologic characteristics of human spermatozoa according to stricter criteria. *Hum Reprod* 5(5):586-92.

PMID 23955672 Gannon JR, Emery BR, Jenkins TG et al [2014] The sperm epigenome: implications for the embryo. *Adv Exp Med Biol* 791:53-66

PMID 24194470 Okabe M [2013] The cell biology of mammalian fertilization. *Development* 140(22):4471-9

PMID 2745673 Barratt CL, Osborn JC, Harrison PE et al [1989] The hypo-osmotic swelling test and the sperm mucus penetration test in determining fertilization of the human oocyte. *Hum Reprod* 4(4):430-4

PMID 2806399 Singh NP, Danner DB, Tice RR et al [1989] Abundant alkali-sensitive sites in DNA of human and mouse sperm. *Exp Cell Res* 184(2):461-70

PMID 2822642 Alvarez JG, Touchstone JC, Blasco L et al [1987] Spontaneous lipid peroxidation and production of hydrogen peroxide and superoxide in human spermatozoa. Superoxide dismutase as major enzyme protectant against oxygen toxicity. *J Androl* 8(5):338-48

PMID 2902165 Ahnstrom G [1988] Techniques to measure DNA single-strand breaks in cells: a review. *Int J Radiat Biol* 54(5):695-707

PMID 3110205 Aitken RJ, Thatcher S, Glasier AF et al [1987] Relative ability of modified versions of the hamster oocyte penetration test, incorporating hyperosmotic medium or the ionophore A23187, to predict IVF outcome. *Hum Reprod* 2(3):227-31

PMID 3135205 Liu DY, Baker HW [1988] The proportion of human sperm with poor morphology but normal intact acrosomes detected with Pisum sativum agglutinin correlates with fertilization in vitro. *Fertil Steril* 50(2):288-93

PMID 6694140 Jeyendran RS, Van der Ven HH, Perez-Pelaez M et al [1984] Development of an assay to assess the functional integrity of the human sperm membrane and its relationship to other semen characteristics. *J Reprod Fertil* 70(1):219-28

PMID 7484449 Cooper TG [1995] Role of the epididymis in mediating changes in the male gamete during maturation. *Adv Exp Med Biol* 377:87-101

PMID 7816062 Auger J, Kunstmann JM, Czyglik F et al [1995] Decline in semen quality among fertile men in Paris during the past 20 years. *N Engl J Med* 332(5):281-5

PMID 8299795 Oehninger S, Blackmore P, Morshedi M et al [1994] Defective calcium influx and acrosome reaction (spontaneous & progesterone-induced) in spermatozoa of infertile men with severe teratozoospermia. *Fertil Steril* 61(2):349-54

PMID 8359932 Zini A, de Lamirande E, Gagnon C [1993] Reactive oxygen species in semen of infertile patients: levels of superoxide dismutase- and catalaselike activities in seminal plasma and spermatozoa. *Int J Androl* 16(3):183-8

PMID 8391465 Gorczyca W, Traganos F, Jesionowska H et al [1993] Presence of DNA strand breaks and increased sensitivity of DNA in situ to denaturation in abnormal human sperm cells: analogy to apoptosis of somatic cells. *Exp Cell Res* 207(1):202-5

PMID 8467513 Gorczyca W, Gong J, Darzynkiewicz Z [1993] Detection of DNA strand breaks in individual apoptotic cells by the in situ terminal deoxynucleotidyl transferase and nick translation assays. *Cancer Res* 53(8):1945-51

PMID 8774300 Menkveld R, Rhemrev JP, Franken DR et al [1996] Acrosomal morphology as a novel criterion for male fertility diagnosis: relation with acrosin activity, morphology (strict criteria), and fertilization in vitro. *Fertil Steril* 65(3):637-44

PMID 8844314 Lindheim SR, Barad DH, Zinger M et al [1996] Abnormal sperm morphology is highly predictive of pregnancy outcome during controlled ovarian hyperstimulation and intrauterine insemination. *J Assist Reprod Genet* 13(7):569-72

PMID 8973665 Sharma RK, Agarwal A [1996] Role of reactive oxygen species in male infertility. *Urology* 48(6):835-50

PMID 9430436 Franken DR, Bastiaan HS, Kidson A et al [1997] Zona pellucida mediated acrosome reaction and sperm morphology. *Andrologia* 29(6):311-7

PMID 9696208 Guzick DS, Sullivan MW, Adamson GD et al [1998] Efficacy of treatment for unexplained infertility. *Fertil Steril* 70(2):207-13

PMID 9780307 Aitken RJ, Gordon E, Harkiss D et al [1998] Relative impact of oxidative stress on the functional competence and genomic integrity of human spermatozoa. *Biol Reprod* 59(5):1037-46

PMID 9886521 Chia SE, Tay SK, Lim ST [1998] What constitutes a normal seminal analysis? Semen parameters of 243 fertile men. *Hum Reprod* 13(12):3394-8

ISBN 978-0721607986 Sigman M, Jarrow JP [2007] Male Infertility. In Wein AJ, Kavouss LR, Novick AC, et al, eds. *Campbell-Walsh Urology*, vol 1. Saunders Elsevier Press, 609-653

Tempest HG, Gillott DJ, Grigorova M et al [2010] P11 Sperm aneuploidy: When to stop counting? *Reprod Biomed Online* 20:S26

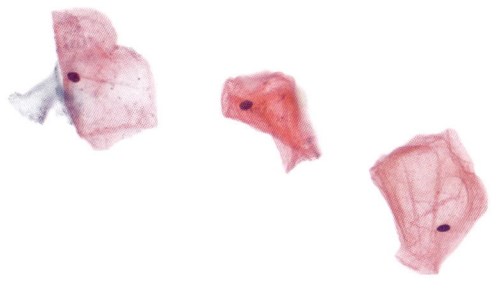

Cohen MB, Couturier MR, Straseski JA, Kjeldsberg CR

Urine
Chapter 9

Anatomy & pathophysiology

The urinary tract plays vital roles, largely through the kidneys, in normal human physiology including homeostasis of volume, electrolyte levels, and maintenance of acid-base balance. It includes the kidneys, ureters, urinary bladder, and urethra **f9.1**. The microscopic anatomy of the kidney is centered on the nephron, of which there are ~1,000,000 per kidney, and its microanatomy is well described in standard histology and anatomy textbooks [ISBN 072-1660290]. As such, the kidney shows remarkable reserve and loss of 50% of renal function is generally well tolerated. The renal pelves all the way to the urethra, with a large reservoir in the urinary bladder, principally serve as the conduit of urine to be excreted. This urinary system is lined by a unique epithelium, urothelium, which is distinct from squamous and glandular epithelium. It should be noted, however, that the distal urethra is lined by squamous cells. The urothelium is composed of 2 major cell types—superficial (sometimes referred to as cap, dome, or umbrella) cells and basal cells. By electron microscopy, the unique nature of this epithelium is readily identified where the intercellular junctions prevent "backflow" of urine.

Like other body fluids, urine may be viewed as an ultrafiltrate of blood (ie, plasma). The kidney is the principal site for this event receiving ~25% of the cardiac output. Normally, the kidneys produce ~1L of urine per day. The functional unit in the kidney is the nephron, which includes the glomerulus and the tubules. Under normal physiologic conditions, the glomerulus filters plasma by retaining proteins and other components. Under abnormal conditions (eg, damage from autoimmune disease) the glomerulus may not be able to properly serve as a filter and leakage occurs, as is the case with the loss of protein in the urine (proteinuria).

The history of urinalysis dates back to at least the Middle Ages [PMID 3048852, ISBN 019-5134958, ISBN 978-0930304874]. At that time, it was referred to as uroscopy and was based on the gross examination of urine for the identification of disease (eg, diabetes). However, it was also referred to as "pisse prophecy." Modern urinalysis coincides with the development of the microscope, almost 200 years ago, and chemical analyses, ~100 years ago; the identification of microorganisms overlaps with these 2 approaches. Today, much of the analysis is automated but laboratorian involvement, especially microscopy, remains key.

A large number of diseases can affect the kidney and result in changes in the urine. Consequently, the examination of urine (urinalysis) can be of vital importance. For example, the identification of proteinuria leads to the development of a distinct differential diagnosis that requires further testing to identify the specific etiology. Similarly, hematuria, azotemia, pyuria, and abnormal urothelial cells requires additional investigation. In short, any of the major disease processes (eg, environmental, genetic, hemodynamic, immunological, inflammatory/infectious, neoplastic, nutritional, and thromboembolic) may affect and involve the urinary system and be detectable in some fashion by urinalysis [PMID 15791892].

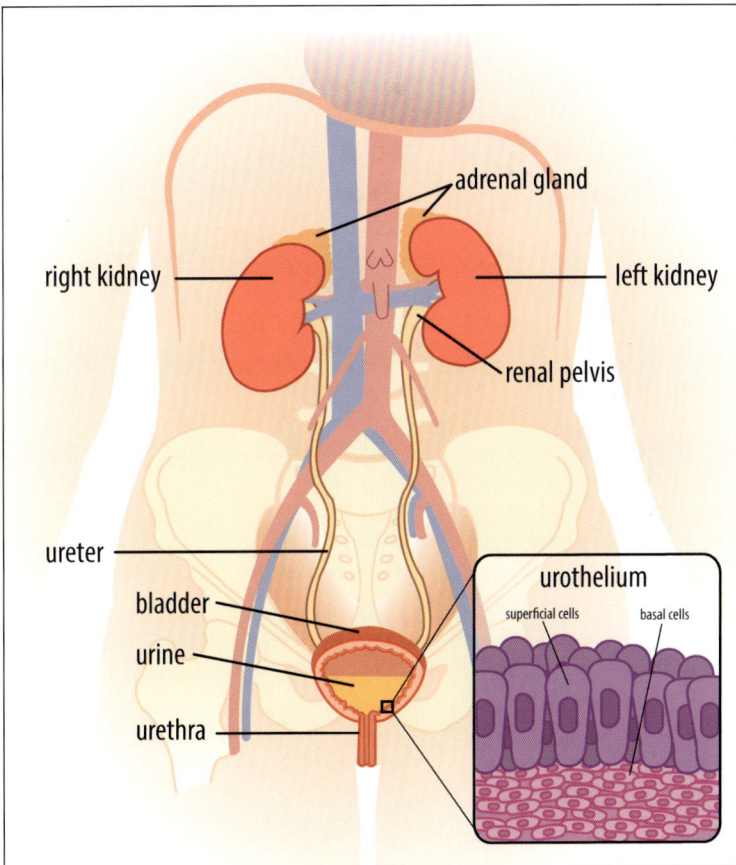

f9.1 Gross anatomy of the urinary tract

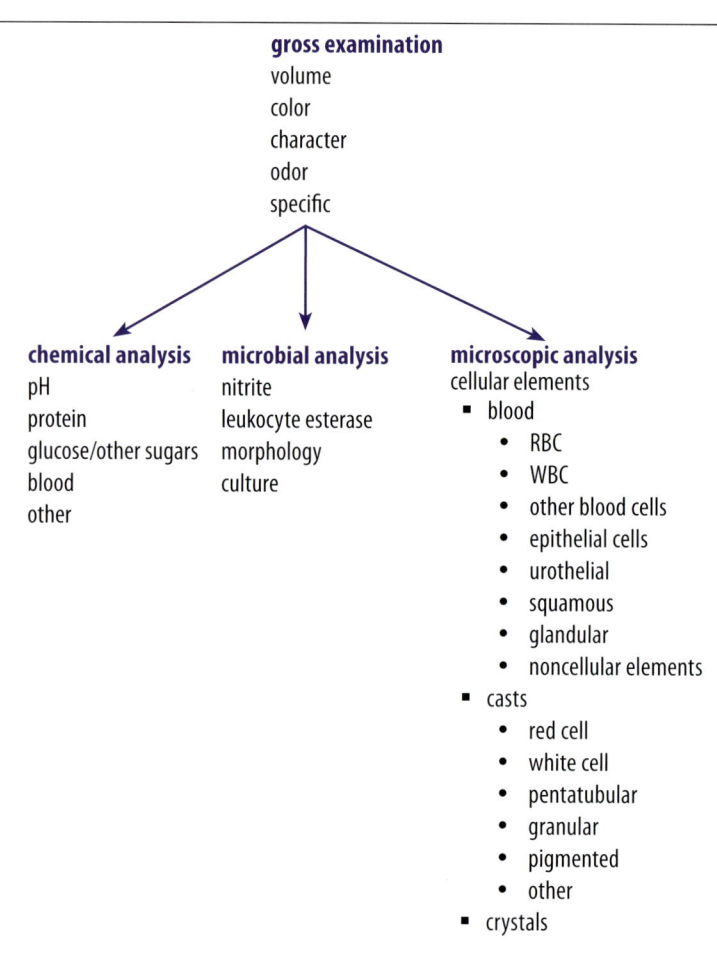

f9.2 Approach for the analysis of urine specimens

Clinical indications & considerations & recommended laboratory studies

Examination of urinary sediment is important in certain clinical settings. Normal sediments either rule out certain diseases or make them very unlikely. Abnormal sediments, principally the identification of cells (eg, red blood cells [RBCs], white blood cells [WBCs]), casts (eg, hemoglobin, granular), or crystals (eg, uric acid, tyrosine) indicates significant disease, many of which involve the kidney. An approach focusing on the most common laboratory studies is presented in f9.2. Generally, a "shotgun" approach is not cost effective and the clinical history and physical findings should be incorporated into the decision making. Obviously, a reagent strip (or "dipstick"), despite its many limitations, is a relatively inexpensive, rapid, and useful way to screen specimens in the physician's office. Based on this, samples may then be sent to the laboratory for more detailed and accurate analyses.

The specific clinical scenario will determine what testing will occur. For example the workup of hematuria, which has a long differential diagnosis, will likely include urinalysis [PMID 9135826]. Some of the diseases that should be considered include coagulopathy, stones, urothelial carcinoma, and glomerulonephritis. If cancer is a likely consideration, then cytology and further workup often by a urologist, is the course. Glomerulonephritis, of which there are many types, is typically evaluated by a nephrologist. However, it is worth noting that extensive workup for asymptomatic microscopic hematuria may not be cost effective.

One of the more common causes of hematuria is infection of the urinary bladder, which is associated with clinical symptoms such as dysuria, increased frequency, and pyuria (neutrophils in the urine). Bladder infections are often caused by Gram– bacilli (eg, E coli).

Careful examination of the sediment for casts and crystals is important to identify a host of diseases that may be renal in origin or systemically based with secondary renal involvement.

There are several common indications for the examination of urine. One would be azotemia, an elevation in blood urea nitrogen (BUN) and an indication of a decrease in the glomerular filtration rate (GFR). There may be abnormalities in the specimen including proteinuria, hematuria, pyuria, casts, or crystals. A change in urinary volume (increased or decreased) warrants further examination. Other clinical indicators suggesting urinary tract disease, notably the kidney, include hypertension (with or without edema), electrolyte abnormalities, acid-base disturbances, as well as fever and pain. In short, there are a large array of diseases and disease processes that can involve the urinary tract, whether as the primary site or as a signal of systemic illness.

Specimen collection, requirements & stability

A variety of urine specimens may be collected and submitted to the laboratory. As one might predict, this is predicated on the clinical setting. Examples include a clean catch urine (often a random collection done in a physician's office), first morning specimen (akin to an 8 hour collection), 24 hour urine specimen, a fasting specimen, a catheterized specimen, a specimen from a suprapubic aspiration (sometimes performed in young children), and a bladder wash (for cytologic evaluation of malignancy) t9.1. Patients must be given detailed instructions for the appropriate collection, which must be done in a sterile manner.

t9.1 Common urinary specimen types used for morphologic analysis

Voided	Catheterized	Bladder wash
Inexpensive	Modest expense	Expensive
Scant cellularity	More cellular	Highly cellular
Poor preservation	Better preservation	Well preserved
Samples entire urinary system	Distal urinary system not sampled	Upper & distal urinary system not sampled
Readily obtained	No	No
Noninvasive	Invasive	Invasive
Contamination	No*	No
Mostly single cells	Clusters	Clusters, fragments
Squamous cells, umbrella cells, inflammatory cells	Umbrella & basal cells	Umbrella & basal cells

*If indwelling, always contaminated

Ideally, specimens should be submitted to the laboratory within 2 hours of collection per Clinical and Laboratory Standards Institute (CLSI) guidelines. For specimens that may be delayed (eg, 24 hour urine or transport issues) refrigeration or preservatives may be used. A common preservative is boric acid and for environmental reasons, nonmercuric preservatives should be utilized; other preservatives that have been used include formalin, toluene, and chlorhexidine.

One recurring problem is ensuring proper labeling of the specimen and the provision of a fully executed laboratory online requisition that includes relevant historical and current clinical information.

Gross examination

Urinalysis begins with gross examination. It is only briefly discussed here; additional information may be found in standard sources [ISBN 978-0891891031, PMID 3048852, ISBN 978-0891896203, ISBN 978-1437709742].

Appearance

The gross examination of urine begins with its appearance, and color is the most notable.

Color

The yellow color of urine is due to urochrome, an end product of hemoglobin catabolism t9.2. Red suggests blood and only a small amount is needed to be identified as gross hematuria. Other colors may be observed including brown (suggesting bile pigments), orange (urobilinogen), and dark brown (suggesting hemoglobin). Certain color changes may also be due to drugs or foods, such as beets.

t9.2	Color analysis of urine
Color	Possible pathologic etiologies
Clear	Diabetes insipidus
Hazy	Casts, crystals, microorganisms, cells
White	Pyuria, lipids, chyle
Yellow	Bilirubin and its metabolic derivatives
Pink-red	Hemoglobin, RBCs, myoglobin, porphyrins, beeturia
Brown	Methemoglobin, myoglobin, porphyrins

Clarity

Normally, urine is clear and free of particulate material. Various states of turbidity may be encountered and the etiologies include crystals, abundant cells (eg, WBCs or epithelial cells), mucin, and lipids.

Odor

There is an odor associated with normal urine but certain conditions can alter this. For example, bacterial overgrowth (fetid odor) and certain metabolic disorders (eg, maple syrup urine disease and phenylketonuria [mousy]) will produce characteristic odors.

Volume

Recording the volume of urine received in the laboratory is a critical part of the gross examination. This is in part an issue of specimen type; a random sample may be 30-60 mL, which will be quite different from a 24 hour urine collection. As noted, the normal daily urine output is ~1 L and there may be either less or more volume depending on the underlying disease process. Polyuria may be seen with diabetes mellitus and diabetes insipidus, the latter due to a deficiency of antidiuretic hormone (ADH). Decreased urine volume may be seen with dehydration or intrinsic renal diseases.

Specific gravity & osmolality

Specific gravity and osmolality both describe the density of a urine sample, which is related to the concentrating ability of the kidney and the patient's state of hydration. Specific gravity is dependent on the number and weight of the total solutes, or dissolved solids, found within the urine. More precisely, it is defined as the ratio of the mass of a solution (eg, urine) to the mass of an equal volume of water. The solutes—urea, sodium chloride, phosphate and sulfate—contribute significantly to the specific gravity of urine in a healthy individual. As it is a ratio, specific gravity is dimensionless and normal values range from 1.003-1.035, with lower values representing dilute urine and higher values associated with very concentrated urine.

Urine with low specific gravity may occur in patients with impaired renal concentrating ability such as glomerulonephritis, diabetes insipidus, or pyelonephritis. Elevated specific gravity values may be associated with diabetes mellitus, dehydration, congestive heart failure, adrenal insufficiency, or liver disease. Increased concentrations of glucose and protein contribute to the density of urine and will therefore elevate the specific gravity. Administration of radiographic dyes or dextran solutions can result in extremely high specific gravity values that may confound interpretation. When the kidney has lost the ability to either concentrate or dilute the urine, the specific gravity will not vary considerably from 1.010 (the specific gravity of plasma) upon repeated analysis, which is known as isosthenuria.

Several methods exist for the measurement of specific gravity. Dipstick pads containing electrolytes along with color dyes that detect hydrogen ion release (pH) as the pKa of the electrolytes change in relation to the ionic concentration of the urine. Since this indirect measurement technique detects only ionic solutes, excess glucose, protein, or dyes reportedly do not interfere. A refractometer may be used to indirectly determine the refractive index of a urine sample as compared to water. The refractive index, or ability of light to bend as it passes through a substance, is directly proportional to the density of particles within the sample and is thus related to specific gravity. This nonspecific technique therefore includes large interfering solutes in the final value. Measurements are determined by viewing the sample through the refractometer as it is directed toward a light source. The refractometer must be precisely calibrated in order to provide accurate results. Urinometer and falling drop techniques also exist for the measurement of specific gravity of urine but are more cumbersome and not commonly performed.

Osmolality defines the number of particles in the sample per unit of solution. Since it is not affected by the density of large solutes, osmolality is often considered a superior measurement over specific gravity to determine the concentrating and diluting capabilities of the kidney. Urea and creatinine concentrations are responsible for the majority of osmotic activity while glucose and protein do not contribute greatly under normal situations. Healthy individuals with normal diets and fluid intake will produce urine with an osmolality of 500-850 mOsm/kg water. The normally functioning kidney should be able to produce dilute urine (40-80 mOsm/kg water) during extreme fluid intake and concentrated urine (800-1,400 mOsm/kg water) during periods of dehydration.

Osmolality is most commonly determined using the freezing point depression method. An osmometer is used to determine the freezing point of a urine sample, which is related to osmolality by the relationship of 1,000 mOsm/kg water lowering the freezing point by 1.86°C below the freezing point of water (0°C). Therefore, lower freezing points are associated with higher osmotic activity.

Cell counts

The determination of cell counts is of limited value in the examination of urinary specimens. At best, semiquantitative values may be reported (eg, 2+ neutrophils) but these do not correlate well with quantitative determinations even if they are performed. That said, the reporting of the presence of red blood cells (RBCs), the various types of white blood cells (WBCs) and epithelial cells (squamous, urothelial, renal tubular) is important. In addition, as noted elsewhere (Microbiologic examination, below), the reporting of bacterial culture results including the threshold for a significant bacterial count is subjective, institutionally driven, and therefore a bit of a quagmire.

Microscopic examination

There are several ways of examining urine sediment. Bright field microscopy of a fresh specimen (<2 hours) is prototypic and may be enhanced with the addition of a supravital dye such as crystal violet-safranin stain. Other forms of microscopy include phase contrast, which is advantageous for crystal identification, and polarized microscopy whose use is especially helpful for crystal identification as well as fibers [http://www.microscopyu.com/articles/phasecontrast/index.html, http://www.microscopyu.com/articles/polarized/index.html].

In approaching slide examination, it is important to have a standard and rigorous approach. First, it is important to know what is normal, from which one can appreciate what is abnormal. Second, it includes both the cellular elements and the background; the latter might include microorganisms, crystals and casts, and other elements that will provide clues as to the etiology of the abnormal urinary sediment t9.3. Careful attention to both is important for a thorough assessment. In addition, it is important to know what kind of specimen one is examining; what is normal in voided urine (and hence abnormal) is not necessarily the same as in a first morning urine or a bladder wash.

t9.3	Morphologic elements encountered in urinary specimens
Cellular	
Epithelial	
Urothelial cells—umbrella, basal	
Squamous cells	
Glandular cells, including renal tubular epithelial cells	
Inflammatory cells	
PMNs	
Macrophages, including giant cells	
Lymphocytes	
Microorganisms	
Bacteria	
Mycobacteria—bacillus Calmette-Guérin (BCG)	
Viruses	
Fungi (yeast)	
Parasites—*Trichomonas vaginalis*, *Schistosoma* ova	
Noncellular	
Crystals	
Casts	
Corpora amylacae	
Artifacts	
Talc	
Fibers	
Pollen	

PMN = polymorphonuclear leukocyte (neutrophil)

Epithelial cells

There are 3 major cell types that may be observed: squamous, urothelial ("transitional"), and glandular [ISBN 019-5134958, ISBN 978-0891896449]. It is worth reiterating that the specimen type will determine what cell type may be observed and whether it is abnormal, and that a "normal" specimen, in the absence of disease, is scantly cellular. In a typical voided clean catch urine, squamous cells are the most abundant. These cells are large, platelike with centrally placed nuclei and a low nuclear:cytoplasmic (N:C) ratio i9.1, i9.2. Squamous cells are usually of superficial or intermediate type, varying only in the N:C ratio and are derived chiefly from the urethra. It is worth noting that women may have squamous metaplasia up to and involving the bladder trigone and that these cells may cycle as under normal physiologic conditions as the estrogen and progesterone levels vary.

Urothelial cells, as previously mentioned, are of 2 major types—superficial or basal. The former are relatively large, although smaller than squamous cells, with abundant cytoplasm and relatively large nuclei; not uncommonly, these cells may be bi-or multinucleated i9.3. The basal cells, which are usually uncommon in voided specimens, are smaller, have a higher N:C ratio, and also lack any nuclear atypia i9.4. Obviously, in catheterized specimens or other instrumented specimens, urothelial cells may be more prevalent. In voided specimens, the identification of clusters of urothelial cells is

9: Urine

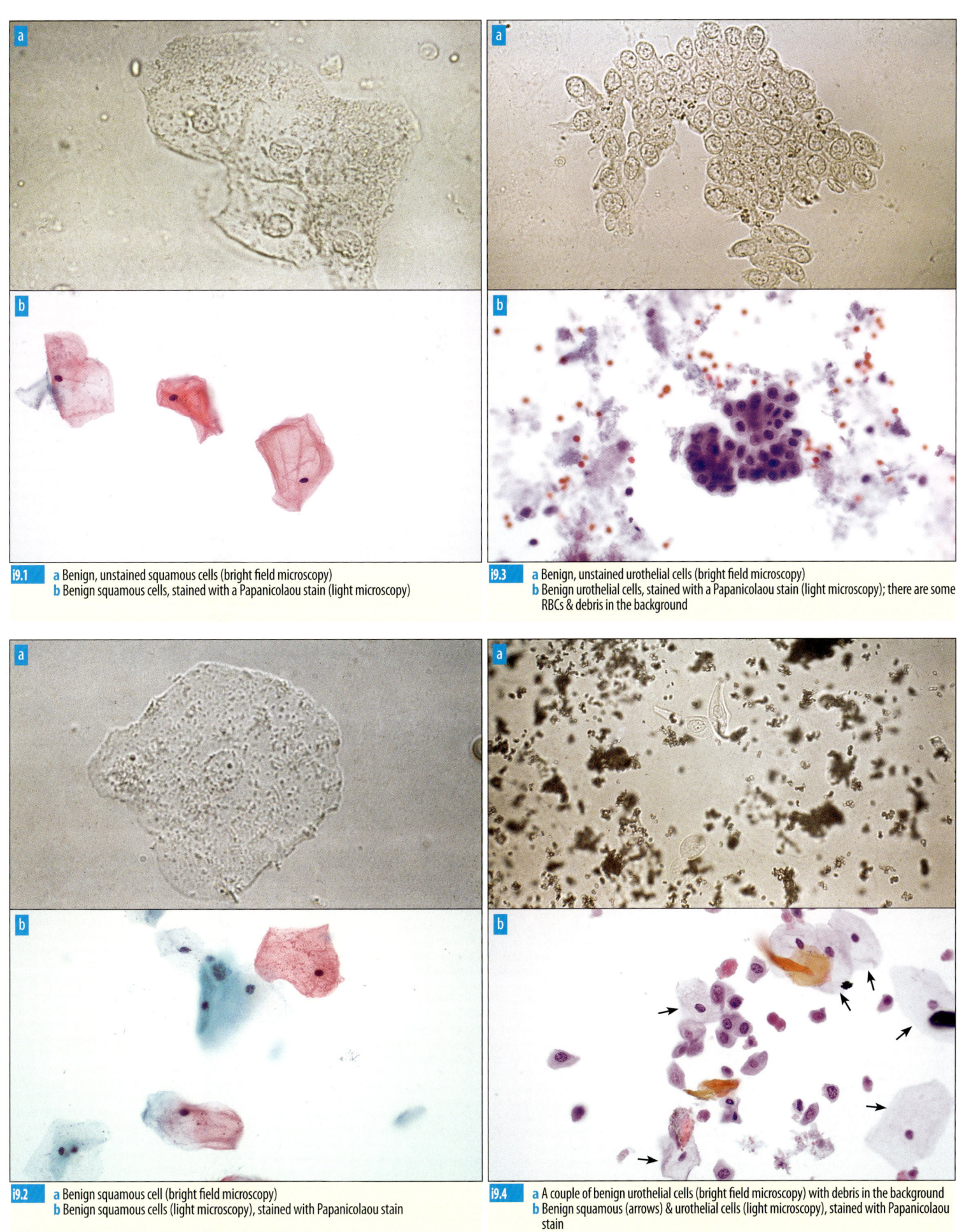

i9.1　a Benign, unstained squamous cells (bright field microscopy)
　　　b Benign squamous cells, stained with a Papanicolaou stain (light microscopy)

i9.2　a Benign squamous cell (bright field microscopy)
　　　b Benign squamous cells (light microscopy), stained with Papanicolaou stain

i9.3　a Benign, unstained urothelial cells (bright field microscopy)
　　　b Benign urothelial cells, stained with a Papanicolaou stain (light microscopy); there are some RBCs & debris in the background

i9.4　a A couple of benign urothelial cells (bright field microscopy) with debris in the background
　　　b Benign squamous (arrows) & urothelial cells (light microscopy), stained with Papanicolaou stain

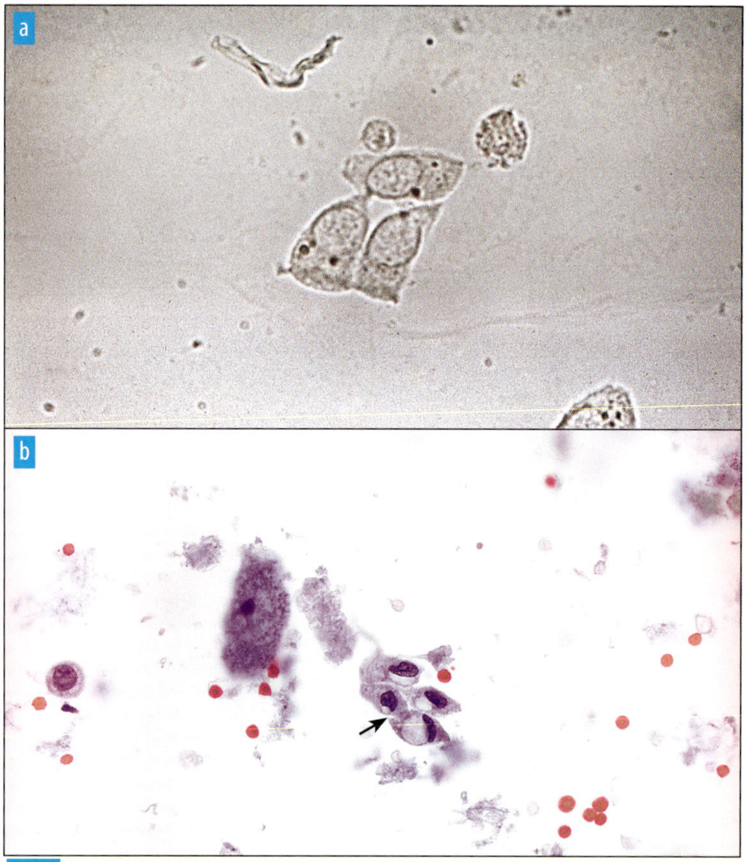

i9.5   **a** Renal tubular epithelial cells (bright field microscopy)
        b Renal tubular epithelial cells (arrow) (light microscopy)

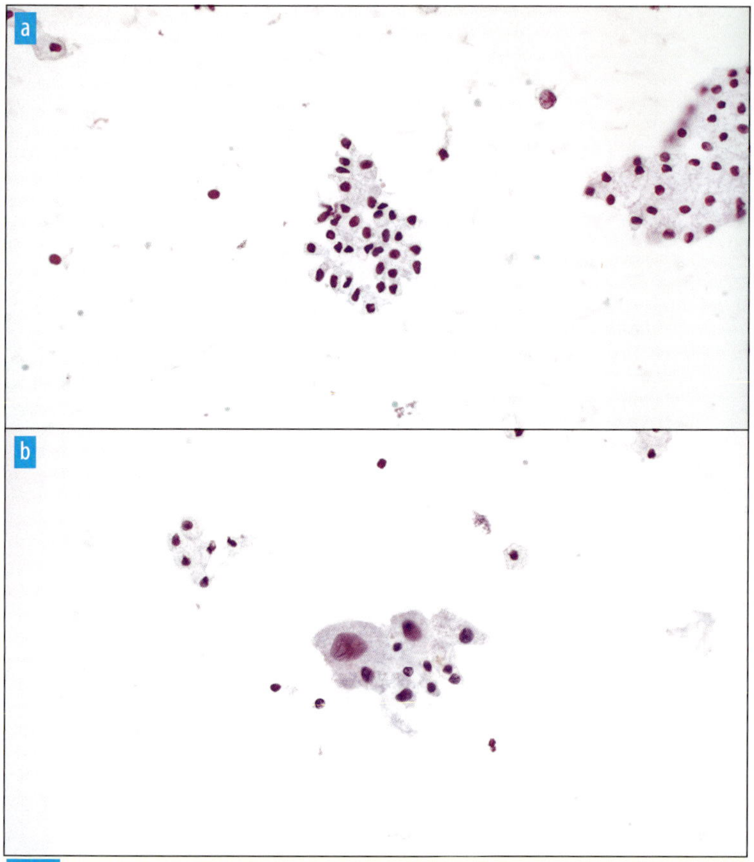

i9.7   Seminal vesicle cells (light microscopy, Papanicolaou stain)

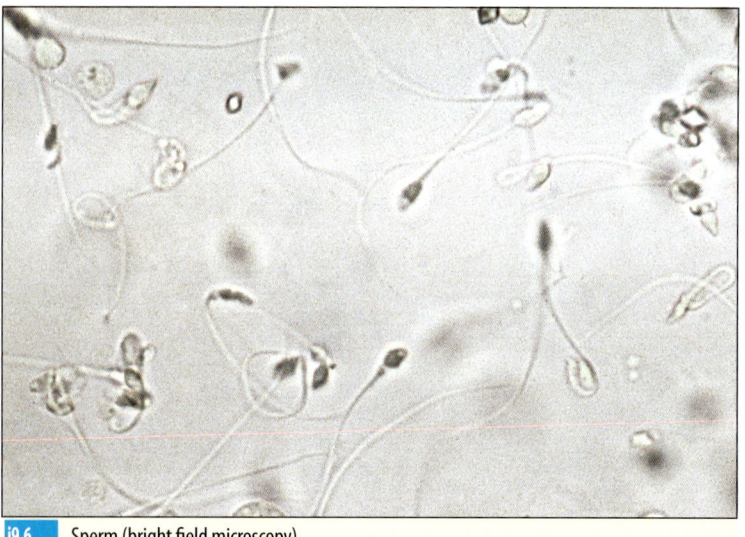

i9.6   Sperm (bright field microscopy)

cells are resident in the adjacent structures of the urethra (eg, prostate, bulbourethral glands), they do not exfoliate (as a general rule). More commonly but still rare are renal tubular cells that are shed. These are typically poorly preserved but are recognizable as glandular cells **i9.5**. Their recognition is important since it is a compelling indication of disease.

As noted above, it is also important to look at the background. For example, the identification of sperm **i9.6**, especially in young females, should be treated as a critical value and immediately reported. Rarely, other cell types may be observed as in the case of seminal vesicle cells in men **i9.7**. Examples of malignancy include low grade urothelial carcinoma **i9.8**, high grade urothelial carcinoma **i9.9**, and squamous cell carcinoma **i9.10**. Finally, there are a number of causes of cellular atypia that may be confused with malignancy **t9.4**.

t9.4	**Pitfalls: causes of cellular atypia**
Lithiasis (stones)	
Drugs: BCG, mitomycin C, thioTEPA, cyclophosphamide	
Radiation	
Conduit: ileal loop, neobladder	

abnormal and may suggest stones, unreported instrumentation, or most significantly, urothelial carcinoma especially low grade. The identification of atypia, nuclear atypia in particular, may also be a sign of urothelial malignancy but this must be separated from degeneration. The identification of high grade urothelial carcinoma is well accepted but the recognition of low grade urothelial carcinoma is more controversial, although specific morphologic features have been identified [PMID 8062194, ISBN 072-1660290, PMID 14696141].

Glandular cells are rarely identified. While glandular

9: Urine

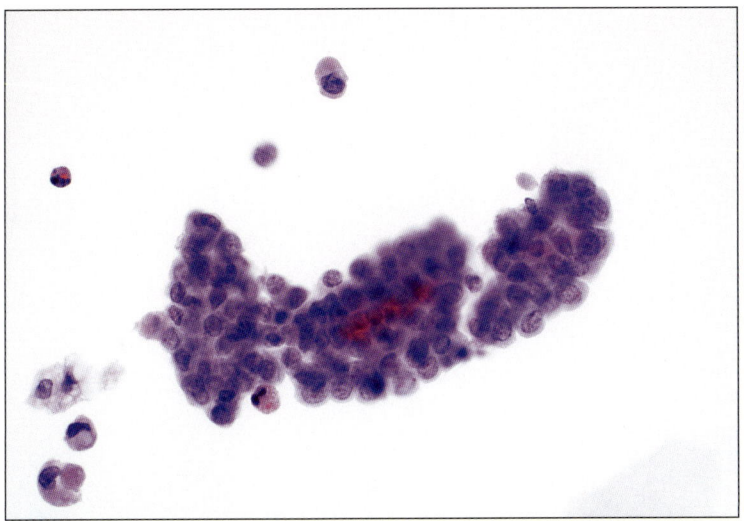

i9.8 A cluster of cells suspicious for a low grade urothelial carcinoma (Papanicolaou stain)

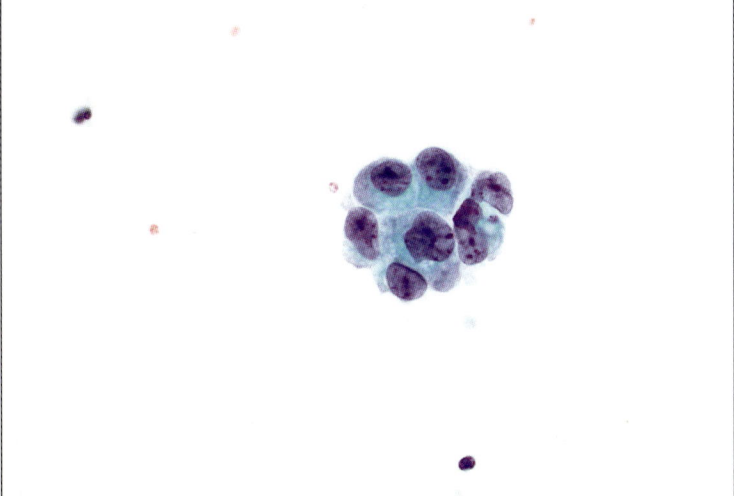

i9.9 High grade urothelial carcinoma (Papanicolaou stain)

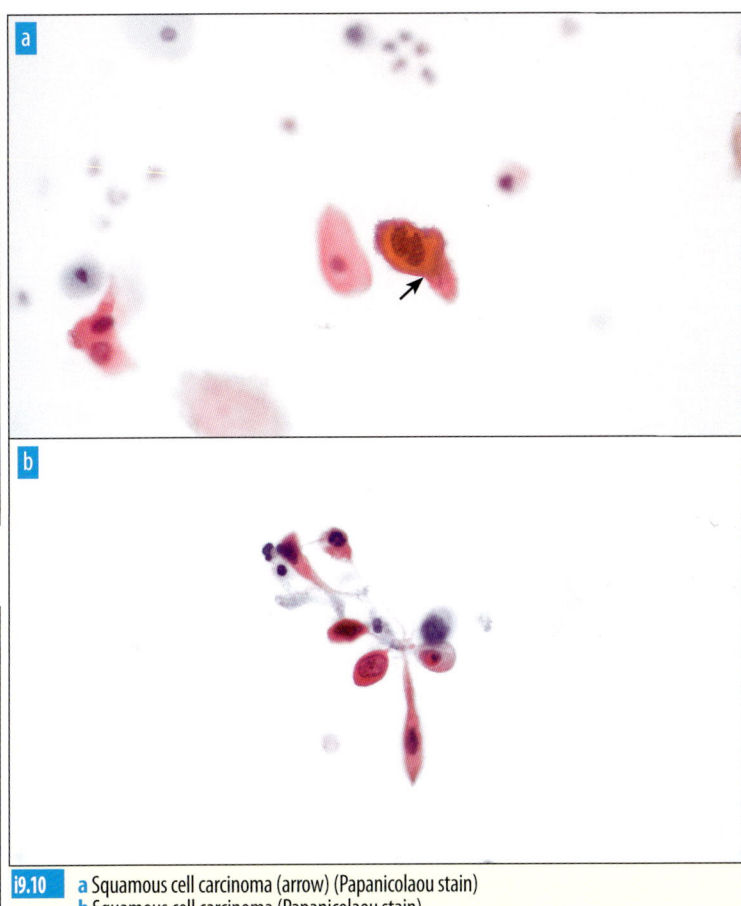

i9.10 **a** Squamous cell carcinoma (arrow) (Papanicolaou stain)
b Squamous cell carcinoma (Papanicolaou stain)

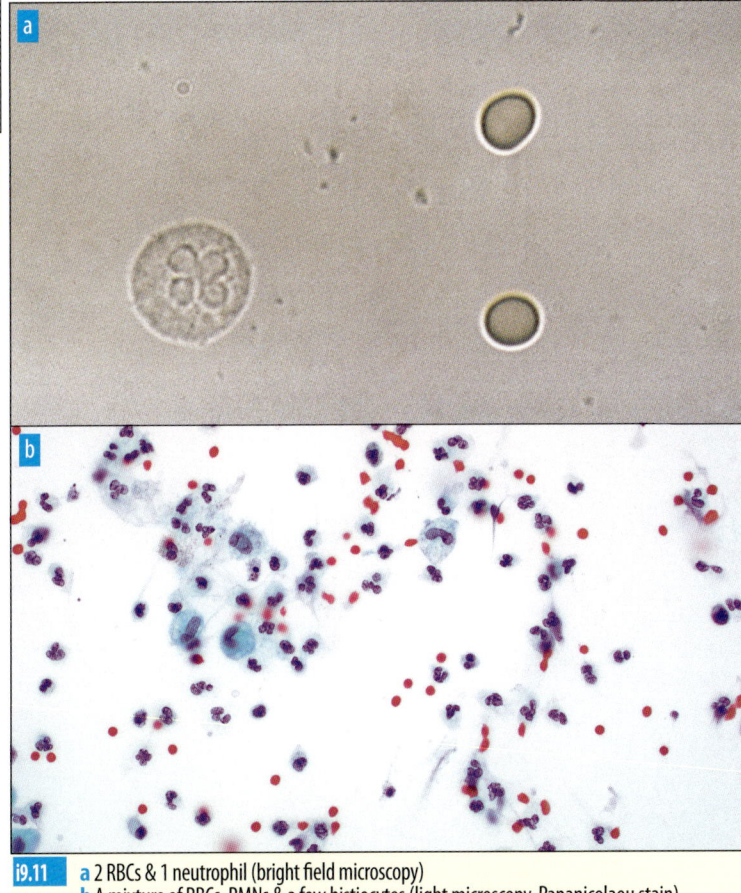

i9.11 **a** 2 RBCs & 1 neutrophil (bright field microscopy)
b A mixture of RBCs, PMNs & a few histiocytes (light microscopy, Papanicolaou stain)

Nonepithelial cells

RBCs may be observed in urine samples although they are often associated with disease including inflammatory, other nonneoplastic diseases (eg, glomerulonephritis, stones), or neoplastic i9.11a; the identification of dysmorphic (eg, crenated) RBCs indicates renal disease i9.12 [ISBN 978-0930304874, ISBN 978-0891896203]. Their number may be semi-quantitated. WBCs of all types may be observed but PMNs are most common i9.11. Clusters of inflammatory cells may also be seen i9.13, i9.14 as well as histiocytes i9.11b, i9.15 and eosinophils i9.16. Careful examination may help in the identification of malignant hematopoietic cells as in acute leukemia i9.17.

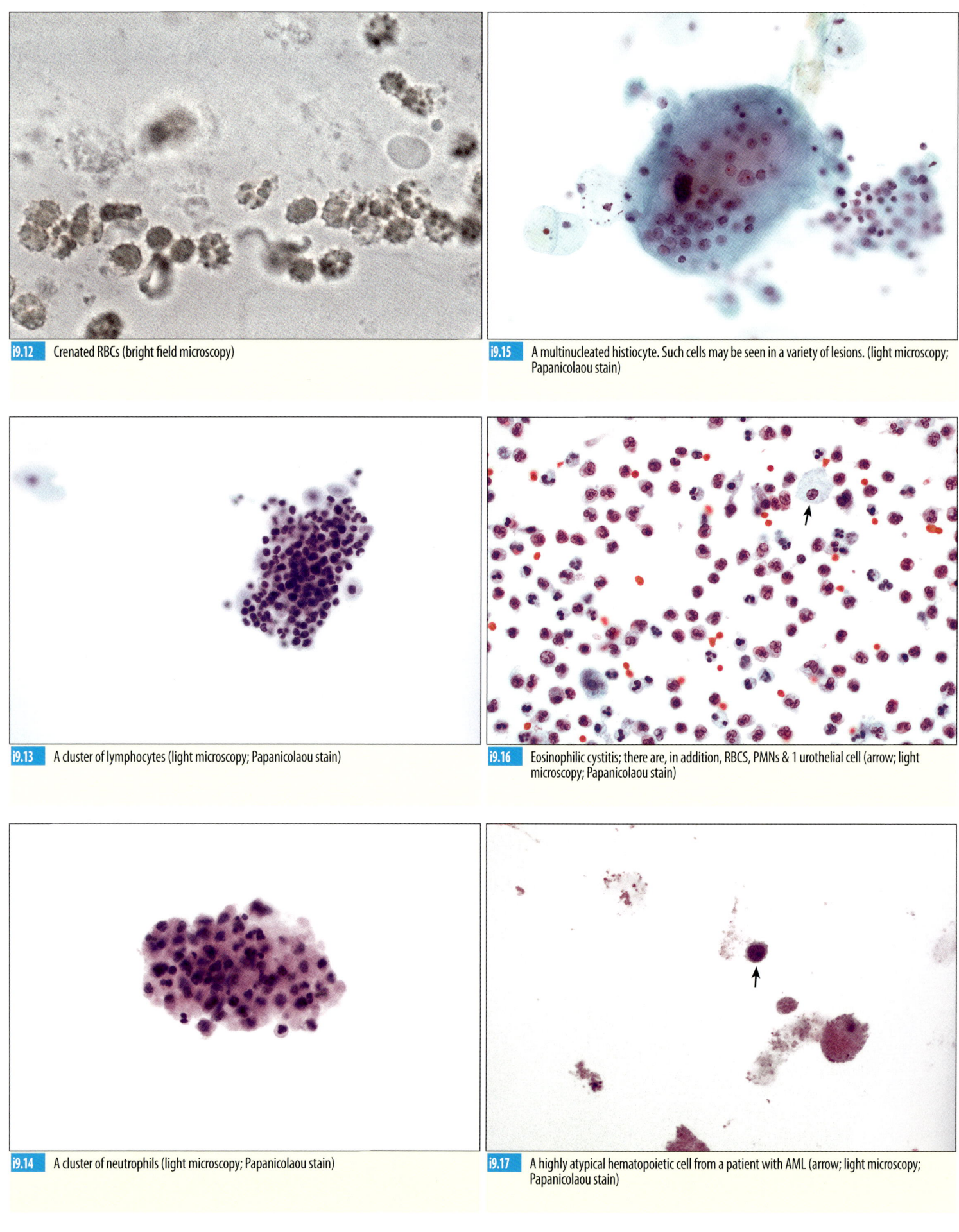

i9.12 Crenated RBCs (bright field microscopy)

i9.15 A multinucleated histiocyte. Such cells may be seen in a variety of lesions. (light microscopy; Papanicolaou stain)

i9.13 A cluster of lymphocytes (light microscopy; Papanicolaou stain)

i9.16 Eosinophilic cystitis; there are, in addition, RBCS, PMNs & 1 urothelial cell (arrow; light microscopy; Papanicolaou stain)

i9.14 A cluster of neutrophils (light microscopy; Papanicolaou stain)

i9.17 A highly atypical hematopoietic cell from a patient with AML (arrow; light microscopy; Papanicolaou stain)

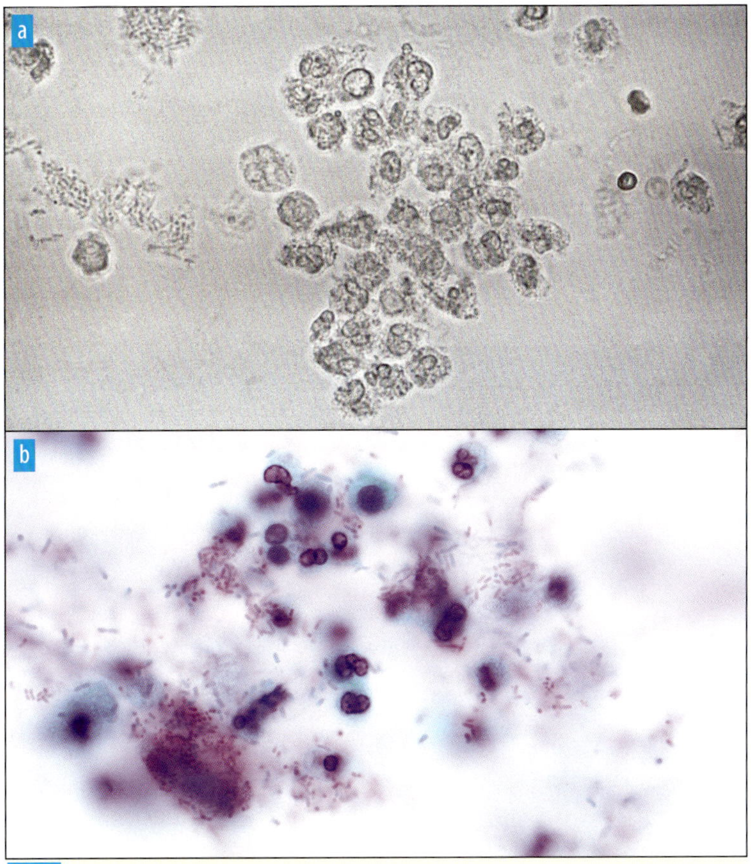

9: Urine

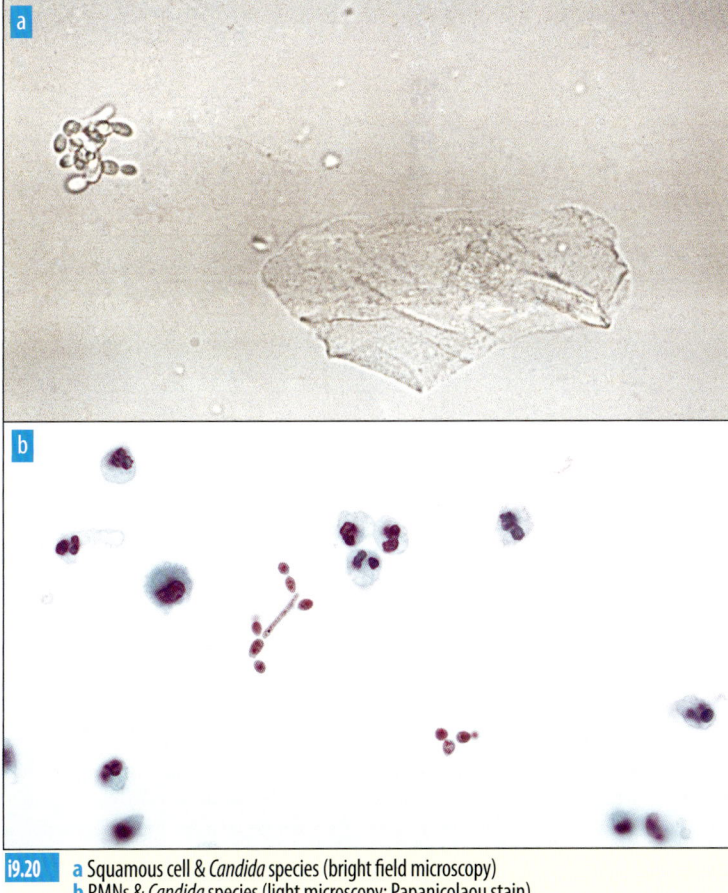

i9.18 PMNs & bacteria from a patient with acute cystitis
a Bright field microscopy
b Papanicolaou stain

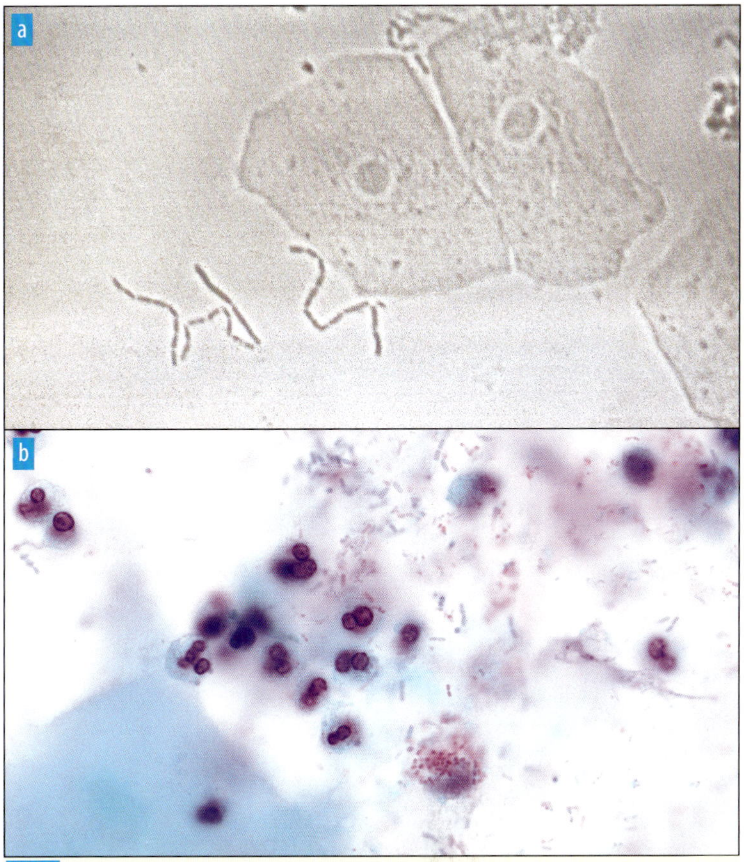

i9.19 **a** 2 squamous cells & bacteria (rods; bright field microscopy)
b 1 squamous cell, numerous PMNs & bacteria (light microscopy)

i9.20 **a** Squamous cell & *Candida* species (bright field microscopy)
b PMNs & *Candida* species (light microscopy; Papanicolaou stain)

Microorganisms

A whole array of microorganisms may be identified in urine and the morphology is best done in concert with culture or other techniques used in the microbiology laboratory (eg, PCR). By far, the most common are bacteria and the Gram– bacilli, such as *E coli*. These are most often due to cystitis and associated with a prominent neutrophilic response i9.18-i9.19. Fungi may also be seen in urine typically *Candida* i9.20, i9.21. The morphologies of bacteria and fungi have been well described in various texts [ISBN 978-0891891031, ISBN 978-0930304874, ISBN 978-0891896449].

Similarly, evidence of viral infection may also be seen. Of particular importance is BK virus (a polyomavirus) that is usually associated with immunocompromised patients such as those who have had a kidney transplant. The infected cells are single and contain rounded nuclei that are very hyperchromatic i9.22-i9.23. The viral nature is best appreciated on Papanicolaou stained preparations. Importantly, these infected cells must be distinguished from nuclear degenerative changes, from whatever cause, and high grade urothelial carcinoma. Hence, the name "decoy cell," which is often used for these virally transformed cells [ISBN 019-5134958, ISBN 978-0891896449].

9: Urine

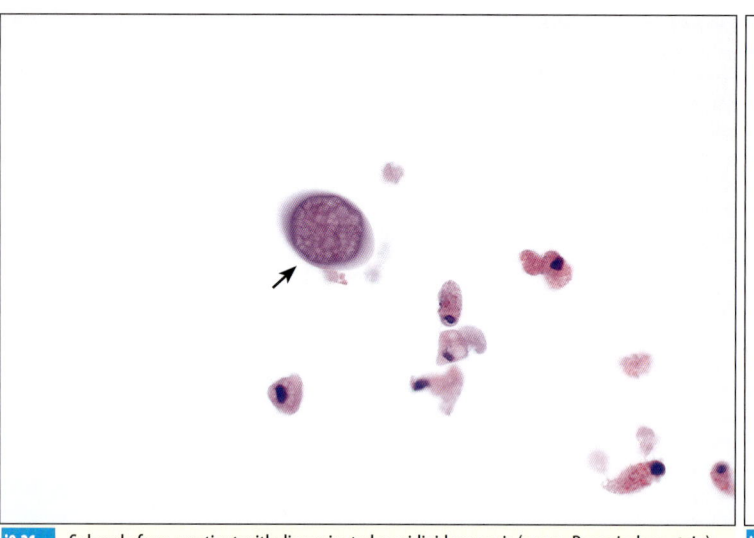

i9.21 Spherule from a patient with disseminated coccidioidomycosis (arrow; Papanicolaou stain)

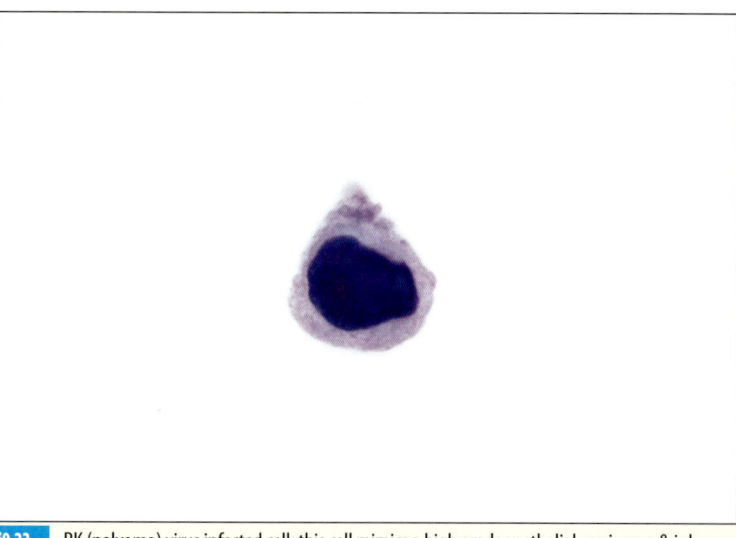

i9.23 BK (polyoma) virus infected cell; this cell mimics a high grade urothelial carcinoma & is hence called a decoy cell (light microscopy; Papanicolaou stain)

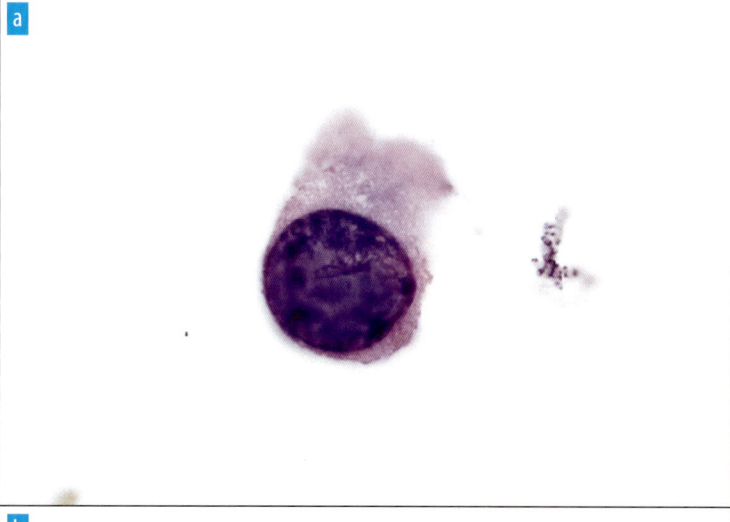

i9.22 BK (polyoma) virus infected cell (light microscopy; Papanicolaou stain)

A variety of parasites may also be seen, including *Trichomonas vaginalis* i9.24 and *Schistosoma* i9.25; the former is often a vaginal contaminant and the latter found in specific patient populations where the flukes are endemic. Pediculosis (lice) i9.26 and pinworms (*Enterobius vermicularis*) i9.27 and are also contaminants that are not uncommonly encountered.

9: Urine

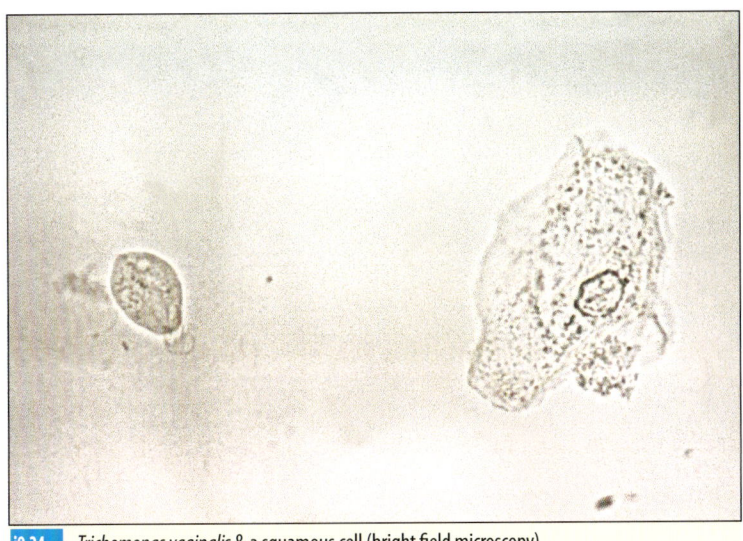

i9.24 *Trichomonas vaginalis* & a squamous cell (bright field microscopy)

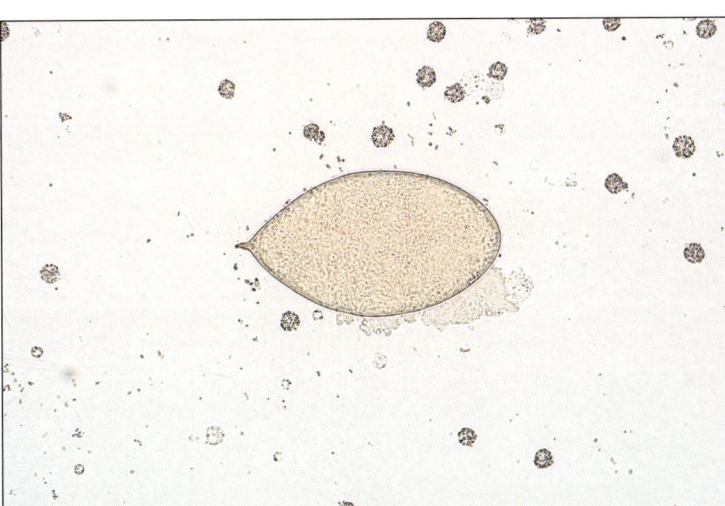

i9.25 *Schistosoma haematobium* ovum (bright field microscopy)

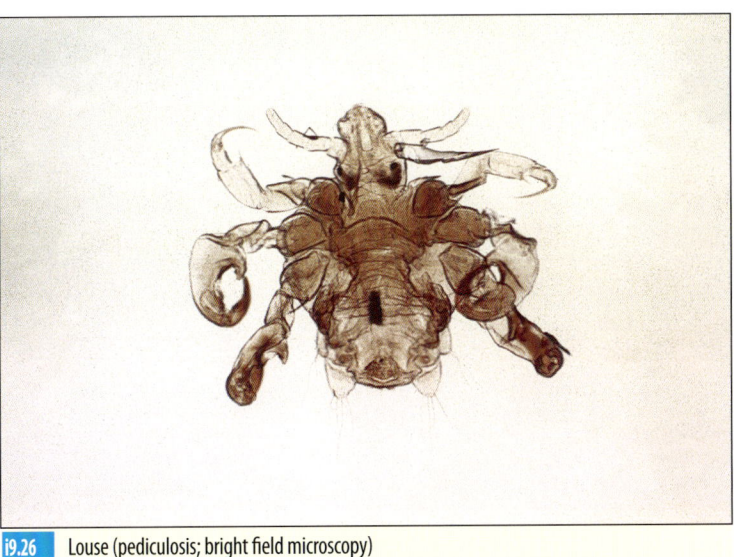

i9.26 Louse (pediculosis; bright field microscopy)

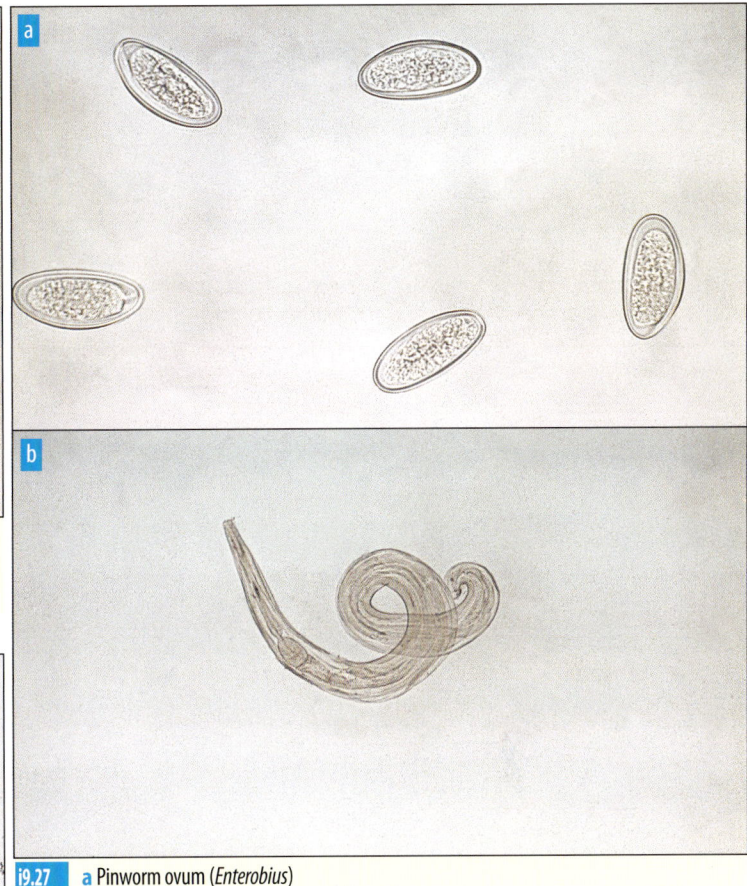

i9.27 **a** Pinworm ovum (*Enterobius*)
b Pinworm (bright field microscopy)

Crystals

The recognition and identification of crystals are one of the most important components of a comprehensive urinalysis t9.5. While many crystals do not indicate significant disease, others do. Consequently, the morphologic distinction is critical. That said, the details of this analysis are beyond the scope of this text. Interested readers are referred to more focused texts on the subject [ISBN 978-0891891031, ISBN 978-0930304874, ISBN 978-0891896203, ISBN 978-1437709742, ISBN 019-5134958]. In addition, formal stone analysis is described below.

t9.5	Morphologic features of select commonly encountered crystals	
Type	**Appearance**	**Significance**
Calcium carbonate	Amorphous	None
Calcium phosphate	Variable	None
Cystine	Flat hexagons	AR disorder
Oxalate	Oval, dumbbell, bipyramidal	May be pathologic
Struvite	Coffin lid, wedge shaped	May be pathologic "infectious" stones (triple phosphate, magnesium ammonium phosphate)
Uric acid	Usually rhomboid; other	May be pathologic hyperuricemia, tumor lysis

AR = autosomal recessive

9: Urine

Crystals typically form as a result of supersaturation, although this does not explain the whole story. Their morphologic identification may require other forms of microscopy (eg, polarized light) in order to make a definitive identification. Finally, examination of first morning urine is best.

An array of crystals is seen and some are illustrated in i9.28-i9.41.

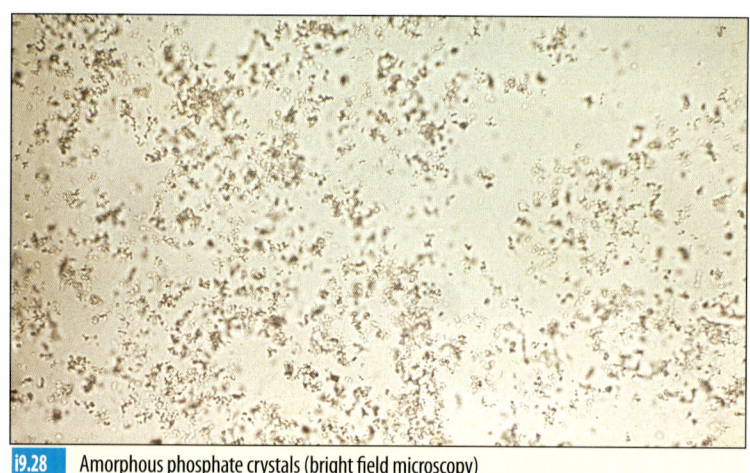

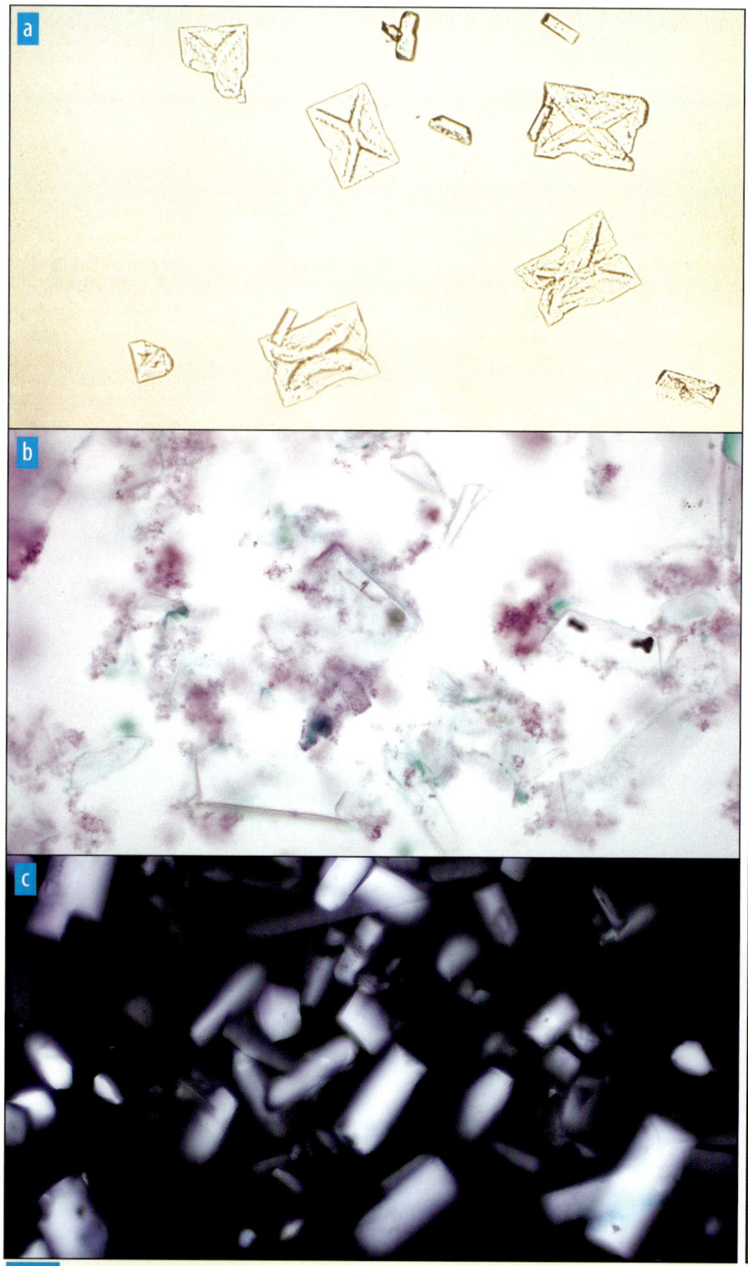

i9.28 Amorphous phosphate crystals (bright field microscopy)

i9.29 Triple phosphate crystals
 a Bright field microscopy
 b Light microscopy
 c Polarized light microscopy

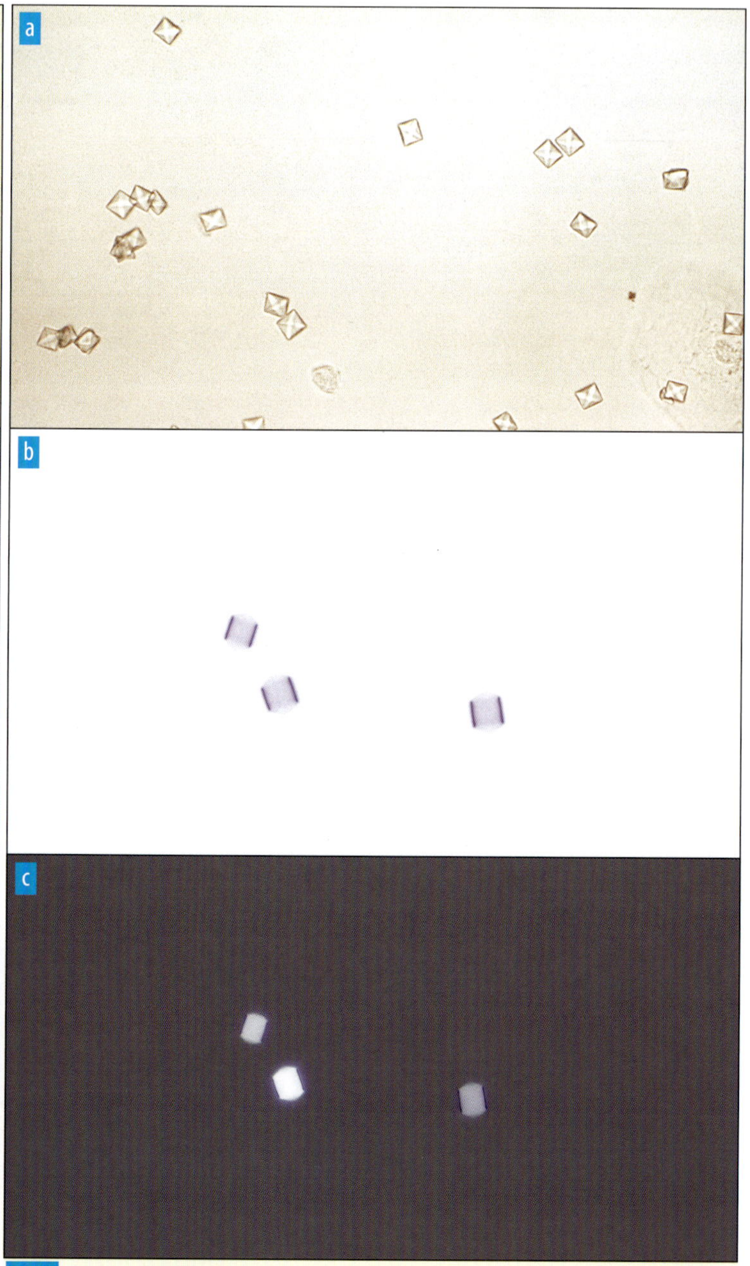

i9.30 Calcium oxalate crystals
 a Bright field microscopy
 b Light microscopy
 c Polarized light microscopy

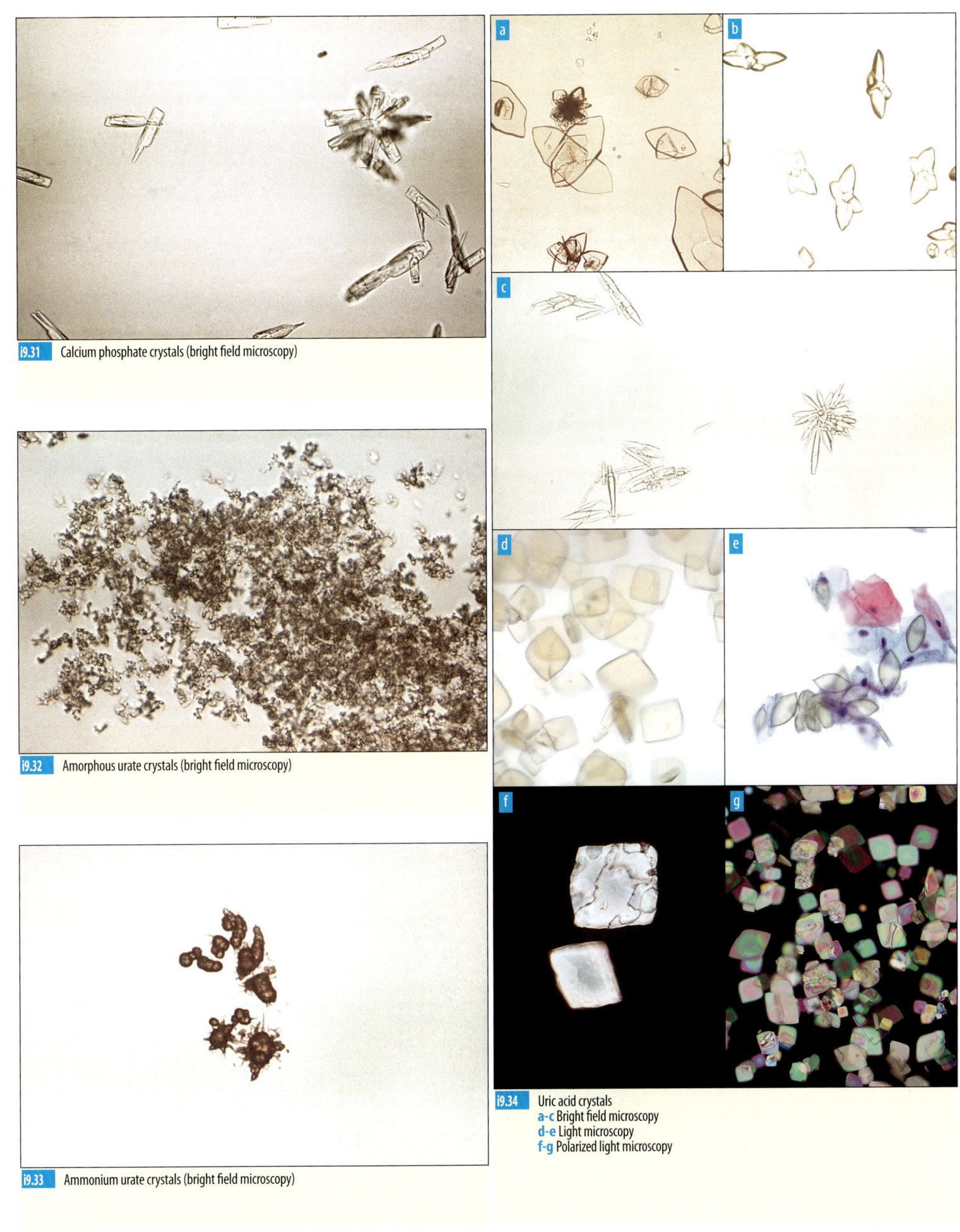

i9.31 Calcium phosphate crystals (bright field microscopy)

i9.32 Amorphous urate crystals (bright field microscopy)

i9.33 Ammonium urate crystals (bright field microscopy)

i9.34 Uric acid crystals
 a-c Bright field microscopy
 d-e Light microscopy
 f-g Polarized light microscopy

9: Urine

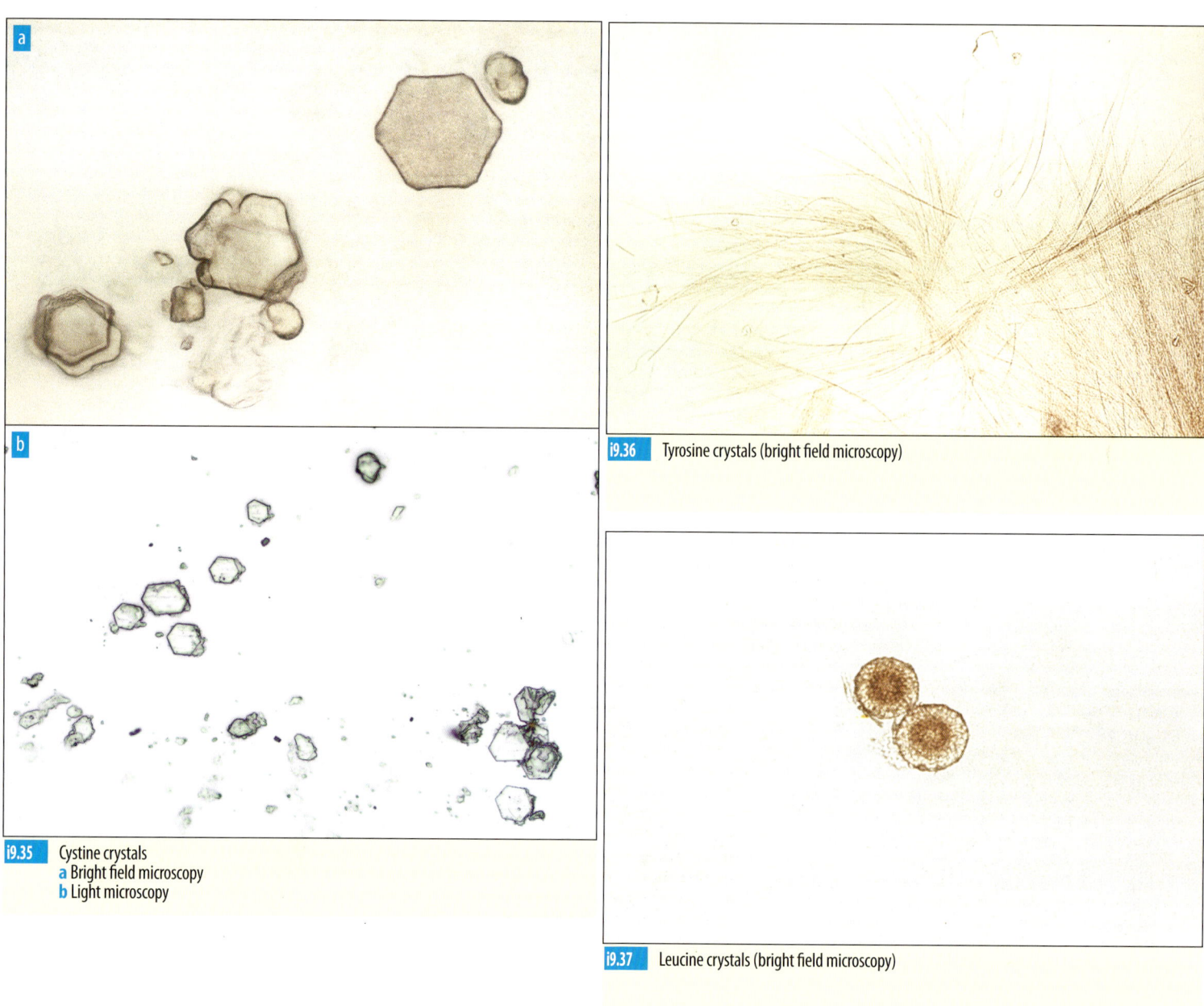

i9.35 Cystine crystals
 a Bright field microscopy
 b Light microscopy

i9.36 Tyrosine crystals (bright field microscopy)

i9.37 Leucine crystals (bright field microscopy)

9: Urine

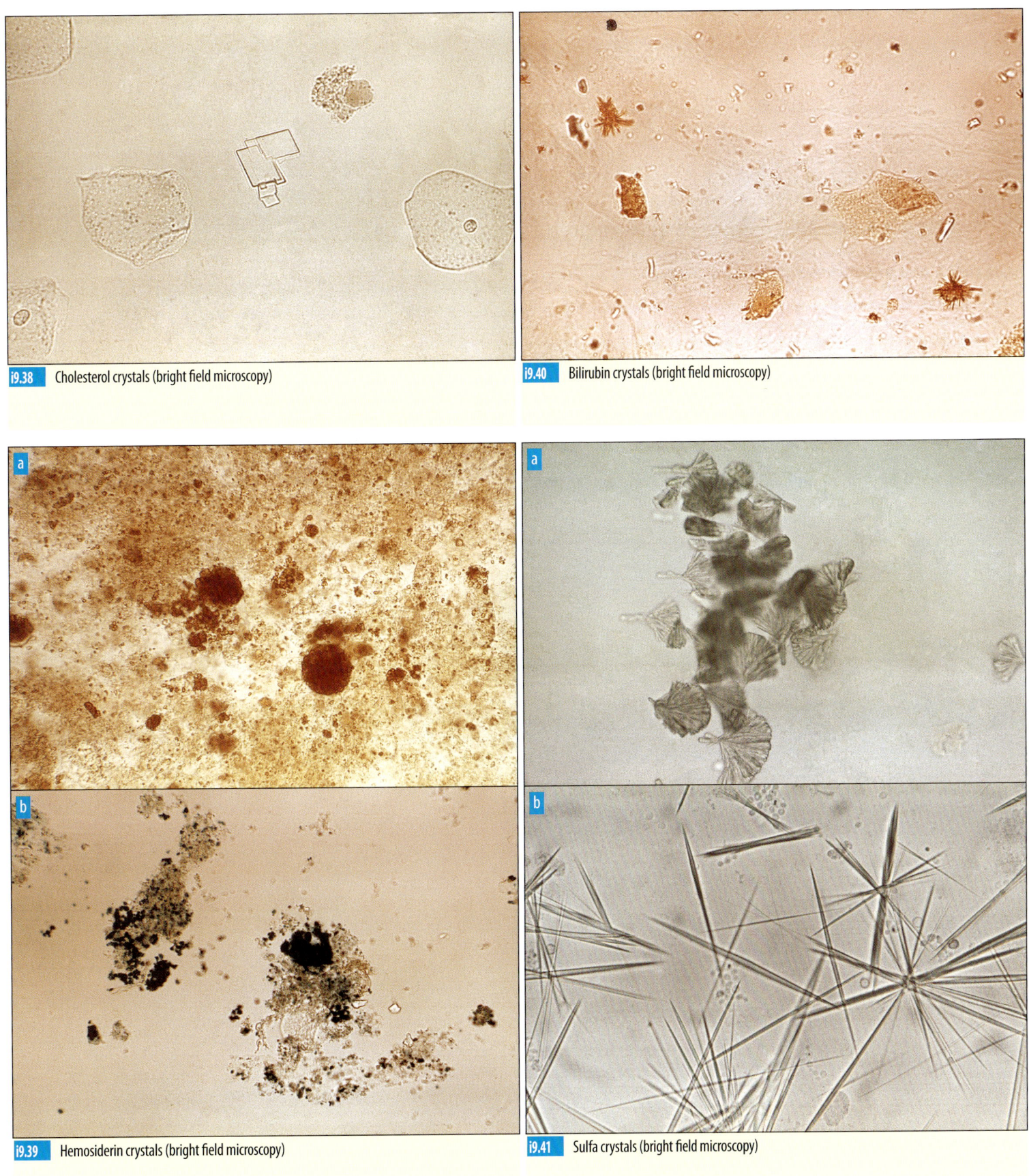

i9.38 Cholesterol crystals (bright field microscopy)

i9.40 Bilirubin crystals (bright field microscopy)

i9.39 Hemosiderin crystals (bright field microscopy)

i9.41 Sulfa crystals (bright field microscopy)

Casts

Casts form in the distal nephron and are an amalgamation of protein, notably Tamm-Horsfall protein, as well as other elements t9.6. Broadly, they are divided into cellular (eg, WBC cast) and noncellular types (eg, granular cast) and do not all indicate renal pathology. Hyaline and granular casts are most often found is healthy patients; most of the rest indicate a variety of disease and indicate underlying renal pathology.

t9.6	Morphologic features of select commonly encountered casts	
Type	**Appearance**	**Occurrence**
Epithelial cell	Single or clusters of tubular cells; variable degeneration	ATN, rejection
Granular	Fine or coarse granules, refractile	May imply disease, including nonrenal
Fatty	Fat globules, refractile	Nephrotic syndrome, ATN
Hyaline	Colorless, translucent	May imply disease
Mixed cell	Variable, composed of epithelial, red and white cells; variable degeneration	Tubular-interstitial disease
Red cell	RBCs, red hue	Glomerular injury
Waxy	Dense, refractile	ESRD, acute glomerular injury
White cell	Mostly PMNs in core	Pyelonephritis, rejection, sepsis

ATN = acute tubular necrosis; ESRD = end stage renal disease; PMN = polymorphonuclear leukocyte (neutrophil); RBC = red blood cell

Their identification is based on morphology that is typically carried out with bright field microscopy. Other forms of microscopy are sometimes used and special stains (eg, Sternheimer-Malbin stain) may be useful in select situations. As with crystals, the detailed analysis of casts is part of the complete urinalysis and is beyond the scope of this text. Readers are also referred to one of the many specialized texts for distinguishing the various types of casts [ISBN 978-0930304874, ISBN 978-0891891031, ISBN 978-0891896203, ISBN 978-1437709742, ISBN 019-5134958]. Examples of the casts are included for illustrative purposes i9.45-i9.54.

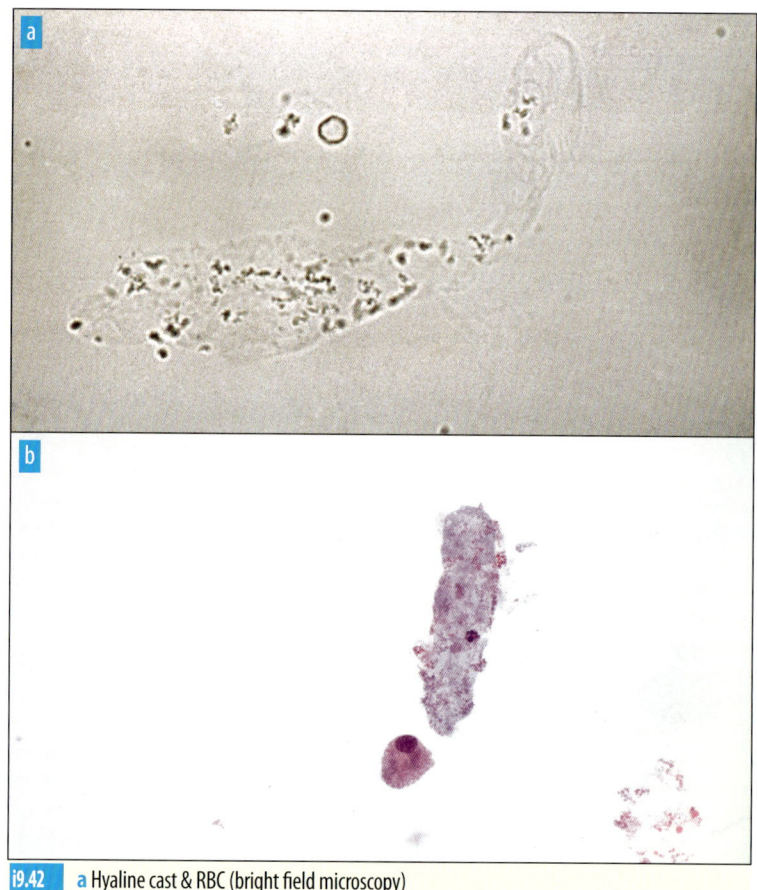

i9.42
a Hyaline cast & RBC (bright field microscopy)
b Hyaline cast (light microscopy; Papanicolaou stained)

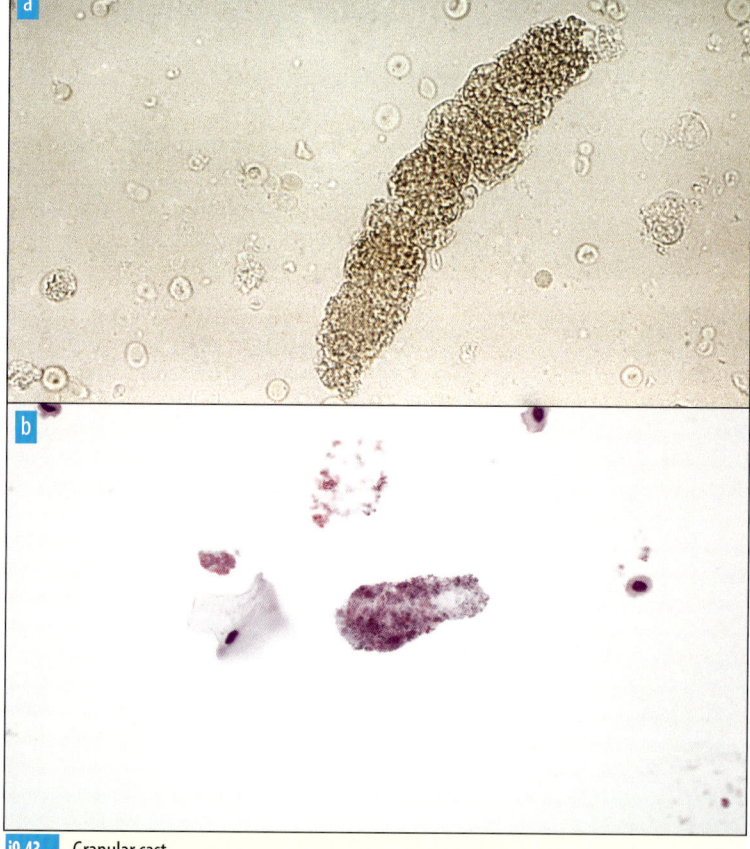

i9.43 Granular cast
a Bright field microscopy
b Light microscopy

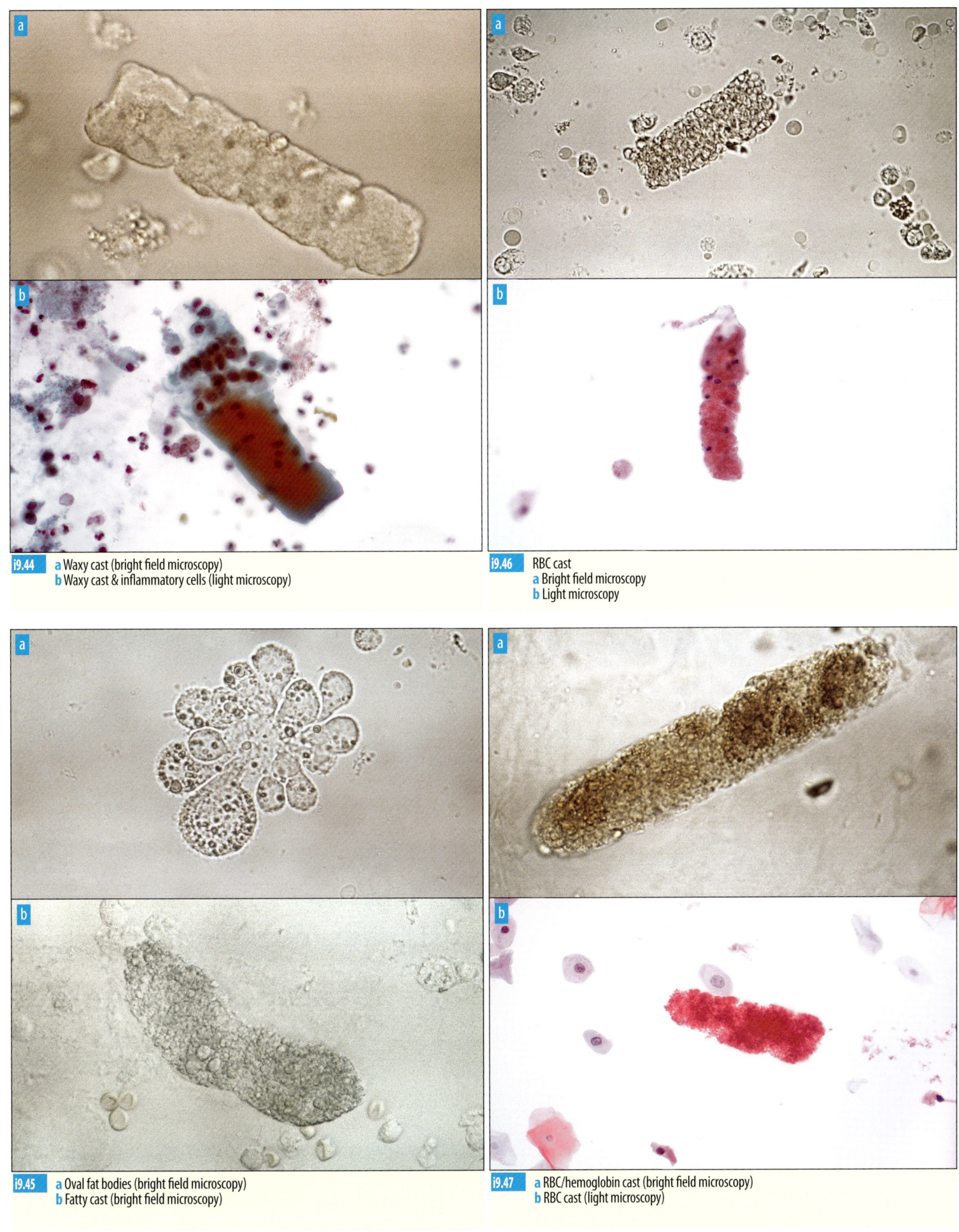

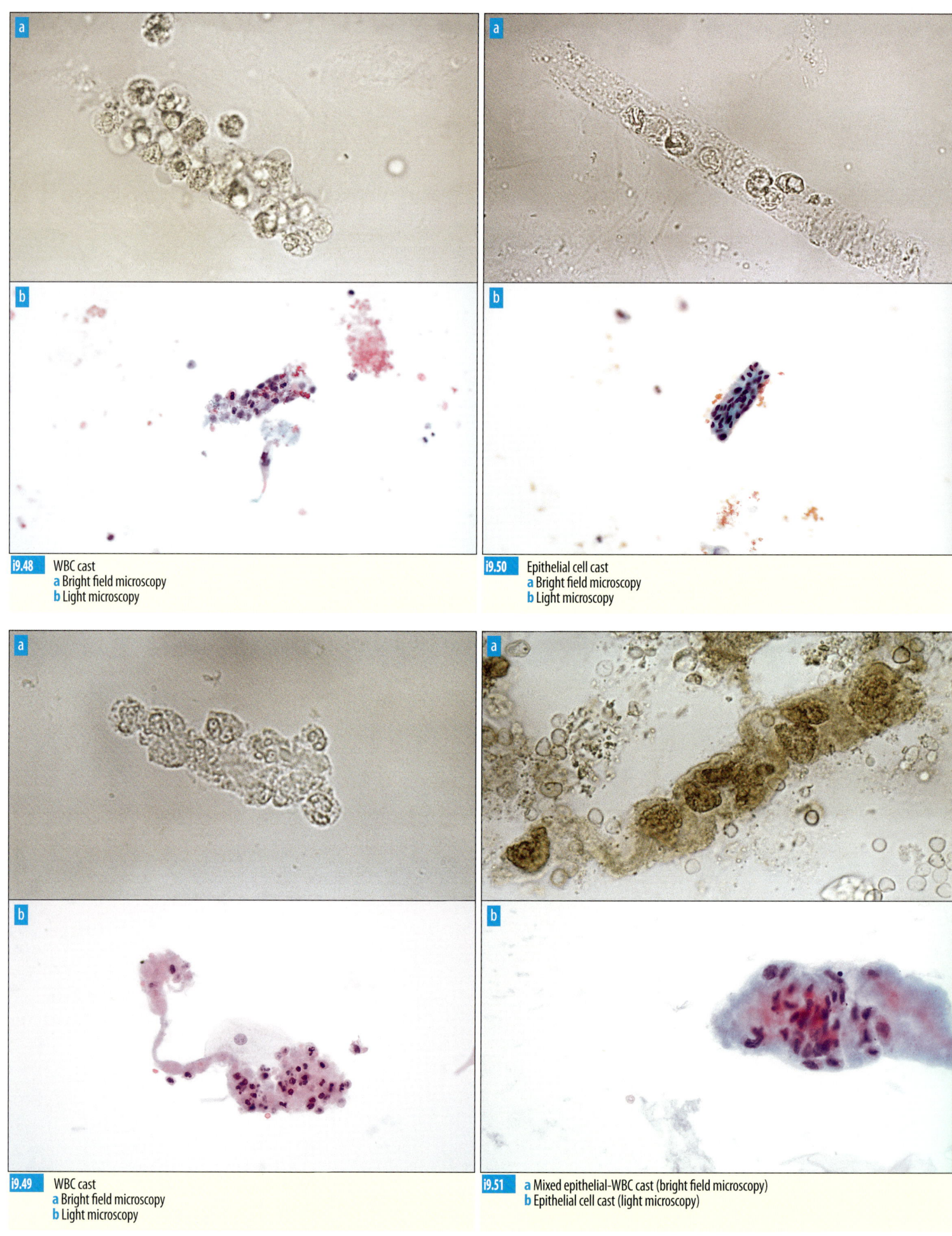

i9.48 WBC cast
a Bright field microscopy
b Light microscopy

i9.50 Epithelial cell cast
a Bright field microscopy
b Light microscopy

i9.49 WBC cast
a Bright field microscopy
b Light microscopy

i9.51 a Mixed epithelial-WBC cast (bright field microscopy)
b Epithelial cell cast (light microscopy)

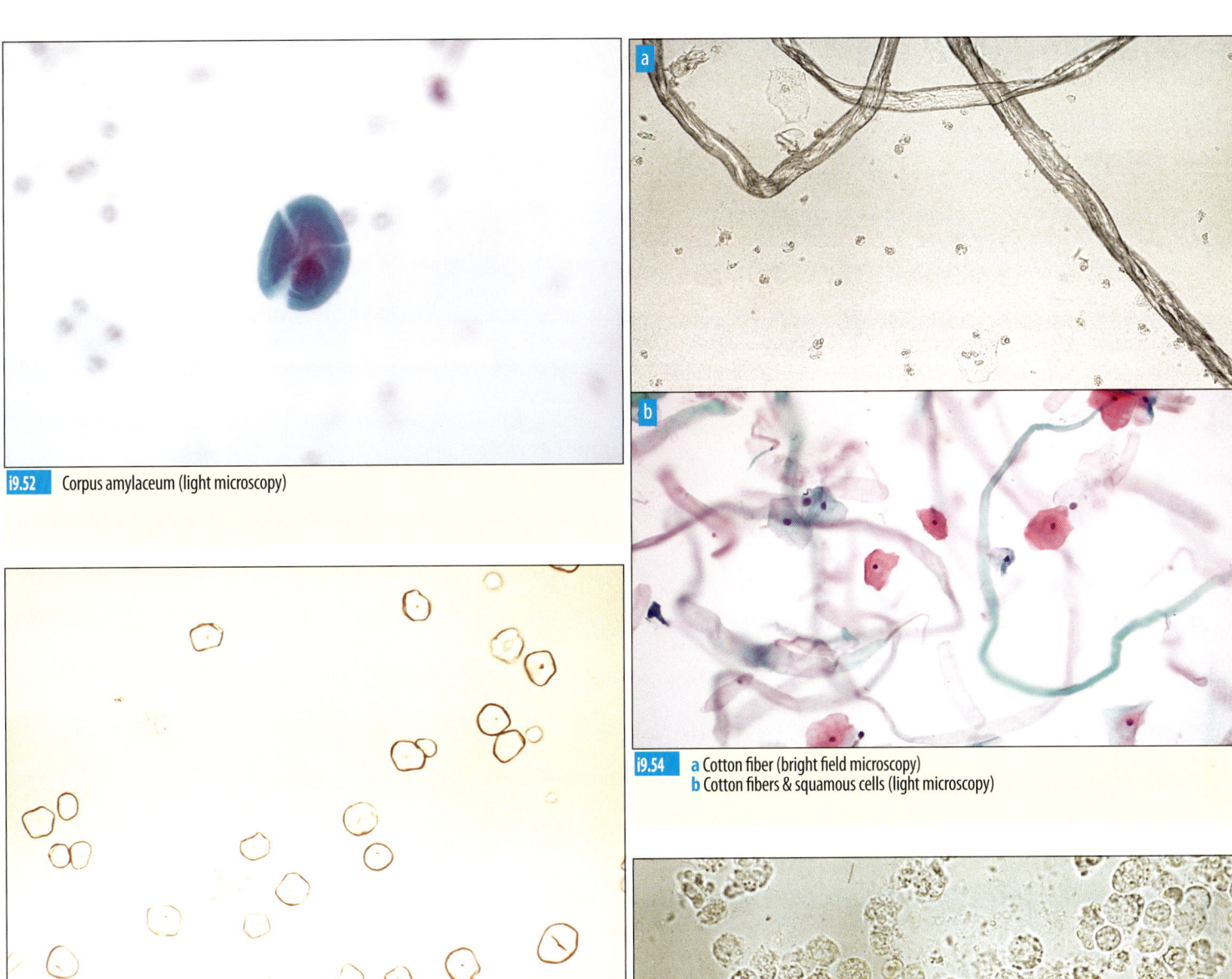

i9.52 Corpus amylaceum (light microscopy)

i9.53 Starch particles (bright field microscopy)

i9.54 a Cotton fiber (bright field microscopy)
b Cotton fibers & squamous cells (light microscopy)

i9.55 Plant cell & WBCs (bright field microscopy)

Other

A variety of other elements may be identified in urine specimens, including corpora amylaceae i9.52; starch, a contaminant i9.53; cotton fibers, another contaminant, usually obtained during preparation i9.54; and plant material i9.55.

Chemical analysis

Routine urinalysis includes an assessment of the physical, chemical and microscopic characteristics of a urine sample. Each component provides information regarding the renal function of an individual. Chemical analyses are often performed using commercially available reagent test strips ("dipsticks") or routine chemistry analyzers. Dipsticks contain a series of individual absorbent pads that contain specific reagents for each analyte. One or more qualitative or semiqualitative measurements can thus be made per strip. Confirmatory tests may be warranted in certain clinical situations. Individual manufacturer instructions should be followed for storage and use of dipsticks, urine testing procedure, and test interpretation. It is also important to note that there are both false positive and false negative interfering agents. For example, vaginal contamination can alter the leukocyte esterase assay on the reagent strip; similarly, proteins other than albumin (eg, immunoglobulin) may affect the protein assay component of the strip.

pH

The kidneys, in conjunction with the lungs, are a primary regulator of acid-base composition. Healthy kidneys work to reabsorb and produce bicarbonate while they secrete free hydrogen or ammonium ions. Deviation from normal pH values indicates a disruption in this regulatory function of the kidney. Urine pH may be between 4.5 and 8.0 in healthy individuals with values commonly near 6.0. Acidosis in the body causes increased excretion of hydrogen ions into the urine, or aciduria, while alkalosis causes the opposite effect.

Urine pH measures free hydrogen ions by determining the reciprocal of the hydrogen ion concentration. Therefore, high concentrations of hydrogen ion are reflected in a low pH (acidic) and low hydrogen concentrations result in a high pH (alkaline).

Aciduria may be produced during metabolic or respiratory acidosis, diabetic ketoacidosis, hypokalemia, or from dietary intake or medications. Alkalinuria may occur during metabolic or respiratory alkalosis, from dietary intake, medications, bacterial contamination or infection, or following a large meal. Urine pH may aid in determining the composition of urine crystals or calculi as different types may preferentially form in acidic or alkaline urine.

Dipstick measurement of urine pH utilizes indicators that change color based on the pH of the sample, such as methyl red and bromothymol blue. pH values may be estimated within half units between 5 and 9 using dipstick technology. If precise measurements are needed, a pH meter with a glass electrode is recommended. It is important to use freshly collected urine to determine pH as samples will alkalinize upon standing.

Protein

The majority of plasma proteins are stopped at the glomerulus or reabsorbed by the tubules. While small amounts of protein may be found in the urine of healthy individuals, increased protein loss into the urine is pathognomonic of kidney damage and warrants further investigation. Proteinuria may also be useful in the assessment of hypertension, heart disease and diabetes. Proteinuria may be transient or persistent and aberrant findings should be followed over time.

Causes of transient proteinuria include strenuous exercise, pregnancy, fever, stress or acute illness. Persistent proteinuria may be due to glomerular damage resulting in increased permeability to large molecular weight proteins (eg, albumin), impaired tubular reabsorption of filtered low molecular weight proteins (eg, β_2 microglobulin, enzymes), or an increase in plasma proteins that can overwhelm the reabsorption capacity of the tubules (eg, myoglobinuria, Bence-Jones proteinuria). It should be noted that there is considerable biological variation in urine protein concentrations and measurements are affected by a variety of extrarenal processes and interferences.

The healthy kidney excretes a small fraction of the total protein found in the plasma, >150 mg of protein per 24 hours. Some proteins, such as the Tamm-Horsfall mucoprotein, are secreted by the renal tubules themselves and are therefore normally found in urine. Tamm-Horsfall protein contributes to the structure of several casts that can be observed on microscopic examination of the urine sediment.

Protein may be measured using dipstick reagent pads or by precipitation by acid or heat. Dipstick measurement is based on the "protein error of indicators" phenomenon, which describes the color change of pH indicators commonly used in reagent pads in the presence of protein. The pH at which the indicator (often tetrabromophenol blue) changes color is different in the presence of protein as protein acts as a hydrogen ion acceptor. Common indicators change from yellow (no protein present) to blue-green (protein present) with a direct relationship between color intensity and protein concentration. Sensitivities may go as low as 6 mg/dL but most dipsticks detect protein down to 15 or 20 mg/dL. Results should be interpreted in context with specific gravity and pH.

Urine protein dipsticks are widely utilized despite certain limitations. Overall, use of dipsticks for detection of total protein in urine is not recommended. These reagents are highly sensitive to albumin; therefore a negative result does not necessarily rule out the presence of smaller molecular weight proteins. Dipsticks lack suitable sensitivity to detect low and significant amounts of protein, do not correct for urine concentration, and provide only semiquantitative results. Alkaline or highly buffered urine may cause false positives as reagents are sensitive to pH. Proteinuria detected by dipstick should be confirmed by quantitative methods preferably in ratio with creatinine.

While manual methods for detection of total protein concentrations exist and have been used for many years, these types of tests are readily available on automated chemistry analyzers. Quantitative methods include turbidimetry and colorimetry. Methods vary in their protein specificity and the detection of multiple proteins in one measurement precludes standardization among methods.

Albumin

Albumin is the most abundant protein found in the plasma and is therefore an early and important indicator of kidney disease when found in the urine. Historically referred to as microalbuminuria, albuminuria is the preferred term for increased albumin concentrations in urine. Albuminuria has been linked to cardiovascular disease, diabetes, and outcomes of chronic kidney disease. Albumin assays are more sensitive and specific than total protein assays and can therefore detect proteinuria earlier. Some clinical practice guidelines recommend the measurement of albumin rather than total protein for the detection of proteinuria [PMID 23732715, PMID 23264422]. The Kidney Disease Improving Global Outcomes (KDIGO) group prefers albumin:creatinine ratio (ACR) measurements to protein:creatinine ratios (PCR) or the use of dipsticks for proteinuria screening for chronic kidney disease [PMID 23732715].

Healthy individuals have ACR values <30 mg/g creatinine. Albuminuria diagnosis varies by society but many such as the American Diabetes Association define the range of 30-300 mg/g creatinine as indicative of early nephropathy that may respond to intervention and >300 mg/g creatinine associated with an increased likelihood of progressing to end stage renal disease [PMID 23264422]. Standards of care and practice guidelines for the diagnosis and monitoring of diabetes mellitus all include routine measurement of albumin in the urine to detect early renal dysfunction in these patients.

First morning urine is preferred for measurement and albumin concentrations correlate well with 24 hour urine specimens. Timed urine specimens can be used if more accurate information is required.

Glucose

In the healthy individual, glucose is filtered by the glomerulus and completely reabsorbed by the renal tubules. Thus, the presence of glucose or other reducing sugars in the urine is often indicative of disease. Plasma glucose concentrations exceeding 180 mg/dL may exceed the renal reabsorptive capacity and induce glycosuria. Glycosuria without concomitant hyperglycemia may be observed in cases of renal tubular dysfunction.

Glycosuria is commonly associated with diabetes mellitus but may also be present in endocrine disorders such as Cushing syndrome, hyperthyroidism, pheochromocytoma, pancreatitis, and cystic fibrosis. Other causes include pregnancy, stroke, liver disease, and some pharmaceutical drugs. Glycosuria should be investigated and incorporated into the clinical context of the patient. Further testing may include fasting blood glucose concentrations. Measurement of urine glucose is not recommended for screening for diabetes mellitus and has been replaced with blood glucose determinations.

Measurement of glucose in urine may be performed several ways. Routine chemistry analyzers provide quantitative results with good precision and accuracy. Glucose oxidase and hexokinase reactions followed by spectrophotometric detection are common methods used by commercial vendors. Dipsticks also commonly employ the glucose oxidase mediated conversion of glucose to gluconic acid and hydrogen peroxide culminating with an oxidized chromogen that allows semiqualitative measurement of glucose concentrations. The chromogen used and the sensitivity of the measurement vary by manufacturer but most provide readings from trace (equating to 100 mg/dL of glucose) to 4+ (2,000 mg/dL of glucose). Reagents within the dipstick pad will continue to react beyond the specified testing interval thus consistent timing is necessary to avoid falsely elevated glucose results. Additional variables such as temperature and urine concentration may also affect dipstick glucose results. Therefore, manufacturer instructions for testing should always be adhered to. False positive glucose results may be caused by oxidizing agents (eg, bleach, microbial peroxides) and low specific gravity (dilute urine). False negative results may be observed in the presence of high concentrations of bacteria, reducing agents (eg, ascorbate), or high specific gravity. The glucose oxidase reaction is specific for glucose; nonglucose sugars are not detected by routine dipstick analysis.

Nonglucose sugars may be present in the urine of individuals with inherited disorders or deficiencies that prevent their metabolism. Examples include galactose, lactose, sucrose, fructose, or pentose. Lactose may also be found normally in the urine of pregnant or lactating women. The majority of nonglucose sugars act as reducing substances and may therefore be detected by measuring their ability to reduce copper (eg, Benedict test, Clinitest). Any reducing substances, including glucose, will produce a positive result with this test. A color change is produced as cupric ions (Cu^{2+}) are reduced to cuprous oxide ($Cu^{1+}O$). This semiquantitative test is less sensitive and specific than the glucose oxidase method and is thus not considered an adequate confirmatory test for a positive glucose dipstick result. The presence of nonglucose reducing substances is of particular concern in pediatric patients, thus performing copper reduction tests on this population has been routine for many years. The need for this testing is decreasing as newborn screening tests are used to detect reducing sugars.

When possible, 24 hour urine collections are preferred for glucose determinations to eliminate variation in concentration throughout the day. Samples should include a preservative or be stored refrigerated prior to testing. Glucose testing should be performed soon after collection to avoid bacterial contamination.

Ketones

The presence of ketones in the urine indicates a defect in carbohydrate metabolism or absorption or an inadequate supply of carbohydrate in the diet. As the body switches to metabolizing fatty acids, the byproducts of incomplete fat metabolism, ketones, may appear in the blood and urine. The predominant ketones found in the urine are β hydroxybutyric acid, followed by acetoacetic (diacetic) acid and acetone. Small amounts of ketones are found in the urine of healthy individuals; however, the concentration is often below the sensitivity of ketone dipsticks. Elevated urine ketone concentrations are most commonly associated with uncontrolled diabetes mellitus, more frequent in type

1 than type 2 diabetes. Ketones may also be associated with inherited metabolic diseases, cachexia, low carbohydrate diet, anorexia, and extreme vomiting and/or diarrhea.

Urine dipsticks and tablets commonly utilize the sodium nitroprusside reaction to detect ketones. Acetone and acetoacetic acid react with sodium nitroprusside under alkaline conditions to produce a colored complex. While some reagent formulations preferentially react with acetoacetic acid and some also detect acetone, no dipstick reagent detects β hydroxybutyric acid. Sensitivities vary for each manufacturer, but are commonly as low as 5 mg/dL acetoacetic acid and 50 mg/dL acetone. Results are semiquantitative and may represent trace (5 mg/dL) up to large (160 mg/dL) concentrations. The detection of either acetoacetic acid or acetone is usually sufficient to diagnose ketonuria.

Nitrite

Bacterial conversion of nitrate to nitrite is an indirect indicator of a urinary tract infection, or bacteriuria. This conversion is dependent upon several crucial factors: the bacteria must possess the enzyme necessary for reducing nitrate, nitrate must be present in the urine sample, and adequate time must be allowed for the conversion to occur. The last point is why first morning urine is preferred for detection of bacteria as the urine has usually been held for an adequate period of time. Therefore, negative dipstick results do not rule out possible infection. Dipstick measurement of nitrite is meant as a screening tool and results should be confirmed with bacteriological culture. Urine specimens should also be tested shortly after voiding in order to eliminate contamination with bacteria.

Dipstick reagents will vary by manufacturer but have traditionally employed sulfanilamide or *p*-arsanilic acid reacting with nitrite to form a diazonium salt. This compound couples with quinolone to produce a colored end product. Results are interpreted as negative or positive for the presence of nitrite. Sensitivities vary but dipsticks can commonly detect nitrite down to 0.05 mg/dL.

Leukocyte esterase

The presence of white blood cells (leukocytes) in combination with positive nitrite results is indicative of urinary tract infection, calculi, or other kidney dysfunction including glomerulonephritis. Neutrophils are the most common leukocyte that would be found in the urine during an infection and these cells contain esterases that can be detected using a dipstick reagent pad. Common substrates include an acid ester, which reacts with the esterase and further complexes with a salt to form a colored end product. Results are semiqualitative and range from negative (sensitivities average 10 leukocytes/µL) up to moderate or large (detecting ~500 leukocytes/µL). Microscopic or automated methods should be used to confirm leukocyte numbers; however leukocyte esterase activity may remain after cells have lysed.

Blood

Blood in the urine (hematuria) is not found in healthy individuals and is indicative of a pathological process. Renal trauma or injury, tumors, calculi, and infection are examples of clinical causes of hematuria all of which necessitate further investigation. Urine samples may range from gross (visual change in urine color) to microscopic (color unchanged) hematuria.

Lysed RBCs cause hemoglobinuria and are associated with trauma, burns, transfusion reactions, or drugs and poisoning. Hemoglobinuria may be due to lysing of RBCs within the urine (commonly due to alkaline pH or low specific gravity) or intravascular hemolysis that causes free hemoglobin to be passed into the urine. Intravascular hemolysis is usually implicated when hemoglobinuria is observed in the absence of hematuria.

Myoglobin is a component of cardiac and skeletal muscle and may also be found in the urine (myoglobinuria) following crush injuries, muscle trauma, or even severely strenuous exercise. Rhabdomyolysis causes myoglobin release from skeletal muscle in quantities sufficient to induce acute renal failure. Myoglobin is rapidly cleared from the plasma filtration through the glomerulus; thus plasma concentrations may be low even in the presence of myoglobinuria. Myoglobin may be measured by immunoassay if quantitation is necessary.

Importantly, dipstick reagent pads are capable of detecting all 3 scenarios described above: RBCs (intact & lysed), hemoglobin, and myoglobin. Modern dipstick pads induce lysis of intact RBCs upon addition of the sample, thereby eliminating false negative results in the presence of intact cells. Reactions are based on the ability of hemoglobin and myoglobin to act as a peroxidase and catalyze the oxidation of a chromogen (often tetramethylbenzidine) in the presence of hydrogen peroxide. A spotted appearance on the test pad is indicative of intact cells while a diffuse color change is usually observed when free hemoglobin or myoglobin is present. Reporting of these 2 different types of results differ; intact RBCs may be reported as negative, trace, or moderate while "hemolyzed" samples may be reported on a scale from trace to 3+. Commonly, dipsticks are capable of detecting down to 5 RBCs/µL and ~0.02 mg/dL hemoglobin. False positive results may occur in the presence of oxidizing agents (eg, bleach, microbial peroxides) or menstrual blood. False negative results may occur in the presence of ascorbic acid, formalin, high specific gravity, or acidic urine.

Bilirubin & urobilinogen

Bilirubin is a byproduct of hemoglobin metabolism. It is conjugated in the liver and excreted as bile; therefore, only very small amounts are found in the urine of healthy individuals. When plasma concentrations of bilirubin are elevated, excess conjugated bilirubin may be excreted into the urine. The most common causes of bilirubinuria are biliary obstruction (eg, gallstones, tumors, inflammation, cholestasis) or hepatocyte dysfunction (eg, hepatitis or congenital disorders). Bilirubin is further converted to urobilinogen in the intestine and excreted into the feces. A small amount of urobilinogen is reabsorbed into the bloodstream and sent back to the liver and eventually, the intestines. This fraction of urobilinogen is finally excreted into the urine, but only in small amounts. Urobilinogen presence exceeding these low concentrations may indicate liver dysfunction or intestinal obstruction.

Both conjugated and unconjugated bilirubin are commonly quantitated using spectrophotometric methods on automated chemistry analyzers. However, dipsticks for the detection of bilirubin and urobilinogen in urine are frequently used as a screening method. Bilirubin dipstick reagent pads couple bilirubin with a diazonium salt to produce azobilirubin in the presence of acid. Urobilinogen detection is based on the Erlich reaction, which produces a colored product when it reacts with an aldehyde. Other reactions exist that have higher specificity for urobilinogen. The actual reaction used will vary by manufacturer. Dipsticks often have sensitivities of 0.5 mg/dL for bilirubin and 0.2-0.4 mg/dL for urobilinogen. Importantly, drug metabolites or imaging compounds may produce color in the urine that can interfere with the dipstick reaction and cause false positive bilirubin results. Because of this, confirmatory tests with lower sensitivities are commonly used for urine samples that produce a positive dipstick result for bilirubin. Ictotest (Bayer) tablets are one example of this second tier testing.

Testing for bilirubin and urobilinogen should be performed on fresh urine specimens. Upon exposure to light, bilirubin is converted into biliverdin. Biliverdin does not react with the dipstick reagent pad for bilirubin, thus a false negative result may occur. Similarly, urobilinogen is converted to urobilin upon exposure to oxygen.

Microbiologic examination
Bacterial urinary tract infections

Urinary tract infections (UTIs) should always be diagnosed initially by clinical signs and symptoms. Urinalysis (UA) and culture serve as adjunct tests to help support the diagnosis of a UTI and generally should not be performed in the absence of symptoms. While most infectious disease testing from urine utilizes commercially available, highly regulated reagents and specimen collection instructions, urine culture and subsequent "workup" does not have equivocally clear standards. As such, the art of urine culture reporting and decision making (as whether to perform antimicrobial susceptibility testing or even organism identification) is largely institutionally driven. In some aspects, urine testing for most applications in infectious disease is akin to orchestral sheet music, whereas urine culture practices better resemble that of free form jazz; in other words, every lab is playing the same song, but with their own variations of the tune.

Urinalysis markers as a screen for UTI

Rapid testing of urine using dipstick or automated analyzers has simplified the approach to screening urine specimens for culture. An ongoing debate has centered on creating an effective, automated, algorithmic approach to reducing urine specimens that are unnecessarily sent for culture (which represents a major burden on the laboratory). Unfortunately, despite decades of efforts to refine these approaches, no effective algorithm or automation has been implemented that both reliably predicts UTIs and reliably determines the appropriateness of culture initiation [ISBN 978-1555816780]. Several measures have been suggested as decision points for whether a culture should automatically reflex from a UA, eg, microscopic identification of >10 WBCs per field of view, a positive leukocyte esterase (LE) test, presence of bacteria on Gram stain of urine sediment, and/or nitrate reduction. Each of these tests has obvious pitfalls that limit its utility for reflexive testing reaffirming the importance of physician instinct/judgment over laboratory based analytical measures.

For both WBC counts and LE, these tests can be predictive for inflammatory processes in the bladder or urethra (typically associated with a UTI); however, in immunosuppressed patients (AIDS, leukopenia, primary immunodeficiency syndromes, pretransplant induction, etc), these tests have practically no value in predicting a UTI. A Gram stain likewise has reasonable negative predictive value in healthy adults; however the presence of bacteria does not necessarily equate to an infection as bacteria may be nonuropathogenic, represent asymptomatic bacteriuria, or be the result of poorly collected specimens that were contaminated by urethral flora, labia flora, and/or urinary meatus flora. Nitrate to nitrite reduction is predictive for infection from members of *Enterobacteriaciae* (eg, *E coli*); however, this test is not helpful for infections caused by nonnitrate reducing uropathogens such as *Enterococcus* [ISBN 978-1555816780].

Culture

Urine cultures represent the most common test performed in a clinical microbiology laboratory and the majority of cultures are negative for uropathogens [ISBN 978-1555816780]. Correspondingly, these cultures consume a considerable amount of the laboratory's work efforts, for low clinical return. The importance of establishing a clinical suspicion or running diagnosis of UTI cannot be overstated in terms of the clinical utility (or disutility as it may be) of urine cultures. This global challenge is the main driving force behind failed attempts to derive an effective triage/reflex algorithm for cultures.

If a urine specimen is submitted for culture after primary screening, it is integral that the laboratory know the precise method for which the urine was collected (ie, clean catch, indwelling catheter collection, straight catheterized collection, suprapubic aspirate, pediatric urine collection bag). The mechanism of urine collection will determine the threshold of bacteria that will be reported, identified, and tested for antimicrobial susceptibility testing. These thresholds are institutionally determined by the laboratory and are not appropriate for discussion in this text. One example of the importance of specimen collection and labeling is when a catheter is involved in the collection. The laboratory will apply a very high stringency to the degree of culture workup for urine collected through an indwelling catheter (which is rarely advisable). In this case, biofilms are known to form on Foley catheters within hours of placement (typically from fecal flora) and therefore the presence of 3 or more potential uropathogens in culture would be considered insignificant [ISBN 978-1555816780]. However, if the specimen was collected via straight catheterization, the presence of 3 or more potentially fecal derived uropathogens (eg, *Enterococcus*, *E coli*, *Candida*) could represent a complicated UTI or a fistula into the bladder from the gastrointestinal tract [ISBN 978-1555816780]. Likewise, a suprapubic aspirate would have a very low threshold for working up the culture (as little as 1 colony). In fact, suprapubic aspirates are the only urine specimen that can be treated as a sterile body fluid from a microbiologic standpoint and as a result, anaerobic cultures may be performed on request (though interpreting the significance of these cultures may be difficult) [ISBN 978-1555816780]. In the case of pediatric urine collection bags, these are generally not appropriate for cultures and should not be submitted due to the immense amount of fecal flora present on a diapered infant's perianal region [ISBN 978-1555816780]. Laboratories should reject these specimens and request a straight catheter or suprapubic aspirate collection. In the case of clean catch urine, the first void urine is most useful for culture as it will contain the most accurate count of bacteria present in the bladder since the bacteria will have been replicating in the bladder for ~8 hours or more [ISBN 978-1555816780]. It is important to remember when gauging the significance of bacteria in a urine sample that the urethra, unlike the rest of the urinary tract, is not sterile and contains resident flora (often derived from the skin or feces) [ISBN 978-1555816780].

Urine cultures are quantitative in that the laboratory uses a calibrated inoculation loop to deliver a precise volume of urine (0.01 µL or 0.001 µL) to each plate. The inoculum is then spread to cover the entire surface, which allows relative quantification after 18-24 hours of growth (sufficient to recover most uropathogens). The resulting colonies are enumerated and the calculated number of colony forming units per mL of urine is reported (if significant). Because these cultures are quantitative, it is imperative that the urine samples are collected and transported immediately to the laboratory to avoid growth of bacteria after collection. Storage of specimens at room temperature in excess of 2 hours will invariably result in inaccurate culture results. In the event that urine specimens cannot be transported to the lab for culture within 2 hours, the specimen may be refrigerated for up to 24 hours. Boric acid tubes can also be used to maintain urine specimens at room temperature for up to 24 hours if refrigeration is not possible though the sample may not be compatible with other urinalysis methods due to the boric acid [ISBN 978-1555816780]. Urine cultures are generally discarded after 48 hours as most pathogens will grow within this time period including slow growing pathogens such as *Corynebacterium urealyticum* and bacteria that are partially treated with antimicrobials in advance of urine collection [ISBN 978-1555816780].

Urine cultures are set up by the laboratory typically using 2 or more media types. The classic approach includes a nonselective blood containing media such as Columbia sheep blood agar, a selective media for Gram– organisms (typically MacConkey agar), and less frequently, CLED agar (cysteine, lactose, and electrolyte deficient). More recently, propriety media using chromogenic colony identification of organisms have been incorporated into many urine cultures due to their comparable performance to traditional media [PMID 11923381]. These media provide presumptive identification of the organisms in ~18-24 hours and can be helpful to guide empiric therapy. These agar plates are generally quite expensive compared to routine media; however, the tradeoff is that many organisms can be identified without additional automated techniques or extra biochemical testing. While these plates do not have perfect specificity, the sensitivity is generally comparable to that of the nonselective blood agar plate for most organisms [PMID 11923381].

Viral detection

There are 2 viruses that have clinical significance for detection in urine samples, albeit for very different reasons: cytomegalovirus (CMV) and BK virus. CMV is shed in high concentrations in the urine of humans infected with the virus including neonates with congenital CMV infection. This urinary shedding of CMV can occur for a year or more in some instances [ISBN 978-0781760607]. This prolonged shedding is particularly problematic in infants with sensorineural hearing loss as testing of the urine cannot definitively determine congenital CMV infection from postnatal CMV infection [PMID 21827433].

A traditional urine based method for diagnosing congenital, primary, or reactivated CMV is viral culture. The rapid "shell vial culture" assay is particularly useful to detect CMV in less time than traditional viral culture and paired with CMV direct fluorescence antibody testing of the shell vial, the infections can often be detected in 24 hours [PMID 12749681, PMID 11986492]. Urine should be collected in a sterile container and transported refrigerated to the laboratory. A sample of the urine is then inoculated into the shell vial and centrifuged to enhance infection of the cell monolayer. CMV can also be detected in urine by PCR. Though rapid culture and PCR have similar specificity, there is improved sensitivity by PCR for both urine samples from congenitally infected babies as well as immunocompromised patients [PMID 22177273]. Though CMV urine PCR has gained traction in the diagnosis of congenital CMV, rapid culture remains the gold standard [PMID 21827433]. In the case of immunocompromised patients, PCR from serum or plasma are considered the new diagnostic gold standard replacing rapid urine culture. PCR has 1 additional crucial advantage over rapid culture in that it can typically be performed and resulted in a matter of hours from the laboratory receiving the specimen.

BK virus is a polyomavirus and though it is unrelated to CMV, it shares many similar clinical characteristics. BK virus is typically acquired during childhood and adults show similar seropositivity rates to CMV (~50%-80%). Also akin to CMV, the virus lays dormant in the human body indefinitely. Reactivation only occurs during periods of severe immunosuppression. BK virus nephropathy is a significant concern in kidney transplant patients. BK virus reactivation occurs in 30%-50% of transplant patients within 3 months of transplant and therefore testing of urine during these periods is most useful [PMID 15996241, PMID 15707414]. The diagnosis of BK virus nephropathy may be made by cytology or biopsy looking for "decoy cells" on a Papanicolaou stain [PMID 19394729, PMID 12099383]. Decoy cells are infected renal tubular epithelial cells with intranuclear basophilic inclusion bodies. This approach has very high sensitivity, but only 20% positive predictive value [PMID 10199744, PMID 10692517]. The virus can be readily detected in urine specimens by PCR, which can then complement the poor positive predictive value exhibited by the Papanicolaou stain. In later stages of infection, both the plasma and eventually the kidney itself will have detectable virus DNA present.

Parasitic evaluation

Schistosoma species and *Trichomonas vaginalis* are the only relevant parasites detected in urine. Though *T vaginalis* is conventionally identified via microscopic examination of a wet mount and/or culture from urethral discharge, an amplified DNA assay is now available for direct testing of female urine specimens (see "Molecular detection of sexually transmitted infections," below).

Detection of urinary schistosomiasis is a relatively simple procedure but should always be performed by experienced parasitologists since identification of ova requires specific expertise. Urine specimens should be collected during peak time of ova excretion (typically midday: noon to 3 PM). Alternatively, urine can also be collected over the course of 24 hours in a single sterile collection container. The laboratory should concentrate or centrifuge the urine at ~1,000× g to obtain a pellet in the bottom of the collection tube; this is integral to detect light infections [PMID 15463638]. A sample of the pellet should then be prepared for wet mount examination. Specimens from patients with urinary schistosomiasis often have hematuria that can be detected microscopically in the sediment and often macroscopically (urine will appear dark brown or red) [PMID 22632645]. *S haematobium* are oblong and measure ~150 µm in length with variable width. The ova are characterized by a prominent terminal spine i9.27. Rarely, ova from *S japonicum* can be seen in urine specimens and these ova are spherical, ~90 µm in diameter, and possess an inconspicuous lateral spine that is often not visible by microscopy.

Urinary antigen testing

Urinary antigen testing has become a standard diagnostic tool for several significant respiratory infections particularly *Legionella pneumophila*, *Streptococcus pneumoniae*, and *Histoplasma capsulatum*. Urinary antigen testing capitalizes on the concentration of shed "antigen" from these pathogens in the kidneys for eventual excretion in the urine. These pathogens are not present in the urine for culture per se, only the target antigen. Excreted antigens can then be detected via an immunoassay such as an enzyme linked immunosorbent assay (ELISA) or an immunochromatographic or lateral flow assay (LFA). The clear benefits of these assays are a noninvasive specimen collection, rapid turnaround time, and improved sensitivity over culture. This allows urinary antigen testing to be used to establish a diagnosis of respiratory infection independent of an invasive collection such as a bronchoalveolar lavage or bronchial washing.

Streptococcus pneumoniae antigen testing is available as an LFA from Alere (BinaxNOW) and the same product can be used to test CSF specimens for suspected CSF involvement (see Chapter 3) or to detect community acquired pneumonia (CAP) via urine testing. According to manufacturer claims, the test has sensitivities of 86%-90% and specificities of 71%-94% and will detect all 23 common serotypes of *S pneumoniae*. Independent evaluations of the product have also yielded similar ranges of specificity and sensitivity as those claimed by the manufacturer and the variability in sensitivity is largely based on the lack of a true "gold standard" for diagnosing pneumococcal CAP [PMID 24886525].

Legionella pneumophila antigen testing is available as both a 96 well microtiter ELISA and LFA. Various manufacturers sell FDA cleared products, each with variable clinical sensitivity and clinical specificity. This variation is largely due to the gold standard used for comparison for each product. One meta-analysis determined that these various assays have a pooled clinical sensitivity and specificity of 74% and 99%, respectively [PMID 19318671]. Therefore, the assays can reliably diagnose *Legionella* infection but cannot rule it out. Another important limitation of this assay is that all commercial products are designed to detect only serogroup 1 of *Legionella pneumophila* with published sensitivities of 5%-40% for nonserogroup 1 *L pneumophila* and other *Legionella* species [PMID 12097254]. Antigen shedding may be detected in the first 24 hours and antigenuria in clinically cured patients may persist for several weeks making this assay inappropriate as a "test of cure" [PMID 17980914].

Histoplasma capsulatum infections can also be diagnosed using urine antigen testing as an adjunct interrogation to culture, histopathology, antibody detection, and PCR. Unlike *Legionella* and *S pneumoniae*, urine antigen testing for *Histoplasma* is most sensitive for detecting disseminated histoplasmosis rather than localized respiratory disease [PMID 17913863, PMID 2794560]. *Histoplasma* antigen testing can be performed in house using an FDA cleared polyclonal antibody based ELISA from Immy, a monoclonal ELISA employing analyte specific reagents for *Histoplasma* galactomannan (also from Immy), or testing can be obtained commercially from MiraVista Diagnostics via a proprietary, though well studied ELISA [PMID 23966508, PMID 17580268, PMID 17913863]. All of these assays have been shown to cross react with other various dimorphic fungi, including *Blastomyces*, *Coccidioides*, *Sporothrix*, and *Paracoccidioides* [PMID 23966508, PMID 17580268, PMID 17913863]. In addition to urine, testing of serum is typically performed as a paired collection in order to maximize the likelihood of antigen detection. Serial testing of urine is helpful to track response to antifungal therapy as the assay has quantitative capabilities, which reflect fungal burden in the body.

Molecular detection of sexually transmitted infections

Several methods are commercially available for molecular detection of *Chlamydia trachomatis* and *Neisseria gonorheae* from urine specimens including DNA hybridization probe, PCR, transcription mediated amplification, and strand displacement amplification [PMID 16044393]. The traditional gold standard for the diagnosis of both of these infections is culture from swabs of the suspected site of infection (eg, vagina, cervix, urethra). Culture for *C trachomatis*, however, lacks adequate sensitivity [PMID 16044393]. *N gonorrheae* culture is sensitive and specific if the required specimen collection and culture conditions are strictly adhered to; however sensitivity is precipitously reduced when the culture is not appropriately performed [PMID 16044393].

An important consideration is that many of these molecular tests can also be performed using swabbed specimens from the urethra or cervix. For *C trachomatis*, either specimen type (swabs or urine) yields equivalent test performance [PMID 15941699]. One caveat to this equivalence is that the sensitivity of molecular assays for *C trachomatis* is affected by the timing of urine collection. Studies have shown reduced sensitivity for midstream, clean catch urine vs first void urine [PMID 10805367, PMID 22230830]. Though the performance of molecular testing from clean catch urine is superior to culture, the optimal test performance for molecular assays should be sought using first void urine specimens. Additionally, *N gonorrheae* molecular tests are more sensitive for women when performed on endocervical specimens rather than urine [PMID 15941699]. When taking these test characteristics together, a female patient being tested for both *N gonorrheae* and *C trachomatis* on a single specimen would be best served using an endocervical or urethral swab rather than urine.

Trichomonas vaginalis can also be detected from urine using FDA cleared molecular testing using transcription mediated amplification. Similar to *C trachomatis*, this molecular testing of urine (as well as endocervical or vaginal swab) is significantly more sensitive than the standard culture method [PMID 21902528]. The assay is currently approved for testing of female urine specimens and can be used in symptomatic and asymptomatic patients. Testing of male patients is currently not FDA cleared, though studies have shown excellent performance using male urine specimens [PMID 16943353, PMID 19185101].

If urine is collected for molecular testing, the manufacturer's recommendations should be strictly adhered to as manufacturers provide a specific collection tube and media that is optimized for their platform. The collection tubes are often specifically designed to be processed and sampled on a particular instrument. Alternative media types and collection tubes may be independently validated by a laboratory; however the laboratory should be consulted before any nonstandardized collection tube is utilized.

Special studies

Calculi and stone composition analysis may be an important adjunct to urinalysis. Crystal identification, at least by morphology, was briefly discussed above. In select instances the chemical composition of the stones, especially if recurrent may provide important information to be used in the management of the patient.

Calculi

Renal calculi, or kidney stones, require specialized laboratory investigation to determine the composition of the stone. Understanding the stone composition may aid in preventing future stone formation. Additional testing can even provide information related to the risk of stone formation given the current concentration of analytes within the urine. These analyses are usually performed in specialized laboratories with expertise in these complex techniques.

Urinalysis in combination with blood tests provides a metabolic evaluation that can aid in investigating renal calculi formation. Crystal formation identified by urine microscopy is another important finding in the patient with renal calculi. If a calculus is passed in the urine, investigations into its composition can be performed often using X ray crystallography or infrared spectroscopy. While calculi may be composed of a variety of different compounds, calcium oxalate is the most common followed by calcium phosphate, uric acid and magnesium phosphate. However, composition will vary by population, age, and geographical region.

Risk of stone formation may also be determined by measuring the concentration of stone promoters and stone inhibitors t9.7. Solubility and energetics of saturation and precipitation are used together to predict the formation of a calculus for a given individual. This information may be useful for patient management and for reducing the risk of future stone formation. Immunohistochemistry, per se, has limited utility in the examination of urine specimens even in the context of urothelial neoplasia.

t9.7	Examples of promoters & inhibitors of renal calculi formation
Promoters	**Inhibitors**
Low urine volume	Citrate
pH <5.5	Magnesium
pH >7.2	
Calcium	
Oxalate	
Sodium	
Sulfate	
Uric acid	

Bladder tumor antigens

Although immunohistochemistry may have limited value in evaluating urothelial neoplasms, there are a number of antibody based, commercially available assays that may be used for the identification of urothelial neoplasia via the detection of "tumor specific" antigens t9.8. As a general rule, they all have tangible limitations with respect to sensitivity and specificity and thus their routine application in the management of suspected, or more commonly with recurrent urothelial carcinoma, is limited and institutionally determined. Numerous reviews have been written about the accuracy of these various assays [ISBN 019-5134958, ISBN 978-0891896449, PMID 11152093]. However, this must be viewed in context. For example, it has been stated that some of these markers are more accurate than cytology, especially for low grade urothelial carcinoma and that cystoscopy remains the gold standard but this is a broad statement and may be true for voided urine specimens and less so for bladder washing samples. Those interested are referred to the more detailed articles.

t9.8	Select biomarkers used for the detection of urothelial carcinoma
BGA (blood group antigens)	
BTA (bladder tumor antigens)	
FISH (fluorescent in situ hybridization); UroVision	
FDP (fibrin/fibrinogen degradation products)	
Hyaluronic acid/hyaluronidase	
Immunologic assays; Immunocyt	
NMP22 BladderChek (nuclear matrix protein)	
Ploidy analysis/cell cycle analysis (by flow cytometry or image analysis)	

FISH

Fluorescence in situ hybridization (FISH) testing for the detection of urothelial cancer, UroVysion is an FDA approved test. The assay identifies multiple chromosomes looking for aneuploidy of chromosomes 3, 7, and 17 and loss of the 9p21 locus. The sensitivity has been reported to be higher than cytology (~75% vs ~50%). There are, predictably, limitations such as the need for adequate cellularity, tumor location (eg, within a diverticulum), and specific morphologic types (eg, nested variant). More importantly, the cost of the test and its need to be sent to laboratories performing the test influence the overall utility of UroVysion [ISBN 019-5134958, ISBN 978-0891896449, PMID 18724101].

Other

There are a number of other tumor markers that are under various stages of investigation. Examples include UBC, which detects certain cytokeratins, the transcription factors BLCA1 and BLCA4, hyalurinidase/hyaluronic acid, microsatellite instability, telomerase, and miRNA.

Artifacts & pitfalls

A number of artifacts can occur in the examination of urine specimens, many of which arise from poor collection and/or preservation i9.56-i9.58. Fibers and other foreign materials (eg, pollen) may be encountered. In addition, poorly preserved specimens may lead to bacterial overgrowth and/or degenerative changes (eg, cellular lysis) precluding a meaningful evaluation. Similarly, the choice of the type of microscopy used can affect the evaluation. Bright field and phase contrast each have their role but each also has its limitations.

There are also limitations in assay methods. For example, there are distinct limitations in reagent strips that are often used for in-office chemical and microbiologic assessments. Relatedly, experience in microscopy is necessary for the proper identification of the various crystals and casts as well as cell types that may be encountered in urine specimens.

There are a broad array of crystals and casts, and their correct identification is important if the laboratory is to help guide further investigation of the patient and their care. It is also important to be able to accurately distinguish the various cell types, both inflammatory and epithelial, since they are often not well preserved.

Finally, the morphologic evaluation of specimens for urothelial malignancy, usually restricted to high grade urothelial carcinoma, requires distinct expertise. Discerning such tumor cells from degenerative changes, especially in voided specimens, and BK virus ("decoy cells") can be a significant pitfall even for the trained cytologist.

Key points

The examination of urine is a key component in the evaluation and management of patients with suspected or known systemic and urinary tract diseases/processes. The information garnered from the examination of this unique fluid is the most diverse of any of the fluids that are routinely evaluated and may suggest diseases such as infection, multiple myeloma, diabetes, staghorn calculus, glomerulonephritis, urothelial malignancy, and dehydration.

- The chemical composition, the evaluation for microorganisms, the microscopic identification of urothelial tumors, casts and crystals, are all part of the urinalysis and can provide important insight to the healthcare provider.
- The meaningful communication of the related laboratory results is critically important for excellent patient care.
- There are certain instances when the results of urinalysis should be reported immediately. These critical results include certain kinds of casts (RBC, bacterial), high levels of glucose and ketones (especially from a patient in the emergency department), and the presence of sperm in a young female or vulnerable adult.

References

PMID 10199744 Binet I, Nickeleit V, Hirsch HH et al [1999] polyomavirus disease under new immunosuppressive drugs: a cause of renal graft dysfunction and graft loss. *Transplantation* 67(6):918-922

PMID 10692517 Nickeleit V, Hirsch HH, Zeiler M et al [2000] BK-virus nephropathy in renal transplants-tubular necrosis, MHC-class II expression and rejection in a puzzling game. *Nephrol Dial Transplant* 15(3):324-332

PMID 11152093 Ross JS, Cohen MB [2001] Biomarkers for the detection of bladder cancer. *Adv Anat Pathol* 8(1):37-45

PMID 11923381 Aspevall O, Osterman B, Dittmer R et al [2002] Performance of 4 chromogenic urine culture media after one or 2 days of incubation compared with reference media. *J Clin Microbiol* 40(4):1500-1503

PMID 11986492 Pass RF [2002] Cytomegalovirus infection. *Pediatr Rev* 23:163-169

PMID 12097254 Fields BS, Benson RF, Besser RE [2002] *Legionella* and Legionnaires' disease: 25 years of investigation. *Clin Microbiol Rev* 15(3):506-526

PMID 12099383 Drachenberg RC, Drachenberg CB, Papadimitriou JC et al Morphologic spectrum of polyomavirus disease in renal allografts: diagnostic accuracy of urine cytology. *Am J Transplant* 1(4):373-381

PMID 12749681 Leung AK, Sauve RS, Davies HD [2003] Congenital cytomegalovirus infection. *J Natl Med Assoc* 95(3):213-218

PMID 14696141 Layfield LJ, Elsheikh TM, Fili A et al [2004] Papanicolaou Society of Cytopathology. Review of the state of the art and recommendations of the Papanicolaou Society of Cytopathology for urinary cytology procedures and reporting : the Papanicolaou Society of Cytopathology Practice Guidelines Task Force. *Diagn Cytopathol* 30(1):24-30

PMID 15463638 de Vlas SJ, Gryseels B [1992] Underestimation of *Schistosoma mansoni* prevalences. *Parasitol Today* 8:274-277

PMID 15707414 Brennan DC, Agha I, Bohl DL et al [2005]Incidence of BK with tacrolimus vs cyclosporine and impact of preemptive immunosuppression reduction. *Am J Transplant* 5(3):582-594

PMID 15791892 Simerville JA, Maxted WC, Pahira JJ [2005] Urinalysis: a comprehensive review. *Am Fam Physician* 71(6):1153-1162

PMID 15941699 Cook RL, Hutchison SL, Østergaard L et al [2005] Systematic review: noninvasive testing for *Chlamydia trachomatis* and *Neisseria gonorrhoeae*. *Ann Intern Med* 142(11):914-925

PMID 15996241 Bressollette-Bodin C, Coste-Burel M, Hourmant M et al [2005] A prospective longitudinal study of BK virus infection in 104 renal transplant recipients. *Am J Transplant* 5(8):1926-1933

PMID 16044393 Olshen E, Shrier LA [2005] Diagnostic tests for chlamydial and gonorrheal infections. *Semin Pediatr Infect Dis* 16(3):192-198

PMID 16943353 Hardick A, Hardick J, Wood BJ, Gaydos C [2006] Comparison between the Gen-Probe transcription-mediated amplification *Trichomonas vaginalis* research assay and real-time PCR for *Trichomonas vaginalis* detection using a Roche LightCycler instrument with female self-obtained vaginal swab samples and male urine samples. *J Clin Microbiol* 44(11):4197-4199

PMID 17580268 Cloud JL, Bauman SK, Neary BP, et al [2007] Performance characteristics of a polyclonal enzyme immunoassay for the quantitation of *Histoplasma* antigen in human urine samples. *Am J Clin Pathol* 128(1):18-22

PMID 17913863 Connolly PA, Durkin MM, Lemonte AM, et al [2007] Detection of histoplasma antigen by a quantitative enzyme immunoassay. *Clin Vaccine Immunol* 14(12):1587-1591

PMID 17980914 Diederen BM [2008] *Legionella* spp and Legionnaires' disease. *J Infect* 56(1):1-12

PMID 18724101 Halling KC, Kipp BR [2008] Bladder cancer detection using FISH (UroVysion assay). *Adv Anat Pathol* 15(5):279-286

PMID 19185101 Nye MB, Schwebke JR, Body BA [2009] Comparison of APTIMA *Trichomonas vaginalis* transcription-mediated amplification to wet mount microscopy, culture, and polymerase chain reaction for diagnosis of trichomoniasis in men and women. *Am J Obstet Gynecol* 200(2):188.e1-7

PMID 19318671 Shimada T, Noguchi Y, Jackson JL, et al [2009] Systematic review and metaanalysis: urinary antigen tests for Legionellosis. *Chest* 136(6):1576-1585

PMID 19394729 Wiseman AC [2009] polyomavirus nephropathy: a current perspective and clinical considerations. *Am J Kidney Dis* 54(1):131-142

PMID 21827433 Ross SA, Novak Z, Pati S et al [2011] Overview of the diagnosis of cytomegalovirus infection. *Infect Disord Drug Targets* 11(5):466-474

PMID 21902528 Chapin K, Andrea S [2011] APTIMA *Trichomonas vaginalis*, a transcription-mediated amplification assay for detection of *Trichomonas vaginalis* in urogenital specimens. *Expert Rev Mol Diagn* 11(7):679-688

PMID 22177273 de Vries JJ, van der Eijk AA, Wolthers KC et al [2012] Real-time PCR vs viral culture on urine as a gold standard in the diagnosis of congenital cytomegalovirus infection. *J Clin Virol* 53(2):167-170

PMID 22230830 Mangin D, Murdoch D, Wells JE et al [2012] *Chlamydia trachomatis* testing sensitivity in midstream compared with first-void urine specimens. *Ann Fam Med* 10(1):50-53

PMID 22632645 Gryseels B [2012] Schistosomiasis. *Infect Dis Clin North Am* 26(2):383-397

PMID 23264422 American Diabetes Association [2013] Standards of medical care in diabetes¬—2013. *Diabetes Care* 36Suppl1:S11-66

PMID 23732715 Stevens PE, Levin A, Kidney Disease: Improving Global Outcomes Chronic Kidney Disease Guideline Development Work Group Members [2013] Evaluation and management of chronic kidney disease: synopsis of the kidney disease: improving global outcomes 2012 clinical practice guideline. *Ann Intern Med* 158(11):825-830

PMID 23966508 Theel ES, Jespersen DJ, Harring J, et al [2013] Evaluation of an enzyme immunoassay for detection of *Histoplasma capsulatum* antigen from urine specimens. *J Clin Microbiol* 51(11):3555-9

PMID 24856525 Couturier MR, Graf EH, Griffin AT [2014] Urine antigen tests for the diagnosis of respiratory infections: legionellosis, histoplasmosis, and pneumococcal pneumonia. *Clinics in Laboratory Medicine* 34(2):219-236

PMID 2794560 Zimmerman SE, Stringfield PC, Wheat LJ, et al [1989] Comparison of sandwich solid-phase radioimmunoassay and 2 enzyme-linked immunosorbent assays for detection of *Histoplasma capsulatum* polysaccharide antigen. *J Infect Dis* 160(4):678-685

PMID 3048852 Haber MH [1988] Pisse prophecy: a brief history of urinalysis. *Clin Lab Med* 8(3):415-430

PMID 8062194 Raab SS, Lenel JC, Cohen MB [1994] Low grade transitional cell carcinoma of the bladder. Cytologic diagnosis by key features as identified by logistic regression analysis. *Cancer* 74(5):1621-1626

PMID 9135826 Rockall AG, Newman-Sanders AP, al-Kutoubi MA, Vale JA [1997] Hematuria. *Postgrad Med J* 73(857):129-136

ISBN 019-5134958 Bardales RH [2002] *Practical Urologic Cytopathology*. Oxford University Press

ISBN 072-1660290 Murphy WM [1997] *Urological Pathology*, 2e. WB Saunders Company

ISBN 978-0781760607 Mocarski ES Jr, Shenk T, Pass RF [2007] Cytomegaloviruses. In: Knipe DM, Howley PM, ed. *Fields' Virology*, 5e. Lippincott Williams & Wilkins, p2702-2772

ISBN 978-0891891031 Haber MH [1981] *Urinary Sediment: A Textbook Atlas*, 1e. American Society for Clinical Pathology

ISBN 978-0891896203 Schumann GB, Friedman MT [2003] *Wet Urinalysis*. American Society for Clinical Pathology

ISBN 978-0891896449 DeMay RM [2012] Exfoliative cytopathology In *The Art & Science of Cytopathology*, 2e. ASCP Press

ISBN 978-0930304874 Haber MH, Blomberg D, Galagan K et al [2010] *Color Atlas of the Urinary Sediment. An Illustrated Field Guide Based on Proficiency Testing.* CAP Press

ISBN 978-1437709742 McPherson RA, Pincus MR [2011] *Henry's Clinical Diagnosis and Management by Laboratory Methods*, 22e. Elsevier Saunders

ISBN 978-1555816780 Baron EJ, Thomson RB Jr [2011] Chapter 16: Specimen collection, transport, and processing: bacteriology. In: *Manual of Clinical Microbiology*. ASM Press, p228-271

[2014] Phase contrast. http://www.microscopyu.com/articles/phasecontrast/index.html (accessed 03/28/2014)

[2014] Polarized light microscopy. http://www.microscopyu.com/articles/polarized/index.html (accessed 03/28/2014)

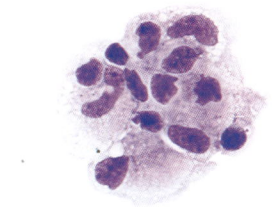

Hussong JW, Straseski JA, Couturier MR

Specialized Body Fluids
Chapter 10

In this chapter we will review some of the basic principles and tests in the evaluation of saliva, vitreous fluid and sweat. There will be an emphasis on chemical analysis and microbiologic testing. For a more complete and in depth review of the evaluation of these specimen types, the reader should refer to specialized texts.

Saliva

Saliva is produced by the salivary glands and is a filtrate of plasma. It consists predominantly (>99%) of water but also contains electrolytes, enzymes, mucus, hormones, antibacterial compounds and cellular elements. Normal saliva is clear, colorless, with a pH ranging from 6.0-7.4. It has a specific gravity between 1.002 and 1.012. The major salivary glands, including the parotid, submandibular and sublingual glands, are responsible for the majority of saliva production f10.1. It is estimated that humans produce 0.75-1.5 L of saliva a day with only minimal production during sleep.

The acini within the salivary glands are either serous, mucous or a mixture of the 2 types t10.1. The serous cells produce watery fluid that contains enzymes, such as amylase, that begin the digestion of starchy and fatty food substances. The mucous cells produce more viscous saliva that is richer in glycoproteins, which serves to lubricate the oral mucosa and protects it from trauma during speaking, swallowing and eating. It also contributes to the maintenance of oral hygiene. Patients with xerostomia, or dry mouth, have reduced production or flow of saliva, and the associated complications of hyposalivation. These include increased dental caries, oral candidiasis, burning or tingling in the mouth, mouth soreness and increased thirst.

t10.1 Salivary gland acinar types	
Salivary gland	**Acinar type**
Parotid	Serous
Submandibular	Serous and mucous
Sublingual	Primarily mucous
Minor	Primarily mucous

Specimen collection, requirements & stability

The method of collection and transport of saliva specimens depends on the testing to be performed. For cytologic examination, fresh specimens are required for preparation of smears/cytospins or cell blocks as previously described. In addition, the use of oral brush collection techniques can produce more cellular specimens for oral cytology examination. The reader is referred to any of the specialized texts for in depth morphologic descriptions.

Saliva specimens for chemical analysis are preferably frozen prior to analysis. Freezing and centrifuging precipitates interfering glycoproteins and provides a less viscous sample for testing. Care should be taken to avoid contamination of saliva samples with blood from the oral cavity (eg, following aggressive brushing or flossing). Most biological analytes are present in higher concentrations in the blood; thus its presence in saliva may invalidate the measurement.

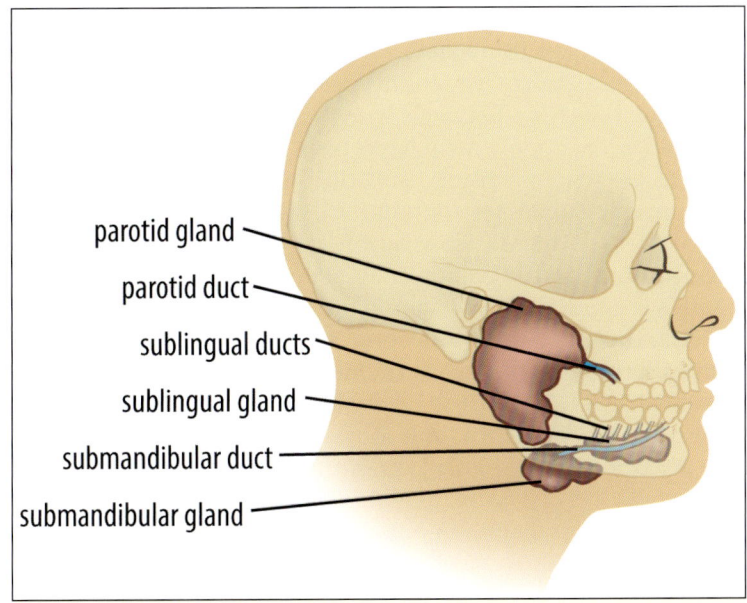

f10.1 Anatomic distribution of the major salivary glands (parotid, submandibular and sublingual)

Time of collection should be noted if analytes that are subject to diurnal variation (eg, cortisol) are to be measured. The pH of saliva and serum differ and may affect the ratio of bound:free drug or hormone. Extremely acidic or basic saliva may compromise analytical measurements.

Chemical analysis

The primary areas of chemical analysis that utilize saliva as a sample type include endocrinology (hormones) and toxicology. It should be noted that saliva testing of these analytes is subject to numerous challenges. Most notably, a correlation between analyte concentrations in blood and saliva must exist in order for saliva testing to be a useful surrogate sample type. This direct relationship does not exist for all analytes. The small concentrations of most analytes found in saliva require assays with very low levels of detection. Reference values from healthy populations are limited and standardized assays and collection devices are not available.

Both hormone and drug concentrations measured in saliva are considered to be free of binding proteins and thus reflect the biologically active (unbound) concentration in blood.

Cortisol

Cortisol concentrations determined from saliva specimens mirror free cortisol concentrations in blood [PMID 17456296], since cortisol binding protein and albumin are not present in saliva. The lack of these binding proteins also eliminates the need for an extraction step prior to analysis. Salivary samples are frozen after collection and centrifuged prior to testing, which aids in precipitating the interfering glycoproteins found in this specimen type. Salivary cortisol is commonly detected using immunoassays with chromatographic and mass spectrometry methods becoming more widely available.

The loss of diurnal cortisol variation is indicative of Cushing syndrome, with the lack of a late night (midnight) cortisol nadir supporting other aspects of the clinical picture. Measurement of the late night cortisol value is the preferred test for Cushing syndrome and saliva collection is often more practical at this late timepoint in the outpatient setting. 2 independent salivary cortisol measurements are recommended, with values >145 ng/dL (4 nmol/L) considered diagnostic for Cushing syndrome with 92%-100% sensitivity and 93%-100% specificity [PMID 18334580]. Salivary cortisol may also be more useful than urinary free cortisol in patients with mild Cushing syndrome [PMID 18057379, PMID 18334580]. Late night salivary cortisol assays are not sensitive enough to provide diagnostic information for suspected cases of Addison disease or hypocortisolism.

Sex steroids

The use of saliva for the measurement of sex steroids has been discussed but not widely adopted due to rapid fluctuations in this sample type [PMID 19176642]. Pulsatile patterns over short time frames have been observed for estradiol [PMID 16002538], progesterone [PMID 7926142], testosterone, dehydroepiandrosterone and aldosterone [PMID 19176642]. Multiple samples would therefore be necessary to provide useful information for these analytes. Saliva concentrations have also proven to be of little value for thyroid and pituitary hormones [PMID 3320544].

Toxicology

Many exogenous analytes, such as drugs, can be detected in saliva. The lack of binding proteins present in the saliva allows for measurement of the pharmacologically active form of many drugs. However, pH greatly affects drug concentrations and extremely acidic or basic samples may provide erroneous results. The correlation between plasma and saliva concentrations will depend on the physicochemical properties of the drug in question. Sensitive methods are required to detect the small concentrations of drug found in this sample type. Immunoassays are often used as an initial screen with chromatographic and mass spectrometry methods used for confirmation. Toxicological applications of saliva testing include monitoring of therapeutic drug concentrations and detection of illicit or abused substances.

Monitoring of therapeutic drugs for arrhythmia, epilepsy, immunosuppression, cancer, viral and microbial infection and others have been described using saliva [PMID 15576290]. Appropriate measurements of therapeutic drug concentrations in saliva are dependent on the relationship between saliva and plasma for each drug. If the saliva:plasma ratio deviates significantly from 1, saliva testing is often not effective [PMID 15576290]. Furthermore, there must be evidence of a correlation between saliva concentrations and clinical and/or pharmacological effects in order for testing to be clinically informative. Saliva testing may be particularly convenient for patient populations that are subjected to routine testing, such as monitoring of immunosuppressants following organ transplant.

Drugs of abuse are readily measured in saliva samples and relationships between saliva drug concentration and behavior or impairment have been described [PMID 1620213]. In cases where sample substitution or adulteration is suspected, saliva testing may be particularly beneficial. However, localized absorption of drugs via smoking, snorting or oral ingestion may confound interpretation of saliva concentrations. It should also be noted that similar to blood, the window of detection for drugs in saliva is short and therefore urine may provide more useful information regarding long term use [PMID 1640691]. Ethanol diffuses rapidly into saliva, as it is not ionized or protein bound, and is often found in higher concentrations in saliva than the blood [PMID 8215090]. Saliva testing may also be performed for amphetamines, cannabinoids, cocaine, opiates, methadone, barbiturates, benzodiazepines and even nicotine.

Microbiologic testing

Saliva is currently not a specimen that has clinical utility in testing for bacterial, mycobacterial, fungal, or parasitic agents of disease. Though some saliva tests do exist in the peer reviewed literature for organisms such as *Borrelia burgdorferi* and *Helicobacter pylori*, they are not conventionally accepted testing methods and are beyond the scope of this text. Saliva testing is currently used primarily in the field of human immunodeficiency virus (HIV), with evolving clinical applications for hepatitis C virus (HCV) and cytomegalovirus (CMV).

HIV

HIV testing from oral fluid is available as a point of care (POC) device and serves as a screen for HIV1 or HIV1 and HIV2 antibodies. These tests are typically performed in acute care settings by a physician or medical assistant, and the results are generally available in ~20 minutes [PMID 23034833]. However, patients can also perform this testing at home using the same POC device, packaged for sale as an over the counter product (analogous to a home pregnancy test). These tests provide instructions to the patient as to how the test is performed and interpreted (including a toll free consultation service to provide resources for follow-up testing and local physician referrals).

Point of care HIV tests only serve as a screen for HIV infection and require follow-up confirmation testing, which must be ordered by a treating physician and performed at a qualified laboratory. The sensitivity and specificity of POC saliva tests for HIV have been shown to be comparable to blood based EIAs for antibody detection [PMID 21288853]. In one study, 6 FDA approved POC HIV tests were shown to have nearly identical clinical agreement among them; essentially allowing for the laboratory to perform the assay that best fits its needs for product stability/storage, workflow, and other technical aspects [PMID 21288853].

The testing algorithm for HIV is constantly evolving and inappropriate for inclusion in this text. It is imperative that the local health authority be contacted to determine the current state of the art algorithm necessary to achieve appropriate diagnostic evidence of infection. Consultation with local infectious disease/HIV experts is strongly recommended in all cases.

CMV

CMV acquired during pregnancy can result in significant birth defects, one of the most common being congenital hearing loss. Congenital infection with CMV may be entirely asymptomatic at birth, with hearing loss only being detected later during infancy. ~10%-15% of children with congenital CMV develop hearing impairment [PMID 1645882].

The gold standard for diagnosing congenital CMV is rapid culture of saliva or urine. Many laboratories no longer perform viral culture, limiting the facilities in which this testing can be performed. CMV culture also requires specific cell culture reagents and considerable experience in viral culture and DFA staining, making it difficult to establish in the laboratory. CMV PCR testing from saliva has recently gained attention as a sensitive and convenient mechanism for testing for congenital CMV infections. One large multicenter study showed equivalent sensitivity for PCR vs rapid culture for both liquid and dried saliva samples [PMID 21631323]. Currently, most major reference laboratories offer CMV PCR testing; however it is critical to confirm that the lab's assay is validated for saliva specimens.

HCV

Salivary testing for HCV is currently not available in the United States; however, there are POC products currently in use in Europe. In 1 study, the saliva POC test showed 97.5% agreement with a standard EIA from serum specimens [PMID 21940910]. This shows great promise and may become available in the future for US markets.

Fluids of the eye

Vitreous fluid

Vitreous is a viscous, clear, colorless fluid, comprised predominantly of water (>90%), that fills the interior of the eye f10.2. It contains inorganic salts, glucose, hyaluronic acid, ascorbic acid and type II collagen fibers. It is typically scantly cellular with only rare macrophages. Vitreous fluid is isolated, resulting in less susceptibility to biochemical changes and contamination. Under pathologic conditions, the vitreous fluid can become opacified due to accumulation of blood, inflammatory cells, tumor cells or amyloid.

Vitrectomy is the surgical removal of vitreous gel (vitreous humor) from the eye. It is performed for a number of indications, including repair of retinal detachments allowing access to the back of the eye, removal of hemorrhagic vitreous fluid, cytologic examination, chemical analysis and microbiologic studies. Commonly, 1.5-2.0 mL of vitreous fluid can be removed. Chemical analysis is particularly useful during postmortem evaluation and can provide important information regarding the time of death or

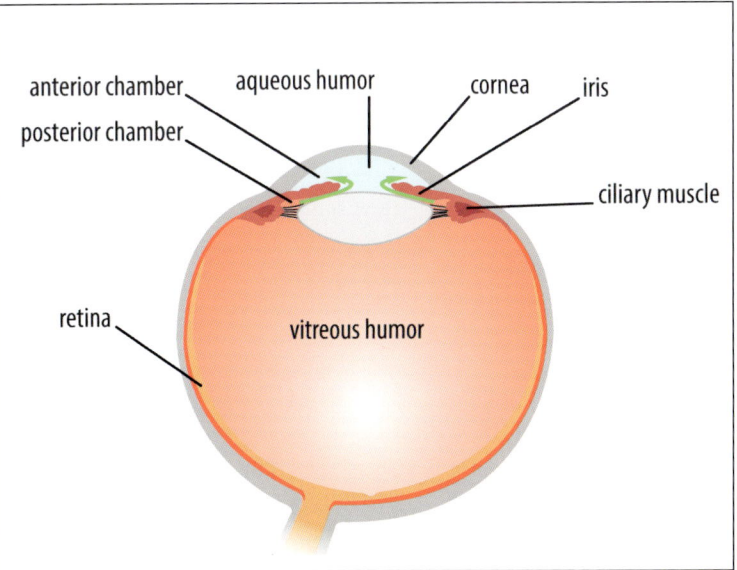

f10.2 Anatomy of the eye. Green arrows show the flow of aqueous humor.

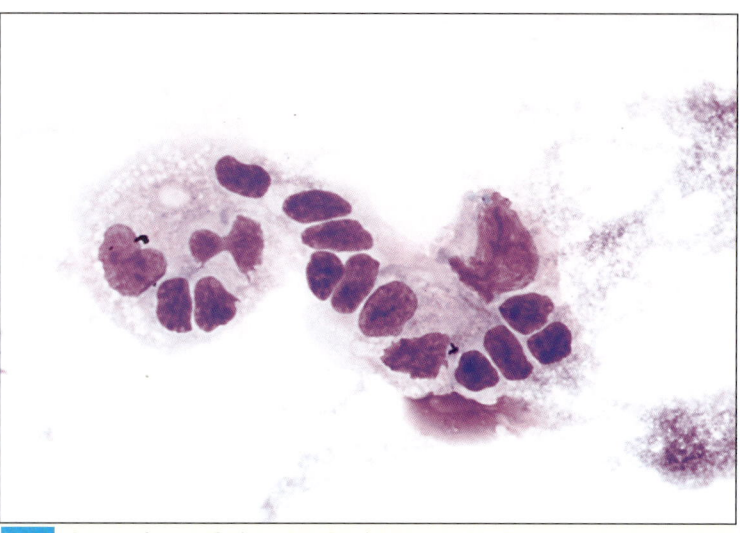

| i10.1 | Cytospin of vitreous fluid containing lymphoma |
| i10.2 | Lymphoma cells in vitreous fluid characterized by irregular nuclear contours and an atypical chromatin pattern |

the presence of disease. Diagnostic vitrectomies or vitreous aspiration taps are performed for posterior uveitis unresponsive to therapy to rule out malignancy as well as when intraocular infection is considered the primary cause of the presence of inflammation. A major indication for vitreous aspiration is to evaluate for lymphoma i10.1, i10.2 [PMID 11307054, PMID 23589676]. Flow cytometric analysis of vitreous fluid can provide additional supporting evidence for the presence of lymphoma.

Fine needle aspirations can be performed to sample localized intraocular lesions or tumors. The aspirated specimen is processed for smear/cytospin preparation and cell block preparation as previously discussed.

Aqueous fluid

Aqueous fluid is formed by the ciliary body behind the iris. It flows into the anterior chamber through the pupillary space. Aqueous fluid then travels into the angle structures and drains out of the eye f10.2.

The region in the anterior chamber at which the cornea and iris meet is known as the angle. Within the angle are some structures that make up the aqueous drainage system of the eye, including the ciliary body, the trabecular meshwork, and the canal of Schlemm.

As the aqueous fluid exits the angle, it passes through the trabecular meshwork that acts as a filter, then travels through a tiny channel in the sclera, the canal of Schlemm. The aqueous flows into minute channels, eventually being absorbed into the blood vessels of the eye.

The balance between production and drainage of aqueous fluid determines intraocular pressure of the eye. Glaucoma results when intraocular pressure rises from inability of the aqueous fluid to flow through the trabecular meshwork (open angle glaucoma) or narrowing of the angle that obstructs flow (angle closure glaucoma).

Specimen collection, requirements & stability

The time between collection and analysis should be as short as possible. While analyte stability may vary, a 4 hour delay in analysis did not affect glucose or lactate measurements in a study of 38 vitreous samples [PMID 19167848]. Glucose and lactate measurements are not affected by fluoride collection tubes [PMID 19167848].

The viscosity of vitreous fluid may hinder chemical analysis, particularly when automated chemistry analyzers are used for measurement. Pretreatment of the sample to liquefy it may be necessary. Hyaluronic acid present in the sample may be catalyzed by the addition of hyaluronidase [PMID 15027566] or heat. Ultrasonification and centrifugation have also been suggested, with comparable results [PMID 19729257, PMID 21511417]. Validation of the pretreatment technique and analytical method should be performed prior to testing.

The entirety of the ocular bulb should be gently aspirated in order to minimize analyte concentration gradients that may exist throughout the eye. Removal of the vitreous fluid, with as little disruption of the surrounding tissue, will provide the best specimen for further laboratory measurements.

It has been reported that concentration differences between the left and right eye may exist for analytes such as electrolytes [PMID 9608696]. However, other reports show no significant difference between the samples [PMID 15894848, PMID 19729257].

Chemical analysis

Chemical analysis of vitreous fluid may provide useful information in specific cases. Its uniquely isolated location delays the autolytic changes that are normally observed in blood postmortem. This makes vitreous fluid valuable in the diagnosis of metabolic diseases such as electrolyte imbalances and diabetes mellitus as well as the investigation of the postmortem interval. It can also provide clues in forensic investigations; however these are outside the scope of this text. A discussion of the more common chemical analyses performed on vitreous fluid is provided.

There are several critical issues that may affect the chemical analysis of vitreous fluid and must be appreciated prior to undertaking any laboratory investigation. Most analytical methods have been calibrated for serum and/or urine, and application of these methods to vitreous samples may not be appropriate [PMID 16781101]. In fact, no standardized methods exist for the measurement of chemical analytes in vitreous fluid [PMID 16781101]. Poor precision has also been reported for multiple analytes with this fluid type [PMID 19729257]. An earlier report revealed significant differences between analytical methods in vitreous fluid measurements for urea nitrogen, glucose, sodium, potassium and chloride [PMID 4031810]. Flame photometry, colorimetry and ion selective electrodes all performed differently in direct comparisons with this fluid type. Different preanalytical treatments of vitreous fluid samples can also affect chemical analysis [PMID 21511417]. Lastly, it is impossible to obtain reference intervals that describe the "normal" biochemical makeup of the postmortem state. Measurements must be related to similar clinical scenarios or, when possible, to antemortem values.

Glucose & glucose metabolism

Blood glucose concentrations decrease precipitously in the immediate postmortem period due to cellular and bacterial consumption. Vitreous fluid has very few cells present and is rarely contaminated with bacteria; therefore it is a preferred sample type for determining the antemortem glycemic state. Vitreous glucose concentrations decrease in the first 24 hours postmortem, but remain stable thereafter [PMID 19167848, PMID 16781101]. Historically, the combination of vitreous lactate and glucose concentrations were considered representative of the antemortem blood glucose concentration, assuming that lactate is produced during anaerobic metabolism of glucose [PMID 7076064]. A more recent study has indicated that the endogenous increase in lactate in the postmortem interval erroneously increases this blood glucose estimation, and vitreous glucose alone is a more appropriate measure of the antemortem glycemic state [PMID 19167848].

The biological decrease in glucose concentrations observed in both serum and vitreous fluid makes postmortem diagnosis of hypoglycemia difficult. Instead, vitreous is the preferred fluid to assess postmortem hyperglycemia. Clinical observations of living patients indicated that vitreous glucose concentrations are <1/2 of those found in the blood [PMID 8157178]. Glucose concentrations exceeding 10 mmol/L in the vitreous compartment may be indicative of nondiabetic hyperglycemia, diabetic ketoacidosis or hyperosmolar nonketotic hyperglycemia [PMID 19167848, PMID 21663468]; however, elevated values may also be found in other clinical situations (eg, asphyxia, congestive heart failure, hypothermia).

Ketoacidotic coma is one of the more frequent complications of uncontrolled diabetes mellitus and may be fatal. Therefore, postmortem diagnosis of ketoacidosis and the undiagnosed antemortem diabetic state are important. 3 endogenous ketone bodies (acetone, acetoacetic acid and β hydroxybutyrate) are produced by the liver as a source of energy in the absence of glucose. β hydroxybutyrate is a specific marker of ketoacidosis in the postmortem state [PMID 19167848, PMID 16139109] and vitreous concentrations correlate well with vitreous glucose concentrations [PMID 16139109]. A study of 453 cadavers assigned to diabetic and nondiabetic diagnostic groups reported that vitreous β hydroxybutyrate concentrations were statistically significantly higher in the diabetic group, indicating this measurement may be useful in cases of a negative or inconclusive autopsy [PMID 16139109]. Beyond diabetic ketoacidosis, ketone bodies may be found in a variety of other clinical situations including starvation, malnourishment, alcoholic ketoacidosis, hypothermia and infection.

Vitreous lactic acid concentrations increase postmortem due to glycolysis [PMID 19167848], which may confound the diagnosis of lactic acidosis at autopsy. However, elevated lactate concentrations may be also found in cases of diabetic or alcoholic ketoacidosis, renal or liver diseases, and toxicity associated with cyanide or iron. A recent study indicated that serum and urine methods for lactate measurement do not apply well to determining concentrations in vitreous samples [PMID 21511417]. The variation in measurement of vitreous lactate exceeded the analytical imprecision of the assay, regardless of the preanalytical treatment applied to the specimen.

Glycated protein concentrations may indicate antemortem glycemic control and aid in assessing diabetes postmortem. Vitreous fructosamine concentrations have correlated well with antemortem serum glucose concentrations [PMID 10460416, PMID 19290382]. Combined elevated vitreous fructosamine and glucose concentrations have been proposed to indicate undiagnosed antemortem hyperglycemia [PMID 19290382]. However, another study reported the sum of vitreous glucose and lactate was a better predictor of antemortem diabetes than fructosamine alone [PMID 11563732].

Insulin & c-peptide

Proinsulin is enzymatically cleaved to produce equimolar concentrations of insulin and c-peptide. This in vivo process allows for the use of c-peptide and the insulin:c-peptide ratio to differentiate between endogenous insulin production and exogenous administration of an insulin analogue. However, peptide hormones do not efficiently cross into the vitreous compartment; thus measurement of insulin and the precursor sequence c-peptide have not routinely yielded adequate results. Efforts to develop assays for the detection of insulin in vitreous fluid using mass spectrometry have only been documented recently [PMID 22102262, PMID 22779084] and are not available for routine clinical use.

Electrolytes

While vitreous fluid is considered a segregated fluid compartment, increased permeability of the retinal cell membrane and loss of active and selective membrane transport contribute to postmortem changes in analyte concentrations in this body fluid. Notably, potassium gradually and linearly diffuses into the vitreous fluid immediately postmortem. Increased potassium concentrations may therefore be useful in estimating the postmortem interval (see "Postmortem interval," below).

Sodium and chloride vitreous concentrations are relatively stable in the early postmortem period and are considered representative of the antemortem state. Values often reflect those found in the serum of healthy individuals; thus electrolyte measurement of the vitreous fluid can be useful for diagnostic purposes. Both sodium and chloride serum concentrations naturally decrease postmortem [PMID 8328447], so elevated concentrations are more often of clinical interest than decreased values. Causes of hypernatremia at autopsy are varied and include conditions of insufficient water intake, excessive fluid loss, or excessive sodium administration [PMID 19782311].

Vitreous calcium and magnesium measurements do not correlate with antemortem concentrations and do not contribute to the determination of the postmortem interval [PMID 8328447, PMID 7175469, PMID 2416687]. Additionally, calcium measurements in vitreous specimens may be affected by preanalytical liquefying steps using heat treatment or hyaluronidase [PMID 21511417].

Creatinine & urea nitrogen

Similar to many electrolytes, creatinine and urea nitrogen values in the vitreous fluid often reflect those found in the serum of healthy individuals; thus vitreous measurements may be useful for diagnostic purposes. Postmortem creatinine and urea nitrogen concentrations are relatively stable and correlate with antemortem concentrations [PMID 8328447]. Their similar stabilities and clinical utilities indicate they can be used interchangeably. Increased concentrations of creatinine and urea nitrogen are associated with disorders of nitrogen retention, primarily associated with renal dysfunction. Elevated values found in conjunction with hypernatremia may be indicative of dehydration among varied other conditions.

Alcohols

Vitreous fluid may prove valuable for the measurement of alcohols in situations where other body fluids are contaminated, diluted, or otherwise unavailable or unsuitable for testing. Ethanol can be detected in the vitreous compartment up to 2 hours after ingestion. Vitreous ethanol concentrations may be compared to blood concentrations to determine whether the individual was in the absorptive or postabsorptive phase at the time of death. However, caution should be used when interpreting vitreous ethanol values and estimations of blood ethanol concentrations from vitreous should not be made [PMID 11533077, PMID 16105262]. It should also be noted that ethanol can be produced postmortem during the decomposition process or by species of bacteria, yeast and mold, which may confound autopsy results [PMID 8838464].

Isopropanol may be present in the vitreous fluid due to ingestion or from the conversion of acetone to isopropanol. Methanol and/or formic acid may be detected if administered or ingested.

Special studies
Postmortem interval

Although several chemical analyses of the vitreous compartment have been proposed for the determination of the postmortem interval (PMI), or "time of death," including vitreous calcium, ammonia, hypoxanthine and creatine, the best investigated analyte remains vitreous potassium [PMID 8328447]. Potassium begins diffusing from the surrounding retinal cells immediately postmortem and vitreous concentrations increase linearly thereafter until equilibrium with plasma is reached. Many regression models describing the linear relationship between PMI and potassium concentrations have been used to establish equations for calculating the PMI [PMID 1452104, PMID 16439082, PMID 8328447]. These equations assume that changes in potassium concentration are proportional with time and that they occur at a constant rate. There are conflicting reports in the literature as to whether these equations are useful or accurate for determining the PMI, and they should be used with caution.

Vitreous calcium, sodium and chloride did not contribute to the PMI determination in studies of 120 [PMID 20666922] and 210 autopsies [PMID 24166687].

Microbiologic examination of vitreous fluid & endophthalmitis

Endophthalmitis is defined as a bacterial or fungal infection within the eye, involving the vitreous fluid and/or aqueous fluid. Patients typically exhibit clinical symptoms during endophthalmitis, including ocular pain, intense conjunctival inflammation, and episcleral inflammation. These infections are considered critical medical emergencies, and if left untreated can result in permanent vision loss or impairment.

Endophthalmitis is typically diagnosed through culture of the vitreous fluid after careful collection via needle aspiration and deposition into a sterile collection tube. Ideally, the specimen should be inoculated to solid media in the ophthalmology clinic, in consultation with the clinical microbiologist, though this rarely happens in practice [ISBN 978-1555816780]. If immediate inoculation is not possible, the specimen should be transported at room temperature and processed within 24 hours [ISBN 978-1555816780]. Typically the fluid yield is quite low (as a reflection of this small anatomic compartment), and as a result the specimen may require allocation to different culture conditions based on the differential diagnosis and probability of a specific classification of pathogen (eg, bacterial, fungal, AFB, parasitic). The specimen is typically diluted during collection with an irrigation fluid, which provides more fluid to use for testing, but correspondingly dilutes the sample, and therefore reduces culture, stain, immunological, and molecular sensitivity [ISBN 978-1555816780]. It is imperative that the specimen is centrifuged and the resulting sediment inoculated to the appropriate solid media to maximize culture sensitivity. Likewise, the Gram stain should be prepared (if volume allows) from a cytocentrifugal preparation (see Chapter 2) or a small sample of the centrifuged pellet (if specimen volume allows). Testing by molecular or immunological assays should be performed from an aliquot of the original specimen.

Bacterial endophthalmitis

The most common agents of bacterial endophthalmitis include *Staphylococcus aureus*, coagulase negative *Staphylococcus*, *Pseudomonas aeruginosa*, *Streptococcus pneumoniae*, viridans streptococci, *Neisseria meningitidis*, *Nocardia* species, *Bacillus cereus*, and *Propionibacterium acnes* [PMID 22173077, PMID 23438028, ISBN 978-1555816780]. The propensity of certain organisms to be found in the vitreous fluid typically is a reflection of the nature of the endophthalmitis (eg, acute postcataract, chronic postcataract, postinjection, posttraumatic, endogenous bacterial) t10.2 [PMID 23438028].

t10.2 Causative agents of different types of endophthalmitis*

Type of endophthalmitis	Known causes
Postcataract	
Acute	Coagulase negative *Staphylococcus*, *Streptococcus pneumoniae*, viridans Streptococci
Chronic	*Propionibacterium* species
Postinjection	Coagulase negative *Staphylococcus*, viridans streptococci, various fungi
Posttraumatic	*Bacillus cereus*, coagulase negative *Staphylococcus*, *Pseudomonas*, various fungi, rapid growing *Mycobacterium* species
Endogenous (hematogenously derived)	*Staphylococcus aureus*, streptococci, *Neisseria meningitidis*, *Candida* species, rapid growing *Mycobacterium* species

*Modified from [PMID 23438028]

Each of these organisms can be readily cultivated on a chocolate agar plate at 35°-37°C in an atmosphere containing 5% CO_2 and frequently a blood agar plate will also be included in the culture for aerobic bacteria if specimen volume is available. The general exception for easily cultured organisms from the aforementioned list is *Propionibacterium*, which includes species that are strictly anaerobic as well as aerotolerant. In order to effectively rule out anaerobic bacteria such as *Propionibacterium*, an anaerobic culture is required on a rich media such as Brucella blood agar.

Mycobacterial endophthalmitis

Nontuberculous mycobacteria (NTM) can also cause endophthalmitis, attributable to both exogenous and endogenous infections. The most common causes of these infections are rapid growing NTM, primarily *Mycobacterium fortuitum* and *Mycobacterium chelonae* [PMID 22173077]. If infections with NTM are suspected, it is crucial to order an acid-fast stain (recognizing the low sensitivity of this approach) as well as culture for acid-fast bacilli (AFB) on solid media such as Lowenstein-Jensen [PMID 22173077]. Rapid growing NTM may grow on standard bacteriologic culture media described above; however the growth often requires up to 7 days and may be missed if the plates are discarded prior to that time. Slow growing NTM require several weeks to grow and would not be detected in routine bacteriologic cultures held for 7 days. The slow growing NTM also are not reliably recovered on standard bacteriologic media, reaffirming the importance of culturing on specific AFB media.

Fungal endophthalmitis

Fungal endophthalmitis is extremely difficult to identify and to treat. The most common causes of fungal endophthalmitis include *Aspergillus* species, *Candida* species, and *Fusarium* species [PMID 22114969, PMID 24381050]. Most cases of *Candida* endophthalmitis are endogenous, and occur as a result of candidemia [PMID 23438028]. Other pathogenic fungi that can cause endophthalmitis, albeit less commonly, includes: the dimorphic endemic mycoses (*Blastomyces dermatitidis*, *Coccidioides* species, *Histoplasma capsulatum*, *Paracoccidioides brasiliensis*, *Sporothrix schenckii*), *Cryptococcus neoformans*, certain zygomycetes (*Rhizopus*, *Mucor*, *Rhizomucor*) and certain hyaline moulds (*Acremonium*, *Paecilomyces*, *Scedosporium*) [PMID 22173077, PMID 24381050].

Specimens should be inoculated onto Sabouraud dextrose agar, inhibitory mold agar, and/or brain heart infusion (BHI) agar with 10% sheep blood at initial setup [ISBN 978-1555816780]. Media containing cycloheximide should always be avoided as it may slow the growth or completely inhibit some fungi [PMID 10832689, PMID 86285586, ISBN 978-0812114638]. In general, selective agents in the media are not required, as the specimens should not contain "contaminants" or normal flora, which typically are a challenge for routine fungal cultures of nonsterile specimens. The plates should be incubated at 30°C for an extended period of time (up to 30 days or more). Several of these fungi listed will grow readily in culture within the first week, while others may require longer periods of incubation for growth to allow for a morphologic identification. Typically, cultures require several weeks to yield growth, and therefore empiric therapy must begin in advance of laboratory test results. Primary staining of specimens is often not performed since vitreous fluid volumes are typically limiting, and stains for fungal hyphae and yeast are generally insensitive.

Viral infections

Though culture or DFA were once the standard diagnostic tests for viral infections of the eye, culture is no longer recommended due to low sensitivity [PMID 23797960]. Vitreous fluids can be tested by PCR to identify several different viral infections with superior sensitivity. For instance, vitreous fluid can be tested by PCR in order to diagnose suspected herpesvirus mediated retinitis, including cytomegalovirus (CMV), varicella zoster virus (VZV), and herpes simplex virus (HSV) [PMID 23797960]. It is important to note that aqueous humor is also acceptable to test for retinitis (preferred for VZV and HSV), while vitreous fluid is primarily recommended for testing CMV rather than aqueous humor. Often all 3 viruses are tested from a single specimen for convenience, and aqueous humor is generally easier to collect than vitreous fluid [PMID 23797960].

Molecular testing should be performed in a laboratory that has thoroughly validated their assay for vitreous and aqueous humor, as both specimen types may inhibit PCR reactions [PMID 8567898]. Thermostable polymerases are impervious to the inhibitory effect elicited by these specimen types, and it is crucial to ascertain from the laboratory whether its assay utilizes thermostable polymerases in advance of testing [PMID 8567898]. In addition to using a thermostable polymerase, all assays should include an internal control amplification target to further control for matrix mediated inhibition.

Parasitic infections

Toxoplasma gondii and *Toxocara* species are the 2 parasitic diseases that can involve the eye and may be tested for using vitreous fluid specimens. In both infections, serological evidence of past or acute infection is typically established before invasive ocular specimens are collected, though these may be negative even in ocular infections with either parasite. Vitreous fluid testing is generally noncontributory for other parasitic infections of the eye such as ocular larval migrans with *Dirofilaria* species, scleral loiasis caused by *Loa loa*, onchocerciasis caused by *Onchocerca volvulus*, or keratitis caused by *Acanthamoeba* or microsporidia.

T gondii can be detected in vitreous fluid by testing with a sensitive molecular assay (most commonly a real time PCR). PCR has been shown to reliably confirm cases of toxoplasmosis that were supported by clinical signs and symptoms as well as serological markers [PMID 10442904]. PCR is also particularly helpful in cases where the symptoms were not typical, such as ocular toxoplasmosis, but *T gondii* was in the differential diagnosis [PMID 10442904]. Testing of serum samples for antibodies is difficult due to the high seroprevalence for *T gondii* in many populations [PMID 22712598]. Typically this testing from serum samples requires multiple IgM and IgG assays to be used on a single sample in order to confidently assign acute/recent infection via seroconversion [PMID 22712598]. This makes testing of volume limited specimens such as vitreous fluid challenging, since intraocular production of antibodies must be confidently established using at least 1 or more IgM and IgG tests [PMID 22712598]. Given the performance of molecular diagnostics in these infections, immunological testing is no longer a necessary pathway of testing, but may provide additional evidence of ocular toxoplasmosis.

Ocular toxocariasis may also be diagnosed through immunological testing of intraocular fluid such as vitreous fluid, but unlike *Toxoplasma*, molecular assays are not readily available. ELISA assays for *Toxocara* can be performed on both serum and vitreous fluid in order to support the diagnosis of ocular toxocariasis [PMID 22938514]. In fact, the vitreous fluid often has higher levels of antibody than the serum specimen [PMID 12498639, PMID 16340531]. Additionally, eosinophils are also typically detected in the vitreous fluid of patients with ocular toxocariasis, which further contributes to the diagnosis and helps to differentiate from other conditions such as cancer.

Sweat

Sweat is a clear, hypotonic solution secreted by the sweat glands in the skin. Sweating is the primary mechanism for temperature regulation of the body with a feedback loop with the hypothalamus. In addition to heat, the sweat glands secrete sweat in response to stress, physical activity and hormones.

Sweat glands consist of 2 primary types. The eccrine sweat glands and the apocrine sweat glands. The eccrine sweat glands develop in utero and are distributed over the entire body surface with a few exceptions, such as the nails, ear canal, lips, glans penis and labia minora. The apocrine sweat glands are primarily located in the armpits, areolae of the nipples, and perineal region. They increase in size and become active after puberty.

The eccrine sweat glands are primarily responsible for thermoregulation. Other important functions include excretion of water and electrolytes and preserving the skin's acidic mantle. Neurotransmitters such as acetylcholine are released in response to heat and cause sweat secretion. The eccrine glands are comprised of tubular structures with long branches. The tubular portion is tightly coiled, responsible for secreting sweat, and located in the deep skin layers. The duct portion is typically straight and is responsible for the transport of the sweat to the skin surface f10.3. Evaporation of sweat from the skin surface causes evaporative cooling.

Humans commonly produce 0.5-1.0 L of sweat per day under normal conditions. This capacity can significantly increase with increased temperature and exercise up to 10 L per day. Excessive sweating can result in significant loss of fluids and important electrolytes.

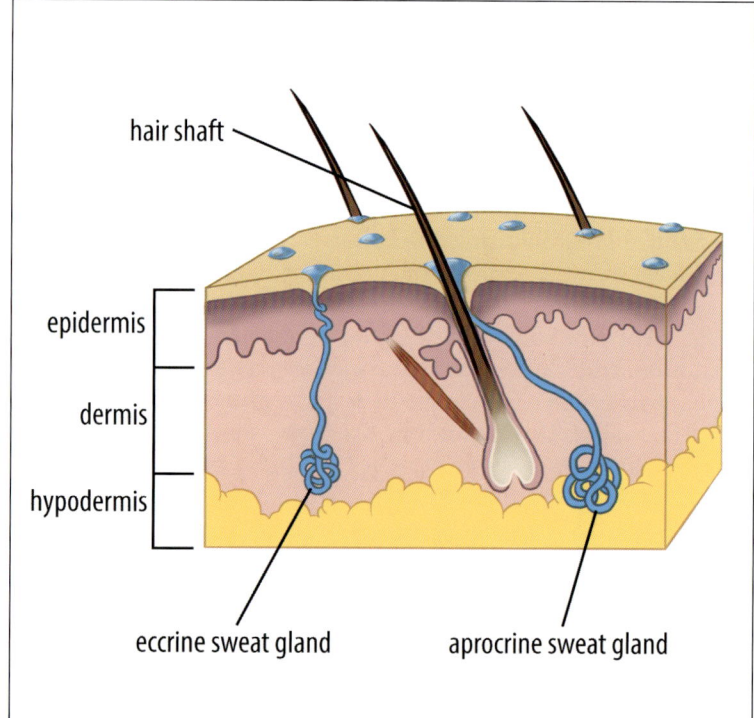

f10.3 Diagram of skin showing the sweat glands in relationship to the skin surface

Sweat is comprised predominantly of water and electrolytes. The primary electrolytes in sweat are sodium and chloride. It also contains potassium, urea, calcium, bicarbonates and a small amount of protein and glycoprotein. Eccrine sweat is hypotonic. It has a pH ranging from ~4.5-7.

Laboratory measurement of sweat chloride levels is often one of the initial tests in the workup of cystic fibrosis. Cystic fibrosis (CF) is an inherited disorder that affects children and young adults. Classic CF is more common in Caucasians with an incidence of 1/3,000. It is caused by mutations in the cystic fibrosis transmembrane conductance regulator (*CFTR*) gene **f10.4**. The defective gene and protein product results in unusually thick and sticky mucous. This abnormal mucus leads to clogging of lung passages resulting in increased infections as well as pancreatic dysfunction due to obstruction of secretion of enzymes needed for food digestion and absorption. Patients with cystic fibrosis may present with salty tasting skin (due to the increased sodium and chloride levels), recurrent lung infections, persistent coughing, shortness of breath, poor growth and weight gain and greasy or bulky stools.

Individual states within the United States have various screening guidelines for cystic fibrosis testing as part of their newborn screening program. This typically involves placing a few drops of the infant's blood onto a Guthrie card for analysis by a state laboratory. This analysis commonly measures immunoreactive trypsinogen (IRT) levels as an indication of pancreatic function. Blood samples from infants with elevated IRT levels are often further analyzed for *CFTR* gene mutations [PMID 14569807, PMID 15173476, PMID 9532980]. The area of newborn screening for cystic fibrosis continues to undergo reevaluation to determine the best newborn screening approaches [PMID 23810505, PMID 23891278]. The reader should check with his or her state for the latest requirements for newborn screening.

Furthermore, as part of the workup for cystic fibrosis, infants with a positive cystic fibrosis newborn screen or patients suspected of having cystic fibrosis due to clinical findings and medical history, often will undergo a sweat chloride test (see below).

Specimen collection, requirements & stability

The collection of sweat for chloride and other testing is highly specialized and is usually limited to centers with adequate expertise. Approved guidelines for collection and analysis are available for reference [PMID 17586196, CLSI C34-A3 CLSI 2009]. Localized sweat production for chemical analysis is induced by applying the cholinergic drug, pilocarpine nitrate, to the skin and usually on the forearm. The drug is delivered directly into the skin via a small electric current in a process referred to as iontophoresis. The current delivers pilocarpine from the positive electrode and a negative electrode containing an electrolyte solution completes the circuit. Following stimulation, the arm is cleaned, dried and sweat is collected onto preweighed sodium chloride free filter paper or gauze or into microbore tubing (Macroduct, Wescor, Inc) that is affixed to the skin. After a maximum of 30 minutes collection time, electrolyte content is determined directly from the filter paper, gauze or tubing. Electrodes and collection devices should be of standard sizes to eliminate variability.

Adequate sweat rates are critical for accurate measurement. Low sweat rates are associated with decreased electrolyte concentrations and increased probability of sample evaporation. Sweat rates of 1 g/m^2/minute minimum are recommended for valid results; however, minimum sweat weights and volumes will vary with the size of the electrodes and stimulation area, the collecting device used and the length of collection time [PMID 17586196]. Typical minimum sample volumes for 30 minute collection protocols are 75 mg on filter paper or gauze, or 15 µL using microbore tubing [CLSI C34-A3 CLSI 2009].

To ensure adequate sample collection, testing of sweat in asymptomatic newborns is not recommended until after 2 weeks of age and a minimum of 2 kg body weight [PMID 18639722]. Symptomatic newborns can be tested as early as 48 hours after birth if adequate sample volume can be obtained [PMID 18639722].

Many institutions employ the practice of obtaining sweat collections from 2 locations from each patient. This not only provides an internal control but also increases the likelihood of obtaining adequate sample volume from at least 1 site. Bilateral samples should not be pooled for a single analysis, but measured independently. Laboratories should determine acceptability criteria for the 2 results, but agreement within 10 mmol/L for values ≤60 mmol/L or within 15 mmol/L for values >60 mmol/L is often recommended [PMID 17586196].

Sweat samples should be tested soon after collection. If delayed testing is necessary, the gauze or filter paper should be weighed immediately after collection and then stored tightly sealed up to 72 hours at 4°C [CLSI C34-A3 CLSI 2009]. Samples collected in microbore tubing should be transferred to another tube, sealed and stored up to 72 hours prior to processing.

Chemical analysis
Sweat chloride

Sweat for the determination of chloride concentrations is collected as described in the section "Specimen collection, requirements and stability" above, often using preweighed filter paper or gauze. After collection, the filter paper or gauze is removed and reweighed to determine the density of sweat obtained. Sweat is eluted from the collection device for further analysis. The recommended detection method for chloride in sweat is coulometric titration using a chloridometer, and duplicate measurements are advised, when possible. Other methods are available, but should be thoroughly validated for this specific sample type. In particular, the lower end of the measurement range should be capable of detecting concentrations as low as 10 mmol/L.

Reference intervals for sweat chloride vary by age. For infants under the age of 6 months, chloride values ≤29 mmol/L are considered normal (cystic fibrosis unlikely), values 30-59 mmol/L are considered intermediate (recommend repeat testing) and values ≥60 mmol/L are indicative of cystic fibrosis. Individuals >6 months of age have slightly higher normal values: chloride values ≤39 mmol/L

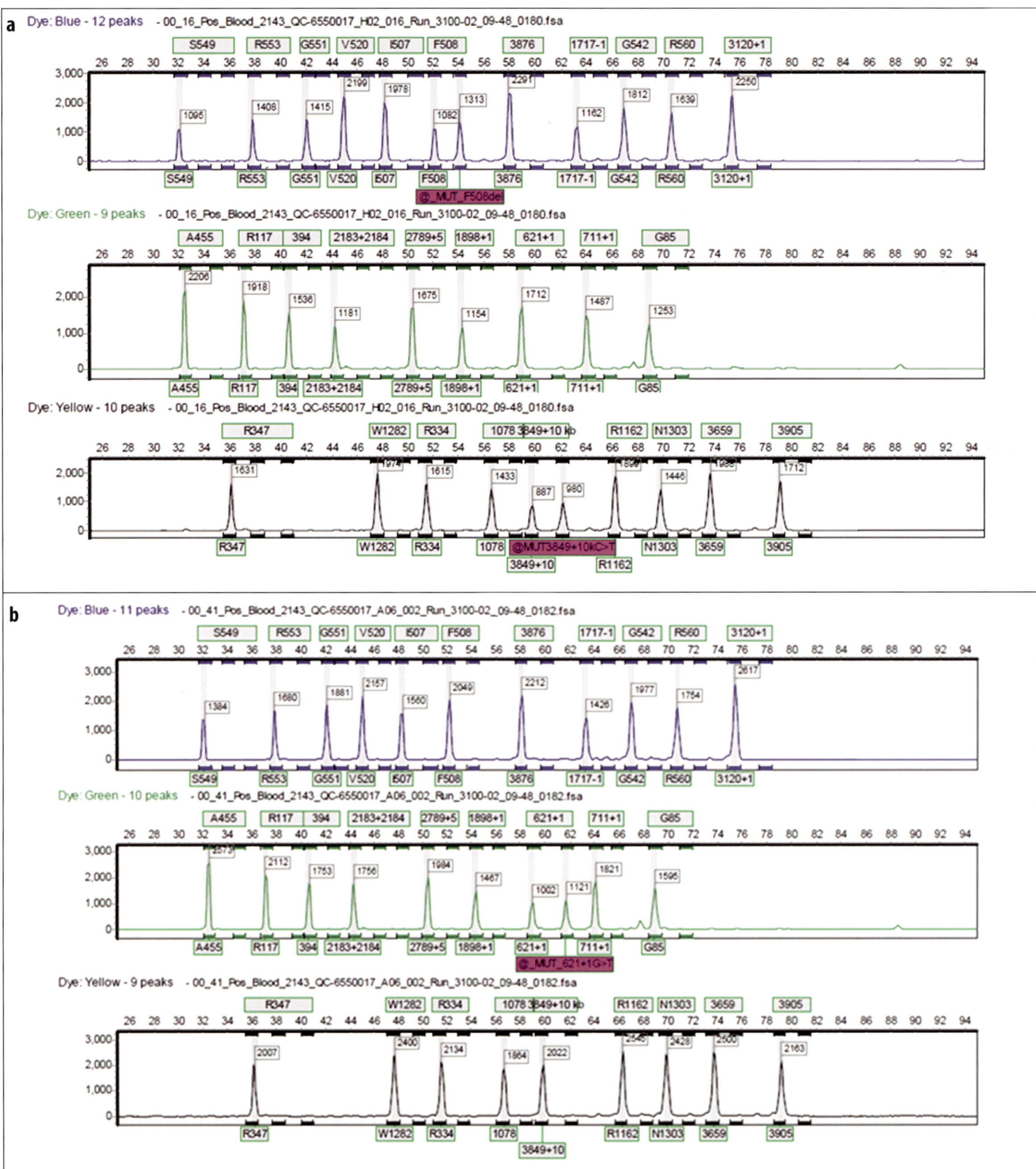

f10.4 Electropheragrams depicting a targeted mutation panel for common cystic fibrosis (CF) mutations; the method performed is an Oligation Ligation Assay (OLA; Abbott Molecular, Abbott Park, Illinois, USA) Purified DNA is amplified by polymerase chain reaction (PCR), followed by probe ligation; products are separately by capillary electrophoresis
a 2 mutations (F508del and 3849+10kb C>T) indicate that this individual is affected with CF
b 1 mutation (621+1G>T) indicates that this individual is at least a CF carrier. If this patient had CF symptoms or a positive sweat chloride test, CFTR gene sequencing may be performed to identify a second mutation not detected by a common mutation panel (images courtesy of Dr Elaine Lyon, ARUP Laboratory/University of Utah, Salt Lake City)

are considered normal (cystic fibrosis unlikely), values 40-59 mmol/L are intermediate (recommend repeat testing) and values ≥60 mmol/L are indicative of cystic fibrosis. Overall, individuals diagnosed with cystic fibrosis as adults have lower chloride values than those diagnosed in infancy. Diagnostic criteria for cystic fibrosis require elevated sweat chloride values on 2 or more occasions [CLSI C34-A3 CLSI 2009].

Measurements for sodium and osmolality in sweat have been performed historically; however these are not recommended and do not provide diagnostic information for cystic fibrosis [CLSI C34-A3 CLSI 2009].

Qualitative tests for sweat conductivity are commercially available as screening tests for cystic fibrosis. These results are not directly equivalent to sweat chloride determinations due to the presence of other ions in sweat such as bicarbonate and lactate. Patients with positive conductivity results should be referred to an accredited center for quantitative sweat chloride testing.

Molecular testing

In addition to sweat chloride testing, CF DNA mutation analysis provides further confirmation or exclusion of a diagnosis of CF. This testing is typically performed on peripheral blood samples. Everyone inherits 2 copies of the *CFTR* gene. Some inherited copies of the gene are mutated. Inheriting 2 mutated copies of the gene in association with clinical symptoms typically indicates the patient has cystic fibrosis. Over 1,500 CF mutations have been identified. Various FDA approved sequencing kits are commercially available for the detection of mutations in the *CFTR* gene f10.4. Genotype testing, though, is not recommended for the general population. It is recommended that patients with a positive family history of cystic fibrosis, expectant couples or those planning pregnancy and individuals with symptoms of cystic fibrosis be considered for testing.

Artifacts & pitfalls

- Hemorrhage within vitreous fluid can affect many chemical analyte values
- A positive newborn screening test for cystic fibrosis (CF) by immunoreactive trypsinogen is not diagnostic of CF and requires confirmation by mutation analysis

Key points

- Saliva is a filtrate of plasma comprised primarily of water
- HIV testing of saliva is used only for screening and requires confirmation testing
- Measurement of potassium levels in vitreous fluid can aid in the determination of the postmortem interval or time of death
- Endophthalmitis is a bacterial or fungal infection of vitreous and/or aqueous fluid
- Cystic fibrosis is an inherited disorder caused by mutations in the cystic fibrosis transmembrane conductance regulator (CFTR) gene

References

PMID 10442904 Montoya JG, Parmley S, Liesenfeld O et al [1999] Use of the polymerase chain reaction for diagnosis of ocular toxoplasmosis. *Ophthalmology* 106(8):1554-63

PMID 10460416 Osuna E, García-Víllora A, Pérez-Cárceles MD et al [1999] Vitreous humor fructosamine concentrations in the autopsy diagnosis of diabetes mellitus. *Int J Legal Med* 112(5):275-9

PMID 10832689 Tanure MA, Cohen EJ, Sudesh S et al [2000] Spectrum of fungal keratitis at Wills Eye Hospital, Philadelphia, Pennsylvania. *Cornea* 19:307-312

PMID 11307054 Buggage R, Chan C, Nussenblatt R [2011] Ocular manifestations of central nervous system lymphoma. *Curr Opin Oncol* 13(3):137-42

PMID 11533077 Jones AW, Holmgren P [2001] Uncertainty in estimating blood ethanol concentrations by analysis of vitreous humour. *J Clin Pathol* 54(9):699-702

PMID 11563732 Osuna E, García-Víllora A, Pérez-Cárceles M et al [2001] Glucose and lactate in vitreous humor compared with the determination of fructosamine for the postmortem diagnosis of diabetes mellitus. *Am J Forensic Med Pathol* 22(3):244-9

PMID 12498639 Magnaval JF, Malard L, Morassin B et al [2002] Immunodiagnosis of ocular toxocariasis using Western-blot for the detection of specific anti-*Toxocara* IgG and CAP for the measurement of specific anti-*Toxocara* IgE. *J Helminthol* 76:335-339

PMID 1452104 Gamero Lucas JJ, Romero JL, Ramos HM et al [1992] Precision of estimating time of death by vitreous potassium—comparison of various equations. *Forensic Sci Int* 56(2):137-45

PMID 14569807 Wang L, Freedman S [2002] Laboratory tests for the diagnosis of cystic fibrosis. *Am J Clin Pathol* 117Suppl:S109-15

PMID 15027566 Garg U, Althahabi R, Amirahmadi V et al [2004] Hyaluronidase as a liquefying agent for chemical analysis of vitreous fluid. *J Forensic Sci* 49(2):388-91

PMID 15173476 Comeau A, Parad R, Dorkin H et al [2004] Population-based newborn screening for genetic disorders when multiple mutation DNA testing is incorporated: a cystic fibrosis newborn screening model demonstrating increased sensitivity but more carrier detections. *Pediatrics* 113(6):1573-81

PMID 15576290 Choo RE, Huestis MA [2004] Oral fluid as a diagnostic tool. *Clin Chem Lab Med* 42(11):1273-87

PMID 15894848 Mulla A, Massey KL, Kalra J [2005] Vitreous humor biochemical constituents: evaluation of between-eye differences. *Am J Forensic Med Pathol* 26(2):146-9

PMID 16002538 Chatterton RT Jr, Mateo ET, Hou N et al [2005] Characteristics of salivary profiles of oestradiol and progesterone in premenopausal women. *J Endocrinol* 86(1):77-84

PMID 16105262 Honey D, Caylor C, Luthi R et al [2005] Comparative alcohol concentrations in blood and vitreous fluid with illustrative case studies. *J Anal Toxicol* 29(5):365-9

PMID 16139109 Osuna E, Vivero G, Conejero J et al [2005] Postmortem vitreous humor β-hydroxybutyrate: its utility for the postmortem interpretation of diabetes mellitus. *Forensic Sci Int* 153(2-3):189-95

PMID 1620213 Kidwell DA [1992] Discussion: caveats in testing for drugs of abuse. *NIDA Res Monogr* 117:98-120

PMID 16340531 Stewart JM, Cubillan LD, Cunningham ET Jr [2005] Prevalence, clinical features, and causes of vision loss among patients with ocular toxocariasis. *Retina* 25:1005-1013

PMID 1640691 Schramm W, Smith RH, Craig PA et al [1992] Drugs of abuse in saliva: a review. *J Anal Toxicol* 16(1):1-9

PMID 16439082 Madea B, Rödig A [2006] Time of death dependent criteria in vitreous humor: accuracy of estimating the time since death. *Forensic Sci Int* 164(2-3):87-92

PMID 1645882 Demmler GJ [1991] Infectious Diseases Society of America and Centers for Disease Control: summary of a workshop on surveillance for congenital cytomegalovirus disease. *Rev Infect Dis* 13:315-29

PMID 16781101 Madea B, Musshoff F [2007] Postmortem biochemistry. *Forensic Sci Int* 165(2-3):165-71

PMID 17456296 Dorn LD, Lucke JF, Loucks TL et al [2007] Salivary cortisol reflects serum cortisol: analysis of circadian profiles. *Ann Clin Biochem* 44(Pt 3):281-4

PMID 17586196 LeGrys VA, Yankaskas JR, Quittell LM et al [2007] Diagnostic sweat testing: the Cystic Fibrosis Foundation guidelines. *J Pediatr* 151(1):85-9

PMID 18057379 Kidambi S, Raff H, Findling JW [2007] Limitations of nocturnal salivary cortisol and urine free cortisol in the diagnosis of mild Cushing syndrome. *Eur J Endocrinol* 157(6):725-31

PMID 18334580 Nieman LK, Biller BM, Findling JW et al [2008] The diagnosis of Cushing syndrome: an Endocrine Society Clinical Practice Guideline. *J Clin Endocrinol Metab* 93(5):1526-40

PMID 18639722 Farrell PM, Rosenstein BJ, White TB et al [2008] Cystic Fibrosis Foundation guidelines for diagnosis of cystic fibrosis in newborns through older adults: Cystic Fibrosis Foundation consensus report. *J Pediatr* 153(2):S4-S14

PMID 19167848 Zilg B, Alkass K, Berg S et al [2009] Postmortem identification of hyperglycemia. *Forensic Sci Int* 185(1-3):89-95

PMID 19176642 Wood P [2009] Salivary steroid assays—research or routine? *Ann Clin Biochem* 46(Pt 3):183-96

PMID 19290382 Vivero G, Vivero-Salmerón G, Pérez Cárceles MD et al [2008] Combined determination of glucose and fructosamine in vitreous humor as a post-mortem tool to identify antemortem hyperglycemia. *Rev Diabet Stud* 5(4):220-4

PMID 19729257 Thierauf A, Musshoff F, Madea B [2009] Postmortem biochemical investigations of vitreous humor. *Forensic Sci Int* 192(1-3):78-82

PMID 19782311 Ingham AI, Byard RW [2009] The potential significance of elevated vitreous sodium levels at autopsy. *J Forensic Leg Med* 16(8):437-40

PMID 20666922 Jashnani KD, Kale SA, Rupani AB [2010] Vitreous humor: biochemical constituents in estimation of postmortem interval. *J Forensic Sci* 55(6):1523-7

PMID 21288853 Delaney KP, Branson BM, Uniyal A et al [2011] Evaluation of the performance characteristics of 6 rapid HIV antibody tests. *Clin Infect Dis* 52(2):257-263

PMID 21511417 Blana SA, Musshoff F, Hoeller T et al [2011] Variations in vitreous humor chemical values as a result of preanalytical treatment. *Forensic Sci Int* 210(1-3):263-70

PMID 21631323 Boppana SB, Ross SA, Shimamura M et al [2011] Saliva polymerase-chain-reaction assay for cytomegalovirus screening in newborns. National Institute on Deafness and Other Communication Disorders CHIMES Study. *N Engl J Med* 364(22):2111-8

PMID 21663468 Boulagnon C, Garnotel R, Fornes P et al [2011] Post-mortem biochemistry of vitreous humor and glucose metabolism: an update. *Clin Chem Lab Med* 49(8):1265-70

PMID 21940910 Drobnik A, Judd C, Banach D et al [2011] Public health implications of rapid hepatitis C screening with an oral swab for community-based organizations serving high risk populations. *Am J Public Health* 101(11):2151-2155

PMID 22102262 Thevis M, Thomas A, Schänzer W et al [2012] Measuring insulin in human vitreous humour using LC-MS/MS. *Drug Test Anal* 4(1):53-6

PMID 22114969 Chhablani J [2011] Fungal endophthalmitis. *J Expert Rev Anti Infect Ther* 9(12):1191-201

PMID 22173077 Garg P [2012] Fungal, mycobacterial, and *Nocardia* infections and the eye: an update. *Eye (Lond)* 26(2):245-51

PMID 22712598 Butler NJ, Furtado JM, Winthrop KL et al [2013] Ocular toxoplasmosis II: clinical features, pathology and management. *Clin Experiment Ophthalmol* 41(1):95-108

PMID 22779084 Sklan A [2012] Bullseye: successful determination of insulin in vitreous humor by LC-MS/MS. *Bioanalysis* 4(9):991

PMID 22938514 Arevalo JF, Espinoza JV, Arevalo FA [2013] Ocular toxocariasis. *J Pediatr Ophthalmol Strabismus* 50(2):76-86

PMID 23034833 Corstjens PL, Abrams WR, Malamud D [2012] Detecting viruses by using salivary diagnostics. *J Am Dent Assoc* 143(10Suppl):12S-8S

PMID 23438028 Durand ML [2013] Endophthalmitis. *Clin Microbiol Infect* 19(3):227-34

PMID 23589676 Matsuoka M, Yoshida H, Kinoshita Y et al [2013] 2 cases of intraocular lymphoma diagnosed by analysis of vitreous and infusion fluid. *Clin Ophthalmol* 7:691-4

PMID 23797960 Newman H, Gooding C [2013] Viral ocular manifestations: a broad overview. *Rev Med Virol* 23(5):281-94

PMID 2416687 Siddamsetty AK, Verma SK, Kohli A et al [2013] Estimation of time since death from electrolyte, glucose and calcium analysis of postmortem vitreous humour in semi-arid climate. *Med Sci Law* Epub ahead of print

PMID 24381050 Buchta V, Feuermannová A, Váša M et al [2014] Outbreak of fungal endophthalmitis due to *Fusarium oxysporum* following cataract surgery. *Mycopathologia* Epub ahead of print

PMID 3320544 Vining RF, McGinley RA [1987] The measurement of hormones in saliva: possibilities and pitfalls. *J Steroid Biochem* 27(1-3):81-94

PMID 4031810 Coe JI, Apple FS [1985] Variations in vitreous humor chemical values as a result of instrumentation. *J Forensic Sci* 30(3):828-35

PMID 7076064 Sippel H, Möttönen M [1982] Combined glucose and lactate values in vitreous humour for postmortem diagnosis of diabetes mellitus. *Forensic Sci Int* 19(3):217-22

PMID 7175469 Dufour DR [1982] Lack of correlation of postmortem vitreous humor calcium concentration with antemortem serum calcium concentration. *J Forensic Sci* 27(4):889-93

PMID 7926142 Delfs TM, Klein S, Fottrell P et al [1994] 24-hour profiles of salivary progesterone. *Fertil Steril* 62(5):960-6

PMID 8157178 Lundquist O, Osterlin S [1994] Glucose concentration in the vitreous of nondiabetic and diabetic human eyes. *Graefes Arch Clin Exp Ophthalmol* 232(2):71-4

PMID 8215090 Cone EJ [1993] Saliva testing for drugs of abuse. *Ann N Y Acad Sci* 694:91-127

PMID 8328447 Coe JI [1993] Postmortem chemistry update. Emphasis on forensic application. *Am J Forensic Med Pathol* 14(2):91-117

PMID 8567898 Wiedbrauk DL, Werner JC, Drevon AM [1995] Inhibition of PCR by aqueous and vitreous fluids. *J Clin Microbiol* 33(10):2643-6

PMID 86285586 Chern KC, Meisler DM, Wilhelmus KR et al [1996] Corneal anesthetic abuse and *Candida* keratitis. *Ophthalmology* 103:37-40

PMID 8838464 O'Neal CL, Poklis A [1996] Postmortem production of ethanol and factors that influence interpretation: a critical review. *Am J Forensic Med Pathol* 17(1):8-20

PMID 9532980 [1997] Genetic testing for cystic fibrosis. *NIH Consens Statement* 15(4):1-17

PMID 9608696 Pounder DJ, Carson DO, Johnston K et al [1998] Electrolyte concentration differences between left and right vitreous humor samples. *J Forensic Sci* 43(3):604-7

ISBN 978-0812114638 Kwon-Chung KJ, Bennett J [1992] *Medical Mycology*. Lea & Febiger, p45-46

ISBN 978-1555816780 Baron EJ, Thomson RB Jr [2011] Specimen collection, transport, and processing: bacteriology. In: *Manual of Clinical Microbiology*, 10e. ASM Press, p228-271

CLSI C34-A3 CLSI [2009] *Sweat Testing: Sample Collection and Quantitative Chloride Analysis; Approved Guideline*, 3e. CLSI document C34-A3. Clinical and Laboratory Standards Institute

Index

Bold pages indicate illustrations; *italic pages* indicate tables

A

Absorption spectrophotometry, detection of cerebrospinal fluid bilirubin by, 72
Acanthamoeba species, 80
Acid-base disturbances, 180
Acid-fast bacilli and fungal culture, 19-20
Aciduria, 198
Acinetobacter baumannii, 75, 76
Acquired immunodeficiency syndrome (AIDS), 115, 201
Acridine orange test, 172
Acrosin, 170
Acrosome reaction, 162
 assays showing, 170, *171*
N-acteyl-D-glucosaminidase, 152
Acute calcific periarthritis, 149
Acute leukemia, 63-65, *64*, *65*
Acute lymphocytic leukemia (ALL), 64
Acute myelogenous leukemia (AML), 64
 involvement of central nervous system by, 65
Acute pancreatitis, 120
Acute pericarditis, 90
Acute peritonitis, 120
Adenocarcinoma
 colon, 128
 distinguishing benign mesothelial cells from cells in, 97, *97*
 metastatic, 92, 110
 rectum, 128
 stomach, **126**, 128
Adenosine deaminase (ADA)
 cerebrospinal fluid and, 72
 peritoneal fluid and, 133
 pleural and pericardial fluids and, 112-113, 115
 synovial fluid and, 152
Agglutination, 164

Albumin, 69, 129
 total protein and, 69
 in urine, 199
Albuminuria, 199
Alcohols, 212
Aldosterone, 208
Alizarin red S staining, 13
Alkaline phosphatase, 131, 152
Alkaline phosphatase-antialkaline phosphatase detection (APAAP) method, 21
Alkalinuria, 198
Alkaptonuria, 145
Aluminum phosphate crystals, 146
Alzheimer disease, 74
Amebic hepatic abscess, 115
American College of Medical Genetics and Genomics (ACMG) Standards and Guidelines for Clinical Genetics Laboratories, 28
American College of Obstetricians and Gynecologists
 on pregnancy loss associated with amniocentesis, 32
 on women undergoing an invasive prenatal procedure, 41
Amniocentesis, 32
 complications of, 32
 in diagnosing premature rupture of membranes, 33
 for genetic analysis, 39
 pregnancy loss associated with, 32
Amniocytes, cell culture of, 39
Amniotic fluid, 31-42
 anatomy and pathophysiology, **31**, 31-32
 chemical analysis, 34-38
  bilirubin, 32, **35**, 35-36, **36**
  cholinesterase, 35
  α fetoprotein, 34-35
  lamellar body count, 37-38
  lecithin to sphingomyelin ratio, 37, **37**

 phosphatidylglycerol, 38
 pulmonary surfactants, 36-37
 chemical markers of ruptured membranes, 38
 clinical indications for testing of, 32, *32*
 composition of, 31
 contamination of, with whole blood, 38
 culture of cells, 27
 discoloration of, 6
 functions of, 31
 gross (macroscopic) examination of, 6
 microbiologic examination, 41-42
  vertically transmitted infections, 41-42, *42*
 premature rupture of membranes, 33-34
 prenatal diagnosis of chromosomal abnormalities, **39**, 39-41
 specimen collection, requirements and stability, 32
  gross examination, 33
  microscopic examination, 33
 spectrum of bacteria found in, 41
 transport of, 27
 volume of, 31-32
Amoebic encephalitis, 80
Amylase, 113, 130
Amyloid arthropathy, 145
Amyloid fragments, 146
Anaerobic transfer tubes, 5
Analytical specificity experiments, 18
Analytic variables, 2
Analyzers, 13
Anaplastic large cell lymphoma, **106**
Anencephaly, 34
Angioedema, 142
Angiostrongylus cantonensis, 81
Ankylosing spondylitis, 151, 154
Anticoagulants, 5
Anti D immune globulin, 35

Index

Antigen detection, 18
Antinuclear antibodies (ANA), 113-114
    detection of, in pleural fluid, 114
Antisperm antibodies, 168
    testing, 168-169
        ELISA assay for antisperm antibodies, 169
        immunobead assay, 169
        mixed agglutination assay, 169
Apatite, 11, 146
Apocrine sweat glands, 214
Aqueous fluid, 210, **210**
Arachnoid mater, 45
Arachnoid villi, 45
Arboviruses, 77
Arenavirus lymphocytic choriomeningitis virus (LCMV), 78
Arthritides, classification of, **138**
Arthritis
    bacterial, 144
    degenerative, 146
    fungal, 144
    gouty, 146
    psoriatic, 141
    rheumatoid, 144
    septic, 144-145, 146, 148-149, 154-155
Arthrocentesis, 138, 139
Artificial insemination (AI), 161
Ascites, 119
    chylous, 121
Ascitic fluid, 119
Aseptic meningitis, 77
Aspartate aminotransferase (AST), 152
Aspergillus, 79, 133
Assisted reproductive technologies (ART), 161
Aureobasidium pullans, 79
Automated cell counters, 141
Automated cell counts, 9
Automated counting methods, 51
Azoospermia, 165
Azotemia, 179, 180
Azurophilic granules, 59

B

Bacillus anthracis, 114
Bacillus Calmette-Guérin (BCG) vaccine, 80
Bacterial arthritis, 144
Bacterial culture, 19
Bacterial encephalitis, 70
Bacterial endophthalmitis, 213, *213*
Bacterial meningitis, 75-77, *76*
    cerebrospinal fluid examination and, 46
Bacterial peritonitis, 119, 123
Bacterial urinary tract infections, 201
Bacteriological techniques, 18-19
    acid-fast bacilli and fungal culture, 19-20
    bacterial culture, 19 g stain, 19
Bacteroides fragilis, 114
Balamuthia mandrillaris, 80
Basic calcium phosphates (BCP) crystals, 149
Basilar skull fractures, 58-59
Basophils, 93, 101
B cell phenotype, 129
B cell populations, flow cytometry in evaluating, 24
Bence Jones proteinuria, 198
Benign mesothelial cells, distinguishing from adenocarcinoma cells, 97, *97*
Bilateral effusions, 110
Bilirubin
    amniotic fluid and, **35**, 35-36, **36**
    cerebrospinal fluid and, 50, 71-72, **72**
    peritoneal fluid and, 129-130
    in urine, 200-201
Biliverdin, 201
Binucleate synovial lining cell, **143**
Biomarkers, 154
Biopsy, pleural, 91
Biotin-avidin conjugation (ABC) method, 21
Birefringent crystal, 13, 16, **16**
BK virus, 202-203
BK virus nephropathy, 202
Black yeasts, 78
Bladder infections, 180
Bladder tumor antigens in urine, 204-205, *205*
Blastomyces dermatitidis, 79
Blood-brain barrier, 45
    breakdown of, 46
Blood culture bottles, 5
Blood in urine, 200
Blood urea nitrogen (BUN), 180
Body fluids
    important indications for evaluation of, 1
    reasons for examination of, 1
    specimen types and transportation of samples, 26-27
Bone marrow cells, presence of, in cerebrospinal fluid, 57
Borrelia burgdorferi, 156
Bradykinin, 154
Brain herniation, 48
Brain injury markers, 73
Breast carcinoma, 109, 128
    immunohistochemical methods for determination of prognosis and choice of therapy in, 22
    metastatic, **103**
    pleural effusions of, 110
Bright field light microscopy, 12, 182
Bronchopneumonia, 89
Brucella species, 19, 114
Brucellosis, 113, 115
Bull's eye rash, 157
Burkitt lymphoma, 66, **107**, **128**

C

Calcific periarthritis, acute, 149
Calcium oxalate crystals, 16, **16**, 150
Calcium oxalate monohydrate/dihydrate, 146
Calcium phosphates, 146
Calcium pyrophosphate deposition disease, 148
Calcium pyrophosphate dihydrate (CPPD) crystals, 11, 13, 15, 146
Calculi in urine, 204, *204*
Cancer antigen 15-3 (CA15-3), 113
Cancer antigen 19-9 (CA19-9), 113, 132
Cancer antigen 125 (CA125), 113, 132
Candida meningitis, 78
Capillary endothelium, 89
Carcinoembryonic antigen (CEA), 73, 113, 132
Carcinoma
    breast, 109, 128
        immunohistochemical methods for determination of prognosis and choice of therapy in, 22
        metastatic, **103**
        pleural effusions of, 110
    colon, metastasis, **126**
    esophageal, **105**
    gastrointestinal, 109
    lung
        metastatic, **103**
        small cell, **103**, 110
        squamous cell, **103**
    metastatic, **104**
        of unknown primary, **103**
    metastatic neuroendocrine, **105**
    metastatic prostate, 106
    ovarian, 109, **126**, **127**, 128
    prostate, **127**

urothelial, 180, 184
    fluorescence in situ hybridization (FISH) for detection of, 205
    Carnoy fixative, 27, 39
Cartilage cells, 144, 145
    in cerebrospinal fluid, 57
Casts, urinary, 194, *194*, **194-197**
Catheterization, 5
Cell block preparations, 11
Cell concentration and cytospin preparation, 9-10
    equipment and reagents, 9
    procedure, 9-10
Cell counts, 1, 51-52, *52*
Cell culture
    of amniocytes, 39
    of amniotic fluid cells, 27
Cell lysis, 52
Cellular atypia, causes of, *184*
Centrifugation, 50
Cerebral herniation, 47
Cerebrospinal fluid (CSF), 45-83
    abnormal cytology, 53, **59**, 59-63, **60**, **61**, *61*, **62**, *62*, *63*
    analysis for malignancy, 63-68
        acute leukemia, 63-65, *64*, *65*
        chronic leukemias, 65
        malignant lymphomas, 65-66, *66*
        metastatic, 67, **68**
        primary central nervous system tumors, 66-67, **67**
    anatomy and pathophysiology, **45**, 45-46, *46*
    changes in, following hemorrhage, 61, *61*
    chemical analysis, 69
        adenosine deaminase, 72
        bilirubin, 71-72, **72**
        brain injury markers, 73
        C reactive protein, 70
        electrolytes and acid-base balance, 73-74
        glucose, 69
        immunoglobulins, 70
        lactate, 70
        myelin basic protein, 71
        neurodegenerative disease markers, 74
        total protein and albumin, 69
        transferrin, 71
        tumor markers, 72-73
    clinical indications and recommended laboratory studies, 46, *46*, *47*
    colors for, 6
    gross examination, 6, *49*, 49-50, *50*
    as laboratory methods, 4, *5*
    macrophages/histiocytes in, 54, **55**
    microbiologic examination, 74-82, *75*
        bacterial meningitis, 75-77, *76*
        free living amoebic infections, **77**, 80-81
        fungal meningitis, **77**, 78-80, **79**
        neuroborreliosis, 81-82
        neurosyphilis, 82
        parasitic meningitis/meningoencephalitis, **75**, 81
        tuberculous meningitis, **77**, 80
        viral meningitis, **77**, 77-78
    microscopic examination, 50-53
        cell counts, 51-52, *52*
        differential count, *52*, 53, *53*
        normal cytology, 54-58, **55**, **56**, **57**, *57*, **58**
    reference values for, *46*
    specimen collection, requirements and stability, *46*, *47*, 47-49, *48*
Chamber differential, 10
Charcot-Leyden crystals, 101, 146, 150
Chemical analysis, 1, 69
    adenosine deaminase, 72
    of amniotic fluid, 34-38
        bilirubin, **35**, 35-36, **36**
        cholinesterase, 35
        α fetoprotein, 34-35
        lamellar body count, 37-38
        lecithin to sphingomyelin ratio, 37, **37**
        phosphatidylglycerol, 38
        pulmonary surfactant, 36-37
    bilirubin, 71-72, **72**
    brain injury markers, 73
    C reactive protein, 70
    electrolytes and acid-base balance, 73-74
    glucose, 69
    immunoglobulins, 70
    lactate, 70
    myelin basic protein, 71
    neurodegenerative disease markers, 74
    total protein and albumin, 69
    transferrin, 71
    tumor markers, 72-73
Chemical markers of ruptured membranes, 38
Chemistry, 17-18
Chlamydophila psittaci, 116
Choleperitoneum, 129-130
Cholesterol, 11, 130, 146
    in pleural effusions, 91
Cholesterol crystals, 15, 121, 150
    in synovial fluid, 149-150
Cholesterol effusion, 108, 153
Cholinesterase, 35
Chondrocalcinosis, 149
Chondrocytes, **144**
    in cerebrospinal fluid, 57
Chordomas, 67
Chorioamnionitis, 41
Choroid plexus, 45
Chromosomal abnormalities, prenatal diagnosis of, 39
Chromosomal microarray analysis (CMA), 28, **40**, 40-41
Chronic exudative effusions, 112
Chronic kidney disease (CKD), 89
Chronic lymphocytic leukemia (CLL), 65
Chronic myelogenous leukemia (CML), 65
Churg-Strauss syndrome, 112
Chylous ascites, 121
Chylous effusions, 109, 153
    causes for, 6
Cirrhosis, 89
CK19 fragments (CYFRA 21-1), 113
Clarity, 6, 7
Clinical and Laboratory Standards Institute guidelines, 51

Clonal B cell populations, 24
Clostridium species, 114
Clotting, 4
Cloudiness, 6
Coagulopathy, 180
Coccidioides immitis, 79, 114
Coccidioides meningitis, 79
College of American Pathologists (CAP), 2
    on centrifugation of body fluids, 10, 19
    cytogenetics checklist, 28
    on dilutions, 8
Columbia blood, 19
Coma, ketoacidotic, 211
Comet assay, 173-174
Communicating hydrocephalus, 45
Complement, 113-114
Complement components, 153
Congenital nephrosis, 34
Congestive heart failure (CHF), 89, 91, 119
    as cause of pleural effusion, 92
Continuous ambulatory peritoneal dialysis (CAPD), 123, 133
Corpora amylacea, 58, **58**

Corticosteroid crystals, 16, **17**, 150
Cortisol, 208
Coxiella burnetii, 90, 114
Coxsackieviruses, 77, 116
C-reactive protein (CRP), 70
Creatinine, 129-130
Creatinine and urea nitrogen, 212
Creutzfeldt-Jakob disease (CJD), 74
Crohn disease, 143, 151
Cryoglobulin crystals, 146, 150
Cryptococcal meningitis, diagnosis of, 78
Cryptococcal pleuritis, 115
Cryptococcus species, 78
Crystals, *189*, 189-190, **191-193**
   aluminum phosphate, 146
   basic calcium phosphates, 149
   birefringent, 13, 16, **16**
   calcium pyrophosphate dihydrate, 11, 13, 15, 146
   Charcot-Leyden, 101, 146, 150
   cholesterol, 15, 121, 150
      in synovial fluid, 149-150
   corticosteroid, 16, **17**, 150
   cryoglobulin, 146, 150
   hematin, 16, **17**
   hydroxyapatite, 15, 149
   monosodium urate, 11, 14, **147**
   starch, 16, **16**
   in synovial fluid crystal identification, 14-17
Cultures of urine, 201-202
Cushing syndrome, 199, 208
Cyanosis, 37
Cystic fibrosis, 199, 215
Cystic fibrosis transmembrane conductance regulator (CFTR) gene, 215
Cytidine deaminase, 152
Cytocentrifuge, 9
   artifact, 59
   preparation in synovial fluid crystal identification, 12-14
Cytogenetics, 1, 26
   body fluid specimen types and transportation of samples, 26-27
   fluorescence in situ hybridization (FISH) analysis, **27**
   harvesting of metaphase cells, 27-28
   reporting of results, 28
   samples for studies in, 32
   specimen processing, 27
Cytokines, 154
Cytomegalovirus (CMV), 22, 202, 209, 213
   infections from, 108
Cytomorphology, 11

D

Degenerative arthritis, 146
Dehydroepiandrosterone, 208
Diabetes insipidus, 181
Diabetes mellitus, 210
Diagnostic peritoneal lavage (DPL), 119-120, *120*
Diarthrodial joints, 137
Differential cell counts, 10-11, *52*, 53, *53*
Diff-Quik stain, 10
DiGeorge syndrome, 28
Dipalmitoylphosphatidylcholine, 36
Dipstick measurement of urine pH, 198
Dipstick reagents, 200
Direct nucleic acid amplification, 26
Direct target sequencing, 26
D-lactic acid, 152
Doppler ultrasonography as noninvasive method of determining fetal anemia, 36
Dressler syndrome, 90
Dura mater, 45
Dysuria, 180

E

Eccrine sweat glands, 214
Echinococcus granulosus, 115
Echinococcus organisms, **101**
Echoviruses, 77, 90, 116
Edema, reexpansion pulmonary, 91
Effusions, 89
   bilateral, 110
   cholesterol rich, 153
   chylous synovial, 153
   exudative, 108
   exudative peritoneal, 121
   parapneumonic, 108, 114
   synovial fluid lipid, 153
   tuberculous, 115
Electrolytes, 131, 211-212
   acid-base balance and, 73-74
   imbalances in, 210
ELISA assay for antisperm antibodies, 169
Embryonal rhabdomyosarcoma, 67
Empyema, 115
Endemic dimorphic mycoses, 79
Endophthalmitis, 212
   bacterial, 213, *213*
   fungal, 213
   mycobacterial, 213
Entamoeba histolytica, 115

Enterobacteriaceae, 75
Enterococcus species, 75
Enteroviruses, 77
Enzymes, synovial fluid and, 152
Eosinophilic pleocytosis, 62-63
Eosinophilic pleural effusion, 100
Eosinophils, 62, 93, **143**
Epithelial cells, 182, **183**, 184, **184**, *184*
Epithelioid histiocytes, 60
Epstein-Barr virus (EBV), 22
   detection of, 26
Erythema migrans, 157
Erythrophagocytosis, 49, 61
Escherichia coli, 114
Estradiol, 208
Ethanol, 212
Ewing sarcoma, 67
Exophiala dermatitidis, 78
Exophiala jeanselmni, 78
Exserohilum rostratum, 79-80
Exudates, 89, *91*, 91-92
Exudative effusions, 108
   chronic, 112
   peritoneal, 121
Eye fluids, 209-214
   alcohols, 212
   aqueous, 210, **210**
   chemical analysis of, 210-211
   creatinine and urea nitrogen, 212
   electrolytes, 211-212
   glucose and metabolism, 211
   insulin and C-peptide, 211
   microbiologic examination of vitreous fluid and endophthalmitis, 212
   postmortem interval, 212
   specimen collection, requirements and stability, 210
   vitreous, **209**, 209-210

F

Fern test, 33
Fetal demise, 34
Fetal lung maturity (FLM) tests, 32
   diagnostic sensitivity of all, 37
Fetal sex, determining, 33
Fetal structural defects, 34
α fetoprotein (AFP), 34-35, 72, 132
   of amniotic fluid, 34-35
Fibronectin, 132, 152, 154
Fine needle aspiration biopsy (FNAB), 10

Flow cytometry
　assays in, 6
　in evaluating body fluids, 1, 2
　immunophenotyping and, 23-24, **24**, **25**, *25*
Fluorescence in situ hybridization (FISH), 2, 27-28, 39
　for detection of urothelial cancer, 205
　sperm aneuploidy testing by, 174, **174**
　in urine, 205
Follicle-stimulating hormone (FSH), 161
Fractalkine, 154
Francisella tularensis, 114
Free living amoebic infections, **77**, 80-81
Fructose, 199
Fungal arthritis, 144
Fungal disease, 115
Fungal endophthalmitis, 213
Fungal infections, 20
Fungal meningitis, 60, **77**, 78-80, **79**
Fungal peritonitis, 123, 133
Fungi, neurotropic, 78
Fusobacterium nucleatum, 114

G

Galactose, 199
Gallstones, 200
Gamete aneuploidy, 174
Gastrointestinal carcinoma, 109
Genetic analysis, amniocentesis for, 39
Giant cells, multinucleated, 60-61
Giant tumor cells, **104**
Glandular cells, 184
Glaucoma, 210
Globozoospermia, 170
Glomerular filtration rate (GFR), 180
Glomerulonephritis, 180, 181
Glucosamine, 154
Glucose, 69, 112, 131
　glucose metabolism and, 211
　synovial fluid and, *146*, 151
　in urine, 199
γ-glutamyltransferase, 152
Glycosuria, 199
Gonadotropin-releasing hormone (GnRH), 161
Gouty arthritis, 146
Gram stain, 19
Granulocytes, 93

Gross examination, 1, 6-7
　amniotic fluid, 6
　cerebrospinal fluid, 6
　serous fluids, 6
　synovial fluid, 6-7
　urine, 7
Guillain-Barré syndrome (GBS), 70
　latex agglutination assays for, 77
Guinea worm infestation, 142

H

Haemophilus influenzae, 114, 154
　latex agglutination assays for, 77
Haemophilus influenzae type B (Hib), 75
Health Insurance Portability and Accountability Act (HIPAA) (1996), 2
Helicobacter pylori, 22
Helminthic meningitis, 81
Hematin, 16
Hematin crystals, 16, **17**
Hematopoietic cells, flow cytometry in evaluating, 24
Hematuria, 179, 180, 200
Hemizona assay, 170-171
Hemoglobinuria, 200
Hemolysis, 18
Hemolytic disease of the newborn (HDN), 35
Hemorrhage
　changes in cerebrospinal fluid following, 61, *61*
　pathologic, 120
　subarachnoid, 49
Hemorrhagic fluid, 92, 140
Hemothorax, 91, 112
Hepatitis C virus (HCV), 209
　salivary testing for, 209
Herpes simplex virus (HSV), 213
Herpes simplex virus type 2 (HSV2), 78, 108
Herpesviruses, 22
Herpesvirus meningitis, 78
Histiocytes, 93, 97, **121**, **122**
Histiocytes in cerebrospinal fluid, 54, **55**
Histoplasma capsulatum, 114
Histoplasma capsulatum infections, 203
Histoplasma capsulatum meningitis, 79
Histoplasma galactomannan, 203
Histoplasma species, 79
Hodgkin lymphoma, 66, 100
　pleural effusions in, 111
Human chorionic gonadotropin (hCG), 73

Human immunodeficiency virus (HIV), 209
Human papillomavirus, detection of, 26
Hunter-Hurler syndrome, 61
Hyaluronic acid, 137, 210
Hyaluronidase, 18, 141, 170
Hybridization/probe based signal amplification, 26
Hydatid disease, 100, 115
Hydramnios, 32
Hydrocephalus, 45
　communicating, 45
　obstructive, 45
Hydroxyapatite crystals, 15, 149
Hyperbilirubinemia, 6, 72
Hypertension, 180
Hyperthyroidism, 199
Hyperuricemia, 149
Hypoosmotic swelling test, 167-168
Hypoproteinemia, 110, 119
Hyposalivation, 207

I

Icterus, 18
IgG, 70
Immunobead assay, 169
Immunoglobulins, 70
Immunohistochemistry, 20-22, *22*, 23
Immunologic analysis, synovial fluid and, 153-154, *154*
Immunophenotyping, 20-24
　flow cytometry, 23-24, **24**, **25**, *25*
　immunohistochemistry, 20-22, *22*, 23
Impedance method, 38
Indirect immunobead test, 169
Infectious disease testing, 26
Infectious pericarditis, 116
Inflammatory arthropathies, 151
In situ hybridization, 26
Insulin and C-peptide, 211
Insulinlike growth factor binding protein-1, 38
Interferon-γ (IFN-γ) levels, 115
Interlaboratory exchange programs, 2
Intraabdominal malignant neoplasms, 119
Intracytoplasmic sperm injection (ICSI), 161, 167
In vitro fertilization (IVF), 161
Isoelectric focusing (IEF) electrophoresis, 70

K

Karyograms, 27, 39
Karyorrhexis, 97
Karyotyping, 2
Ketoacidotic coma, 211
Ketones in urine, 199-200
Kidney Disease Improving Global Outcomes (KDIGO) group, 199
Kidneys, 179
Kidney stones, 204, *204*
Kingella kingae, 154
Kinyoun stain, 20
Klebsiella pneumoniae, 114
Kleihauer-Betke stain, 6
Klinefelter syndrome, 165

L

Laboratory methods, 1, 3-28
   chemistry, 17-18
   general principles, *3*, 3-4
   gross (macroscopic) examination, 6-7
      amniotic fluid, 6
      cerebrospinal fluid, 6
      serous fluids, 6
      synovial fluid, 6-7
      urine, 7
   immunophenotyping, 20-24
      flow cytometry, 23-24, **24**, **25**, *25*
      immunohistochemistry, 20-22, *22*, *23*
   microbiology
      bacteriological techniques, 18-19
         acid-fast bacilli and fungal culture, 19-20
         bacterial culture, 19 g stain, 19
      microbiologic methods, 18
   microscopic examination, 7-17
      automated cell counts, 9
      cell concentration and cytospin preparation, 9-10
      differential cell counts and cytomorphology, 10-11
      manual cell count, 7-8
      slide staining, 10, *10*
      synovial fluid crystal identification, *11*, 11-17, **12**, *12*, **13**, **14**, **15**, **16**, **17**
   molecular testing, 26-28
      cytogenetics, 26
         body fluid specimen types and transportation of samples, 26-27
         harvesting of metaphase cells, slide preparation, and chromosome and fluorescence in situ hybridization (FISH) analysis, **27**, 27-28
         reporting of results, 28
         specimen processing, 27
   specimen collection, requirements and stability, 4-6
      amniotic fluid, 4, *4*
      cerebrospinal fluid, 4, *5*
      serous fluids, 5, *5*
      synovial fluid, 5, *5*
      urine, 5-6, *6*
La Crosse virus (LCV), 77
Lactate, 70, 131
   synovial fluid and, 152-153
Lactate dehydrogenase, 152
   total protein and, 111
Lactic acid, 70
Lactic dehydrogenase (LDH), 130
Lactose, 199
Lamellar bodies, 36
Lamellar body count (LBC), 37-38
Large cell lymphomas, 111
Latex agglutination, 78
Lecithin, 36
Lecithin to sphingomyelin ratio (L:S), 37, **37**, 38
Legionella pneumophila, 114
Legionella pneumophila antigen testing, 203
Leptin, 154
Leptotrichia species, molecular studies of, 41
Leukemia, 90
   acute, 63-65, *64*, *65*
   acute lymphocytic, 64
   acute myeloid, 22, *53*
   chronic lymphocytic, 65
   chronic myelogenous, 65
Leukocyte count, 110, 141
Leukocyte esterase in urine, 200
Leukocytes and immature germ cells, 168
Leukocytospermia, 168
Leukopenia, 201
Liley chart, 36, **36**
Lipase, 130
Lipemia, 18
Lipids, 16, **16**, 112
   synovial fluid and, 153
Lipophages, 61, 97-98
Lipoprotein electrophoresis, 112
Listeria monocytogenes, 75, 76
L-lactic acid, 152
Löffler syndrome, 100
Lubricin, 154
Lumbar puncture, 47
   contraindications to performance of, 47-48
   headache as complication of, 48
   indications for, 46, *46*
Lumbar tap, traumatic, 49
Lung cancer, 109, 115
Lupus erythematosus, 101, **101**, 124, **144**
Lupus pleuritis, 112
Luteinizing hormone (LH), 161
Lyme arthritis, 156-157, **157**
Lyme disease, 81-82, 142
Lymphatic resorption, 89
Lymphoblastic lymphoma, 66, **107**
Lymphoblasts in cerebrospinal fluid, 59
Lymphocytes
   in cerebrospinal fluid, 54, **54**, 59, **59**
   nucleated cells and, 11
   peritoneal fluid and, **122**
   plasmacytoid, 60
   pleural and pericardial fluids and, 93, 98-99, **99**
   synovial fluid and, 141, **143**
Lymphocytic nucleoli, 99
Lymphocytic pleocytosis, 59
   cause of cerebrospinal fluid, *53*
Lymphocytic pleural effusions, 100
Lymphocytosis, 100
Lymphoid pleocytosis, benign, 59
Lymphoma/leukemia studies, 27
Lymphomas
   adenosine deaminase and, 115
   chylous effusion associated with, 109
   large cell, 111
   malignant, 65-66, *66*, 128
   malignant pericardial effusions and, 90
   Non-Hodgkin B cell, 100, **128**
   Non-Hodgkin large cell, **106**
   pleural fluid and, 113
   T cell, 66

M

Macrophages, 93, 97
   in cerebrospinal fluid, 54, **55**
Magnesium in cerebrospinal fluid, 74
Makler Counting Chamber, 164, 165
MALDI-TOF mass spectrometry, 20
Male infertility, accurate diagnosis of, 161
Malignancy
   as cause of pleural effusion, 92
   cerebrospinal fluid analysis for, 63-68
Malignant cells, 93
Maltese crosses, 16
Manual cell count, 7-8
   equipment and reagents in, 7
   procedure (using improved Neubauer hemocytometer), **7**, 7-8, *8*
Maple syrup urine disease, 181
Markers of malignancy, 131-132
Mast cells, 101
Maternal cell contamination testing, 39-40
Maternal sensitization, 35
Matrix effect, 17, 18
Maximum extinction, 13
May-Grunwald-Giemsa (MGG) stain, 10
Meconium aspiration syndrome, 6
Medulloblastoma, 66-67
Megakaryocytes, 57, 102
Melanoma, 67
Meningeal carcinomatosis, 68, 70
Meningitis
   aseptic, 77
   bacterial, 75-77, *76*
   Candida, 78
   Coccidioides, 79
   fungal, 60, **77**, 78-80, **79**
   helminthic, 81
   Histoplasma capsulatum, 79
   tubercular, 60
   tuberculous, **77**, 80
   viral, **77**, 77-78
Meningitis/meningoencephalitis, parasitic, **75**, 81
Meningoencephalitis
   bacterial
   syphilitic, 60
   viral, 70
Mesothelial cells
   malignant, **104**
   pleural and pericardial fluids and, 93, 94, **94**, **95**, **96**, 96-97, **104**

Mesothelin, 113
Mesothelioma, 90
Mesothelium, 89
Metaphase cells, 27
Metastatic carcinomas, **104**
   adenocarcinoma, 92, **104**, 110
   breast carcinoma, **103**
   colon, **126**
   esophageal carcinoma, **105**
   lung carcinoma, **103**
   melanoma, 6, **105**
   neuroendocrine carcinoma, **105**
   prostate carcinoma, **106**
Metastatic malignancies, 67, **68**
Metastatic sarcomas, 111
Microalbuminuria, 199
Microarray analysis, 39-40
Microbiologic examination, 18, 74-82, *75*
   of amniotic fluid, 41
   bacterial meningitis, 75-77, *76*
   free living amoebic infections, **77**, 80-81
   fungal meningitis, **77**, 78-80, *79*
   neuroborreliosis, 81-82
   neurosyphilis, 82
   parasitic meningitis/meningoencephalitis, **75**, 81
   of saliva, 209
   tuberculous meningitis, **77**, 80
   viral meningitis, *77*, 77-78
   of vitreous fluid and endophthalmitis, 212
Microbiology, 1
   bacteriologic techniques, 18-19
      acid-fast bacilli and fungal culture, 19-20
      bacterial culture, 19
   microbiologic methods, 18
ß$_2$-microglobulin, 73
Microorganisms, 187-188
Microorganism viability, 18
Microscopic examination, 1, 7-17
   automated cell counts, 9
   cell concentration and cytospin preparation, 9-10
   of cerebrospinal fluid, 50-53
      cell counts, 51-52, *52*
      differential count, 52, 53, *53*
   differential cell counts and cytomorphology, 10-11
   manual cell count, 7-8
      equipment and reagents in, 7
      procedure (using improved Neubauer hemocytometer), **7**, 7-8, *8*
   slide staining, 10, *10*
   synovial fluid crystal identification, 11, 11-17, **12**, *12*, **13**, **14**, **15**, **16**, 17

Mitochondrial reactive oxygen species (ROS), 171
Mixed agglutination assay, 169
Molecular amplification of nucleic acids, 26
Molecular analysis, 1
   polymerase chain reaction in, 64
Molecular detection of sexually transmitted infections, 203-204
Molecular testing, 2, 26-28
   cytogenetics, 26
      body fluid specimen types and transportation of samples, 26-27
      harvesting of metaphase cells, slide preparation, and chromosome and fluorescence in situ hybridization (FISH) analysis, **27**, 27-28
      reporting of results, 28
      specimen processing, 27
Monocytes, 93, **143**
   in cerebrospinal fluid, 54, **55**
   in synovial fluid, **142**
Monocytic pleocytosis, 60
Monocytosis, chronic, 142
Mononuclear cells, 11
Mononuclear phagocytes, 60, 93, 97, 121
Monosodium urate (MSU) crystals, 11, 14, **147**
Monosodium urate (MSU) monohydrate, 146
Morphologic evaluation, 1
Multinucleated giant cells, 60-61
Multiple gestation, 34
Multiple macrophages, **97**
Multiple of the median (MoM), 34
Multiple sclerosis, 70
Mumps virus, 77
Muramidase (lysozyme), 152
Mycobacterial endophthalmitis, 213
Mycobacterium tuberculosis, 80
Mycoplasma, culture of, 41
Mycoplasma pneumoniae, 114
Myelin basic protein (MBP), 71
Myoglobin, 200

N

Naegleria fowleri, 80
Neisseria gonorrhoeae, 19, **145**, 154, 155, **155**, 156
Neisseria meningitides, 75
   latex agglutination assays for, 77
Neonatal hypoxia, 37

Neonatal tachypnea, 37
Nephron, 179
Neubauer hemocytometer, procedure using improved, **7**, 7-8, *8*
Neubauer hemocytometer counting chamber, 164
Neural tube defect (NTD), 34
    screening for, 34
Neuraminidase, 170
Neuroblastoma, 67, 111
Neuroborreliosis, 81-82
Neurodegenerative disease markers, 74
Neuron specific enolase (NSE), 73
Neurosyphilis, 70, 82
Neurotropic fungi, 78
Neutrophilia, 93
Neutrophilic pleocytosis, 62, *62*
Neutrophils
    in cerebrospinal fluid, 52, 53, 55, **55**, 62
    in peritoneal fluid, 123
    in serous fluids, 100
    in synovial fluid, 141, **142**
    in urine, 200
Next generation sequencing (NGS), 26
Nile Blue dye, 33-34
Nitrite in urine, 200
Nocardia, 114
Nonepithelial cells, 185, **185-187**
Non-Hodgkin B cell lymphomas, 100, **106**, **128**
Non-Hodgkin large cell lymphomas, **106**
Non-Hodgkin lymphoma (NHL), 66, 129
    pleural effusion in, 111
Nuclear:cytoplasmic ratio, 110
Nucleated cells, 8
Nucleated red blood cells (nRBCs), 11
Nucleic acids, molecular amplification of, 26
Nucleic acid sequencing, 26
5'-nucleotidase, 152

O

Obstructive hydrocephalus, 45
Ochronosis, 145
Ochronotic fluid, 140
Ocular larval migrans, 214
Ocular toxocariasis, 214
Ocular toxoplasmosis, 214
Oligoclonal bands, 70
Oligohydramnios, 32
Oligozoospermia, 165
Omphalocele gastroschisis, 34
Open neural tube defects, tests for assessment of, 32
Optical counting, 38
Osmolality, 182
Osteoarthritis, 143, 145, **145**, 149
Ovarian carcinoma, **105**, 109, **126**, **127**, 128
Oxalate, 11

P

Pancreatitis, 199
    acute, 120
Papanicolaou stain, 10, *10*, 33, 53
Paracentesis, 119
    indications for, 119
Paragonimiasis, 112
Paragonimus westermanni, 115
Parapneumonic effusion, 108, 114
Parasitic evaluation of urine, 203
Parasitic infections, 214
Parasitic meningitis/meningoencephalitis, **75**, 81
Parietal pericardium, 89
Parietal pleura, 89
Parotid gland, 207
Pasteurella peritonitis, 133
Pentose, 199
Periarteritis nodosa, 100
Pericardial effusions, 90
    causes of, *90*
    infectious agents responsible for, 90
Pericardial fluid, 5, *5*. *See also* Pleural and pericardial fluid
Pericardiocentesis, 90
Pericarditis, 90
    acute, 90
    infectious, 90, 116
Pericardium
    parietal, 89
    visceral, 89
Peritoneal cavity, 119
Peritoneal effusions
    causes of, 119, *119*
    exudative, 121
Peritoneal fluid, 5, *5*, 119-134
    anatomy and pathophysiology, 119, *119*
    cell counts, 121
    chemical analysis, 129-132
        alkaline phosphatase, 131
        amylase and lipase, 130
        bilirubin, urea nitrogen and creatinine, 129-130
        cholesterol and triglycerides, 130
        electrolytes, 131
        glucose, 131
        lactate, 131
        lactic dehydrogenase, 130
        markers of malignancy, 131-132
        pH of ascitic fluid, 131
        protein and albumin, 129
    gross examination, *120*, 120-121
    microbiologic examination, *132*, 132-133
    microscopic examination and clinical considerations, 121, **121**, **122**, **123**, 123-124, **125**, **128**
    malignancies, 124, *128*, 128-129
    recommended tests, 120, *120*
    special studies, 133-134
    specimen collection and clinical indications, 119-120, *120*
Peritoneal fluid eosinophilia, 123
Peritoneal washings, 120, 129
Peritoneum, 119
Peritonitis, 133
    acute, 120
    bacterial, 119, 123
    fungal, 123
    Pasteurella, 133
    spontaneous bacterial, 132
    tuberculous, 133
Peroxidase/anti-peroxidase (PAP) detection method, 21
pH
    of ascitic fluid, 131
    of pleural fluid, 112
    of semen, 164
    of synovial fluid, 153
    of urine, 198
Phagocytes, mononuclear, 121
Phagocytic cells, 61
Phagocytosis, 97
Phenylketonuria, 181
Pheochromocytoma, 199
Phosphate, 11
Phosphatidylglycerol, 38
Phosphatidylinositol, 36

Index

Pia mater, 45
Pigmentation, 6
Pigmented villonodular synovitis, 145
Pinealoblastomas, 67
Placental α microglobulin-1 (PAMG-1), 38
Plasmablastic lymphoma, **106**
Plasma cell myeloma, 66
Plasma cells, 93
Plasmacytoid lymphocytes, 60
Plasma osmotic pressure, 89
Pleocytosis, 50, 53
    eosinophilic, 62-63
    lymphocytic, 59
    lymphoid, 59
    monocytic, 60
    neutrophilic, 62
Pleura, 89
Pleural and pericardial fluid, 89-116
    anatomy and pathophysiology, *89*, 89-90, *90*
    biopsy, 91
    cell count, 93
    chemical analysis, 111-114
        adenosine deaminase, 112-113
        amylase, 113
        complement, rheumatoid factor and antinuclear antibody, 113-114
        glucose, 112
        lipids, 112
        pH, 112
        total protein and lactate dehydrogenase, 111
        tumor markers, 113
    clinical considerations, 108-109
    gross examination, *92*, 92-93
    malignant disorders, *109*, 109-111
    microscopic examination, 93-94, **94**, **95**, **96**, 96-102, **97**, *97*, **98-108**, 114-116, **116**
    recommended tests, *91*, *92*, 92
    specimen collection, 90-91
    transudates and exudates, *91*, 91-92
Pleural biopsy, 91
Pleural cavity, 89
Pleural effusions, 89, *89*
    causes of, *90*, 92
    cholesterol levels in, 91
    due to viral infection, 108-109
    eosinophilic, 100
    laboratory tests in, *92*
    lymphocytic, 100
    neoplastic cells in, 110
    unilateral, 108
Pleural eosinophilia, **101**
Pleural fluid, 5, *5*
    gross appearance and clinical significance, *92*
    pH of, 112
Pleural fluid eosinophilia, 100-101
Pleuritis
    cryptococcal, 115
    tuberculosis, 91
Pneumonia as cause of pleural effusion, 92
Pneumothorax, 91
Polarized microscopy, 13, 14
Polarizing lenses, 13
Poliovirus, 77
Polyacrylamide gel electrophoresis, 35
Polyhydramnios, 32
Polymerase chain reaction (PCR), 26
    molecular analysis using, 64
Polymorphonuclear leukocytes, 108
Polymorphonuclear neutrophils, 11, 93, 139
Polyomavirus, 202
Polyuria, 181
Postinfarction syndrome, 90
Postmortem interval, 212
Postpenetration sperm functions, 162
Postpericardiotomy syndrome, 109
Postvasectomy semen analysis, 168
Potassium in cerebrospinal fluid, 73-74
Premature rupture of membranes (PROM), 33-34
    chemical markers of, 33
    preterm (PPROM), 32, 33
Prenatal diagnosis of chromosomal abnormalities, 39
Prenatal testing, indications for invasive, 40
Pretransplant induction, 201
Prevotella melaninogenicus, 114
Primary central nervous system tumors, 66-67, **67**
Primary immunodeficiency syndromes, 201
Primitive germinal matrix cells in cerebrospinal fluid, 58
Proficiency testing, 18
Progesterone, 208
Propionibacterium acnes, 19
Protein, 129
    synovial fluid and, 151-152
    in urine, 198

14-3-3 Protein, 74
Proteinuria, 179, 180, 198
    Bence Jones, 198
Pseudocholinesterase (PChE), 35
Pseudochylothorax, 93, 108
Pseudochylous effusion, 93
Pseudochylous fluid, 121
Pseudogout, 146
Pseudomonas aeruginosa, 75, 114
Psoriasis, 151
Psoriatic arthritis, 141, 154
Pulmonary embolism, 109
    as cause of pleural effusion, 92
Pulmonary surfactants, 36-37
Pulse amplitude, 38
Pyelonephritis, 181
Pyknosis, 97
Pyospermia, 168
Pyuria, 179, 180

Q

Q fever, 113
Quality control measurements, 2
Queenan chart, 36, **36**

R

Reactive arthritis, 142
Reactive oxygen species (ROS), 168
    assessment of, 171-172
    mitochondrial, 171
Real time polymerase chain reaction (PCR), 18, 26
Recovery experiments, 18
Red blood cells (RBCs), 7, 8
Reed-Sternberg (RS) cells, 111
    in Hodgkin lymphoma, **107**
Reexpansion pulmonary edema, 91
Refractive index, 181
Refractometer, 181
Reiter cells, 144, **144**
Reiter disease, 144
Reiter syndrome, 141, 151, 154
Renal calculi, 204, *204*
Reporting of results, 28
Respiratory distress syndrome (RDS), 37
Retinoblastoma, 66-67
Retrograde ejaculations, 164
Reverse transcription (RT), 26
Rhabdomyolysis, 200

Rhabdomyosarcoma, **127**
   embryonal, 67
Rheumatoid arthritis (RA)
   adenosine deaminase and, 113, 115
   pleural effusions and, 109
   seronegative, 154
   seronegative juvenile, 154
   synovial fluid and, 143, 144
Rheumatoid factor, 113-114
Rice bodies, 140
Romanowsky stain, 10, *10*
rosebud, 228

S

St Louis encephalitis, 77
Saliva, **207**, 207-209
   chemical analysis, 208
   cortisol, 208
   cytomegalovirus (CMV), 209
   Hepatitis C virus (HCV), 209
   Human immunodeficiency virus (HIV), 209
   microbiologic testing, 209
   sex steroids, 208
   specimen collection, requirements and stability, 207-208
   toxicology of, 208
Salivary glands, 207
Sappinia pedata, 80
Sarcomas, 109, **127**
   Ewing, 67
   metastatic, 111
S100B, 73
Schistosoma species, 188, **189**, 203
Scleral loiasis, 214
Semen analysis, 161, *162-163*, 162-163
   gross examination of, 164
   microscopic examination, 164-168
   pH of, 164
   postvasectomy, 168
Seminal fluid, 161-175
   antisperm antibody testing, 168-169
      ELISA assay for antisperm antibodies, 169
      immunobead assay, 169
      mixed agglutination assay, 169
   assays of sperm functional ability, 169-171
      acrosome reaction assays, 170, *171*
      sperm penetration assay, 169-170, *170*
   assessment of reactive oxygen species, 171-172
   gross examination of, 164
   microscopic examination of, 164
      leukocytes and immature germ cells, 168
      sperm count, 164-165
      sperm morphology, 166-167
      sperm motility, 165-166
      sperm viability, 167-168
   normal human reproductive physiology, **161**, 161-162
   postvasectomy analysis, 168
   semen analysis, 162-163, *162-163*
      preanalytic considerations, 163
   sperm deoxyribonucleic acid damage assays, 172-174
      acridine orange test, 172
      comet assay, 173-174
      sperm aneuploidy testing by fluorescence in situ hybridization (FISH), *162*, *163*, 174, **174**
      sperm chromatin dispersion (SCD), 172-173
      sperm chromatin structure assay, 172
      terminal deoxynucleotidyl transferase mediated dUTP nick end labeling (TUNEL) assay, 172
Septic .arthritis, 144-145
   microbiologic examination of, 154-155
   monosodium urate (MSU) crystals in, 146
   pseudogout and, 148-149
   synovial fluid and, 144-145
Septic joint fluid, 6-7
Seronegative juvenile rheumatoid arthritis (RA), 154
Seronegative rheumatoid arthritis (RA), 154
Serous effusions, 89
Serous fluids
   gross (macroscopic) examination of, 6
   as laboratory methods, 5, *5*
Serratia marcescens, 140
Serum ascites albumin gradient (SAAG), 119, 129
Sex steroids, 208

Sexually transmitted infections (STIs), molecular detection of, 203-204
Siderophages, 61
Signet ring cell, 97
Slide staining, 10, *10*
Small cell carcinoma of lung, **103**, 110
Sneathia sanguinigenes, molecular studies of, 41
Sodium in cerebrospinal fluid, 73
Soluble mesothelin related peptides (SMRP), 113
Specialized body fluids, 207-217
   eye fluids, 209-214
      alcohols, 212
      aqueous, 210, **210**
      chemical analysis of, 210-211
      creatinine and urea nitrogen, 212
      electrolytes, 211-212
      glucose and metabolism, 211
      insulin and C-peptide, 211
      specimen collection, requirements and stability, 210
      vitreous, **209**, 209-210
   saliva, **207**, 207-209
      chemical analysis, 208
      cortisol, 208
      cytomegalovirus (CMV), 209
      Hepatitis C virus (HCV), 209
      Human immunodeficiency virus (HIV), 209
      microbiologic testing, 209
      sex steroids, 208
      specimen collection, requirements and stability, 207-208
      toxicology of, 208
   special studies
      microbiologic examination of vitreous fluid and endophthalmitis, 212
      postmortem interval, 212
   sweat, **214**, 214-217, **216**
      chemical analysis, 215, 217
      molecular testing, 217
      specimen collection, requirements and stability, 215
Special studies of urine, 204-205
Specimen processing, 27

Index

Sperm aneuploidy testing by fluorescence in situ hybridization (FISH), 174, **174**
Sperm chromatin dispersion (SCD), 172-173
Sperm chromatin structure assay, 172
Sperm count, 164-165
Sperm deoxyribonucleic acid damage assays, 172-174
   acridine orange test, 172
   comet assay, 173-174
   sperm aneuploidy testing by fluorescence in situ hybridization (FISH), 174, **174**
   sperm chromatin dispersion (SCD), 172-173
   sperm chromatin structure assay, 172
   terminal deoxynucleotidyl transferase mediated dUTP nick end labeling (TUNEL) assay, 172
Sperm functional ability, assays of, 169-171
   acrosome reaction assays, 170, *171*
   sperm penetration assay, 169-170, *170*
Sperm morphology, 166-167
Sperm motility, 165-166
Sperm penetration assay, 169-170, *170*
Sperm viability, 167-168
Sphingomyelin, 36
Spina bifida, 34
Spina bifida cystica
   with meningocele, 34
   with meningomyelocele, 34
Spina bifida occulta, 34
Spontaneous bacterial peritonitis (SBP), 132
Sporothrix schenckii, 79
Squamous cell carcinoma of lung, **103**
Squamous cells in cerebrospinal fluid preparations, 58
Staphylococcus aureus, 114, 140, 154, 155, **155**
Starch crystals, 16, **16**
Steroid, 11
Streptococcus agalactiae, 75, 154
Streptococcus bovis, 75
Streptococcus pneumoniae, 75, 114, 155
   antigen test for cerebrospinal fluid, 77, 203
   latex agglutination assays for, 77
Streptococcus pyogenes, 154
Streptomyces, 114
Strongyloides stercoralis, 75

Subacute sclerosing panencephalitis, 70
Subarachnoid hemorrhage, 49
   diagnosis of, 6
Sublingual glands, 207
Submandibular glands, 207
Sucrose, 199
Supersaturation, 190
Suprapubic aspiration, 5
Sweat, **214**, 214-217, **216**
   chemical analysis, 215, 217
   molecular testing, 217
   specimen collection, requirements and stability, 215
Sweat chloride, 215, 217
Sweat glands, 214
   apocrine, 214
   eccrine, 214
Synovial effusions, artifacts in, 17
Synovial fluid, 5, *5*, 137-157
   adult reference values for, **138**
   anatomy and pathophysiology, **137**, 137-138, *138*
   cell counts, *140*, 141
   chemical and immunologic analysis, 151-154
      enzymes, 152
      glucose, *146*, 151
      immunologic analysis, 153-154
      lactate, 152-153
      lipids, 153
      pH, 153
      protein, 151-152
      uric acid, 152
   cholesterol crystals in, 149-150
   crystal examination in, 1, 146, *146*, **147**, **148**, 148-150, **149**, **150**
   crystal identification in, *11*, 11-17, **12**, *12*, **13**, **14**, **15**, **16**, **17**
      cytocentrifuge preparation, 12-14
      types of crystals, 14-17
      wet prep, 12
   gross examination, 6-7, 139-140, *140*
   laboratory studies, 139, *139*
   Lyme arthritis, 156-157, **157**
   microbiologic examination, 154-156, **155**
   microscopic examination of, 141-145, **142**, **143**, *143*, **144**, **145**
   specimen collection, requirements and stability, 138-139
Synovial fluid eosinophilia, 142
   causes of, *143*

Synovial fluid lipid effusions, 153
Synovial lining cells, 142, **143**
Syphilis, 82
Syphilitic meningoencephalitis, 60
Sysmex-5000, 9
Sysmex XE-5000, 141
Systemic lupus erythematosus (SLE), 143
   adenosine deaminase (ADA) and, 115
   pleural effusions and, 109
   pleural fluids and, 113
   synovial fluid and, 144

T

Tamm-Horsfall protein, 194, 198
Tart cells, 101
Tay-Sachs disease, 61
T cell lymphomas, 66
Terminal deoxynucleotidyl transferase mediated dUTP nick end labeling (TUNEL) assay, 172
Testosterone, 208
Thin layer chromatography (TLC), 37
Thoracentesis, 89, 90-91
Total ascitic leukocyte count, 121
Total hemolytic complement (CH50), 153
Total nucleated cell (TNC) count, 7, 8
Total protein
   albumin and, 69
   lactate dehydrogenase and, 111
Toxicology of saliva, 208
Toxocara species, 214
Toxocariasis, ocular, 214
Toxoplasma gondii, 214
Transabdominal amniocentesis, 4
Transferrin, 71
Transudates, 89, *91*, 91-92
Trauma, 100
Traumatic pericardial effusions, 90
Traumatic tap, 49
Treponema pallidum, 82
Trichomonas vaginalis, 188, **189**, 203, 204
Triglycerides, 130
Tube collection
   for amniotic fluid, 48, *48*
   for cerebrospinal fluid, 4, *4*
   order of, 48
   for serous fluids, 4, *5*
   for synovial fluid, 5, *5*
   for urine, 5-6, *6*

Tubercular meningitis, 60
Tuberculosis, 99-100
Tuberculosis pleuritis, 91
Tuberculous effusions, 115
Tuberculous meningitis, **77**, 80
Tuberculous peritonitis (TBP), 133
Tuberculous pleurisy, 97, 108
Tuberculous pleuritis, 108, 113
Tumor cell phagocytosing, **103**
Tumor markers, 72, 113
Tumors, Wilms, 67
TUNEL assay, 172
Turbidity, 6

U

Ulcerative colitis, 151
Undifferentiated leptomeningeal cells in cerebrospinal fluid, 58
Unilateral pleural effusion, 108
Urea nitrogen, 129-130
Ureaplasma, culture of, 41
Ureters, 179
Urethra, 179
Uric acid, synovial fluid and, 152
Urinalysis (UA), 5
   history of, 179
   markers as screen for urinary tract infection (UTI), 201
   routine, 198
Urinary antigen testing, 203
Urinary bladder, 179
Urinary schistosomiasis, 203
Urinary tract, 179
Urinary tract infections (UTIs)
   bacterial, 201
   urinalysis markers as screen for, 201
Urine, 179-205
   anatomy and pathophysiology, 179, *179*
   blood in, 200
   cell counts, 182
   chemical analysis, 198-201
      albumin, 199
      bilirubin and urobilinogen, 200-201
      blood, 200
      glucose, 199
      ketones, 199-200
      leukocyte esterase, 200
      nitrite, 200
      pH, 198
      protein, 198
   clinical indications and considerations, 180, **180**
   cultures, 201-202
   dipstick measurement of pH, 198
   gross examination, 181-182
      appearance, 181
      clarity, 181
      color, 181, *181*
      odor, 181
      specific gravity and osmolality, 181-182
      volume, 181
   gross examination of, 7
   as laboratory methods, 5-6, *6*
   microbiologic examination, 201-204
      bacterial urinary tract infections, 201
      cultures, 201-202
      molecular detection of sexually transmitted infections, 203-204
      parasitic evaluation, 203
      urinalysis markers as screen for urinary tract infection (UTI), 201
      urinary antigen testing, 203
      viral detection, 202-203
   microscopic examination, 182, *182*
      casts, 194, *194*, **194-197**
      crystals, *189*, 189-190, **191-193**
      epithelial cells, 182, **183**, 184, **184**, *184*
      microorganisms, 187-188
      nonepithelial cells, 185, **185-187**
   special studies, 204-205
      bladder tumor antigens, 204-205, *205*
      calculi, 204, *204*
      fluorescence in situ hybridization (FISH), 205
   specimen collection, requirements and stability, *180*, 180-181
Urine protein dipsticks, 198
Urinometer, 181
Urobilinogen in urine, 200-201
Urothelial carcinoma, 180, 184
   fluorescence in situ hybridization (FISH) for detection of, 205
   UroVysion for detection of, 205
Urothelial cells, 182
Urothelium, 179
UroVysion for detection of urothelial cancer, 205
Urticaria, 142
Uteroplacental insufficiency, 32

V

Varicella-zoster virus (VZV), 78, 213
Vas deferens, obstructions of, 164
Velo-cardio-facial syndrome, 28
Vernix caseosa, 31
Vertically transmitted infections, *41*, 41-42
Viral detection, 202-203
   in urine, 202-203
Viral infections, 213-214
   pleural effusions due to, 108-109
Viral meningitis, *77*, 77-78
Viral meningoencephalitis, 70
Visceral pericardium, 89
Visceral pleura, 89
Vitrectomy, 209
Vitreous aspiration, 210
Vitreous fluid, **209**, 209-210
   viscosity of, 210

W

West Nile virus (WNV), 77
Wet prep in synovial fluid crystal identification, 12
Wet smears, 10
Whipple disease, 145
Wilms tumor, 67
Wright-Giemsa staining, 9, 10-11
Wright stain, 53

X

Xanthochromia, 6, 50, 140
Xerostomia, 207

Y

Yeasts, fungal meningitis caused by, 78-79

Z

Ziehl-Neelson stain, 20
Zygomycetes, 133